CARDIOPULMONARY PHARMACOLOGY

A Handbook for Cardiopulmonary Practitioners
and Other Allied Health Personnel

2nd edition

Cardiopulmonary Pharmacology

A Handbook for Cardiopulmonary Practitioners and Other Allied Health Personnel

Cynthia L. Howder, B.S.Ed., R.R.T., C.P.F.T.
Respiratory Care Instructor
Vincennes University
Vincennes, Indiana

SANS TACHE
Williams & Wilkins
A WAVERLY COMPANY
BALTIMORE • PHILADELPHIA • LONDON • PARIS • BANGKOK
BUENOS AIRES • HONG KONG • MUNICH • SYDNEY • TOKYO • WROCLAW

1996

Editor: Rhonda Kumm
Manager Editor: Cathy Lee
Production Coordinator: Barbara J. Felton
Designer: Rita Baker-Schmidt
Typesetter: Peirce Graphic Services
Printer/Binder: Victor Graphics

351 West Camden Street
Baltimore, Maryland 21201-2436 USA

Rose Tree Corporate Center
1400 North Providence Road
Building 11, Suite 5025
Media, Pennsylvania 19063-2043 USA

Printed in the United States of America

First Edition, 1992

Library of Congress Cataloging-in-Publication Data
Howder, Cynthia L.
Cardiopulmonary pharmacology: a handbook for cardiopulmonary practitioners and other allied health personnel/Cynthia L. Howder. —2nd ed.
p. cm.
Includes bibliographical references and index.
ISBN 0-683-16313-2
1. Pulmonary pharmacology—Handbooks, manuals, etc.
2. Cardiopulmonary system—Effect of drugs on—Handbooks, manuals, etc. I. Title.
[DNLM: 1. Respiratory Tract Diseases—drug therapy. 2. Heart Diseases—drug therapy. 3. Allied Health Personnel. WF 145 H854c 1996]
RM388.H68 1996
616.1'2061—dc20
DNLM/DLC
for Library of Congress 96–686
CIP

The publishers have made every effort to trace the copyright holders for borrowed material. If they have inadvertently overlooked any, they will be pleased to make the necessary arrangements at the first opportunity.

To purchase additional copies of this book, call our customer service department at **(800) 638-0672** or fax orders to **(800) 447-8438**. For other book services, including chapter reprints and large quantity sales, ask for the Special Sales department.

Canadian customers should call **(800) 268-4178**, or fax **(905) 470-6780**. For all other calls originating outside of the United States, please call **(410) 528-4223** or fax us at **(410) 528-8550**.

Visit Williams & Wilkins on the Internet: **http://www.wwilkins.com** or contact our customer service department at **custserv@wwilkins.com.** Williams & Wilkins customer service representatives are available from 8:30 am to 6:00 pm, EST, Monday through Friday, for telephone access.

96 97 98 98 00
1 2 3 4 5 6 7 8 9 10

This book is affectionately dedicated to all my students,
past and present, who have taught me well.

Preface

An extremely large number of drugs are used in the practice of cardiopulmonary medicine. They cannot be administered intelligently or safely without a sound knowledge base and understanding of their mechanisms of action, physiologic effects, side effects, toxicity, and kinetics. The primary purpose of ***Cardiopulmonary Pharmacology*** is to lay the foundation from which the student and practitioner can then build a safe and effective practice of administering drugs.

In Section I, the first seven chapters introduce the learner to drug therapy: principles and administration, phases of pharmacologic action and effect, drug interactions and modifications, evaluation, dosages and calculations, and drug preparation. Chapter 2, *Divisions of and Actions within the Autonomic Nervous System,* has been extensively revised with many new illustrations and tables. A new chapter has been added to this section: *Special Aspects of Neonatal, Pediatric, and Geriatric Drug Therapy.* These special population groups present a unique challenge to the practitioner because of their comparative physiologic variances to the normal adult population for which drugs are prescribed.

In Section II, the major portion of this handbook, Chapters 8 through 19 present the individual pharmacologic agents with criteria for use, administration, mechanisms of action and physiologic effects, contraindications, and adverse effects. A brief preparatory review of basic physiology and anatomy is included in many chapters to help the learner fully understand how a particular drug or drug class affects the body. Some chapters have been rearranged for clarity and consistency. For example, all of the bronchodilators have been placed in one chapter instead of three. A new topic has been added in Section II, *The Therapeutic Gases* (Chapter 8). This chapter details those gases that are uniquely administered through inhalation for their beneficial therapeutic properties.

To enhance the learner's awareness, each chapter has a list of learning outcomes, emphasizing the primary points and goals of the chapter.

Accompanying this handbook is a computer-assisted instruction (CAI) diskette that contains a self-assessment quiz for each chapter. A final comprehensive examination is also included. This should help the learner not only in mastering the subject content but also in being able to do so at his/her own pace.

I believe that students, instructors, and practitioners will find that this handbook and the accompanying computer program are practical and useful and provide an up-to-date reference for accurate cardiopulmonary drug information.

Cynthia L. Howder, B.S.Ed., R.R.T., C.P.F.T.

CONTENTS

INTRODUCTION TO DRUG THERAPY I

Chapters 1 through 7 present the pharmacologic principles upon which the safe and effective administration of cardiopulmonary drugs is based. A thorough, solid understanding of these basic principles is necessary before preceding to Section II—The Individual Pharmacologic Agents.

GENERAL PRINCIPLES OF PHARMACOLOGY 1

Comprehending drugs and their actions and effects is the basis of pharmacology. All drugs alter or enhance the body's own natural system through biochemical and physiological effects. The dose of a drug and the selectivity of a drug's effect are of special importance and are major considerations in therapeutics. Pharmacology is unique not only because it plays a significant part in medicine but also because it deals substantially with the mechanisms of action of biologically active substances.

The role of the practitioner in drug therapy mandates a sound foundation in pathophysiology and pharmacology. The practitioner must fully recognize the principles governing how drugs act upon the body and the various factors that alter a drug's action and effect and the consequences of any alteration. In addition, the practitioner should understand the legal and ethical issues that impact drug therapy.

LEARNING OUTCOMES

Upon completion of this chapter, the learner will be able to:

1. Define the following terms: drug, pharmacology.
2. Specify the five types of drug sources and give an example of each.
3. List and define the various types of drug names.
4. Name the official publication for drug standards.
5. Identify the major sources of drug information.
6. Describe the various legislative acts that pertain to the sale and manufacture of drugs.
7. List and describe the four legal categories of drugs.
8. Identify the seven major components that should be included in a medication order.

9. Explain the major parts of the written prescription and define the following terms: superscription, inscription, subscription, and signature.
10. Associate a standard medical abbreviation used in drug orders with its meaning.
11. Discuss the process and procedures involved in the research and clinical testing of drugs.

KEY TERMS

(The following key terms are highlighted in **bold** when they first occur in the text of this chapter.)

Drug—A chemical substance that exerts a biological effect. A drug may modify one or more of the body's functions and is used to diagnose, treat, or prevent a disease. The terms *medication* and *pharmacologic agent* are synonyms for the term *drug*.

Pharmacology—The study of drugs. Comprehensively, pharmacology is the study of drugs and their:

- origin
- chemical and physical properties
- sites of action within the body and physiologic effects
- influence within the body (mechanism of action)
- absorption, distribution, metabolism, and excretion from the body
- safe and effective dosage regimens and routes of administration
- adverse reactions and toxic effects

DRUG SOURCES

Medicines have been known to man since the days of antiquity. Naturally derived sources of **drugs** used for medicinal purposes originated in the pre-Christian era, when remedies for common illnesses were treated with hot and cold applications, counterirritants, and medicinal herbs. The oldest known written record of drug mixtures dates from 2100 B.C. and is a legacy left by the ancient Sumerians. Significant discoveries were made by the ancient Egyptians, who used belladonna and narcotics such as mandrake and opium. Knowledge about these drugs was relatively limited and gained primarily from empirical observation. Over the centuries, the number of available drugs has increased tremendously and the knowledge of these drugs has become correspondingly more scientific. Currently, drugs originate from five major sources:

Animal sources—Examples include thyroxine (a purified compound obtained from the thyroid gland of an animal), used for the treatment of hypothyroidism, and insulin (an antidiabetic hormone), obtained from the pancreata of hogs, sheep, and cattle. Many vaccines also originate from animal sources.

Vegetable or plant sources—Examples include digitalis, which originates from the dried leaves of the purple foxglove plant, used in the treatment of congestive heart failure and cardiac arrhythmias. Another antiarrhythmic, quinidine sulfate, is the sulfate of an alkaloid obtained from cinchona bark. Atropine and scopolamine are obtained from the plant *Atropa belladonna.* Also, morphine sulfate, cocaine, nicotine, and caffeine all originate from parts of plants.

Mineral sources—These drugs are usually formed from acids, bases, and salts found in food. Calcium, potassium chloride, copper sulfate, and magnesium sulfate originate from mineral sources.

Synthetic sources—The most common sources of drugs today. This group is composed of compounds formed from the natural elements. Examples include meperidine (Demerol), an analgesic; diphenoxylate (Lomotil), an antidiarrheal medication; and the synthetic steroids and sulfonamides.

Genetic engineering—This relatively new and exciting source of drugs has opened a new concept to **pharmacology.** The most recent advances include the cloning and production of human insulin and tissue plasminogen activator (TPA). TPA is the newest thrombolytic agent used to treat myocardial infarction. Initially, TPA was isolated from blood and various tissues. However, the amounts that could be purified were not sufficient for any extensive use. TPA is now produced through genetically engineered cells in culture.

DRUG NOMENCLATURE

Individual drugs may have many names. The formal name given to a drug is its *chemical* name, which consists of the drug's structural formula. A *code* name is given to a drug by a manufacturer while it is still in the development or research phase. If the drug appears therapeutically useful and the manufacturer wishes to market the drug, a *United States Adopted Name* (USAN) is selected by the USAN Council. The name assigned to the drug by the USAN Council is the drug's *nonproprietary* name, which is often referred to as the generic name. If the drug becomes fully approved for use and is admitted to *The United States Pharmacopeia* (see below), the USAN becomes the *official* name. Often, the nonproprietary and official names of a drug are the same; however, older drugs may differ in these names. The manufacturer, or legal owner, will also issue a *trade name,* or *proprietary* name, to the drug. A drug may be marketed by more than one manufacturer; therefore, one drug may have several proprietary names.

The nonproprietary, or generic, name of the drug should be referred to whenever possible because it leads to less confusion when a drug has several proprietary names. For purposes of identification, the generic name will be used throughout this text; if the proprietary name is mentioned, it will be in parentheses following the generic name.

Example: albuterol, salbutamol in Europe (Ventolin, Proventil, Respolin)

Chemical name: α^1-{(*tert*-Butylamino)methyl}-4-hydroxy-*m*-xylene-α, α'-diol
Code name: AH 3365
Generic name: albuterol (international generic name: salbutamol)
Official name: albuterol
Proprietary names: Proventil (Schering), Ventolin (Glaxo), Respolin (available in Australia only)
Chemical Structure:

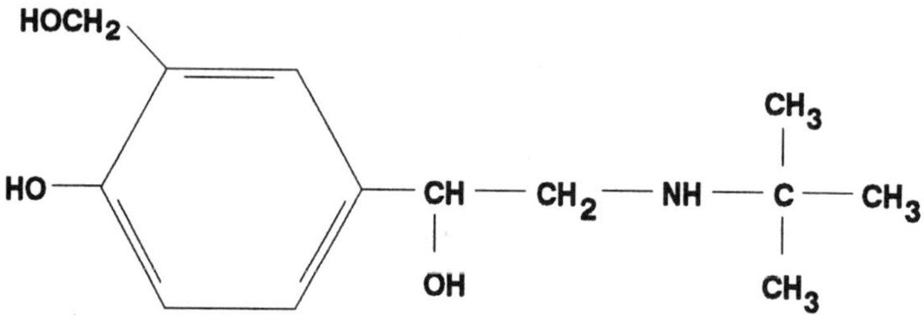

DRUG STANDARDS

The *United States Pharmacopeia* (USP) is an authoritative book that sets drug standards to ensure uniformity of strength for drugs and standards for identification and purity of drugs. Drugs listed in this pharmacopeia are official drugs that legally conform to the standards and are marked "USP." The *National Formulary* (NF) is sponsored by the American Pharmaceutical Association and contains formulas for drug mixtures or single drugs. In 1980, these two official compendia, the USP and NF, were consolidated into a single volume, the USP-NF. A committee of pharmacologists, physicians, and pharmacists reviews and revises this book every 5 years.

SOURCES OF DRUG INFORMATION

Several publications, in addition to the official compendia listed above, are available that provide information on the clinical use and prescription specifications of drugs:

United States Pharmacopeia Dispensing Information (USPDI): First published in 1980, the USPDI comes in two volumes: *Drug Information for the Health Care Provider* (contains drug monographs detailing clinically significant information regarding risks and benefits of drugs) and *Advice for the Patient* (consists of short informational notes written for lay persons' use in understanding the drugs they are given).

United States Pharmacopeia Dispensing Information
USP Drug Information Division
12601 Twinbrook Parkway
Rockville, MD 20852

AMA Drug Evaluations: This publication details current drugs and also new drugs that have not yet been included in the USP. This book also describes accepted therapeutic practices on the use of drugs in special settings (i.e., pediatrics, geriatrics, renal insufficiency, cardiovascular compromise, etc.)

AMA Drug Evaluations
535 North Dearborn Street
Chicago, IL 60610

Physicians' Desk Reference (PDR): The PDR contains an annual listing of drugs from various manufacturers. The volume is arranged in five sections, including a section containing full-size color photographs of various capsules and tablets. It gives useful information on brand name products and a list of manufacturers with their products. Also included is information on action, uses, administration, dosage, contraindications, and composition of each drug.

Physicians' Desk Reference
Box 2017
Mahopac, NY 10541

Drug Facts and Comparisons: This book organizes drugs by pharmacological class and contains a broad range of information approved by the Food and Drug Administration (FDA).

Drug Facts and Comparisons
J.B. Lippincott Co.
111 West Port Plaza, Suite 423
St. Louis, MO 63146

Goodman and Gilman's The Pharmacological Basis of Therapeutics: This book gives in-depth information regarding each facet of pharmacology and makes an excellent source of study.

Goodman and Gilman's The Pharmacological Basis of Therapeutics, 8th ed.
McGraw-Hill, Inc.
Health Professions Division
1221 Avenue of Americas
New York, NY 10020

In addition to the above-mentioned publications, periodicals such as *The New England Journal of Medicine* and *The Medical Letter on Drugs and Therapeutics* contain especially useful, current information about drugs and drug-related research.

The New England Journal of Medicine
10 Shattuck Street
Boston, MA 02115

The Medical Letter on Drugs and Therapeutics
56 Harrison Street
New Rochelle, NY 10801

The FDA has recently opened a computer bulletin board service (BBS) that carries information about new drug approvals, withdrawals, warnings, etc. This BBS can be reached at 800–222-0185. Requirements for using the BBS are a personal computer equipped with communications software and a standard modem.

DRUG LEGISLATION

Twentieth-century drug therapy has seen some remarkable changes that affect the control, distribution, and use of drugs. Among these are the improvement and promotion of legislation regarding the sale and manufacture of drugs. Some of the more important acts of legislation regarding the manufacture and sale of drugs are:

- The Federal Food, Drug, and Cosmetic Act (FFDCA) of 1906 (amended 1938, 1962, 1972, 1976)—designated the USP and NF as official standards and empowered the FDA to enforce those standards. Specifically, the FDA has the authority to:

    1. Establish which drugs require prescriptions.
    2. Mandate proper manufacturing, labeling, shipping, and storing of drugs.
    3. Require drugs to be safe and effective by ensuring adequate testing of a compound to prevent premature marketing and possible drug toxicity.
    4. Monitor investigational studies in humans and determine the adequacy of pharmacologic and animal-toxicologic information before and during clinical trials.
    5. Grant approval for use of an investigational new drug (IND).
    6. Identify therapeutically equivalent drugs.

- The Harrison Narcotic Act of 1914—governs the importation, sale, and distribution of all narcotics.
- Durham-Humphrey Amendment of 1952—first law to recognize over-the-counter (OTC) drugs, allowing certain drugs to be sold without a prescription. All other drugs must have a prescription and must be sold by a pharmacist.
- Kefauver-Harris Law of 1962—requires proof of safety and efficacy of all drugs introduced since 1938.
- The Controlled Substances Act of 1971—the federal government imposed further restrictions on prescription drugs that have a high potential for abuse. The distribution and use of these medications—narcotics, depressants, stimulants, and hallucinogens—are rigidly controlled by the Drug Enforcement Administration (DEA). These "controlled substances" or "schedule drugs" are placed in different categories according to which regulations apply (see below). The pharmacist is required to label controlled drugs by placing the letter "C" and the Roman numeral for the schedule in the upper right corner of the prescription label.

Schedule I—potential for abuse is high; all nonresearch use is forbidden. These drugs have no accepted medical use and lack accepted safety as drugs. Examples include heroin, lysergic acid diethylamide (LSD), peyote, marijuana, and mescaline. Owing to the antiemetic properties of marijuana for patients undergoing cancer chemotherapy, this agent may soon be transferred to schedule II.

Schedule II—potential for abuse is high; no telephone prescriptions or refills are allowed. These drugs have accepted medical use with severe restrictions. Abuse may lead to psychologic or physical dependence. Examples are narcotics (opium, morphine, codeine, etc.), stimulants (amphetamine, cocaine), and depressants (amobarbital, pentobarbital, secobarbital).

Schedule III—potential for abuse is less than that of drugs in schedule I or II. There is a 5-refill maximum; no refills are available after 6 months from the date of the initial order. These drugs have accepted medical use. They have moderate to low potential for physical dependence and high potential for psychologic dependence. Examples are codeine combinations, glutethimide, and phendimetrazine.

Schedule IV—potential for abuse is less than that of schedule III drugs; prescriptions must be rewritten after 6 months or 5 refills. Schedule IV differs from schedule III in penalties for illegal possession. Examples are phenobarbital, paraldehyde, chloral hydrate, pentazocine (Talwin), propoxyphene (Darvon), benzodiazepines such as diazepam (Valium), lorazepam (Ativan), chlordiazepoxide (Librium), triazolam (Halcion), and flurazepam (Dalmane).

Schedule V—potential for abuse is less than that of schedule IV drugs; can be treated as any other (nonnarcotic) prescribed drug. These drugs may also be dispensed without a prescription unless state regulations apply. These drugs have current accepted medical use, and potential for dependence is low. Examples are diphenoxylate (in restricted dosages and with atropine, as in Lomotil) and restricted concentrations of codeine, dihydrocodeine, ethylmorphine.

There are several severe criminal penalties for violation of the Controlled Substances Act. The most frequent violations are illegal possession, use, or distribution of the drugs by a physician, pharmacist, or health care practitioner responsible for administering these drugs. In addition to prosecution and a possible fine and/or imprisonment, a practitioner in violation of this act may lose his/her license to practice the profession.

- Orphan Drug Amendments of 1983—provides incentives for development of drugs that treat diseases with a less than 200,000 patient population in the USA.
- Drug Price Competition and Patent Restoration Act of 1984—abbreviated new drug applications for generic drugs and required bioequivalence data. Patent life extended by amount of time drug delayed by FDA review process.

- Expedited Drug Approval of 1992—allowed accelerated FDA approval for drugs of high medical need. Required detailed postmarketing patient surveillance.

LEGAL FACTORS

In the USA, the manufacture and use of legal and illegal drugs are controlled by the FDA and the DEA. Drugs are often classified according to their legal status into four categories:

1. *Over-the-counter* (OTC), or *nonlegend,* drugs are those such as aspirin, antacids, diet aids. Cough and cold remedies require no prescription and may be safely administered by the lay person without the supervision of a health care practitioner.
2. *Prescription,* or *legend,* drugs are those drugs that are not considered safe for unsupervised use. These drugs can only be dispensed by the order of practitioners licensed by law to prescribe (i.e., physicians, dentists, veterinarians, and in a few states, podiatrists, nurse practitioners, and physician's assistants). Prescription drugs can be identified by the following statement: "Caution: Federal law prohibits dispensing without a prescription." All prescription drugs require this statement as well as a package insert. The package brochure lists the indications, contraindications, warnings, and dosing regimen for the drug.
3. *Controlled substances* are classified with respect to their physical properties or psychological abuse potential and accepted medical use (see *Drug Legislation:* Controlled Substances Act of 1971). As noted previously, special prescription procedures apply to controlled substances. *Social drugs* are drugs that are used for their subjectively pleasant psychologic or physical effects. Caffeine, ethanol, and tobacco are currently accepted as legal social drugs that do not need a prescription for use. Controlled-substance prescription drugs obtained illegally and used for nontherapeutic purposes are considered *illicit* social drugs. *Street,* or *designer,* drugs are adjectives that describe illicit social drugs.
4. *Investigational new drugs* (IND) are those agents currently under FDA evaluation for possible approval for commercial use. Prior to approval by the FDA, the use of these drugs requires informed consent from the patient and typically involves extensive data collection regarding therapeutic and adverse effects.

Medication Orders and Prescription Writing

A prescription is an order for medication written by a practitioner licensed by law to prescribe. The drug may be prescribed by its nonproprietary (generic) name, the official name, or a manufacturer's trade name.

The Medication Order (Fig. 1.1*a*)

In the hospital setting, medications are prescribed in the patient's chart on a particular page (usually the physician's order pages). This type of prescription order is known as a medication order or chart order. The medication order should be carefully screened for accuracy and legibility. Questions that may arise regarding the in-

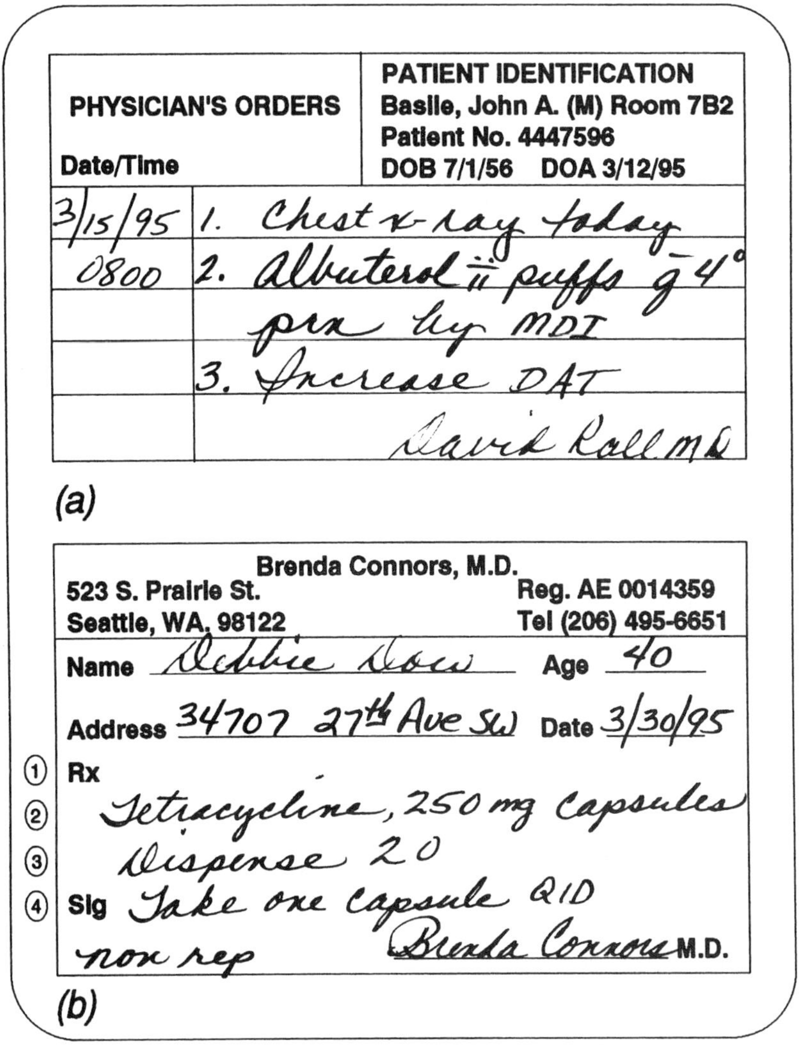

PHYSICIAN'S ORDERS Date/Time	PATIENT IDENTIFICATION Basile, John A. (M) Room 7B2 Patient No. 4447596 DOB 7/1/56 DOA 3/12/95
3/15/95	1. Chest x-ray today
0800	2. Albuterol ii puffs q 4°
	prn by MDI
	3. Increase DAT
	David Roll MD

(a)

Brenda Connors, M.D.
523 S. Prairie St. Reg. AE 0014359
Seattle, WA, 98122 Tel (206) 495-6651

Name Debbie Dow Age 40

Address 34707 27th Ave SW Date 3/30/95

① Rx

② Tetracycline, 250 mg capsules

③ Dispense 20

④ Sig Take one capsule QID

non rep Brenda Connors M.D.

(b)

Figure 1.1. The inpatient medication order (*a*) and the outpatient prescription (*b*). The typical prescription contains: *1*, superscription; *2*, inscription; *3*, subscription; *4*, signature. See text for explanation.

tent of the order should be immediately clarified with the prescriber before the drug is administered. A medication order usually includes seven important components:

1. Name of the patient—a name stamp is often used. In addition to the patient's full name, the name stamp usually includes the patient's hospital number, age, sex, date of birth, and date of hospital admission.
2. Date and time of the medication order.
3. Name of the drug—either the generic or trade name will be specified. The dosage form may also be indicated if more than one form is available.
4. The dose of the drug.
5. The route of administration.
6. The frequency of administration.
7. The signature of the prescriber.

The Outpatient Prescription (Fig 1.1.*b*)

The contents of a hospital medication order and an outpatient prescription are similar. Normally, an outpatient prescription is written in a certain order and consists of four primary parts:

Superscription: This is simply the Rx (the abbreviation for "recipe," meaning "take thou") informing the pharmacist to prepare the medication.
Inscription: This indicates the drug's ingredients and its amounts. If a drug contains several ingredients, it is customary to list the principal ingredient first.
Subscription: This contains the directions for dispensing.
Signature: Usually abbreviated as "sig," this contains instructions for the patient, such as take 1 teaspoonful four times daily.

In addition to these four parts, the prescription should have the date on which the prescription was written, the patient's name, whether refills are allowed, and the identity of the prescriber (name, license [DEA Registration Number], and professional degree).

To interpret the medication order or prescription, the practitioner should become familiar with the officially approved medical symbols and abbreviations used within their institution. Common medical symbols and abbreviations used in drug orders are listed in Table 1.1. Appendix A contains a comprehensive listing of standard medical abbreviations and symbols as well as common cardiopulmonary abbreviations and symbols.

RESEARCH AND CLINICAL TESTING OF DRUGS

The process and procedures by which new drugs are developed and evaluated before they are released for public use are quite extensive, may require several

Table 1.1
Standard Abbreviations and Symbols Used in Drug Orders.

ā	before	elix, el	elixir
$\overline{aa}$	of each	emuls	emulsion
a.c.	before meals	et	and
ad	to, up to	ext	extract
AD	right ear	°F	Fahrenheit
ad lib	as desired	f/b	followed by
agit	shake, stir	fl, fld	fluid
ah (alt hor)	ever other hour	g, gm	gram
alt noc	every other night	gal	gallon
a.m.	morning	garg	gargle
amp	ampule	gr	grain
amt	amount	gtt	drops
aq	water	h, hr	hour
aq. dist.	distilled water	h.n.	tonight
AS	left ear	h/o	history of
ASA	aspirin	h.s.	at bedtime
asap	as soon as possible	IA	intra-arterial
AU	both ears	IM	intramuscular
bib	drink	inhal	inhalation
b.i.d.	twice daily	inj	injection
b.i.n.	twice a night	IV	intravenous
c̄	with	IVPB	intravenous piggyback
°C	Celsius	°K	Kelvin
cal	calorie	kg	kilogram
cap	capsule	L, l	liter
cc	cubic centimeter	LA	long acting
cm	centimeter	lb., #	pound
c.n.	tomorrow night	lin	liniment
comp	compound	liq	liquid, solution
conc, [ ]	concentration	lot	lotion
D	dose	M	mix
d	day	mcg, μg	microgram
/d	per day	m. et n.	morning and night
d/c	discontinue	mEq, meq	milliequivalent
dil	dissolve, dilute	mg	milligram
disp, dis	dispense	mixt	mixture
dist	distilled	ml	milliliter
dL	deciliter	mm	millimeter
DS	double strength	mmole	millimole
EC	enteric coated	MR ×1	may repeat once

nebul	a spray, nebulize
ng	nanogram
no	number
noct, noc	of the night
non rep	do not repeat
NPO	nothing by mouth
NR	no refill, do not repeat
NS, N/S	normal saline
nsq	not sufficient quantity
od	once a day
OD	right eye
os	mouth
OS, OL	left eye
OTC	over the counter
OU	both eyes
oz	ounce
p̄	after
p.a.a.	let it be applied to the affected region
Paren	parenterally
p.c.	after meals
per	by, through
p.m.	afternoon
p.o.	by mouth
p.r.	per rectum
premed	pre medication
p.r.n.	as needed
pt, o	pint
q	every
q.a.m., q.m.	every morning
q.d.	every day
q.h.	every hour
q.2h., q.3h.	every 2 hours, every 3 hours, etc.
q.h.s., q.n.	every night (hour of sleep)
q.i.d.	four times daily
q.n.s.	quantity not sufficient
q.o.d.	every other day
q.s.	quantity sufficient
qt	quart
rep	may be repeated
Rx	take
s̄	without
SC, SQ	subcutaneous
SD	skin dose
sig, S	write, label
SL	sublingual
sol	solution
solv	solvent
s.o.s.	if necessary, if needed
sp, spt	spirits
SR	sustained release
s̄s̄	one-half
stat	immediately
supp	suppository
susp	suspension
syr	syrup
tab	tablet
Tbsp, Tbl, T	tablespoon
t.i.d.	3 times a day
t.i.n.	3 times a night
tinct, tn	tincture
TO	telephone order
top	topically
tsp, t	teaspoon
U	unit
UD	unit dose
ung	ointment
ut dict	as directed
vag	vaginal
vin	wine
VO	verbal order
w/	with
ws	water soluble
i, ii, iii, iv, v	Roman numerals 1, 2, 3, 4, 5
♏	minim
℈	scruple
ʒ	dram
fʒ	fluidram
℥	ounce
μ	micro

years, and cost the pharmaceutical manufacturer several million dollars. Extensive laboratory and clinical testing benefits the public. Risk-to-benefit ratios are developed, as well as relatively safe and useful drugs, although none of the drugs available are completely without risk.

Once a potentially useful chemical is isolated, the pharmacology of the new substance must be extensively studied. These studies will establish the effective dosage range, the dose at which side effects occur, and the lethal dose. In addition, the safety and toxicity of a drug are evaluated after administration of a single dose as well as during extended, long-term use.

Preclinical Research

Two types of preclinical tests are used to verify drug activity: in vitro (test tube studies) and in vivo (living organisms). Drugs must be tested on animals before being used with humans. Owing to the inherent differences in animal species, pharmacology studies are usually performed on at least three different animal species. Drug efficacy and toxicity are carefully evaluated, as well as the safe therapeutic dose. In addition, pathology studies are performed to determine whether any unusual or harmful organ changes occurred. Pathology studies also include teratology (potential of the drug to induce birth defects) and carcinogenicity (potential of the drug to produce cancer).

All information gained from the animal studies is evaluated, and if the drug seems safe and promising, an *investigational new drug application* is submitted to the FDA. Upon approval by the FDA, the sponsor of the drug will begin the clinical phase of drug development in which human studies will be initiated.

Clinical Research

The protocol for study of drugs in humans is divided into four phases. Each phase is designed to progressively evaluate a drug's therapeutic and adverse properties:

Phase I studies—a small number of healthy volunteers (20 to 100) are given a single dose of the drug. The objectives of phase I are to determine the best route of administration, the safe dosage range, and the rate of absorption, metabolism, and excretion of the new drug.

Phase II studies—in the early stage of phase II, a small number of patients who have the symptoms or diseases for which the drug is purported to be effective are sampled. Dosage ranges and potential usefulness are evaluated. The late stage of phase II includes a larger number of clinical patients and longer periods of therapy. Further evaluation of drug activity and toxicity is made.

Phase III studies—large-scale clinical trials, usually involving 1000 or more patients, are initiated at selected centers for a prolonged period (1 to 3 years). The primary objective of phase III is to determine whether chronic use provides a favorable benefit-to-risk ratio.

Phase IV studies—if a drug survives phase III, a new drug application (NDA) is filed with the FDA. If the FDA approves the drug for marketing and public use, the safety and efficacy of the drug must still be monitored, especially during long-term therapy. This postmarketing surveillance is usually referred to as phase IV.

REFERENCES/RECOMMENDED READING

Fredd S. The FDA and the physician. Am J Gastroenterol 83:1088, 1988.

Joint Commission on Prescription Drug Use. The Final Report of the Joint Commission of Prescription Drug Use, Inc. Washington, DC: US Government Printing Office, 1980.

Kessler DA. The regulation of investigational drugs. N Engl J Med 320:281, 1989.

Miller HI, Young FE. The drug approval process at the Food and Drug Administration: new biotechnology as a paradigm of a science-based activist approach. Arch Intern Med 149:655, 1989.

Sheiner LB, Benet LZ. Premarketing observational studies of population pharmacokinetics of new drugs. Clin Pharmacol Ther 38:481, 1985.

Task Force on Prescription Drugs. Final Report. Department of Health, Education, and Welfare. Washington, DC: US Government Printing Office, 1969.

Young FE, et al. The FDA's new procedures for the use of investigational drugs in treatment. JAMA 259:2267, 1988.

DIVISIONS OF AND ACTIONS WITHIN THE AUTONOMIC NERVOUS SYSTEM 2

Because the primary site for pharmacological manipulation of cardiopulmonary drugs is the autonomic nervous system, familiarity with its system and activities is essential.

LEARNING OUTCOMES

Upon completion of this chapter, the learner will be able to:

1. Define the terms listed in *Key Terms*.
2. Identify and describe the component parts of a neuron.
3. Explain the purpose of the synaptic junction and identify the factors that may affect the relay of impulses through the synapse.
4. List the four mechanisms that may abort a neurotransmitter's action.
5. Identify the systems and subsystems that comprise the nervous system.
6. List the principal organs that the autonomic nervous system (ANS) regulates.
7. Explain why the ANS is also known as the visceral or vegetative system.
8. Describe the two basic types of neurons of the ANS.
9. State the component parts of efferent neurons and explain the purpose of each.
10. Explain why the sympathetic system is also known as the "fight or flight" system and why the parasympathetic system is associated with the SLUD syndrome.
11. Compare/contrast the sympathetic neural pathway with that of the parasympathetic neural pathway.
12. Identify the opposing neural pathway to the parasympathetic system in the airways.
13. Discuss the factors involved in adrenergic, cholinergic, and nonadrenergic noncholinergic neurotransmission as well as the types of neurotransmitters released by each system.

14. Explain what is meant by cotransmitters.
15. List the steps involved in the synthesis of norepinephrine and acetylcholine.
16. Identify the three endogenous catecholamines and their specific locations.
17. Explain the processes involved in terminating the actions of a catecholamine as well as the specific enzymes that deactivate catecholamines. Identify the metabolic by-products formed when norepinephrine and epinephrine are acted upon by these enzymes.
18. Explain the processes involved in terminating the actions of acetylcholine as well as the specific enzyme that deactivates acetylcholine.
19. Identify the three primary types of adrenoceptors, each primary's subtypes, their specific locations within the body, and their particular biological responses. List an agonist agent and antagonist agent for each type of α-adrenoceptor and β-adrenoceptor and state the purpose for administering such an agent.
20. Explain the molecular basis of adrenoceptor function.
21. State the purpose for administering a phosphodiesterase inhibitor.
22. Differentiate between indirect- and direct-acting sympathomimetics.
23. Identify the two primary types of cholinoceptors, each primary's subtypes, their specific locations within the body, and their particular biological responses. List an agonist agent and antagonist agent for each type of cholinoceptor.
24. Explain the molecular basis of cholinoceptor function.
25. Compare/contrast cAMP with cGMP and the physiologic effects produced from each.
26. Differentiate between direct- and indirect-acting cholinergic agents. State the purpose for administering a direct-acting agent and the purpose for administering an indirect-acting agent.
27. Describe the nonadrenergic noncholinergic receptor types and physiologic mechanism of action.
28. List the substances known as autacoids, the factors that mediate their release or synthesis, and the biologic response induced from each.
29. Identify the types of drugs that inhibit the synthesis of prostaglandins, thromboxane, and leukotrienes.
30. Explain why the hypothalamus is considered the major integration center for the ANS.
31. Identify the primary sites and modes of action of the various agents used in autonomic pharmacology.

KEY TERMS

(The following key terms are highlighted in **bold** when they first occur in the text of this chapter.)

acetylcholinesterase (AChE)—An enzyme that destroys acetylcholine.

acetyltransferase—Enzymes that have the ability to catalyze the transfer of an acetyl group from one entity to another (e.g., choline acetyltransferase is an enzyme that brings about the synthesis of acetylcholine).

adrenergic—Epinephrine-like effects; the name of the nerve fibers that synthesize, store, and release norepinephrine or epinephrine.

adrenergic receptors (adrenoceptors)—The chemical sites in organs and tissues that respond to circulating catecholamines such as norepinephrine, epinephrine, or agents that act in a similar manner to catecholamines. The adrenoceptors are subdivided into α-adrenoceptors and β-adrenoceptors. Dopaminergic receptors are also a type of adrenoceptor.

afferent—Conducting inward or to an organ.

agonist—Drug affinity to a specific receptor site. The drug has the ability to produce an effect.

anaphylaxis—An exaggerated or unusual reaction of an organism to a foreign substance. The resultant reaction may be life threatening.

antagonist—Drug affinity to a specific receptor site. The drug does not produce a physiological effect itself. The drug blocks the action and effect of an agonist.

antiadrenergic—Blocking an adrenergic response.

antibodies (Ab)—Substances within the body that react with a specific antigen.

anticholinesterase (anti-AChE)—Any drug that has the ability to inhibit the enzyme acetylcholinesterase, thereby potentiating the effects of acetylcholine at the postsynaptic receptor site.

antigen (Ag)—Any substance that leads to the development of antibodies, inducing a specific immune response.

autacoid—Gk "self remedy;" various endogenous substances that function as a type of local hormone or messenger.

autonomic—Capable of self function; self-governing.

blocker—Any agent that has the ability to inhibit a neurotransmitter's action at the effector organ.

catalyst—A substance that has the ability to increase the reaction of a chemical process without being consumed in the reaction.

catecholamines—A group of sympathomimetic amines (neurohormones) produced by the adrenal medulla and adrenergic nerve endings that cause an adrenergic response on the autonomic nervous system. Endogenous catecholamines include dopamine, epinephrine, and norepinephrine. These agents contain a *catechol* nucleus with an *amine* side chain.

cholinergic—Acetylcholine-like effects; the nerve fibers that synthesize, store, and release acetylcholine.

cholinergic receptors (cholinoceptors)—The chemical sites in organs and tissues that respond to circulating acetylcholine or agents that act in a manner similar to acetylcholine. The cholinoceptors are subdivided into nicotinic and muscarinic types.

competitive inhibition—A term used to describe any substance that has the ability to challenge a neurotransmitter for its receptor site and, once bound to the receptor, causes a blockade effect in which there is no biological response from the receptor.

degradation—Making a chemical compound less complex by separating one or more groups of its atoms.

degranulation—The breaking up of a substance into smaller particles (e.g., the splitting open of the mast cell).

efferent—Conducting outward or away from a given organ.

eicosanoids—All by-products formed from arachidonic acid metabolism.

endogenous—Produced from within the body.

exogenous—Originating or produced outside the body.

glycogenolysis—A reaction produced in the liver by which glucose is formed from the splitting of glycogen.

kinins—Peptides that cause increased vascular permeability, induce hypotension, and cause contraction of smooth muscle (e.g., bradykinin).

mediator—A substance that has the ability to affect a process or produce a reaction.

neuroeffector site—A structure (muscles, glands) that is innervated by the terminal portion of a nerve fiber and that, when stimulated by nerve impulses, produces a reaction.

neurotransmitter—An endogenous substance that is released when the axon terminal of a presynaptic neuron receives an impulse. The substance then travels across the synaptic cleft to act on the target cell (receptor) to either excite or inhibit it. Synonym: neurohormone.

phosphodiesterase—An enzyme that degrades cAMP or cGMP.

protein kinases—Enzymes important in regulating various cellular processes.

stimulus—Any agent that produces a reaction in a receptor.

viscera—Internal organs enclosed within a cavity; body organs.

REVIEW OF NEURONS, SYNAPSES, AND NEUROTRANSMITTERS

Nervous tissue is the fundamental element of the nervous system and consists of two cell types: neurons (nerve cells that direct impulses to and from all parts of the body) and neuroglia (supporting and protecting cells to the neuron). Each neuron (Fig. 2.1.) consists of a nerve cell body (soma) and nerve fibers (one axon and one or more dendrites). An axon extends from the nerve cell body and conducts impulses away from (**efferent**) the cell body. Dendrites are generally shorter than axons and serve to conduct impulses toward (**afferent**) the cell body.

Because each neuron is separate in and of itself, a synaptic junction exists between neurons (Fig. 2.2). The synapse controls the passage and direction of impulses through **neurotransmitter** chemicals. The neurotransmitter chemical is stored in the axon terminals of a neuron. When an impulse is generated, the neurotransmitter substance is liberated from the presynaptic neuron into the synaptic cleft. A transient change in the membrane permeability of the postsynaptic neu-

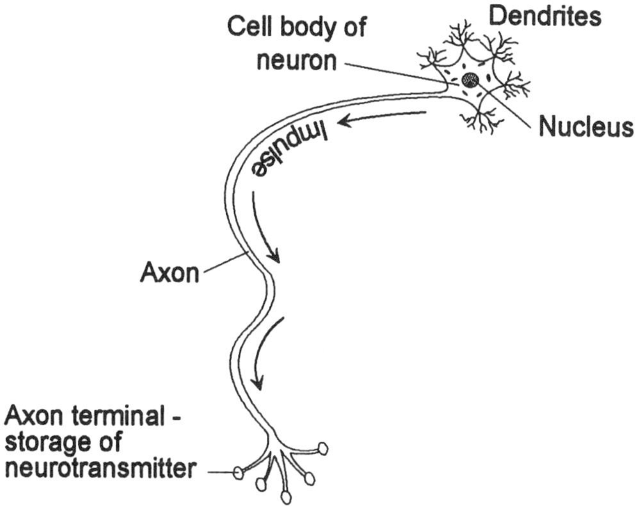

Figure 2.1. The neuron.

ron is generated, allowing the neurotransmitter to bind to a receptor on the post-synaptic cell membrane. Neurotransmitter action is rapidly aborted by one or more medians: 1) enzymatic metabolism of the neurotransmitter by the effector organ; 2) enzymatic **degradation** of the neurotransmitter in the synaptic cleft; 3) if reuptake of the neurotransmitter into the presynaptic neuron occurs, it may be degraded by an enzyme there; or 4) the neurotransmitter may be taken back into the storage site. Also, a small amount of neurotransmitter action is carried away in the blood.

Two types of neurotransmitter substances have been documented: those that cause excitation (such as norepinephrine, acetylcholine, dopamine, histamine, and serotonin) and those that cause inhibition (such as glycine and γ-aminobutyric acid [GABA]). Synapses are sensitive to pH, a lack of oxygen, fatigue, and drugs. When these factors are present, the relay of impulses may be affected.

DIVISIONS OF THE NERVOUS SYSTEM

The nervous system integrates communication and unification throughout the body. Composed of the brain, spinal cord, and a network of nerves, the nervous system is the most complex organ system in the body.

Organized into two main subdivisions (Fig. 2.3), the nervous system consists of the central nervous system (CNS), composed of the brain and spinal cord, and the peripheral nervous system (PNS), composed of the somatic nervous system and the **autonomic** nervous system. The autonomic nervous system is further

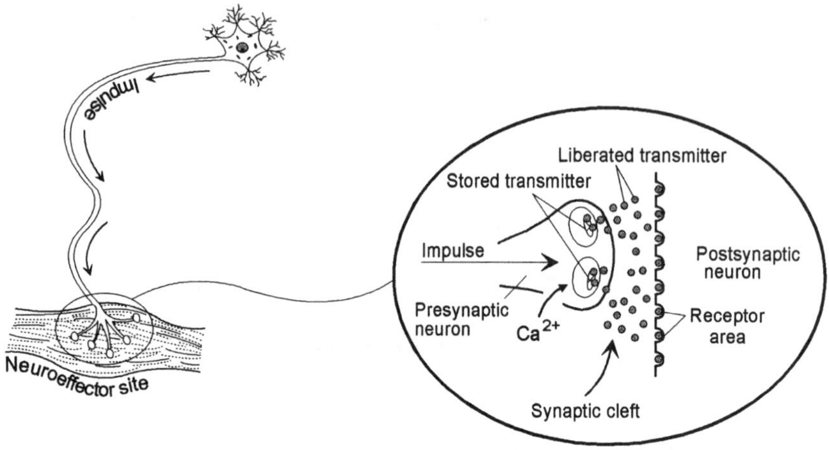

Figure 2.2. Schematic representation of neurohormonal transmission. Impulse transmission through the presynaptic neuron initiates depolarization of the axonal terminal resulting in calcium ion influx through voltage-sensitive calcium channels. Ionic calcium promotes the liberation of the neurotransmitter into the synaptic cleft. The neurotransmitter diffuses across the synaptic cleft and binds with receptors of the postsynaptic neuron. By this mechanism, a biological response from the neuroeffector site (i.e., the organ or tissue being stimulated) results.

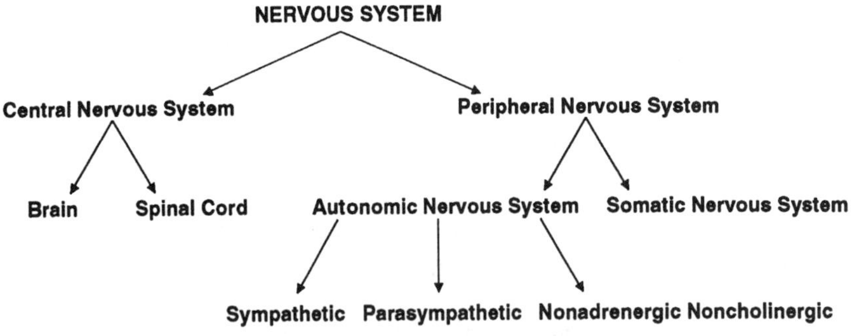

Figure 2.3. The divisions of the nervous system.

subdivided into the sympathetic, parasympathetic, and nonadrenergic noncholinergic nervous systems. The interconnecting functions of the nervous system and its component parts are instrumental in maintaining homeostasis throughout the body. This chapter details the autonomic nervous system; Chapters 14 and 15 present the somatic nervous system and the central nervous system, respectively.

THE AUTONOMIC NERVOUS SYSTEM

Functionally, the autonomic nervous system (ANS) operates at the subconscious, involuntary level in regulating the activities of smooth muscle, cardiac muscle, and certain glands.

Because the ANS is concerned primarily with **visceral** functions (cardiac output, blood flow to various organs, digestion, etc.), it is also known as the visceral or vegetative system. With practice, it is possible to exert some voluntary control over the ANS. Biofeedback is one such example that provides evidence for controlling some autonomic responses. However, we normally do not have voluntary control over the function of organs innervated by the autonomic nervous system. This is why the ANS is called the *involuntary* system, differentiating it from the *voluntary* or *somatic motor system,* which innervates skeletal muscles and can be controlled at will.

Autonomic Neural Pathways

The activities of the visceral effectors (smooth muscle, cardiac muscle, glands) of the ANS are regulated through three neural pathways—the sympathetic (**adrenergic**), the parasympathetic (**cholinergic**), and the nonadrenergic noncholinergic (NANC) systems. Although comparatively little is known about the third neural pathway, the NANC nervous system, its presence has been established through electrical field stimulation of the autonomic tissues (Richardson and Beland 1976).

Generally, the ANS is thought of as a specific *output* or efferent system transmitting messages from the CNS out to the visceral effector sites (cardiac muscle, smooth muscle, glands). However, for the ANS to maintain homeostasis, it depends on the feedback provided from sensory input from the visceral organs and blood vessels. Thus, these sensory neurons should be considered components of the ANS neural pathway. Structurally, then, the ANS consists of two basic types of neurons: general visceral sensory (afferent) neurons and general visceral motor (efferent) neurons. The afferent neurons (input component of the ANS) serve to carry impulses from the viscera to the spinal cord and brain. The efferent neurons (output component of the ANS) serve to carry impulses from the brain and spinal cord to the viscera. The autonomic motor (efferent) neurons regulate visceral activities by either inducing *excitation* or *inhibition* of the visceral tissues they innervate, which are cardiac muscle, smooth muscle, and glands.

As shown in Figure 2.4, the efferent neural pathway is subdivided into preganglionic, ganglionic, and postganglionic neurons. The preganglionic neurons transmit impulses from the CNS (brain and spinal cord) to the ganglion. Postganglionic neurons transmit impulses from the ganglion to the visceral effector, or what is commonly known as the **neuroeffector site** (cardiac muscle, smooth muscle, or gland).

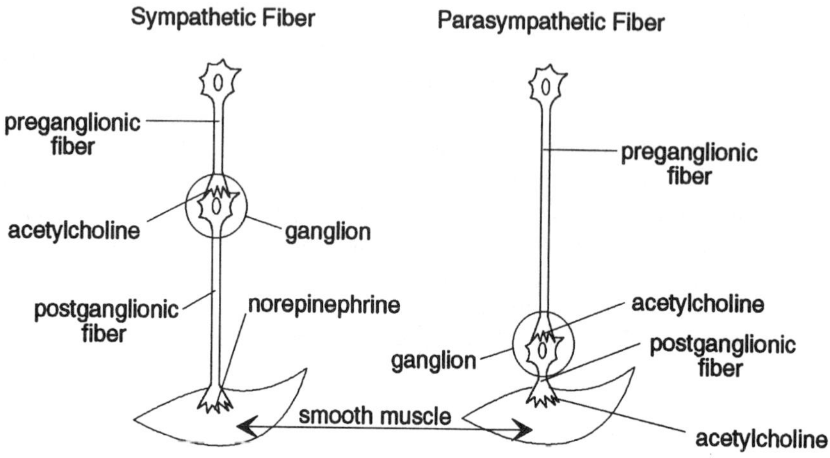

Figure 2.4. The sympathetic and parasympathetic fibers innervating smooth muscle.

Generally, there is dual innervation of ANS organs by the sympathetic and parasympathetic systems. To maintain homeostasis, these subsystems of the ANS produce opposite physiological effects. Under normal circumstances, these two systems maintain harmony and consistency toward bodily functions. However, when the sympathetic system dominates, the body prepares for maximal exertion, the so-called "fight or flight" system: the heart rate increases, the blood pressure rises, blood sugar rises, and the bronchi dilate. When the parasympathetic system dominates, the bodily functions slow down: heart rate decreases and blood pressure drops. In addition, overstimulation of the parasympathetic system activates its excretory and secretory functions, or what is known as the SLUD syndrome: salivation, lacrimation, urination, and defecation. Overall, the parasympathetic system is essential to life whereas the sympathetic system is not. Additional activities of the sympathetic and parasympathetic systems are presented later in this chapter.

Figure 2.5 details the sympathetic and parasympathetic efferent neural pathways and the various organs dually or individually innervated by these systems.

Sympathetic Neural Pathway

In the sympathetic system, the preganglionic neurons originate in the 12 thoracic segments and the first two or three lumbar segments of the spinal cord (Fig. 2.5). For this reason, the sympathetic system is also called the *thoracolumbar* system. Because the sympathetic ganglia are so near the spinal cord, the sympathetic preganglionic neurons tend to be short, whereas the postganglionic neurons are long. One sympathetic preganglionic fiber may synapse with

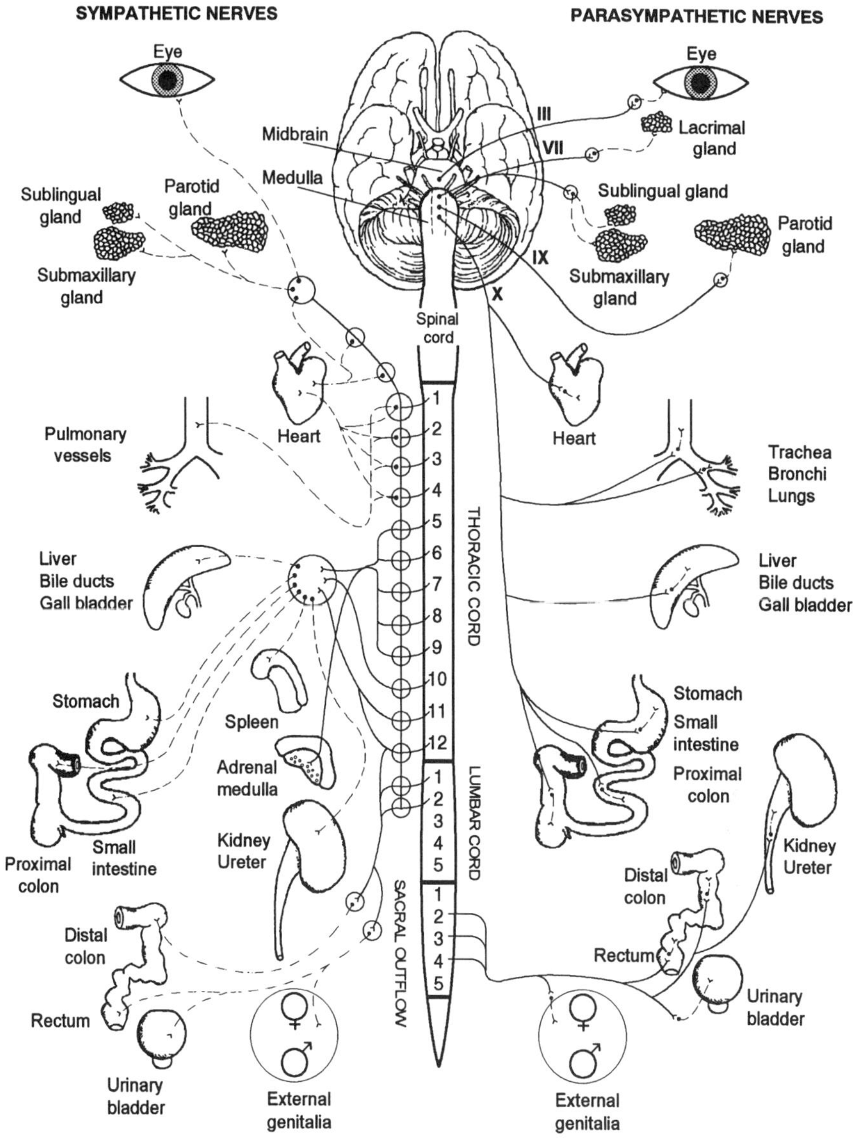

Figure 2.5. The sympathetic and parasympathetic nerves.

20 or more postganglionic neurons, which then innervate several neuroeffector sites. Owing to this arrangement, sympathetic responses tend to be diffuse and widespread throughout the body. Not all sympathetic efferent neurons consist of all three components (preganglionic neurons, ganglion, and postganglionic neurons). The noticeable exception to this pattern is the sympathetic innervation of the adrenal medulla. Notice in Figure 2.5 that one long sympathetic preganglionic neuron extends to the adrenal medulla. Developmentally, the adrenal medulla is a modified sympathetic ganglion in which its cells modulate the sympathetic postganglionic neuron (i.e., the cells of the adrenal medulla secrete a sympathetic neurotransmitter).

Recent studies of electrical field stimulation to autonomic nerves have shown that there is minimal, if any, sympathetic fibers innervating the airways. Thus, the counterpart neural pathway to the parasympathetic system in the airways is believed to be the nonadrenergic noncholinergic system. Neural mapping of the NANC system is ongoing and continues to be an area of interesting possibilities.

Parasympathetic Neural Pathway

The preganglionic neurons of the parasympathetic system originate in the nuclei of the oculomotor (III), facial (VII), glossopharyngeal (IX), and vagus (X) cranial nerves in the brain stem and in the second through fourth sacral segments of the spinal cord (Fig. 2.5). For this reason, the parasympathetic system is also known as the *craniosacral* system. Notice in Figure 2.5 how the parasympathetic preganglionic neurons are extremely long and tend to terminate near or within a neuroeffector site. In contrast to the sympathetic system, the parasympathetic preganglionic neuron usually synapses with only four or five postganglionic neurons, all of which innervate a single neuroeffector site (the exception to this arrangement is the parasympathetic innervation by the vagus nerve). Thus, parasympathetic effects tend to be very localized and discrete.

Autonomic Transmission

When an axon terminal of a neuron receives an impulse, it releases its neurotransmitter substance into the synaptic cleft. The substance then travels across the synapse to act on the target cell to either excite or inhibit it. Autonomic neurons are classified as either adrenergic or cholinergic or nonadrenergic noncholinergic. Whether the autonomic neuron is an adrenergic neuron, a cholinergic neuron, or a nonadrenergic noncholinergic neuron depends on the neurotransmitter it produces and liberates.

Adrenergic Transmission

All neurons that produce and liberate norepinephrine (NE-noradrenaline), epinephrine (Epi-adrenaline), or dopamine are called adrenergic neurons, a term that is derived from the word *adrenaline*. Most, but not all, sympathetic postganglionic neurons are adrenergic neurons because they secrete norepinephrine. The adrenal medulla modulates sympathetic postganglionic fibers by releasing norepinephrine and epinephrine into the blood. All target cells or receptors that respond to the neurotransmitters norepinephrine and epinephrine, or even dopamine, are known as **adrenergic receptors (or adrenoceptors).**

Cholinergic Transmission

All neurons that produce and liberate acetylcholine (ACh) as a neurotransmitter substance are known as cholinergic neurons. All target cells or receptors that respond to ACh are known as **cholinergic receptors (or cholinoceptors).** Neurons that secrete ACh, and therefore are cholinergic neurons, include the following:

1. all autonomic ganglia
2. all parasympathetic postganglionic neurons
3. a few sympathetic postganglionic neurons (most sweat glands and blood vessels in skeletal muscles). Because these sympathetic postganglionic neurons secrete acetylcholine, not all sympathetic postganglionic neurons can be classified as adrenergic neurons.
4. all neuromuscular junctions of skeletal muscle (somatic nervous system).

Figure 2.6 summarizes the above information on adrenergic and cholinergic neural transmission and the labeling of adrenergic and cholinergic fibers.

Nonadrenergic Noncholinergic Transmission

The neurotransmitter substance of the third neural pathway, the NANC system, remains to be clearly defined; however, certain studies suggest that vasoactive intestinal peptide (VIP), peptide histidine methanol, or neuropeptide Y (NPY) may be a primary **mediator** of the NANC system (Barnes 1984, Matsuzaki et al. 1980, Lazarus et al. 1986). The studies seem to favor VIP as the neurotransmitter of the NANC system; however, investigation of this area is ongoing.

Cotransmitters in Autonomic Nerves

Evidence has accumulated in recent years indicating that the most autonomic nerves not only contain a primary neurotransmitter but also secondary transmitter substances. For example, in addition to the primary transmitter norepinephrine, adrenergic nerve terminals also release adenosine triphosphate (ATP),

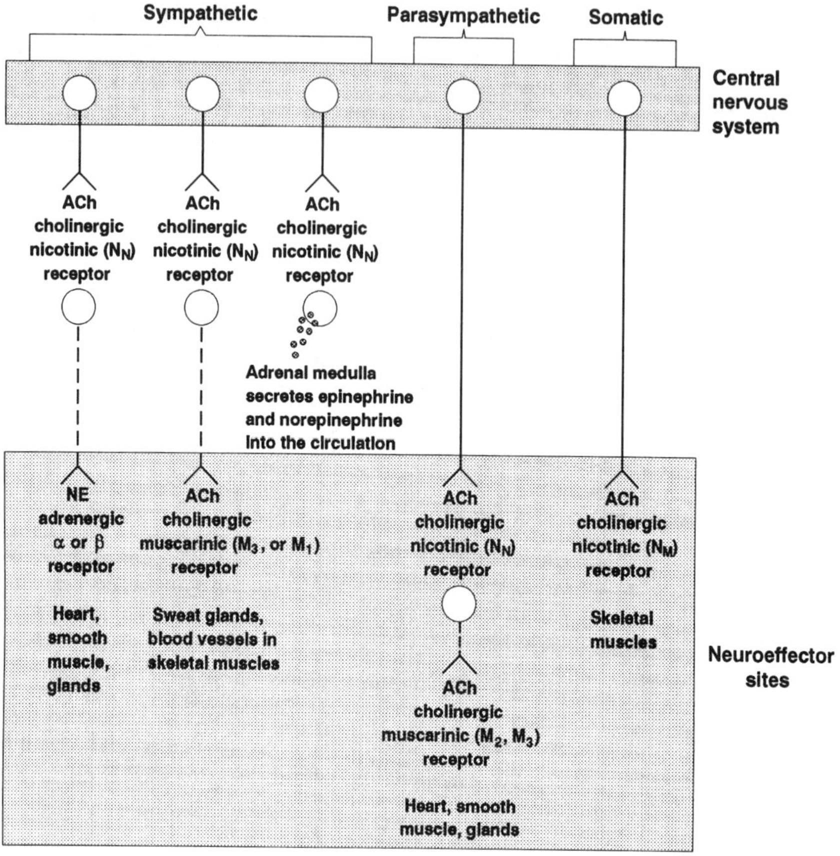

Figure 2.6. Comparison of the sympathetic, parasympathetic, and somatic nervous systems. The central nervous system is represented by the box at the top of the diagram. The neuroeffector sites (cardiac muscle, smooth muscle, glands, skeletal muscle) are represented by the box at the bottom of the diagram. Preganglionic neurons = solid lines; postganglionic neurons = dashed lines. NE = norepinephrine; ACh = acetylcholine.

dopamine-β-hydroxylase, and certain peptides upon impulse stimulation. ATP is also believed to be a transmitter between nonadrenergic noncholinergic nerves as well as the neuropeptides listed above. Stimulation of the preganglionic sympathetic nerve innervating the adrenal medulla produces the release of substance P as well as acetylcholine. The functional role these cotransmitters play in autonomic neurotransmission is not fully understood and is currently under investigation.

Synthesis, Storage, and Release of the Neurotransmitters

Several natural processes occur within the postganglionic fiber before the sympathetic neurotransmitter norepinephrine and the parasympathetic neurotransmitter acetylcholine are evolved and thereby taken into their specific storage sites in the postganglionic fiber.

Synthesis of Norepinephrine

The first step in the synthesis of norepinephrine involves phenylalanine, which is converted to tyrosine by a hydroxylase enzyme. Tyrosine is transported into the cytoplasm of the axon, where it is converted by cytoplasmic enzymes to dopa and then to dopamine. Dopamine is then transported into membrane-bound vesicles (storage vesicles), in which the synthesis and ultimate storage of norepinephrine take place. In the adrenal medulla and certain areas of the brain, norepinephrine is further converted to epinephrine. The synthesis of norepinephrine in the sympathetic postganglionic axon terminal is depicted in Figure 2.7.

Figure 2.8 identifies the chemical steps involved in the enzymatic synthesis of dopamine, norepinephrine, and epinephrine. As can be seen in Figure 2.8, the nuclear structure of these three substances contain a benzene ring with hydroxyl groups at the third and fourth carbon sites. This specific nuclear arrangement is known as a *catechol* nucleus. Each of these substances also contain an *amine* side chain attached at the first carbon position. Thus, by nature of their chemical arrangement, dopamine, norepinephrine, and epinephrine are the body's natural **catecholamines.** Epinephrine is the major hormone secreted by the cells of the adrenal medulla, whereas norepinephrine is the primary transmitter of the sympathetic postganglionic fiber. Dopamine is predominantly located in the basal ganglia of the CNS (see Chapter 15). Dopaminergic fibers and specific receptors for this catecholamine have also been identified in postsynaptic effectors of renal and mesenteric vessels.

Synthesis of Acetylcholine

The enzyme that initiates the synthesis of acetylcholine in the parasympathetic postganglionic fiber is choline **acetyltransferase.** Choline acetyltransferase is produced within the cell body of the neuron and then transported to the terminal portion of the axon. Already located in the terminal portion of the axon are a large number of mitochondria, in which the synthesis of acetyl coenzyme A (CoA) takes place. When choline is brought into the cytoplasm (by active transport) from the extracellular fluid, choline acetyltransferase catalyzes the acetylation of choline with acetyl CoA. This final merging of enzymes takes place within the cytoplasm, after which acetylcholine is taken into the storage vesicles. The synthe-

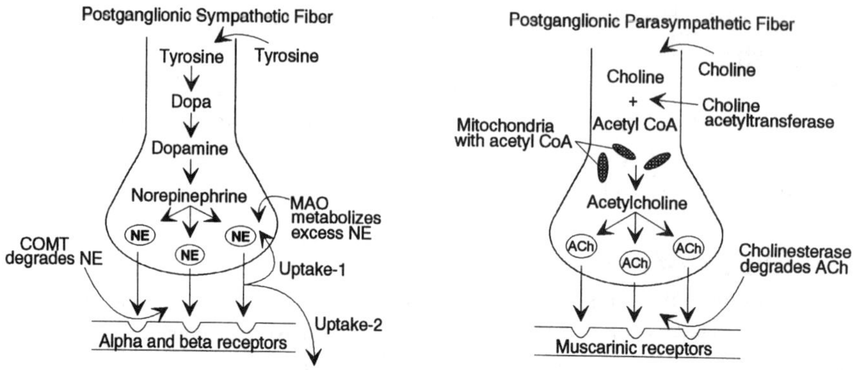

Figure 2.7. The synthesis, storage, release, and inactivation of norepinephrine (NE) and acetylcholine (ACh).

sis of acetylcholine in the parasympathetic postganglionic axon terminal is depicted in Figure 2.7.

Termination of a Neurotransmitter's Actions

As noted previously, different medians act to terminate the action of a neurotransmitter.

Termination of a Catecholamine's Action

The actions of the catecholamines norepinephrine and epinephrine may be aborted by one of four mechanisms: 1) reuptake by adrenergic nerve terminals, 2) uptake at extraneuronal sites, 3) enzymatic transformation, or 4) simple diffusion away from the receptor site with eventual metabolism in the plasma or liver.

Reuptake or recapture of norepinephrine by the adrenergic nerve terminals (Fig. 2.7) is the major route of inactivation of this transmitter. This neuronal uptake process is known as uptake-1 and can be inhibited by cocaine and tricyclic antidepressants, resulting in a potentiation of norepinephrine's activity in the synaptic cleft.

Extraneuronal uptake, termed uptake-2, is a mediated transport system for inactivation of catecholamines that occurs in the postjunctional cell (e.g., perisynaptic glia and smooth muscle cells). This uptake process has a very low affinity for norepinephrine, a high affinity for epinephrine, and an even higher affinity for **exogenous**ly administered catecholamines (e.g., isoproterenol). Uptake-2 is not blocked by cocaine and tricyclic antidepressants, as with uptake-1, but by certain corticosteroids (see Chapter 12), resulting in an increased catecholamine responsiveness.

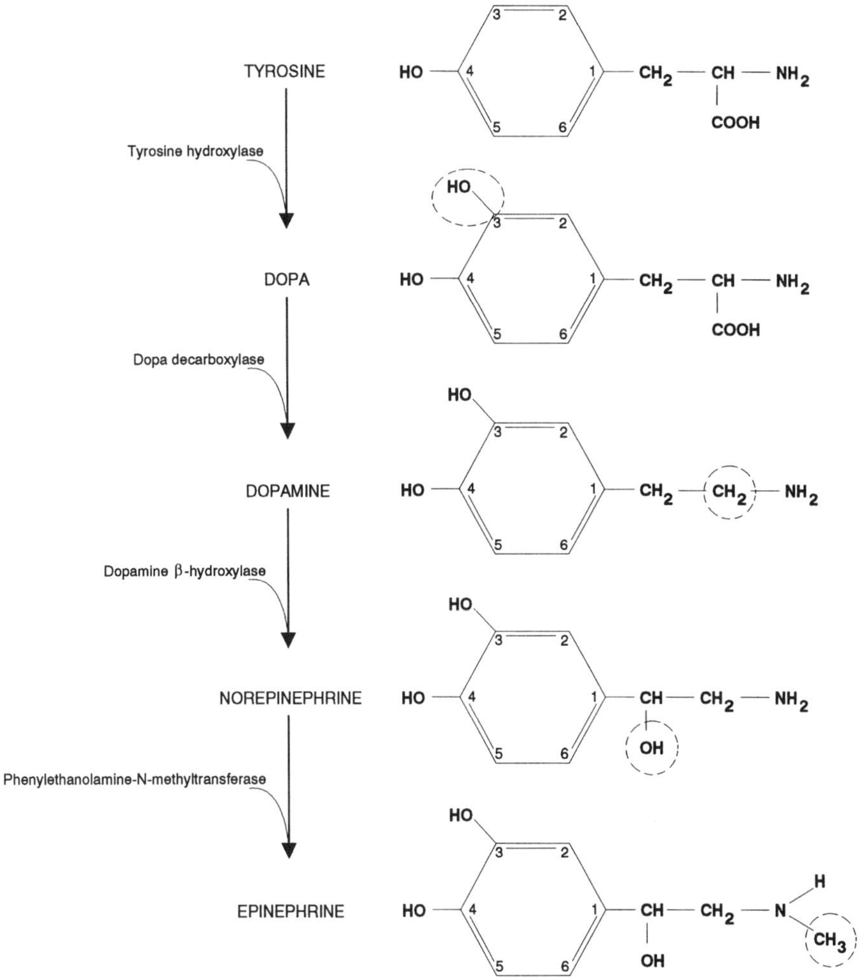

Figure 2.8. The chemical steps involved in the enzymatic synthesis of dopamine, norepinephrine, and epinephrine. The dashed circles represent the primary structural change from the previous agent.

Any circulating catecholamine is subject to rapid enzymatic degradation by either monoamine oxidase (MAO) or, more commonly, by catechol-O-methyltransferase (COMT). Figure 2.9 depicts the metabolic by-products of norepinephrine and epinephrine. Both MAO and COMT are widely distributed throughout the body, including the brain; the highest concentrations of each are found in the liver and kidney. In addition, monoamine oxidase is found within the

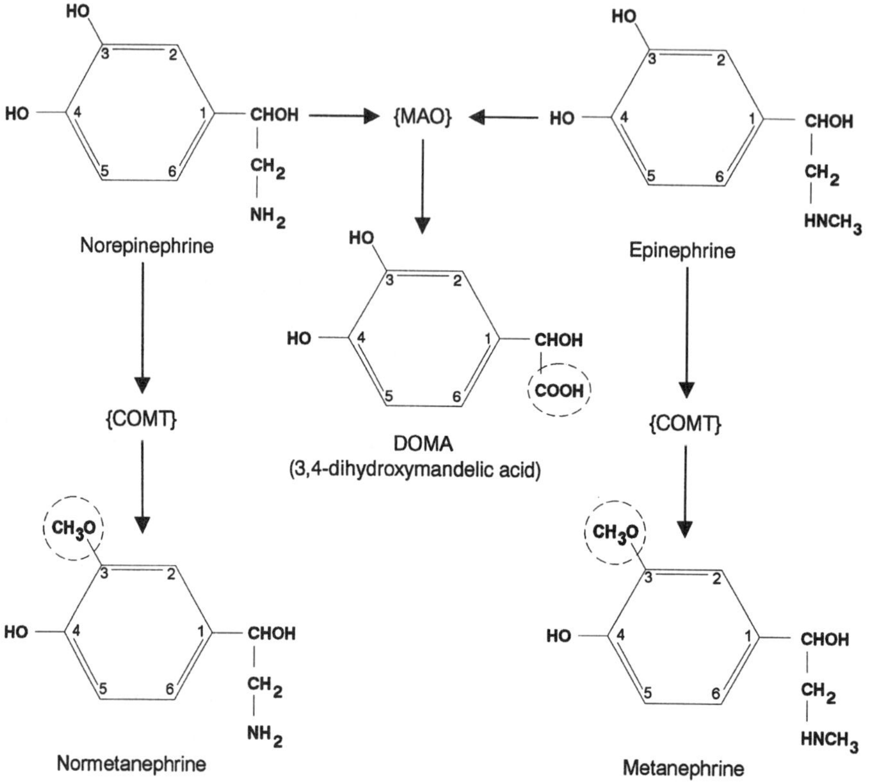

Figure 2.9. Metabolic degradation of the sympathetic neurotransmitters norepinephrine and epinephrine by catechol-O-methyltransferase (COMT) and monoamine oxidase (MAO). The former attacks the carbon-3 hydroxy position, whereas the latter attacks the terminal amino group. The by-products of these reactions have no adrenoceptor activity.

axon terminal of adrenergic neurons, which results in a significant turnover of norepinephrine even in the resting terminal. The metabolic by-products of catecholamines are not able to interact at receptor sites and are eventually excreted in the urine. Because all catecholamines have a relatively short duration of activity owing to their rapid degradation by COMT or MAO, of clinical interest are the catecholamine derivatives (such as the resorcinols and saligenins; see Chapter 10), which are not acted upon by COMT or MAO and therefore have a longer duration of activity.

Termination of Acetylcholine's Action

Acetylcholine is subjected to a number of inactivation processes following its release from the cholinergic neuron. Some of these processes include 1) diffusion from the synaptic cleft, 2) dilution in extracellular fluids, 3) binding to nonspecific sites, and 4) enzymatic degradation. For most cholinergic junctions, the neurotransmitter acetylcholine is rapidly hydrolyzed to acetate and choline by the **catalyst acetylcholinesterase (AChE).** Acetylcholinesterase is found in cholinergic neurons (dendrites and axons), in autonomic ganglionic and postganglionic cholinergic synapses, and in other tissues (e.g., red blood cells). In addition, AChE is highly concentrated at the neuromuscular junction.

Autonomic Receptor Types and Physiologic Mechanism of Action

A great deal has been learned about the chemical nature of the autonomic receptors and this particular area is one of the most active in detailing drug interventions for cardiopulmonary pharmacology. Virtually all neurotransmitters and drugs initiate their physiologic actions by binding to specific receptors (see Chapter 3, Part III). Receptors of the ANS are named after the specific neurotransmitter that they respond to and are of three primary types: adrenergic receptors (adrenoceptors), which respond to norepinephrine, epinephrine, dopamine, and any drug that mimics these substances; cholinergic receptors (cholinoceptors), which respond to acetylcholine and any agent that mimics the action of acetylcholine; and nonadrenergic noncholinergic receptors, which are believed to respond to vasoactive intestinal peptide. Receptors may or may not have direct innervation from autonomic neural fibers. For example, the tracheobronchial tree has numerous adrenoceptors, but there are virtually no, if any, sympathetic fibers that innervate the airways.

Adrenergic Receptor Types and Physiologic Mechanism of Action

The term adrenoceptor is widely used to describe receptors that respond to the **endogenous** catecholamines norepinephrine, epinephrine, dopamine, or any agent that has properties similar to these catecholamines. Adrenoceptors are classified according to the distinct, physiological pathways that they regulate. Three primary types of adrenoceptors have been isolated: α, β, and dopaminergic. Each of these primary adrenoceptors have two or more subtypes.

Identification of each adrenoceptor subtype is based on both **agonist** and **antagonist** selectivity, in addition to functional and anatomical considerations. Synonymous names for those agents that stimulate these adrenoceptors, thereby producing a biological response, are adrenoceptor agonists, sympathomimetic agents, and adrenergic agents. In contrast, synonymous names for those agents that inhibit or block these adrenoceptors from initiating a biological response are adrenoceptor antagonists, sympatholytic agents, **antiadrenergic** agents, and adrenergic blocking agents.

Alpha-Adrenoceptors: α-adrenoceptor subtypes include α_1-adrenoceptors and α_2-adrenoceptors. α_1-adrenoceptors are located at postsynaptic effector sites, especially those of smooth muscle (vascular, genitourinary, intestinal, small bronchioles), whereas α2-adrenoceptors are found on presynaptic nerve terminals, platelets, lipocytes, vascular smooth muscle, as well as postjunctional sites in several tissues such as the brain, uterus, and parotid gland.

Activation of α_1-adrenoceptors by the body's natural catecholamines or by drugs that are considered α_1-adrenoceptor agonists (α_1 sympathomimetics) induces excitation (constriction) in the target organ (i.e., peripheral vasoconstriction, genitourinary contraction, bronchiolar constriction, mucosal constriction). An exception to this is noted in the intestine, where α_1-adrenoceptor activation causes relaxation. α_1-adrenoceptor agonists are used for their hypertensive and mucosal constrictor properties. For example, phenylephrine administered parenterally is a powerful postsynaptic α_1-adrenoceptor stimulant that effectively increases systolic and diastolic blood pressures by peripheral vasoconstriction (see Chapter 18). Phenylephrine also effectively relieves membrane congestion when administered nasally as a spray directly to swollen membranes. Most may not be familiar with the generic name—phenylephrine—but may be familiar with the trade names: Neo-Synephrine, Duration, or Sinex (see Chapter 9). α_1-adrenoceptor blocking agents (antagonists) produce biological responses opposite to those mentioned above. Prazosin (Minipress) is an α_1-adrenoceptor antagonist used for its antihypertensive effects. By blocking the α_1-adrenoceptor, prazosin produces peripheral vasodilation, thereby lowering the blood pressure (see Chapter 18).

Activation of presynaptic α_2-adrenoceptors located on nerve terminals by the body's natural catecholamines or by drugs that are considered α_2-adrenoceptor agonists (α_2 sympathomimetics) produce a negative feedback control mechanism by which adrenergic neurotransmitter release is inhibited. This mechanism is illustrated in Figure 2.10. Norepinephrine released into the synaptic cleft activates postsynaptic α_1-adrenoceptors as well as presynaptic α_2-adrenoceptors. The result of presynaptic α_2-adrenoceptor activation is further inhibition of intraneuronal release of norepinephrine.

In the central nervous system, activation of postjunctional α_2-adrenoceptors in the brain is associated with a diminished sympathetic outflow from the CNS, which results in significant antihypertensive effects on the body. Therefore, α_2-adrenoceptor agonists are used for their antihypertensive effects. Such agents include clonidine (Catapres) and methyldopa (Aldomet) (see Chapter 18). α_2-adrenoceptor antagonists, such as yohimbine, readily enter the CNS and effectively block α_2-adrenoceptor stimulation, thereby producing a rise in blood pressure. α_2-adrenoceptor antagonists also potentiate the release of norepinephrine from nerve endings, which also helps to elevate the blood pressure.

Nonselective α-adrenoceptor agonists, such as the natural catecholamines norepinephrine, epinephrine, and dopamine, are considered vasopressor agents and

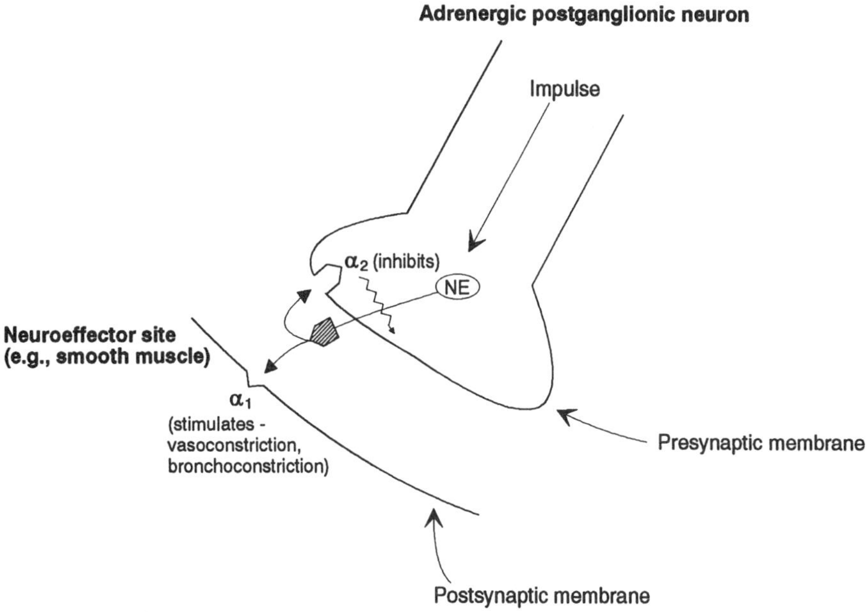

Figure 2.10. Subtypes of α-adrenoceptors. Postsynaptic α_1-adrenoceptors stimulate a reaction whereas presynaptic α_2-adrenoceptors inhibit further release of the neurotransmitter.

are used for their hypertensive effects. Epinephrine is a potent and powerful α agonist, which is why it is a first-line cardiopulmonary resuscitative (CPR) drug used to restore the blood pressure. Nonselective α-adrenoceptor antagonists, such as phenoxybenzamine and phentolamine, are used to control hypertension, especially in patients with pheochromocytoma. Pheochromocytomas are tumors of the adrenal medulla and sympathetic neurons that secrete large amounts of catecholamines (norepinephrine and epinephrine) into the circulation, the result of which is episodic and severe hypertension.

Overall, α_1-adrenoceptor stimulation generally produces *excitation* (constriction) in the target organ, whereas α_2-adrenoceptor stimulation produces *inhibition* (reduced sympathetic and neurotransmitter outflow) in the target organ. Table 2.1 summarizes the characteristics of α-adrenoceptor subtypes as presented in this section.

Beta-Adrenoceptors: β-adrenoceptor subtypes include β_1-adrenoceptors, β_2-adrenoceptors, and β_3-adrenoceptors. β_1-adrenoceptors are located on postsynaptic effector cells, especially the heart, lipocytes, and brain and presynaptic adrenergic and cholinergic nerve terminals, as well as the juxtaglomerular cells

Table 2.1
Characteristics Of α-Adrenoceptor Subtypes

Receptor	Location	Response
α_1	Vascular smooth muscle	Contraction
Epi≥NE>>Iso	Intestinal smooth muscle	Relaxation
	Genitourinary smooth muscle	Contraction
Agonist: Phenylephrine	Bronchiolar smooth muscle	Contraction
(hypertensive agent,	Liver	Glycogenolysis; gluconeogenesis
decongestant)	Heart	Increased contractile force; arrhythmias
Antagonist: Prazosin		
(antihypertensive agent)		
α_2	Nerve terminals	Inhibitory autoreceptor; inhibits further release of NE
EPI≥NE>>Iso	Vascular smooth muscle	Contraction
Agonist: Clonidine	Platelets	Aggregation
(antihypertensive agent)	Pancreatic islets (β cells)	Decreased insulin secretion
Antagonist: Yohimbine	Brain	Decreased sympathetic outflow—decreased blood pressure
(hypertensive agent)		

Epi = epinephrine; NE = norepinephrine; Iso = isoproterenol.

of the kidney. In addition, autoradiographic studies have isolated β_1-adrenoceptors in the lungs (primarily in the bronchial submucosal glands and alveolar walls) (Carstairs et al. 1985). The importance of these particular receptors in the lungs remains to be determined. β_2-adrenoceptors have been identified in the postsynaptic effector cells of smooth muscle (vascular, bronchial, gastrointestinal, and genitourinary) as well as in skeletal muscle and the liver. The airways are well populated with β_2-adrenoceptors; a high density of these receptors is in the smaller, peripheral airways. β_2-adrenoceptors have also been isolated in airway epithelium, alveolar walls, submucosal glands, and bronchial mast cells. A human gene that encodes a third β-adrenoceptor, designated β_3, has recently been identified. β_3-adrenoceptors have been isolated in the postsynaptic effector cells of lipocytes (Emorine et al. 1989). Stimulation of these receptors causes breakdown and destruction (lipolysis) of fat cells. Functionally, β_3-adrenoceptors coexist with β_1-adrenoceptors and β_2-adrenoceptors in a number of fat cells.

Activation of β_1-adrenoceptors by the body's natural catecholamines or by drugs that are considered β_1-adrenoceptor agonists initiates a series of events that lead to excitation of the effector organ, which results in cardiostimulation (increased rate and force of contraction, increased automaticity and atrioventricular nodal conduction velocity), lipolysis, and secretion of renin by the kidney (renin is an enzyme that acts on angiotension to form angiotension I, a pressor substance). Consequently, β_1-adrenoceptor agonists are administered for their ability to increase the cardiac output, the blood pressure, and/or the heart rate. An example of an agent given primarily for its β_1-adrenoceptor activation property is dobutamine (Dobutrex). On the other hand, β_1-adrenoceptor antagonists (**blockers**), such as metoprolol (Lopressor) and atenolol (Tenormin), are antihypertensive agents administered to patients with hypertension. In addition, these agents are used for the treatment of angina pectoris and acute myocardial infarction.

Activation of the β_2-adrenoceptors by the body's natural catecholamines or by drugs that are considered β_2-adrenoceptor agonists produce inhibition or relaxation (dilation) of smooth muscle (vascular, bronchial, gastrointestinal, and genitourinary), enhanced **glycogenolysis** in liver and muscle, and uptake of potassium in skeletal muscle. In addition, inhibition of mast cell **degranulation** and the subsequent secretion of inflammatory mediators is mediated by β_2-adrenoceptors. Sympathomimetic drugs that preferentially activate the pulmonary β_2-adrenoceptors are widely used as bronchodilators to treat bronchospastic disorders. Such drugs include albuterol (Proventil, Ventolin) and salmeterol (Serevent) (see Chapter 10). Selective β_2-adrenoceptor agonists such as ritodrine and terbutaline are used as uterine relaxants to delay or prevent premature labor. Peripheral vascular resistance is reduced via β_2-adrenoceptor mediated vasodilation from vascular smooth muscle β_2-adrenoceptors. Specific β_2-adrenoceptor blocking agents (antagonists) generally have no therapeutic use owing to the potential of eliciting severe bronchoconstriction, especially for patients with hyperreactive airway disease.

Nonselective β-adrenoceptor agonists include the natural catecholamines and isoproterenol (Isuprel). Isoproterenol is a potent β-adrenoceptor agonist that equally stimulates β_1-adrenoceptors and β_2-adrenoceptors. Thus, isoproterenol has powerful cardiostimulatory properties as well as bronchodilatory properties. However, isoproterenol is not commonly used as a bronchodilator owing to its unwanted side effect of increasing the heart rate. Current therapeutic practice regarding bronchodilators leans toward very β_2-adrenoceptor specificity with minimal to no β_1-adrenoceptor stimulation. The prototypic nonselective β-adrenoceptor blocking agent is propranolol (Inderal). Propranolol is used to treat hypertension, cardiac arrhythmias, and myocardial infarction. Because of the β_2-adrenoceptor blockade that results, propranolol is generally contraindicated for patients with hyperreactive airway disease.

Overall, β_1-adrenoceptor stimulation produces *excitation* in the target organ, whereas β_2-adrenoceptor stimulation produces *inhibition* (relaxation) in the target organ. Table 2.2 summarizes the characteristics of β-adrenoceptors as presented in this section.

Dopaminergic Receptors: five subtypes of dopaminergic receptors have been identified: D_1, D_2, D_3, D_4, and D_5. All subtypes are found in relatively high concentrations in the brain (see Chapter 15). Vascular D_1-dopaminergic receptors have been identified in the renal, mesenteric, and coronary beds, whereas D_4-dopaminergic receptors are found in the cardiovascular system.

The distinct locations and functions of the various dopaminergic receptors are not fully known; however, it is known that D_1-dopaminergic receptor stimulation

Table 2.2
Characteristics Of β-Adrenoreceptor Subtypes

Receptor	Location	Response
β_1	Heart	Increased force and rate of contraction; increase atrioventricular nodal conduction velocity
ISO>Epi = NE	Juxtaglomerular cells	Increased renin secretion
Agonist: Dobutamine (inotropic agent—increase cardiac output)		
Antagonist: Metoprolol (antihypertensive agent)		
β_2	Vascular smooth muscle	Relaxation
Iso>Epi>>NE	Intestinal smooth muscle	Relaxation
	Genitourinary smooth muscle	Relaxation
Agonist: Albuterol (bronchodilator)	Bronchiolar smooth muscle	Relaxation
	Liver	Glycogenolysis; gluconeogenesis
	Skeletal muscle	Glycogenolysis; uptake of K^+
β_3 Iso=NE>Epi	Adipose tissue	Lipolysis

Epi = epinephrine; NE = norepinephrine; Iso = isoproterenol.

results in vasodilation and an increase in glomerular filtration rate, renal blood flow, and sodium excretion. Exogenous administration of dopamine is especially useful for patients with low cardiac output associated with compromised renal function, such as occurs in cardiogenic, septic, and hypovolemic shock.

Molecular Basis of Adrenoceptor Function: primary messengers, such as drugs or the natural neurotransmitters, will initially activate a receptor. A series of events will then ensue, during which a secondary messenger is activated. The role of the secondary messenger is to ensure that the desired biological response occurs. A drug or neurotransmitter (primary messenger) that binds to and stimulates a β-adrenoceptor activates a membrane-bound protein, one of a family of guanine nucleotide-binding regulatory proteins known as *G proteins*. The particular G protein activated upon β-adrenoceptor stimulation is designated as G_s ("s" stands for stimulatory). Stimulated G_s, in turn, activates the intracellular enzyme adenyl cyclase (also called adenylyl or adenylate cyclase). Activated adenyl cyclase catalyzes the conversion of adenosine triphosphate (ATP) to cyclic 3′,5′-adenosine monophosphate (cyclic AMP, cAMP). The rise in cAMP (secondary messenger) levels and the resultant activation of cAMP-dependent protein kinase initiate a cascade of events that are ultimately responsible for the β response of cardiostimulation (β_1), increased myocardial contractility (β_1), vasodilation (β_2), and bronchodilation (β_2). The rise in intracellular cAMP also initiates a series of events in the mast cells that leads to inhibition of the release of histamine (a bronchoconstrictor) by suppressing mast cell degranulation.

cAMP is metabolized by the intracellular enzyme **phosphodiesterase** (PDE) into the inactive nucleotide 5′-adenosine monophosphate (5′-AMP). It follows then that drugs that prevent the degradation of cAMP by competitively inhibiting phosphodiesterase will prolong the effect and concentration of cAMP. Phosphodiesterase inhibitors constitute a category of drug therapy that do prevent the degradation of cAMP into its inactive form by phosphodiesterase, thus prolonging the activity of cAMP. Phosphodiesterase inhibitors that act on the myocardial β_1-adrenoceptors cAMP/phosphodiesterase system include Amrinone (Inocor) and Milrinone (Primacor). These drugs act on the heart by increasing the amount of intracellular cAMP, which brings about an increase in calcium ion movement into myocardial cells. The resulting increased force of contraction improves stroke volume, cardiac output, and blood pressure (see Chapter 18). For many years, theophylline was believed to be a potent phosphodiesterase inhibitor. However, it is now suspected that theophylline exerts its bronchodilating effect through a different mechanism of action (see Chapter 10). Figures 2.11 and 2.12 depict β_1- and β_2-adrenoceptor activation/inhibition with their associated biological responses.

Stimulation of α_2-adrenoceptors opposes the production of cAMP by interacting with membrane-bound G proteins termed G_i ("i" stands for inhibitory). Stimulation of α_1-adrenoceptors initiates a series of events that leads to increases in intracellular concentrations of Ca^{2+} as well as causing an influx of extracellular Ca^{2+} in many tissues. In most smooth muscles (the exception being gastrointestinal smooth muscle), the increased concentrations of intracellular Ca^{2+} ultimately causes contraction.

Adrenergic drugs primarily work in one of two ways: the drug either stimulates the release of the natural neurotransmitter norepinephrine from its storage site in the postganglionic fiber (indirectly acting sympathomimetic) or exerts its influence on the β-adrenoceptor by mimicking the action of the natural neurotransmitter (direct-acting sympathomimetic). Most adrenergic drugs are direct acting. The only indirect-acting compound discussed here is tyramine. Tyramine has no action other than to cause the release of norepinephrine from its storage vesicles and is rapidly inactivated by intraneuronal monoamine oxidase. A few adrenergic drugs are mixed-acting agents, in that they have a tyramine-like effect in addition to direct adrenoceptor activation. Such drugs include dopamine (Chapter 18), ephedrine (Chapters 9 and 10), phenylpropanolamine (Chapter 9), and amphetamine.

Table 2.3 summarizes the most important effects of adrenergic stimulation.

Cholinergic Receptor Types and Physiologic Mechanism of Action

The term cholinoceptor is used to describe all receptors that respond to the neurotransmitter acetylcholine or any agent that mimics acetylcholine's action. Because there are many peripheral efferent nerves that are cholinergic, it is helpful as well as convenient to group the cholinoceptors into three categories:

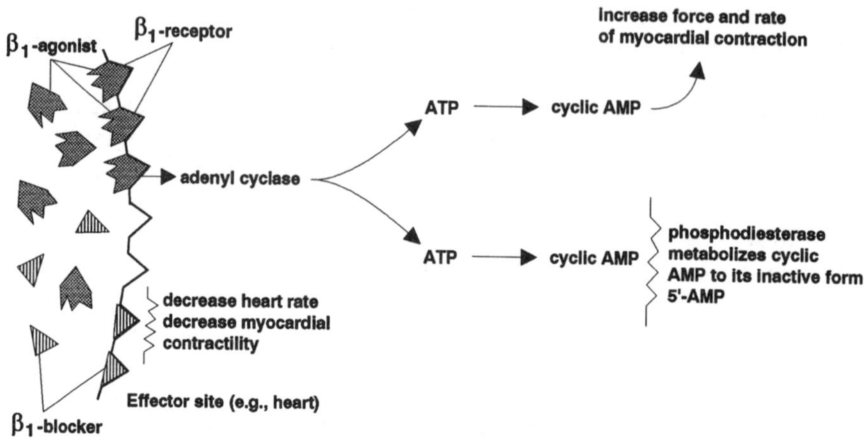

Figure 2.11. Beta receptor stimulation/inhibition. Beta agonists are agents that have the ability to bind to the beta receptor and activate the adenyl cyclase system. Beta blockers (antagonists) are agents that have the ability to bind to the beta receptor but do not activate the adenyl cyclase system. Phosphodiesterase is an enzyme that inactivates cyclic AMP.

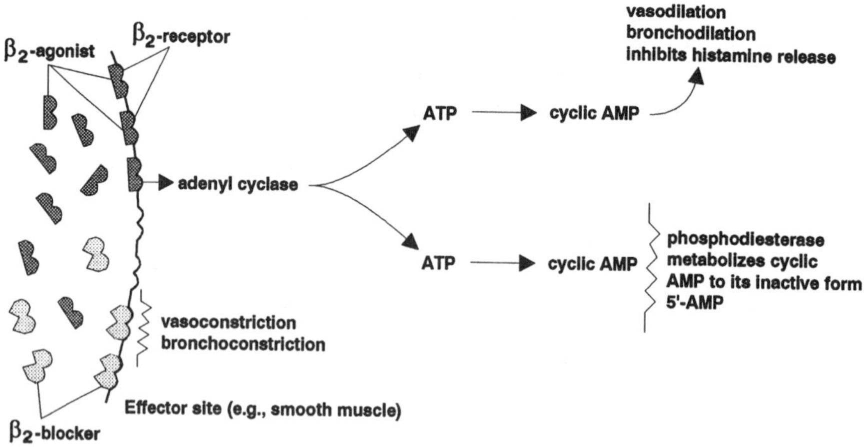

Figure 2.12. Beta receptor stimulation/inhibition. Beta agonists are agents that have the ability to bind to the beta receptor and activate the adenyl cyclase system. Beta blockers (antagonists) are agents that have the ability to bind to the beta receptor but do not activate the adenyl cyclase system. Phosphodiesterase is an enzyme that inactivates cyclic AMP.

Table 2.3.
Responses Of Effector Organs To Adrenergic And Cholinergic Stimulation

Visceral Effector	Adrenergic Response (α_1, α_2, β_1, β_2 β_3)	Cholinergic Response (M_1, M_2, M_3, N_N, N_M)
Adrenal medulla	*	Secretion of epinephrine and norepinephrine (N_N)
Eye		
Radial muscle (iris)	Contraction—mydriasis (α_1)	*
Sphincter muscle (iris)	*	Contraction—miosis (M_3)
Ciliary muscle	Relaxation for far vision (β_2)	Contraction for near vision (M_3)
Fat cells	Lipolysis (primarily β_3, but also α, β_1, β_2)	*
Gastrointestinal tract		
Motility and tone	Decrease (α, β_1 β_2)	Increase (M_3)
Secretion	*	Stimulation (M_3)
Smooth muscle:		
Walls	Relaxation (α_2,β_2)	Contraction (M_3)
Sphincters	Contraction (α_1)	Relaxation (M_3)
Genitourinary smooth muscle		
Bladder wall	Relaxation (β_2)	Contraction (M_3)
Sphincter	Contraction (α_1)	Relaxation (M_3)
Uterus	Pregnant: contraction (α_1) Relaxation (β_2) Nonpregnant: relaxation (β_2)	Contraction (M_3)
Sex organs (male)	Ejaculation (α_1)	Erection (M)
Heart	Increased rate and force of conduction; increased atrioventricular nodal conduction velocity (β_1)	Decreased rate and force of conduction; decreased atrioventricular nodalconduction velocity; vagal arrest (M_2)
Kidney	Renin release (β_1)	*
Lacrimal glands	Increased secretion (α)	Increased secretion (M_3)
Liver	Glycogenolysis and gluconeogenesis (α, β_2)	*
Lung		
Airways	Contraction (α_1)[a]	Contraction (M_3)
Submucosal glands	Decreased secretion (α_1) Increased secretion (β_2)	Increased secretion (M_3)
Nasopharyngeal glands	*	Increased secretion (M_3)
Pancreas	Decreased secretion (α) Increased secretion (β_2)	Increased secretion (M_3)
Pineal gland	Melatonin synthesis (β)	*
Posterior pituitary	Antidiuretic hormone secretion (β_1)	*
Salivary glands	K+ and water secretion (α_1) Amylase secretion (β)	K+ and water secretion (M_3)
Skeletal muscle	Increased contractility; glycogenolysis; K+ uptake (β_2)	Contraction (N_M—somatic nervous system)
Skin		
Pilomotor muscles	Contraction (α_1)	*
Sweat glands	Localized secretion (α_1)	Generalized secretion (M_3)
Spleen capsule	Contraction (α_1) Relaxation (β_2)	*
Vascular smooth muscle	Contraction (α_1, α_2) Relaxation (β_2)	Relaxation (M_3)[b]

[a] These adrenoceptors are not innervated by sympathetic fibers, they respond only to circulating adrenoceptor agonists.
[b] The endothelium of most blood vessels releases endothelium-derived relaxing factor (EDRF), which produces marked vasodilation in response to muscarinic stimuli. These muscarinic receptors are not innervated by parasympathetic fibers; they respond only to circulating muscarinic agonists.

1. preganglionic fibers of the autonomic nervous system (autonomic ganglia and adrenal medulla)
2. postganglionic fibers of the parasympathetic division and a select few postganglionic fibers of the sympathetic division (because they store and release acetylcholine)
3. somatic motor neurons

See Figure 2.6 for illustration of these cholinoceptor locations.

Cholinoceptors are classified according to the physiologic response that is produced when they are stimulated. Two primary types of cholinoceptors have been isolated: muscarinic and nicotinic. Muscarinic receptors have been so named because the cholinergic response at these particular receptors is similar to the effects produced by muscarine (an alkaloid obtained from various mushrooms, e.g., *Amanita muscaria*). Nicotinic receptors have been so named because the biological response from these particular cholinoceptors is similar to the effects produced by the drug nicotine. These two primary cholinoceptors have two or more subtypes.

Identification of each cholinoceptor subtype is based on the basis of both agonist and antagonist selectivity, in addition to functional and anatomical considerations. Synonymous names for those agents that stimulate cholinoceptors, thereby producing a biological response, are cholinoceptor agonists, cholinergic muscle stimulants (those that stimulate the cholinergic nicotinic somatic receptors), parasympathomimetic agents (those that stimulate the muscarinic cholinoceptors), and cholinomimetic agents. On the other hand, synonymous names for those agents that inhibit cholinoceptors, thereby preventing a biological response, include anticholinergic agents, cholinergic antagonists, and parasympatholytic or antimuscarinic agents (those that inhibit the muscarinic cholinoceptors).

Muscarinic Cholinergic Receptors: five subtypes of muscarinic cholinoceptors have been identified: M_1, M_2, M_3, M_4, and M_5. All five subtypes are found in the CNS; however, only three of these five subtypes (M_1, M_2, and M_3) have been defined pharmacologically. Information on the cellular locations of these muscarinic subtypes is somewhat fragmentary and not clearly defined; however, a few generalizations can be made. M_1 receptors are found in some sympathetic postganglionic neurons, some presynaptic sites, autonomic ganglia, CNS neurons, and various secretory glands; M_2 receptors predominate in the myocardium and presynaptic sites; and M_3 receptors are located in various secretory glands, smooth muscle, and vascular endothelium. Autoradiographic mapping of the pulmonary muscarinic receptors (M_3) has shown that these receptors predominate in the large central airways with little to no receptors in the smaller bronchioles. The locations of these muscarinic receptors are differentiated in Figure 2.6.

Overall, activation of muscarinic receptors results in a decrease in the heart rate, a decrease in the force of contraction (which acts to lower cardiac output and blood pressure), and an increase in glandular secretion, vasodilation, and nonvascular smooth muscle contraction. These parasympathetic effects are primarily mediated via impulse transmission through the X cranial nerve (vagus nerve). The exception to this is the vasodilatory effect that results from muscarinic stimuli. Vasculature muscarinic receptors are generally not innervated by parasympathetic fibers (exceptions are vessels in the heart, limb muscles, facial skin, and others); thus, they respond pharmacologically only to circulating muscarinic agonists.

The muscarinic subtypes in the airways appear to serve different physiological functions. M_1 receptors facilitate parasympathetic neurotransmission, thereby enhancing cholinergic reflexes. Presynaptic M_2 receptors located on nerve terminals act as autoreceptors; they inhibit further release of acetylcholine (this is similar to the negative feedback control mechanism of the α_2-adrenoceptors). Pulmonary M_3 receptors mediate the bronchoconstrictive response in airway smooth muscle and the increased secretion noted from stimulating submucosal glands.

Methacholine is a parasympathomimetic agent that works in a manner similar to acetylcholine at the parasympathetic neuroeffector site. It is used in bronchial challenge tests via the inhalation route to assess the degree of airway hyperreactivity in patients with asthma. Inhaled methacholine will produce bronchoconstriction (sometimes severe, depending on the degree of responsiveness in the bronchi to methacholine) in patients who have hyperreactive airway disorders. Atropine is a nonselective muscarinic antagonist (i.e., an *antimuscarinic* agent) that equally blocks all subtypes of muscarinic receptors through **competitive inhibition.** Atropine's effect is to competitively block acetylcholine from binding to the muscarinic receptor. By this action, atropine negates (blocks) vagal nerve impulses. As a result, there is an increase in the heart rate, a reduction in glandular secretions, and bronchodilation. Atropine and its derivative ipratropium bromide (Atrovent) are currently the antimuscarinic bronchodilators of choice when faced with cholinergic mediated bronchospasm (see Chapter 10). Because of its ability to increase the heart rate, atropine is considered a resuscitative drug when a patient experiences hypotensive bradycardia (see Chapter 19). In addition, because of atropine's ability to reduce salivary secretions, atropine is a preoperative drying agent.

Current research pertaining to the use of antimuscarinic bronchodilators indicates that selective M_1 and/or especially M_3 antagonists (inhibitors) would be more useful as bronchodilators over the nonselective antimuscarinic agents, such as atropine. This is because M_2 receptor inhibition is not a desired outcome of antimuscarinic bronchodilators. Agents that inhibit the myocardial M_2 receptors cause an increase in the heart rate, which is an unwanted side effect when only bronchodilation is desired. In addition, inhibition of presynaptic M_2 receptors results in a loss of the negative feedback control mechanism. By this action, there is nothing to prevent further intraneuronal release of acetylcholine.

Nicotinic Cholinergic Receptors: there are two subtypes of nicotinic receptors: N_N (neuronal) and N_M (muscle). N_N receptors are located at all autonomic ganglia and the adrenal medulla, whereas N_M receptors are found at skeletal muscle neuromuscular endplates of the somatic system (Fig. 2.6).

Activation of N_N receptors results in depolarization and firing of postganglionic neurons and secretion of catecholamines (norepinephrine and epinephrine) by the adrenal cells. Selective ganglionic blocking agents, such as trimethaphan (Arfonad), occupy ganglion receptors, thereby preventing acetylcholine from stimulating the receptor. By this action, postganglionic firing is inhibited. These agents are considered antihypertensive agents and are used for hypertensive emergencies to quickly lower the blood pressure.

Activation of N_M receptors elicits neuromuscular endplate depolarization, which results in skeletal muscle contraction. Neuromuscular blocking agents, such as tubocurarine (curare), pancuronium (Pavulon), and succinylcholine (Anectine), effectively block acetylcholine from stimulating the neuromuscular endplate. As a result, total muscle paralysis ensues. It must be remembered that these specific receptors are part of the somatic nervous system, not the autonomic nervous system. The structure and function of these receptors are further detailed in Chapter 14.

Table 2.4 summarizes the characteristics of cholinoceptor subtypes.

Molecular Basis of Cholinoceptor Function: two pathways have been established that account for the basic functions of muscarinic receptors. Both pathways are mediated by interactions with members of the family of G proteins. In one pathway, muscarinic receptors (M_1, M_3, and M_5 subtypes) activate the G_q protein, which leads to a series of events that causes the release of intracellular Ca^{2+}. Thus, these receptors are responsible for the Ca^{2+}-induced contraction of smooth muscle and stimulation of secretory glands. The second pathway for inducing a biological response from muscarinic receptors involves the activation of M_2 and M_4 receptors. These receptors interact with the G_i protein that blocks the activity of adenyl cyclase, thereby lowering intracellular levels of cAMP. The consequences of these effects are most notable on the myocardium, where inhibition of adenyl cyclase accounts for the negative chronotropic and inotropic effects mediated by muscarinic stimulation.

Other cellular events, such as the activation of guanyl cyclase, also result from stimulation of muscarinic receptors. Activated guanyl cyclase catalyzes the conversion of guanosine triphosphate (GTP) to 3′5′-guanosine monophosphate (cyclic GMP, cGMP). Structurally, cGMP is similar to cAMP; nevertheless, cGMP produces opposite physiological effects on smooth muscle (e.g., whereas cAMP produces bronchodilation, cGMP mediates bronchoconstriction). In the mast cell, the rise of intracellular cGMP enhances the release of histamine by al-

Table 2.4.
Characteristics Of Cholinoceptor Subtypes

Receptor	Location	Response
Muscarinic	CNS	Memory function (?)
M_1	Autonomic ganglia	Facilitates ganglionic transmission; enhances cholinergic reflexes
Agonist: Pilocarpine		
Antagonist: Nonselective: Atropine;	Secretory glands	Increased secretion
Partially selective: Pirenzepine		
M_2	CNS	Undefined
Agonist: Oxotremorine-M	Heart	Decreased force and rate of contraction; decreased atrioventricular conduction velocity
Antagonist: Nonselective: Atropine;	Nerve terminals	Inhibitory autoreceptor; inhibits further release of ACh
Partially selective: Methoctramine		
M_3	CNS	Undefined
Agonist: Methacholine	Nonvascular smooth muscle	Contraction [a]
	Secretory glands	Increased secretion
Antagonist: Nonselective: Atropine;	Vascular smooth muscle	Relaxation
Partially selective: 4-DAMP		
Nicotinic	Autonomic ganglia	Depolarization; firing of post-ganglionic neuron
N_N		
Agonist: Nicotine	Adrenal medulla	Secretion of epinephrine and norepinephrine
Antagonist: Trimethaphan (ganglionic blocking agent—antihypertensive agent	CNS	Undefined
N_M	Neuromuscular junction	Endplate depolarization; skeletal muscle contraction
Antagonist: Tubocurarine, Pancuronium (neuromuscular blocking agents—muscle paralyzing agents))		

[a]Relaxation occurs in the sphincters in the urinary and gastrointestinal tracts. CNS = central nervous system; ACh = acetylcholine.

lowing mast cell degranulation. Pertaining to the respiratory system, normal bronchomotor tone is mediated when cAMP and cGMP are in equal balance (Fig. 2.13).

The vascular relaxant effects of muscarinic receptor stimulation are mediated by the release of endothelium-derived relaxing factor (EDRF) from vascular endothelial cells. Upon release from the endothelial cells, EDRF binds to guanyl cyclase, which then rapidly produces cGMP. Whenever cGMP levels rise in vascular smooth muscle, they relax. In 1987, Palmer and colleagues demonstrated that the endothelium-derived relaxing factor emitted from endothelial cells may possibly be nitric oxide (NO). When inhaled as a gas at low levels, NO selectively dilates the pulmonary circulation. Significant systemic vasodilation does not occur owing to nitric oxide's rapid inactivation by coupling with hemoglobin. In patients with marked pulmonary hypertension, inhaled nitric oxide has

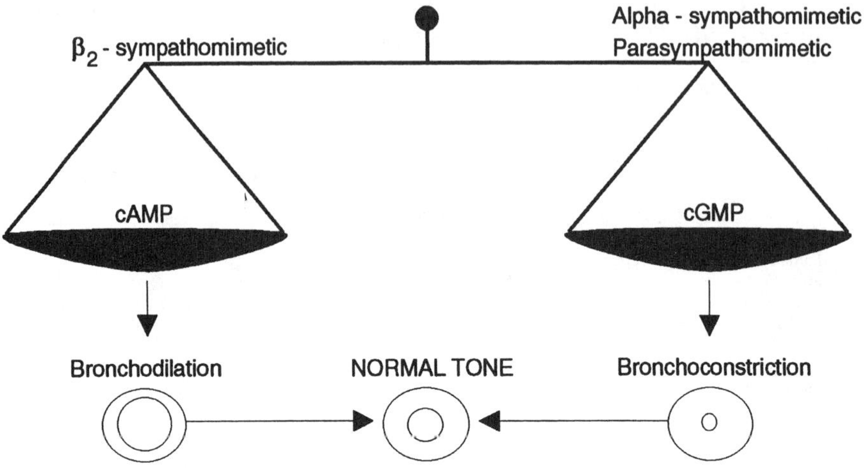

Figure 2.13. Mechanism of bronchial tone.

been shown to reduce pulmonary hypertension and improve arterial oxygenation (see Chapter 8: The Therapeutic Gases, *Nitric Oxide*). The safety and efficacy of exogenously administered nitric oxide is currently being examined in multicenter trials.

cGMP has its own phosphodiesterase system that metabolizes cGMP to its inactive nucleotide 5′-guanosine monophosphate (5′-GMP). Figure 2.14 depicts parasympathetic stimulation/inhibition with its associated biological response in the respiratory system.

Cholinergic drugs primarily work in one of two ways. Either the drug is structurally similar to acetylcholine and it occupies the cholinoceptor to elicit a biological response (direct acting cholinergic) or the drug causes an increase in the concentration and effect of acetylcholine at the receptor site by inhibiting acetylcholinesterase from deactivating acetylcholine (indirect acting cholinergic). Direct-acting cholinergics include such agents as methacholine, carbachol, pilocarpine, and bethanechol. As mentioned previously, methacholine is used in bronchial challenge tests. The last three direct-acting agents listed exert their influence on the muscarinic receptors in the eye and are used for their ability to treat glaucoma. Indirect-acting cholinergics are broadly categorized as acetylcholinesterase inhibitors or, more commonly, cholinergic muscle stimulants. These agents enhance acetylcholine's activity at the neuromuscular junction by preventing acetlycholinesterase from inactivating acetylcholine and are employed in the treatment of myasthenia gravis, either to diagnose its presence or to give maintenance therapy and include such drugs as

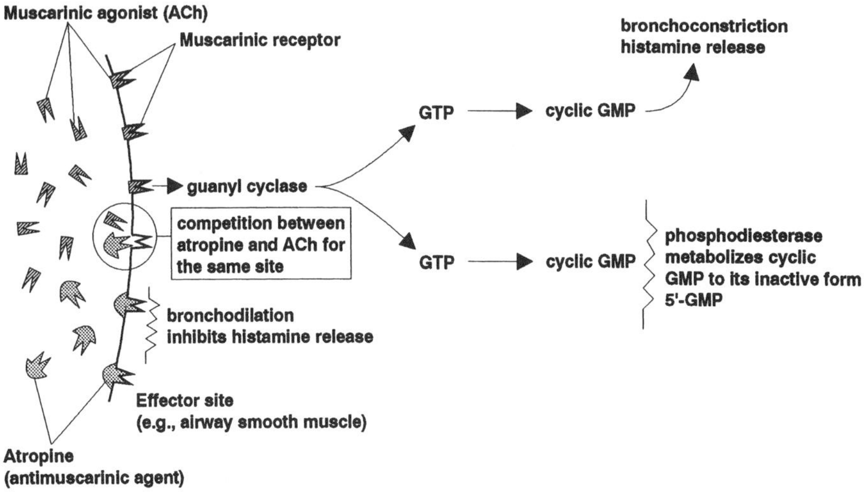

Figure 2.14. Muscarinic receptor stimulation/inhibition. Muscarinic agonists are agents that have the ability to bind to the muscarinic receptor and activate the guanyl cyclase system. Antimuscarinic agents (antagonists) are agents that have the ability to bind to the muscarinic receptor but do not activate the guanyl cyclase system. Phosphodiesterase is an enzyme that inactivates cyclic GMP.

edrophonium (Tensilon), ambenonium (Mytelase), and neostigmine (Prostigmin) (see Chapter 14).

Table 2.3 summarizes the most important effects of cholinergic stimulation.

Nonadrenergic Noncholinergic (NANC) Receptor Types and Physiologic Mechanism of Action

Although relatively little is known about the NANC system and the primary neurotransmitter remains to be clearly defined, several studies indicate that activation of the NANC system produces vasodilation, enhanced cardiac contractility, stimulation of glycogenolysis, and relaxation of smooth muscle in the gastrointestinal and respiratory tract. Most of this action is brought about by the NANC neurotransmitter's ability to activate the adenyl cyclase system and from suppression of acetylcholine release from vagus nerve terminals.

Endogenous vasoactive intestinal peptide (VIP), the substance believed to be the neurotransmitter of the NANC system, is a highly potent airway smooth muscle relaxant; however, studies in which subjects inhaled VIP to potentially produce bronchodilation have shown that exogenously applied VIP has little efficacy as a bronchodilator and exhibits minimal protective effects against histamine-induced bronchoconstriction (Barnes and Dixon 1984). The absence of a bronchodilating effect from inhaled VIP is believed to be caused by either enzymatic breakdown of the peptide or its inability (because of its relatively large size) to gain access to its receptors in airway smooth muscle. Some investigators have suggested that a defect or disturbance in the NANC system might provide an explanation for the hyperreactive airways of asthma and chronic bronchitis caused by the loss of control of normal smooth muscle tone (Richardson and Beland 1976). Because the sympathetic neural pathway does not innervate the airways, the NANC system is believed to be the counterpart and opposing neural system to the parasympathetic system in the airways, which makes the NANC system the major neural inhibitor (relaxer) of airway smooth muscle.

LOCAL CONTROL SUBSTANCES

This section presents an array of substances that are normally present in the body or may be formed within the body that have diverse physiological effects on the visceral organs of the autonomic nervous system. The known biological responses elicited from these substances provide numerous possibilities for therapeutic intervention by the use of agents that mimic, inhibit, or interfere with the synthesis or metabolism of these substances. Collectively, these local control substances are known as **autacoids** (Gk "self remedy") or *local hormones* and include histamine, bradykinin, serotonin (as well as prostaglandins, thromboxane, and related **eicosanoids**), and platelet-activating factor.

Histamine, Bradykinin, and Serotonin

The discovery of histamine dates back to more than 80 years ago, when it was first synthesized and isolated from mammalian tissues. This naturally occurring amine is widely distributed throughout the body and is implicated in a variety of physiologic processes. The profound biological activity of histamine is closely linked to **anaphylaxis.** Both are characterized by smooth muscle constriction, increased capillary permeability, edema, vasodilation (which results in a decrease in blood pressure), and other shock-like symptoms. Thus, histamine is an important mediator of immediate hypersensitivity and allergic reactions and is intimately involved in inflammatory responses. In addition, histamine has an important role in gastric acid secretion.

Following its synthesis, histamine is distributed and stored in tissue mast cells (predominant storage site for histamine) and in the basophils of the circulatory system (the cytologic counterpart of the tissue mast cell). Histamine is stored within the secretory granules of these cells along with heparin, eosinophil chemotactic factor (ECF), neutrophil chemotactic factor (NCF), and enzymes such as peroxidase, neutral proteases, and superoxide dismutase. Those tissues that contain an abundant supply of mast cells, and therefore histamine, include the skin, intestinal mucosa, and the mucosa of the bronchial tree. Smaller amounts of mast cells are found in the heart, liver, neural tissue, and reproductive mucosa. Non-mast cell sites of histamine formation or storage include the cells of the epidermis, cells in the gastric mucosa, neurons within the CNS (where histamine functions as a neurotransmitter), and cells in regenerating or rapidly growing tissues.

Generally, histamine becomes pharmacologically active only upon release from storage sites. Degranulation of the mast cell and subsequent liberation of endogenous histamine can be brought about by a variety of physical and chemical stimuli such as exercise, trauma, tissue injury, chemical irritation, as well as certain drugs (e.g., morphine, tubocurarine). Although these factors are key issues in regulating histamine release, perhaps the most important physiologic mechanism of mast cell and basophil degranulation and subsequent mediator release is immunologic. As part of the allergic response to an **antigen** (Ag), **antibodies** (Ab), in this case immunoglobulin E (IgE), are generated and bound to the surface membrane of mast cells and basophils. Upon subsequent exposure, the antigen bridges with IgE. This event triggers a cascade of biochemical responses that lead to mediator release from mast cells and basophils.

Cromolyn sodium and nedocromil sodium are drugs that are presently employed as adjunct therapy in the management of allergic bronchial asthma. These agents behave as mast cell stabilizers by inhibiting mast cell degranulation. Thus, cromolyn and nedocromil are used prophylactically to decrease the frequency and intensity of asthmatic attacks. The pharmacology of these agents are presented in detail in Chapter 11.

Released histamine exerts its biologic actions by combining with specific histamine-type receptors. At least three distinct classes of receptors that are histamine specific have been isolated in tissues; they are designated as H_1, H_2, and H_3. All three receptors are found in the brain (where histamine is believed to function as a neurotransmitter). Additionally, H_1 receptors are present in endothelial and smooth muscle cells and H_2 receptors are present in gastric mucosa, cardiac muscle cells, and some immune cells. H_3 receptors seem to be localized only to the CNS.

Activation of H_1 receptors by histamine or histamine-like substances elicits bronchial and intestinal smooth muscle contraction, increased capillary permeability, and the formation of edema and wheal, whereas activation of H_2 receptors by histamine mediates an increase in gastric acid secretion and cardiac acceleration as well as inhibiting lymphocyte function. There are some effects of histamine that are brought about by combined H_1 and H_2 stimulation. These include vasodilation, flushing, and headache. Although vascular dilation is considered a combined effect of both H_1 and H_2 receptor activation, it is primarily mediated by H_1 stimulation. H_1 activation initiates a series of events that causes the release of EDRF by endothelial cells, which, as mentioned previously, produces marked vasodilation.

The effects of histamine released in the body can be reduced by one of three mechanisms or by a combination of these mechanisms. *Physiologic antagonists,* such as epinephrine, counteract the biological responses produced by histamine. This is especially important clinically because intravenous injection of epinephrine is the lifesaving drug of choice for systemic anaphylaxis and in other conditions in which massive release of inflammatory mediators occurs.

Histamine receptor antagonists (antihistamines) effectively block histamine from binding to its receptors. For over 45 years, the H_1 antagonists have had a valued place in the treatment of various immediate hypersensitivity reactions. Such agents include diphenhydramine and pyrilamine (see Chapter 9, *Antihistamines*). Specific H_2 antagonists (e.g., cimetidine, ranitidine) are used extensively in the treatment of peptic ulcers. Antagonists that inhibit histamine from binding to the H_3 receptor, such as thioperamide, are not yet available for clinical use. Although the potential use of this agent has yet to be defined, the availability of this selective H_3 antagonist will help define the physiologic role of H_3 receptors.

Release inhibitors are the third mechanism by which the effects of histamine can be reduced. These agents include cromolyn and nedocromil, which have already been discussed. β_2-adrenoceptor agonists also appear capable of reducing histamine release from mast cells (see Chapter 10, *Sympathomimetic Bronchodilators*).

The characteristics of histamine receptor subtypes are summarized in Table 2.5.

Serotonin (5-HT) and bradykinin (Gk "slow moving") are autacoids that have considerable biological activity. These agents, like histamine, are capable of influencing smooth muscle contraction, inducing hypotension, increasing the blood flow and permeability of small blood capillaries, and inciting pain and itching. In addition, serotonin promotes hemostasis upon release from platelets and is the substance secreted by carcinoid tumors. A variety of factors, including vascular injury, tissue damage, allergic reactions, viral infections, and other inflammatory events, activate a series of reactions that enhance the activity of these highly inflammatory mediators.

The actions of serotonin, like those of histamine, can be antagonized in a variety of ways. However, serotonin receptor blockade is the mainstay for therapeutic intervention. Several serotonin receptors (designated as 5-HT receptors) have been identified: 5-HT_1 through 5-HT_7. Competitive 5-HT receptor-blocking agents are used for their ability to prevent nausea and vomiting associated with cancer chemotherapy; to prevent 5-HT-induced smooth muscle contraction; for the prophylactic treatment of migraine and other vascular headaches; to relieve hypertension associated with vasospastic conditions; and to block platelet aggregation promoted by serotonin.

Therapeutic intervention with bradykinin antagonists has produced encourag-

Table 2.5.
Characteristics Of Histamine Receptor Subtypes

Receptor	Location	Response
H_1	Vascular system	Vasodilation; systemic hypotension; increased capillary permeability; edema
Agonist: Betahistine	Gastrointestinal smooth muscle	Contraction
Antagonist: Diphenhydramine; Pyrilamine	Bronchiolar smooth muscle	Contraction
	Skin	Inflammatory response—pain, itching, flushing, wheal
	Brain	Regulates body temperature, antidiuretic hormone secretion, control of blood pressure
H_2	Vascular system	Vasodilation; systemic hypotension
Agonist: Impromidine	Cardiac muscle cells	Increased force and rate of contraction
Antagonist: Cimetidine; Ranitidine	Gastric mucosa	Increased gastric acid secretion
	Immune cells	Inhibition of lymphocyte function
	Brain	Regulates body temperature, antidiuretic hormone secretion, control of blood pressure
H_3	Brain	Inhibitory autoreceptor: regulates the synthesis and interneuronal release of histamine
Agonist: (R) α-methylhistamine		
Antagonist: Thioperamide		

ing results in the relief of cold symptoms caused by the rhinovirus, in the suppression of pain caused by burns, and in the treatment of allergic asthma.

Prostaglandins and Related Eicosanoids

Other mediators influencing the visceral organs of the autonomic nervous system include the by-products of arachidonic acid metabolism, which include the prostaglandins, thromboxane, and the leukotrienes. Collectively, these substances are known as eicosanoids. No other autacoids show more varied effects than these agents of arachidonic acid metabolism.

Various stimuli—including mast cell degranulation, ischemia, hormones, and drugs—activate the release of arachidonic acid from the cell membrane. Once arachidonic acid is released by the cell membrane, it is oxidized by either cyclooxygenase or lipoxygenase.

The lipoxygenase reaction results in the formation of the highly active leukotrienes (Fig. 2.15). Currently, five primary groups of leukotrienes have been identified: LTA through LTE. LTA_4 is an intermediate in the synthesis of the remaining leukotrienes.

Before their structure was fully known, the leukotrienes were identified in perfusates of the lung and designated as the active components of *slow reacting*

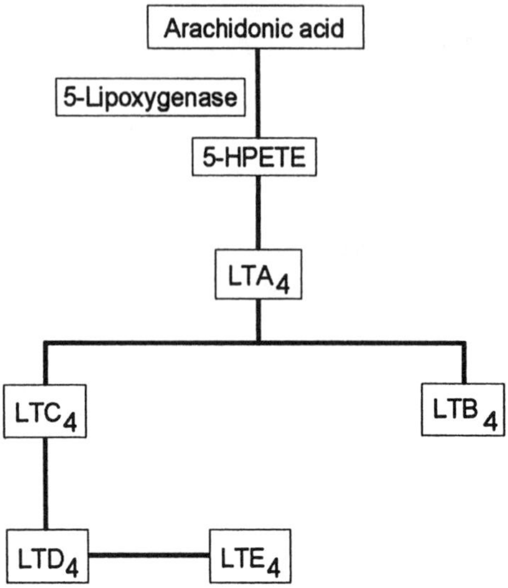

Figure 2.15. Leukotriene synthesis from arachidonic acid.

substance of anaphylaxis (SRS-A) because of their release after an immunologic challenge. SRS-A is a mixture of the highly inflammatory leukotrienes LTC_4, LTD_4, and LTE_4. These leukotrienes exert a prominent bronchoconstrictive effect (they act principally in peripheral airways and are approximately 1000 times more potent than histamine), enhance the responsiveness of bronchi to histamine (LTD_4), induce contraction of gastrointestinal and vascular smooth muscle (LTC_4 and LTD_4), and constrict coronary arteries and skin vessels (also LTC_4 and LTD_4).

Leukotriene B_4 (LTB_4) is a potent chemotactic agent for neutrophils and eosinophils. The mast cell contains, in granule form, both neutrophil and eosinophil chemotactic factors (NCF and ECF), which are released upon mast cell degranulation. LTB_4 from eosinophils is a prominent mediator of inflammation and can be released during an anaphylactic reaction.

Arachidonic acid oxidized by the cyclooxygenase mechanism results in the formation of the prostaglandins and thromboxane (Fig. 2.16). Prostaglandin activity is quite diverse. These agents act on smooth muscle receptors that are not blocked by autonomic blocking agents (such as atropine, propranolol, and phenoxybenzamine). Many actions of the prostaglandins are associated with one of the cyclic nucleotides (cAMP or cGMP).

Prostaglandins $F_{2\alpha}$ ($PGF_{2\alpha}$), D_2 (PGD_2), and thromboxane (TXA_2) exert potent vaso- and bronchoconstrictor effects, whereas the E series of prostaglandins

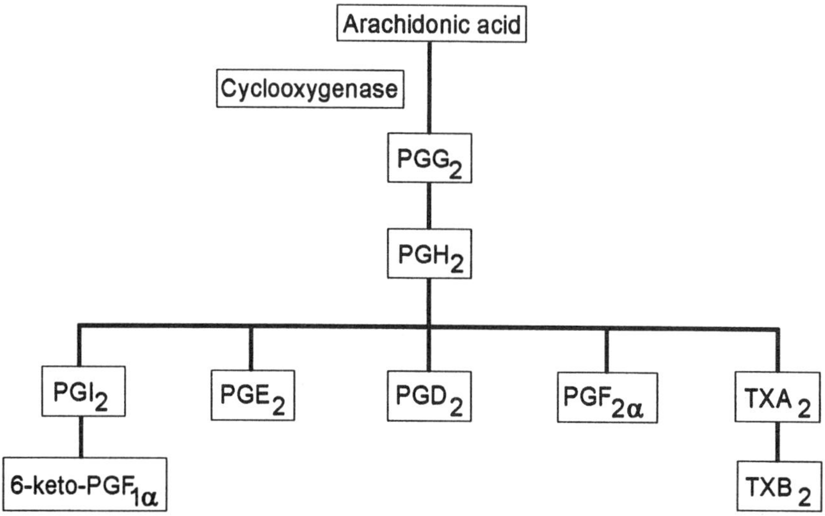

Figure 2.16. Prostaglandin and thromboxane synthesis from arachidonic acid.

(PGE_1, PGE_2) and PGI_2 (prostacyclin) have the ability to relax smooth muscle and suppress the antagonizing effects of bradykinin, histamine, acetylcholine, and serotonin. Table 2.6 summarizes the physiologic effects of prostaglandins and related eicosanoids.

Nonsteroidal anti-inflammatory drugs (NSAIDS) such as aspirin, indomethacin, naproxen, and ibuprofen have the ability to block the synthesis of prostaglandins and thromboxane through the inhibition of arachidonic acid metabolism by the cyclooxygenase pathway. It is important to note that NSAIDS only inhibit prostaglandin and thromboxane synthesis and not that of the leukotrienes. Thus, it is believed that NSAIDS can actually increase the production of leukotrienes by diverting arachidonic acid to the lipoxygenase pathway. However, corticosteroids (see Chapter 12) have the ability to inhibit the synthesis of both prostaglandins and leukotrienes and are therefore of interest as potent anti-inflammatory agents.

Platelet-Activating Factor

A unique type of substance that causes platelets to aggregate is released from leukocytes. This substance has been designated as *platelet-activating factor* (PAF). Like the eicosanoids, PAF is not stored in cells but is synthesized in response to stimulation.

Table 2.6.
Physiologic Effects Of Prostaglandins And Related Eicosanoids

Eicosanoid	Physiologic Effect
PGE_1, PGE_2, PGI_2	Vasodilation, bronchodilation Inflammatory: increases local blood flow, increases vascular permeability
$PGF_{2\alpha}$, PGD_2 TXA_2	Vasoconstriction, bronchoconstriction
PGE_1, PGD_2, PGI_2	Inhibits platelet aggregation
PGG_2, PGH_2, TXA_2	Stimulates platelet aggregation
PGE_1, PGE_2	Stimulates gastric secretion of bicarbonate
$PGF_{2\alpha}$, LTC_4, LTD_4	Gastrointestinal smooth muscle contraction
LTC_4, LTD_4	Bronchoconstriction, vasoconstriction of coronary arteries and skin vessels Inflammatory: increases vascular permeability
LTB_4	Inflammatory; chemotactic agent for neutrophils and eosinophils

PAF is a potent pathophysiologic mediator of asthma and shock. PAF exerts its influence to induce significant vasodilation, stimulate platelet aggregation, and cause contraction of gastrointestinal, uterine, and bronchiolar smooth muscle, as well as to promote the accumulation of eosinophils in the lung, stimulate the secretion of mucus, and cause tracheal and bronchial edema. Although several compounds have been described that selectively block the actions of PAF, the clinical utility of these agents has not been fully established and is still in the early stages of development.

Figure 2.17 presents a graphic summary of the primary agents and mediators described in this chapter that, in one form or another, influence airway activity.

AUTONOMIC CONTROL BY HIGHER CENTERS

Although the ANS usually operates independently without conscious control, it is not a separate nervous system. Many of the regulatory activities of the ANS are brought about by feedback from certain brain centers, such as the hypothalamus. The hypothalamus is considered the major integration center of the ANS in which the balance of sympathetic versus parasympathetic activity or tone is maintained. Output from the hypothalamus influences the autonomic centers in the medulla and spinal cord because anatomically the hypothalamus is connected to both the sympathetic and parasympathetic systems. The posterior and lateral portions of the hypothalamus connect with the sympathetic system. When these areas of the hypothalamus are stimulated, the sympathetic response is to increase the heart rate, increase the blood pressure, increase the body temperature, increase the rate and depth of ventilation, dilate the pupils, and inhibit gastrointestinal secretion and motility. The anterior and medial portions of the hypothalamus connect with the parasympathetic system. Stimulation of these areas result

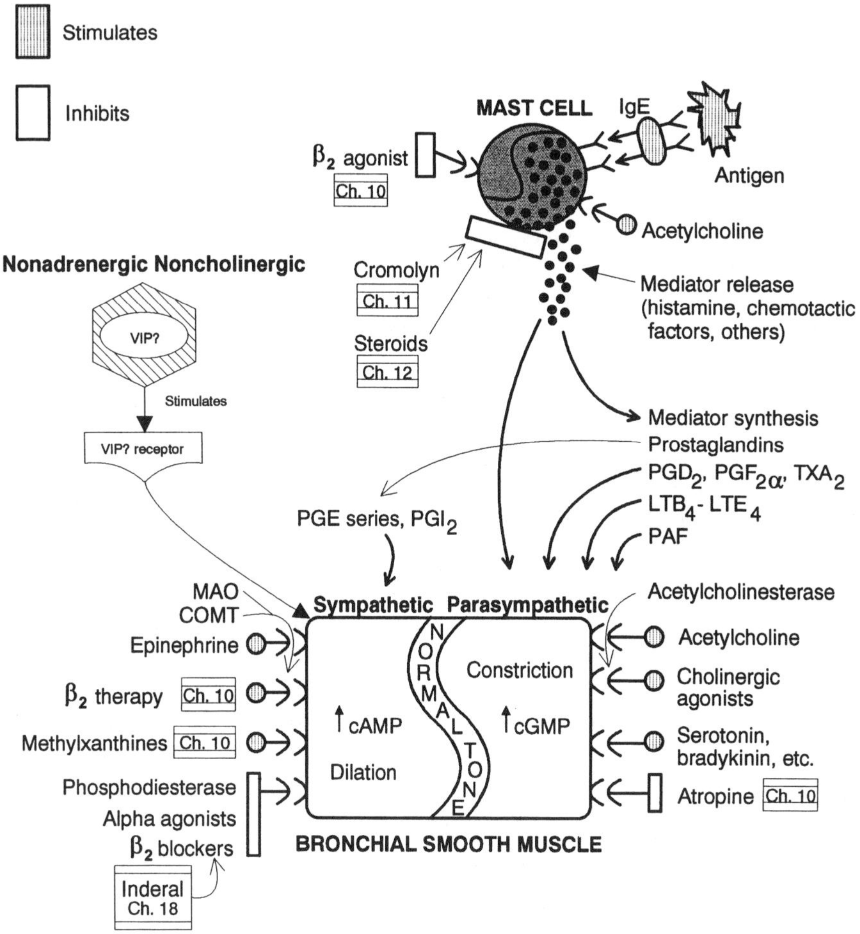

Figure 2.17. Primary agents and mediators that influence airway activity.

in the parasympathetic response of decreasing the heart rate, decreasing the blood pressure, constricting the pupils, and causing an increase in gastrointestinal secretion and motility.

The cerebral cortex can also play a regulatory role in autonomic responses. During extreme emotional stress or anxiety, the cortex can stimulate the hypothalamus as part of the limbic system (see Chapter 15). This stimulatory action results in activation of the cardiac and vasomotor centers of the medulla, which increases the heart rate and blood pressure. On the other hand, stimulation of the cortex may induce vasodilation, which would result in a decrease in blood pressure and fainting, such as might occur when experiencing an extremely unpleasant sight or hearing bad news.

PHARMACOLOGIC MODIFICATION OF AUTONOMIC FUNCTION

This chapter has detailed the divisions and mechanisms of action of the ANS as well as the various mediators that influence the visceral organs of the ANS. Familiarity with *how* the ANS regulates visceral functions leads to an essential understanding of *why* autonomic drugs are effective pharmacologic agents. Most drugs that act in the ANS produce their effects by interacting with, and thus modifying, some step in chemical synaptic transmission. Figure 2.18 illustrates some of the steps that can be altered. Drugs acting on autonomic nerve endings (presynaptic agents) may either enhance or inhibit the synthesis, storage, metabolism, or release of neurotransmitters. Once in the synaptic cleft, the amount of neurotransmitter available for receptor binding may be increased or decreased by drugs that act upon its reuptake or degradation (synaptic agents). Drugs acting on autonomic receptors at neuroeffector sites or at ganglionic passages (postsynaptic agents) can interact either as neurotransmitter agonists or they can block receptor function. Many of these agents offer maximum flexibility and selectivity of effect whereas others are much less selective in their effects.

In addition to the mechanisms listed above, all of which interact in regulating the primary messenger system (i.e., some aspect of neurotransmitter activity), there are autonomic drugs that affect the secondary messenger system (e.g., cAMP and cGMP). Agents affecting the secondary messenger system bring about a change that either cause an increase or a decrease in its intracellular level.

For purposes of understanding *where* and *how* these agents interact, classification of autonomic drugs is based on their site of action (*where*) and mode of action (*how*). Thus, pharmacologic agents that act in the ANS can be categorized into four primary groups:

1. Agents acting on autonomic receptors at the neuroeffector site.
2. Agents acting on autonomic nerve endings.
3. Agents acting on autonomic ganglia.
4. Agents acting on secondary messenger systems.

This classification scheme is presented in Table 2.7. Some of the agents listed in Table 2.7 have been introduced in this chapter and will be further detailed in subsequent chapters of this book.

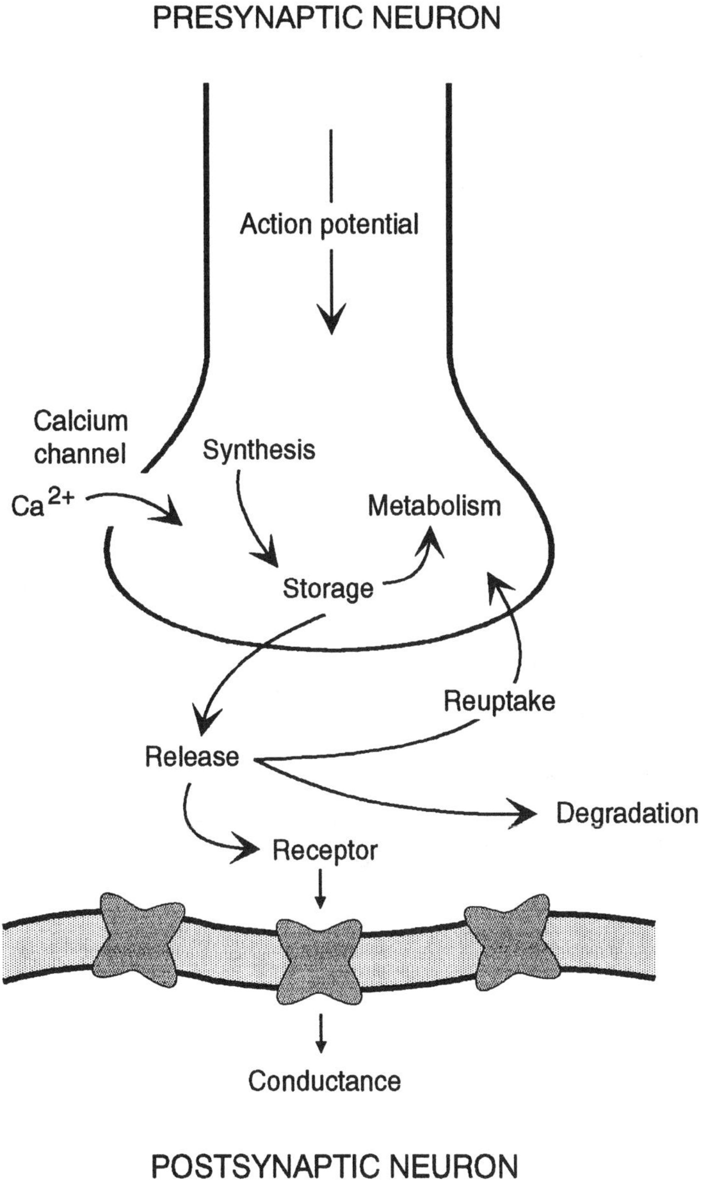

Figure 2.18. Various sites of drug action. Drugs can affect any one or more of the steps involved in the neurohormonal transmission of impulses, leading to inhibition or stimulation at the neuroeffector site.

Table 2.7.
Classification of Autonomic and Related Drugs by Site and Mode of Action

I. Drugs acting on autonomic receptors at the neuroeffector site
- A. *Agonists*
  - 1. Parasympathomimetics (cholinomimetics, cholinoceptor agonists, cholinergic agonists, muscarinic agents)
    - *a) Direct-acting parasympathomimetics: drugs that stimulate cholinoceptors—acetylcholine, methacholine, pilocarpine*
    - *b) Indirect-acting aprasympathomimetics: drugs that potentiate endogenous acetylcholine through inhibition of acetylcholinesterase—physostigmine (cholinergic muscle stimulants [anticholinesterases]—Chatper 15)*
  - 2. Sympathomimetics (adrenoceptor agonists, adrenergic agents)
    - *a) Direct-acting sympathomimetics: drugs that stimulate adrenoceptors*
      - (1) α_1-adrenoceptor agonists: phenylephrine (nasal decongestants—Chapter 9; vasoconstrictors—Chapter 18)
      - (2) α_2-adrenoceptor agonists (CNS): clonidine, methyldopa (antihypertensive agents—Chapter 18)
      - (3) β_1-adrenoceptor agonists: dobutamine (inotropic agents, hypertensive agents—Chapter 18)
      - (4) β_2-adrenoceptor agonists: albuterol, salmeterol (bronchodilators—Chapter 10)
      - (5) Nonselective α-agonists: epinephrine, norepinephrine, (vasoconstrictors—Chapter 18; cardiopulmonary resuscitative agents—Chapter 19)
      - (6) Nonselective β-agonists: isoproterenol (bronchodilators—Chapter 10; inotropic agents—Chapter 18; cardiopulmonary resuscitative agents—Chapter 19)
    - *b) Indirect-acting sympathomimetics: cause the release of norepinephrine from adrenergic nerve terminals—tyramine*
    - *c) Mixed action: cause the release of norepinephrine from adrenergic nerve terminals and can stimulate adrenoceptors—ephedrine, phenylpropanolamine (nasal decongestants—Chapter 9) dopamine (inotropic and hypertensive agent—Chapter 18)*
    - *d) Monoamine oxidase (MAO) inhibitors (CNS): drugs that prevent the degradation of norepinephrine or epinephrine by MAO: tranylcypromine (antidepressants—Chapter 15)*
- B. *Antagonists*
  - 1. Parasympatholytics (cholinoceptor blocking agents, antimuscarinics): drugs that block the stimulation of muscarinic receptors
    - *a) Competitive inhibitor at muscarinic receptors: atropine (bronchodilator—Chapter 10, cardiopulmonary resuscitative agent—Chapter 19), ipratropium (bronchodilator—Chapter 10)*
  - 2. Sympatholytics (adrenoceptor blocking agents): drugs that block the stimulation of adrenoceptors
    - (1) α_1-adrenoceptor blockers: prazosin (antihypertensive agents—Chapter 18)
    - (2) α_2-adrenoceptor blockers (CNS): yohimbine (hypertensive agents—Chapter 18)
    - (3) β_1-adrenoceptor blockers: metoprolol (antihypertensive agents—Chapter 18)
    - (4) β_2-adrenoceptor blockers: no therapeutic usefulness
    - (5) Nonselective α-adrenoceptor blockers: phenoxybenzamine, phentolamine (antihypertensive agents—Chapter 18)
    - (6) Nonselective β-adrenoceptor blockers: propranolol (antihypertensive agents—Chapter 18)

II Drugs acting on autonomic nerve endings
- A. *Agonists that cause the release of neurotransmitters*
  - 1. Cholinergic neurons: carbachol (agents for glaucoma)
  - 2. Adrenergic neurons: indirect and mixed acting sympathomimetics (see above)
- B. *Drugs that inhibit the release of neurotransmitters*
  - 1. Cholinergic neurons: botulinum toxin (agents for cervical dystonia)
  - 2. Adrenergic neurons: bretylium (agents for ventricular arrhythmias—Chapter 19), guanethidine (antihypertensive agents—Chapter 18)
- C. *Drugs that inhibit the synthesis of neurotransmitters*
  - 1. Cholinergic neurons (inhibits synthesis of acetylcholine): hemicholinium (not in clinical use)
  - 2. Adrenergic neurons (depletes norepinephrine): metyrosine (antihypertensive agent for pheochromocytoma—Chapter 18)
- D. *Drugs that inhibit the storage of neurotransmitters in presynaptic neurons*
  - 1. Cholinergic neurons: vesamicol (not in clinical use)
  - 2. Adrenergic neurons: guanethidine, reserpine (antihypertensive agents—Chapter 18, antipsychotic agents [CNS]—Chapter 15)

Table 2.7.—*continued*

- E. Drugs that block the uptake of the neurotransmitter after release
  1. Cholinergic neurons: none
  2. Adrenergic neurons (inhibits uptake-1): cocaine (local anesthetic—Chapter 15), tricyclic antidepressants (antipsychotic agents [CNS]—Chapter 15)
  3. Adrenergic neurons (inhibits uptake-2): corticosteroids (anti-inflammatory agents, increased catecholamine responsiveness—Chapter 12)

III. Drugs acting on autonomic ganglia
- A. *Ganglionic stimulators: stimulates the nicotinic (N_N) receptors at autonomic ganglia*
  1. Stimulates the release of acetylcholine: nicotine
  2. Potentiates endogenous acetylcholine through inhibition of acetylcholinesterase: anticholinesterases (see Chapter 14)
- B. *Ganglionic blockers: inhibits the nicotinic (N_N) receptors at autonomic ganglia*
  1. Blocks acetylcholine from binding to nicotinic receptors (competitive antagonists): mecamylamine (used for severe essential hypertension—Chapter 18), neuromuscular blocking agents (not a desired effect of these agents—see Chapter 14)

IV. Drugs acting on secondary messenger systems
- A. *Secondary messenger activated or degradation is prevented*
  1. cAMP: β-adrenoceptor stimulation (initiates the production of cAMP, see above), phosphodiesterase inhibitors (prevents the degradation of cAMP—amrinone [inotropic agents—Chapter 18]), adenosine receptor antagonists (increases intracellular levels—theophylline [bronchodilator—Chapter 10])
  2. cGMP: muscarinic receptor stimulation (see above), nitric oxide (pulmonary antihypertensive agent—Chapter 8)
  3. Ca^{2+}: α_1-adrenoceptor stimulation (see above), stimulation of nonvascular muscarinic receptors (see above)
- B. *Secondary messenger inhibited*
  1. cAMP: α_2-adrenoceptor stimulation (see above), beta blocking agents (see above)
  2. cGMP: antimuscarinic agents (see above)
  3. Ca^{2+}: calcium channel blockers—verapamil (negative inotropic agents—Chapter 18)

V. Drugs acting on nicotinic (N_M) receptors at the neuromuscular junction
- A. *Agonists*
  1. Direct-acting cholinergic agents (stimulates the cholinoceptor): acetylcholine
  2. Indirect-acting cholinergic agents (potentiates endogenous acetylcholine through inhibition of acetylcholinesterase): neostigmine, physostigmine (cholinergic muscle stimulants [anticholinesterases]—Chapter 14)
- B. *Antagonists*
  1. Depolarizing neuromuscular blocking agents: succinylcholine—Chapter 14
  2. Nondepolarizing neuromuscular blocking agents: tubocurarine, pancuronium—Chapter 14.

VI. Drugs acting on all nerves to block conduction
- A. *Local anesthetics: procaine, lidocaine—Chapter 15*

VII. Other endogenous biologically active compounds
- A. *Inflammatory mediators: histamine, serotonin, bradykinin, prostaglandins, leukotrienes, platelet-activating factor*

REFERENCES/RECOMMENDED READING

Barnes PJ. The third nervous system in the lung: physiology and clinical perspectives. Thorax 39:561, 1984.

Barnes PJ, Dixon CMS. The effect of inhaled vasoactive intestinal peptide on bronchial reactivity to histamine in humans. Am Rev Respir Dis 130:162, 1984.

Barnes PJ, Basbaum CB, Nadel JA. Autoradiographic localization of autonomic receptors in airway smooth muscle: marked differences between large and small airway. Am Rev Respir Dis 127:758, 1983.
Brain SD, Williams TJ. Leukotrienes and inflammation. Pharmacol Ther 46:57, 1990.
Blank ML, et al. Antihypertensive activity of an alkyl ether analog of phosphatidylcholine. Biochem Biophys Res Commun 90:1194, 1979.
Bolton TB. Mechanisms of action of transmitters and other substances on smooth muscle. Physiol Rev 59:606, 1979.
Bonner TI. The molecular basis of muscarinic receptor diversity. Trends Neurosci 12:148, 1989.
Buga GM, et al. Endothelium-derived nitric oxide relaxes nonvascular smooth muscle. Eur J Pharmacol 161:61, 1989.
Burnstock G. Evolution of the autonomic innervation of visceral and cardiovascular systems in vertebrates. Pharmacol Rev 21:247, 1969.
Burnstock G. The changing face of autonomic neurotransmission. Acta Physiol Scand 126:67, 1986.
Carstairs JR, Nimmo AJ, Barnes PJ. Autoradiographic visualization of beta-adrenoceptor subtypes in human lung. Am Rev Respir Dis 132:541, 1985.
Cohen ML, et al. Role of 5-HT2 receptors in serotonin-induced contractions of nonvascular smooth muscle. J Pharmacol Exp Ther 232:770, 1985.
Darin J. The mode of action of cyclic AMP. Respir Care 26:228, 1981.
Emorine L, et al. Molecular characterization of the human β3-adrenergic receptor. Science 245:1118, 1989.
Fahrenkrug J. VIP and autonomic neurotransmission. Pharmacol Ther 41:515, 1989.
Gilman AG. G proteins: transducers of receptor-generated signals. Ann Rev Biochem 56:615, 1987.
Goodman L, Gilman A. The Pharmacologic Basis of Therapeutics. 8th ed. New York: McGraw-Hill, Inc., 1993.
Haaksman EEJ, Leirs R, Timmerman H. Histamine receptors: subclasses and specific ligands. Pharmacol Ther 47:73, 1990.
Hill SJ. Distribution, properties, and functional characteristics of three classes of histamine receptors. Pharmacol Rev 42:45, 1990.
Hokfelt T, et al. Cellular locations of peptides in neural structures. Proc R Soc Lond B Biol Sci 210:63, 1980.
Holtzman MJ. Arachidonic acid metabolism in airway epithelial cells. Annu Rev Physiol 54:303, 1992.
Julius D. Molecular biology of serotonin receptors. Annu Rev Neurosci 14:335, 1991.
Katzung BG. Basic & Clinical Pharmacology. 6th ed. Norwalk: Appleton & Lange, 1995.
Lands AM, et al. Differentiation of receptor systems activated by sympathomimetic amines. Nature 214:597, 1967.
Lands WEM. Biochemistry of Arachidonic Acid Metabolism. Boston: Martinus Nijhoff, 1985.
Lazarus SC, et al. cAMP immunocytochemistry provides evidence for functional VIP receptors in trachea. Am J Physiol 251(1, Part 1):C115, 1986.
Limbird LE. Receptors linked to inhibition of adenylate cyclase: additional signaling mechanisms. FASEB J 2:2686, 1988.
MacGlashan DW, et al. Comparative studies of human basophils and mast cells. Fed Proc 42:2504, 1983.
Mancia G, Zanchetti A. Hypothalamic control of autonomic function. In: Morgane G, Panksepp J. Handbook of the Hypothalamus. Vol 3, Pt B, Behavioral Studies of the Hypothalamus. New York: Marcel Dekker, Inc., 1981, pp 147–202.

Matsuzaki Y, Hamasaki Y, Said SI. Vasoactive intestinal peptide: a possible transmitter of nonadrenergic relaxation of guinea pig airways. Science 210:1252, 1980.

Palmer RM, Ferrigo AG, Moncada S. Nitric oxide release accounts for the biological activity of endothelium-derived relaxing factor. Nature 327:524, 1987.

Parsons SM, et al. Acetylcholine transport: fundamental properties and effects of pharmacological agents. Ann N Y Acad Sci USA 493:220, 1987.

Rees DD, Palmer RM, Moncada S. Role of endothelium-derived nitric oxide in the regulation of blood pressure. Proc Natl Acad Sci U S A 86:3375, 1989.

Richardson J, Beland J. Nonadrenergic inhibitory nervous system in human airways. J Appl Physiol 41:764, 1976.

Rocklin RE, Beer DJ. Histamine and immune modulation. Adv Intern Med 28:225, 1983.

Saxtena PR, Ferrari MD. 5-HT1-like receptor agonists and the pathophysiology of migraine. Trends Pharmacol Sci 10:200, 1989.

Sebaldt RJ, et al. Inhibition of eicosanoid biosynthesis by glucocorticoids in humans. Proc Natl Acad Sci U S A 87:6974, 1990.

Starke K. Presynaptic α-autoreceptors. Rev Physiol Biochem Pharmacol 107:73, 1987.

Surprenant A, North RA. Mechanism of synaptic inhibition by noradrenaline acting at α2-adrenoceptors. Proc R Soc Lond B Biol Sci 234:85, 1988.

PHASES OF DRUG EVENTS 3

To enhance the comprehension of drug administration, action, and effect, a three-phase sequence of events has been developed (Ariens and Simonis 1974). This chapter focuses on these three phases. The pharmaceutical phase (drug administration) is presented in Part I. The pharmacokinetic phase, which involves the movement of a drug within the body from the initial absorption by the bloodstream to excretion from the body, is presented in Part II of this chapter, and the pharmacodynamic phase, the actual mechanism of drug action and effect, is presented in Part III (see also Chapter 2, which presents the actual mechanism of drug action and effect within the autonomic nervous system). Figure 3.1 presents an overview of these three phases of drug events. This chapter concludes with a discussion of the nonrespiratory functions of the lungs as they pertain to synthesis, filtration, metabolism, and elimination.

LEARNING OUTCOMES

Upon completion of this chapter, the learner will be able to:

1. Define the terms listed in *Key Terms.*
2. Identify the primary factors involved when determining the route of drug administration.
3. List the major routes of drug administration. Compare/contrast the intravenous route with the inhalation route.
4. Discuss the advantages and disadvantages associated with each route of drug administration.
5. State the ideal aerosol particle size for optimal bronchiolar and alveolar deposition.
6. Describe the factors influencing aerosol deposition and the ideal ventilatory pattern to achieve maximal aerosol deposition.

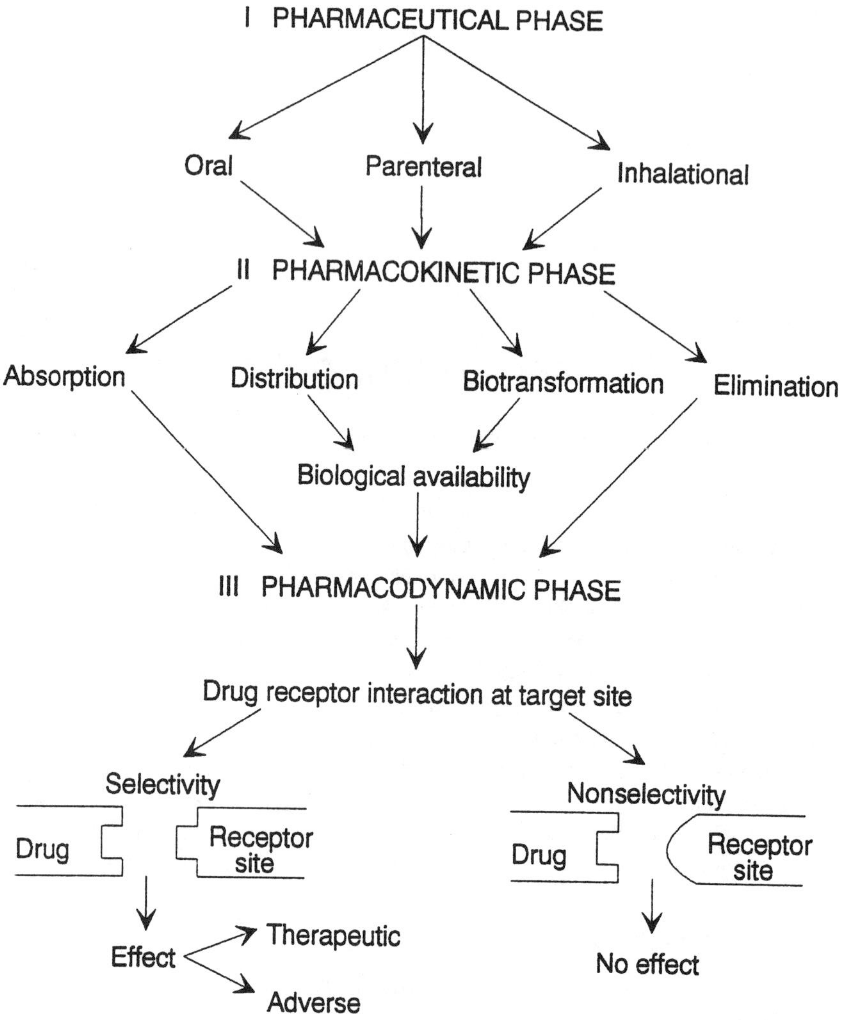

Figure 3.1. The major phases of drug administration, action, and effect, given in sequence.

7. Identify the various aerosol devices, listing the indication for use and any advantages or disadvantages that may apply.
8. Describe the proper technique for administering a metered-dose inhaler (MDI).
9. State the criteria that meets the protocol for administering a small-volume nebulizer (SVN), for administering or changing to an MDI, and for administering a dry-powder inhaler (DPI).

10. Explain the processes of absorption, distribution, redistribution, biotransformation, and elimination. Identify the factors that affect each process.
11. List the five transport mechanisms and give a brief explanation of each.
12. List the primary organ for drug biotransformation and for drug elimination.
13. Explain the drug-receptor interaction and drug specificity.
14. Describe the various aspects of the lung's nonrespiratory functions as they pertain to synthesis, filtration, metabolism, and elimination.

KEY TERMS

(The following key terms are highlighted in **bold** when they first occur in the text of this chapter.)

acidic—Any substance that liberates hydrogen ions; has a pH less than 7.

aerosol deposition—The removal from suspension, or rainout, of aerosol particles.

aerosol penetration—The depth at which an aerosol particle reaches within the lungs.

aerosol stability—The ability of an aerosol particle to remain in suspension.

alimentary canal—The gastrointestinal tract; includes the mouth, pharynx, esophagus, stomach, small and large intestines, and rectum.

base—Any substance that combines with hydrogen ions; has a pH greater than 7.

bioavailability—A measure of the speed and completeness of absorption; the *rate* at which an administered dose reaches the general circulation.

biotransformation—A chemical alteration from the original compound. The by-product of transformation is termed a "metabolite."

blood-brain barrier—A specialized membrane barrier that exists between circulating blood and the brain.

diffusion—The tendency of molecules to move from a region of high concentration to a region of low concentration until an equilibrium exists.

infiltration—Refers to the process in which a substance passes into and deposits within a cell, tissue, or organ.

ionization—The dissociation of compounds (acids, bases) into a particle carrying an electric charge (ion). Ions that carry a positive charge are termed "cations," whereas ions that carry a negative charge are termed "anions." Ionized drug molecules are generally not lipid-soluble, which makes it difficult for these molecules to diffuse into cellular membranes.

osmosis—The passage of a substance through a semipermeable membrane that separates solutions of different concentrations. The substance passes through the membrane from a region of lower concentration to the region of higher concentration.

oxygen-derived free radicals—Reactive oxygen metabolites that are released by neutrophils and macrophages during an inflammatory process.

parenteral—Denotes any medication route other than through the alimentary canal. Usually refers to injectable routes.

pharmaceutical phase of drug therapy—Refers to the administration of drugs; includes all routes of medication administration.
pharmacodynamic phase of drug therapy—Refers to the mechanism of action and effects of drugs.
pharmacokinetic phase of drug therapy—Refers to the movement of drugs within a living organism; includes the processes of drug absorption, drug distribution, drug redistribution, drug metabolism, and drug elimination. Of special importance is the time required for the above processes to occur.
pharmacotherapeutics—Refers to the use of medications to treat diseases.
physiochemical—Pertains to the chemical nature or properties of a substance.
pK_a—The pH at which a drug is 50% ionized and 50% nonionized.
solubility—Capability of being dissolved.

PART I: PHARMACEUTICAL PHASE (DRUG ADMINISTRATION)

Naturally, for a drug to be accessible to the body, it must have a route of entry. The dosage form of a drug usually determines the method of administration. For example, pills, tablets, and capsules are inherent to the oral route. When a drug's action and effect are needed immediately, the intravenous route is used. Figure 3.2 compares the various routes of administration with their respective onsets of action.

Other factors to consider pertaining to a drug's route of administration include the extent to which the drug is absorbed and whether either a systemic or a local effect is desired.

A local effect is one in which the effects of the medication are confined to one area of the body. Local medications come in various forms, such as aerosols, ointments, creams, paste, powders, and lotions. Sprays, aerosols, nebulizers, and gases (such as oxygen, air, or gas mixtures) are methods of introducing local medications into the respiratory tract, which delivers the drug directly to its desired site of action. Local medications can be water-based (aqueous) or oil-based preparations. Water-based medications are absorbed quite rapidly, whereas oil-based medications are absorbed more slowly. Oil-based medications should never be used in the upper or lower respiratory tract, because the oil may be carried to the alveolar region and the patient may develop a lipoid pneumonia.

A systemic effect is one in which the medication is absorbed and delivered to one or more tissue groups by way of the vascular system. Systemic medications can be administered either orally, **parenterally,** or by inhalation.

A patient's age and physical condition also influence the decision regarding the route of drug administration. An unconscious or debilitated patient or a patient who cannot swallow would not be given a tablet or capsule; likewise, an intravenous injection would not be given if another form of drug administration would

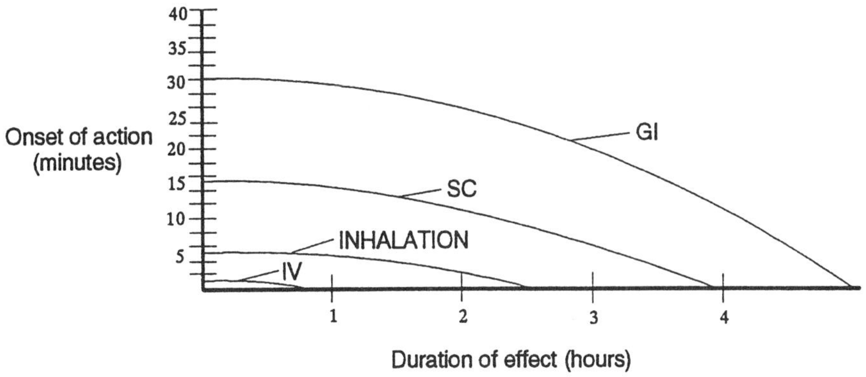

Figure 3.2. Comparison of equal doses of a drug administered by different routes. The intravenous (IV) route achieves the fastest onset of action, followed closely by the inhalation route. The gastrointestinal (GI) and subcutaneous (SC) routes have the slowest onset of drug action; however, drug levels are maintained for a longer period of time.

be more practical, either for economic or emotional reasons. The main and final concern in all routes of administering a drug is the safety of the patient.

Topical Administration

There are two types of topical administration: through the mucous membranes and through the skin.

Topical administration of drugs that are absorbed by the mucous membranes include ophthalmic (eye), nasal (nose), and otic (ear) solutions; sublingual (placed under the tongue) and buccal (placed between the teeth and cheek) tablets; suppositories (rectal, vaginal, or urethral); and lozenges (solid discs that dissolve in the mouth). Absorption of drugs through the mucosa occurs by **diffusion, infiltration,** and **osmosis.** The advantages of mucous membrane absorption include the following:

- Provides quick drug effect—Because the mucous membranes are the thinnest, most vascular dermal surface, the drug is absorbed directly into the bloodstream.
- The medication is not damaged by gastric secretions.
- Prevents gastrointestinal (GI) tract irritation.
- May be used if the patient cannot swallow or if he/she is intubated.
- Avoids degradation by the liver.

The primary disadvantage to topical mucous membrane application is that it may irritate the mucosa. In addition, patients who are given sublingual or buccal tablets must be alert and cooperative because the tablet must be held under the tongue or between the teeth and cheek until the medication is dissolved.

Topical administration of drugs through skin absorption include lotions, ointments, liniments, powders, pastes, jellies, and creams. These types of drugs are usually given for their local effect at the site of application. Advantages of this form of drug administration include:

- Ease of administration;
- Quick relief for itching and pain;
- Fewer allergic or adverse reactions compared to systemic routes.

The primary disadvantage of skin application is adverse reactions to the drug if it becomes systemically absorbed when only a local effect was desired.

A few topical drugs are commonly applied to the skin for systemic absorption via the *transdermal patch.* The transdermal patch uses a unique medicated disk that is applied to the skin, much like a Band-aid. This system provides a continuous release of the drug from a reservoir through a semipermeable membrane. Systemic drug absorption is largely determined by the thickness of the skin layer, the underlying vascular access, and the density of the drug. A precaution to use is that fever will enhance the release and uptake of the drug and may necessitate removal of the patch. Medications that are currently available via these long-acting transdermal patches include nitroglycerin, estrogen, scopolamine, and nicotine.

Oral Administration

Oral ingestion of drugs is the most ancient method known and is still the most commonly used method today. Although the onset of drug action is slow (Fig. 3.2), oral ingestion is considered to be the safest, most convenient, and most economical form of drug administration. Oral drugs may be given as solids or liquids. Solid preparations include tablets, capsules, caplets, pills, and powders. Tablets, pills, or capsules may be enteric coated, which allows the drug to pass through the **acidic** pH of the stomach or protect the stomach from drug irritation. These oral drugs may also be controlled-release, timed-release, sustained-release, or prolonged-action preparations. These specific preparations are designed to produce slow absorption of the drug for 8 hours or longer by controlling the rate of dissolution in the gastrointestinal tract.

Liquid oral medications include solutions (usually consists of the drug dissolved in water that may be colored and flavored), elixirs (a mixture of the drug with a hydroalcoholic solution and glycerin or other sweetening agents), suspensions (consists of drug particles or powders suspended in liquid), syrups (medication that is based in a sugar syrup), and emulsions (a mixture of two liquids that are not mutually soluble—e.g., water and oil). Because liquid medications are already in solution, they tend to be absorbed more rapidly than those given in solid form. Oral administration of drugs requires an alert and cooperative patient with an intact swallowing reflex.

Advantages to oral administration of drugs include:

- Simplicity and convenience—Most often, the patient may self-administer the drug.
- Safety—Gastric lavage is available in the event of overdose.
- Economy.

The major disadvantages to oral administration are:

- Slow absorption rate—This factor makes the oral route unsuitable for emergent situations.
- Erratic and incomplete absorption of the drug—Tablets and pills may pass through the GI tract and be excreted in feces undissolved, or form with food substance in the stomach.
- Irritation of the GI tract, emesis—Some forms of liquids and tablets irritate the esophageal mucosa or GI tract, causing emesis. Others may discolor teeth or have an unpleasant taste.
- Possible aspiration—If the patient is debilitated or extremely combative, he/she may accidentally aspirate the drug.
- Drug abusers—Patients with a history of drug abuse may not be able to manage their own therapy and control intake.

Parenteral Administration

Parenteral administration pertains to all injectable drugs given by any route other than through the alimentary canal. Several injectable parenteral forms of drug administration exist. Parenteral medications may be given just under the surface of the skin (intradermal); into a joint (intra-articular); into the heart muscle (intracardiac); into the bone (intraosseous); into an artery (intra-arterial); into the spinal column (intraspinal); into the pleural space of the lung (intrapleural); into the spinal subarachnoid space (intrathecal); into the vein (intravenous [IV]); into the muscle tissue (intramuscular [IM]); and into the subcutaneous tissue (subcutaneous [SC or SQ]). The three most commonly used parenteral routes indicated for cardiopulmonary drug administration—IV, IM, and SC—are presented here (Fig. 3.3).

Intravenous Injection

Intravenous (IV) injection is the most reliable and fastest method of administering drugs directly into the bloodstream. Absorption factors are circumvented, allowing accurate control and titration of drugs. Medications given intravenously should be considered as the route of choice:

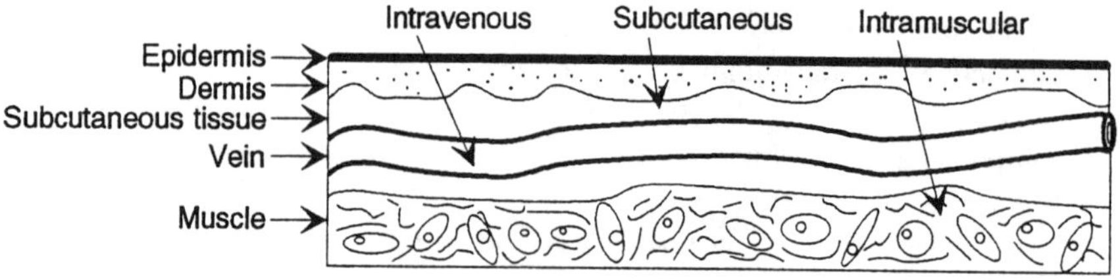

Figure 3.3. The three major injection routes.

- To immediately treat life-threatening conditions and in all emergent situations.
- For patients who need long-term, repeated drug infusions.
- To deliver medications that cannot be given by any other route (e.g., dopamine hydrochloride).
- To delay drug deactivation by the liver.
- To deliver large doses of medication.
- To treat patients who cannot receive medications by any other route (one who is unconscious, patients with gastric ulcers).

Two common access sites for IV catheters include:

IV Central (also referred to as a central line)—The IV catheter is placed in the subclavian, internal, or external jugular vessels. The more central the access, the greater the potential for life-threatening infections. Central lines are usually reserved for patients who have limited venous access or who are critically ill.

IV Peripheral—The veins of the hands or forearms are usually the preferred vessels for peripheral IV catheters. The lower extremity veins are not used owing to the increased risk of thrombophlebitis.

There are three methods of IV administration:

IV Push (direct IV or IV bolus)—The drug is delivered rapidly over several minutes. The drug becomes effective immediately. This is the method of choice in emergent situations; it is also used to deliver drugs that cannot be diluted.

IV Continuous (continuous drip administration or primary line infusion)—Drug delivery is maintained at a constant rate to maintain a therapeutic drug level. This method is preferred to sustain the desired action of a short-acting drug.

IV Intermittent (intermittent administration or additive set infusion)—This method is also referred to as IV piggyback (see Fig. 3.4). The dosage of a drug is intermittently infused over a period of time or given as a one-time dose. This method is used to maintain therapeutic serum levels of longer-acting drugs. In a piggyback administration, the patient may receive a con-

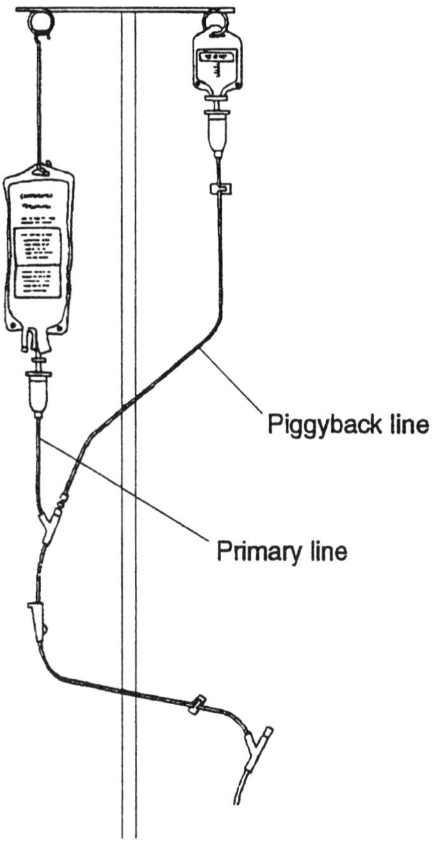

Figure 3.4. Method of intravenous administration in which a patient receives a continuous infusion of fluid to which an additional agent (the piggyback medication) has been added.

tinuous infusion of fluid to which an additional agent (the piggyback medication) is added.

IV drug administration has several advantages:

- Immediate **bioavailability**—The drug is injected directly into the bloodstream.
- Dosage is complete and accurate.
- Large drug doses can be delivered.
- Metabolism of the drug by the liver is avoided.

The primary disadvantage of IV drug administration is increased adverse reactions owing to the total direct systemic effect. IV drug administration is the most dangerous of all routes of drug administration because of the speed of onset of pharmacologic action. IV drug administration may cause life-threatening reactions if the drug is delivered too rapidly, if the flow rate is not carefully monitored, or if incompatible drugs are mixed together. Complications such as air embolism, systemic infection, or vein irritation may also occur.

Intramuscular Injection

Intramuscular (IM) injection produces a slower onset of drug action than the intravenous route; however, drug levels are preserved for longer periods of time. If the general circulation is patent, effective dosages are more predictable. Medications administered through the IM route are usually aqueous suspensions, solutions in oil, or medications that are not available in oral form. An advantage of the IM route over other parenteral routes is that muscles have a greater supply of blood vessels and fewer sensory nerve endings. Other advantages of using the IM route include:

- Allows long-term absorption of medications.
- Allows large doses to be administered (up to 5 ml).
- Does not require an IV injection site.
- Allows medication delivery to a patient who is unconscious, uncooperative, or unable to swallow.

Although IM drug administration is generally considered safe, inexpensive, and effective, certain patient populations should not be given IM injections. Those patients who are elderly, emaciated, or otherwise lack adequate muscle mass should not be given IM injections. In addition, IM injection is contraindicated for patients with decreased peripheral perfusion resulting from disorders such as shock, edema, and peripheral vascular disease. Any patient with a poor blood supply to the muscle should not be given IM injections. Some other disadvantages of the IM route of administration include:

- Slow absorption rate if the medication precipitates in the muscle.
- Local pain and tissue irritation.
- Possible injection into a nerve, vein, or bone, which may result in damage to the nerve, vein, or bone.

Subcutaneous Injection

Subcutaneous (SC) injection produces the slowest onset of drug action found in the parenteral system, yet this enhances a sustained effect of the drug's level. Only drugs that do not irritate tissue are used subcutaneously. Most subcutaneously delivered medications are isotonic, nonviscous, and soluble. The primary advantage of the SC route is easy self-administration (e.g., insulin injection). Factors that affect the absorption rate are exercise and heat (increases blood supply to the area, thereby increasing the absorption rate) and injection site trauma (causes the release of histamine, which in turn decreases blood flow and slows the absorption rate).

Patients with compromised perfusion (conditions such as shock, edema, peripheral vascular disease) are not good candidates to receive SC injections. In addition, SC injections should not be administered to obese patients, patients with dermatologic problems, burns, or otherwise diseased tissue.

Inhalation Administration

Inhalational drug therapy is the administration of a drug into the respiratory tract. Drugs may be administered as gases, sprays, aerosols, or powders. Typically, inhalants are administered for their local effect on the respiratory tract. Exceptions are the systemically absorbed anesthetic gases (nitrous oxide and halothane) and various other therapeutic gases (see Chapter 8, The Therapeutic Gases).

Nasal decongestants, bronchodilators, corticosteroids, mucolytics, and antiallergy agents are commonly administered through oral or nasal inhalation. Owing to the large surface area of the pulmonary system, drugs are rapidly absorbed through the mucous membranes and pulmonary epithelium. Because the drug is inhaled directly into the airway at its desired site of action, adverse reactions are minimal compared to other routes of administration. Because most inhaled medications must be delivered throughout the tracheobronchial tree to be effective, patients must have reasonable ventilatory capabilities and patent pulmonary capillary blood flow.

Primary advantages of giving drugs by the inhalation route include:

- As mentioned, the lung's large surface area allows rapid drug absorption and distribution.
- Potent drugs may be given in small doses, minimizing side effects.
- The respiratory route is easily accessible.

There are two primary disadvantages of giving drugs by the inhalation route:

- Patients must cooperate by inspiring deeply, unless they are mechanically ventilated.
- It is impossible to regulate precise dosages owing to the rainout of drug particles. Some drug particles may be deposited in the oropharynx or swallowed.

Aerosol Therapy

The most common method of delivering medications by the inhalation route lies with aerosol therapy. An aerosol consists of solid or liquid particles that are suspended in a gas. Inhalation aerosol therapy, therefore, is a suspension of a drug that is dispensed in a spray or mist.

Several factors must be considered when using inhalational drugs by way of aerosol therapy. As mentioned above, the patient must cooperate by inspiring deeply. For an effective treatment, the patient should inspire slowly and deeply through the mouth with a 5- to 10-second inspiratory hold if possible (for maximum drug **deposition** and distribution throughout the lungs).

The patient's degree of lung congestion, or bronchospasm, is also a major factor when giving inhalational drugs. Naturally, the more congested the lungs, or the more severe the bronchospasm, the more difficult it is for the inhaled drug to penetrate the deeper recesses of the lung. In these situations, much larger doses than would ordinarily be given may be required to achieve satisfactory results (Morgan et al. 1982).

A third factor to consider when giving aerosol drugs is the size of the aerosol drug particles, which affects the **stability** of the particle and drug deposition within the lung. Aerosolized drug particles approximately 5 to 10 μm are inhaled and then deposited into the patient's upper airway (pharynx, larynx, trachea), while particles 2 to 5 μm are deposited proximal to the alveoli. Drug particles between 1 and 2 μm can enter the alveoli, with 95 to 100% retention of those particles down to 1 μm. Particles 0.25 to 1 μm are generally stable, with minimal settling. Drug particles less than 0.1 μm are inhaled and exhaled without deposition. The ideal respirable range of aerosol particles is considered to be 1 to 5 μm, because such particles can penetrate and be deposited into the lung periphery. Figure 3.5 illustrates **aerosol deposition** according to drug particle size.

The devices used in aerosol therapy that aid the practitioner in administering medications to the patient's tracheobronchial tree include various types of nebulizers (many are based on the Babington, ultrasonic, Bernoulli, or Venturi principle), which produce aerosol particles for inhalation. A baffle placed within the device reduces the larger particles into smaller ones, thereby producing the respirable range of aerosol particles. If larger particles (>5 μm) are desired for deposition into the upper airways, an *atomizer* is used, which is basically a nebulizer without any baffles. Nebulizers are generally powered by a compressed gas source (either oxygen or air). The exception is the ultrasonic nebulizer, which is electrically powered.

Each nebulizer has its own specific indication for use:

- Small-volume jet nebulizer (SVN): The SVN is also known as a handheld nebulizer (HHN), an updraft nebulizer, or an acorn nebulizer (primarily because of its shape). This device has a reservoir capacity of <20 ml and is indicated for medication delivery (e.g., bronchodilators, corticosteroids, mucolytics, antiallergy medications). There are a few disadvantages to the use of the SVN. One is medication waste during exhalation. This disadvantage can be eliminated with the use of a finger valve placed in line before the nebulizer. By occluding the orifice during inhalation, nebulization is permitted. Releasing the port during exhalation shunts the gas flow to the atmosphere. Another disadvantage of this device

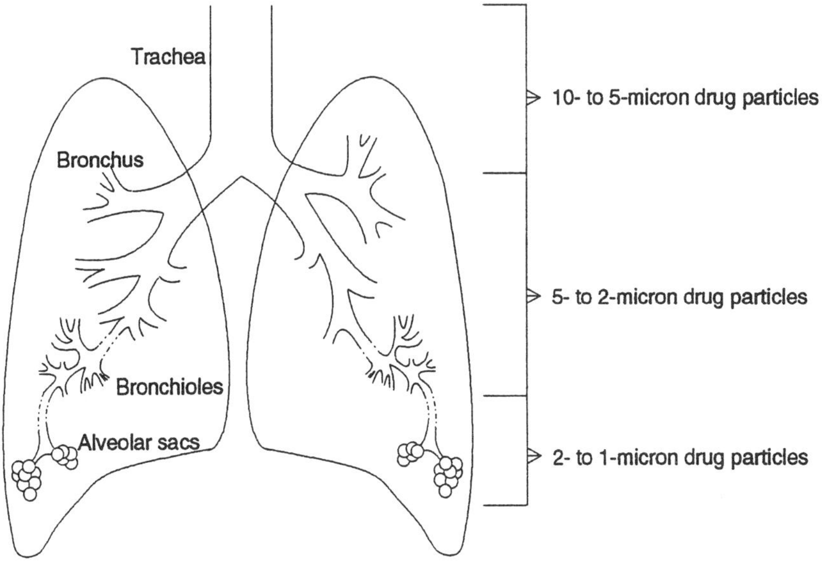

Figure 3.5. Inhaled drug particle deposition. The smaller the drug particle, the better its deposition into the deeper recesses of the lungs.

is that, even with an ideal ventilatory pattern, approximately 10 to 12% of the dose is retained within the lungs (Lewis and Fleming 1985, Zainudin et al. 1990). The ideal flow rates at which to power the SVN are between 6 and 8 L/min. A final precaution for using the SVN concerns patients with chronic airflow obstruction who are also CO_2 retainers. For these patients, the SVN should be powered by compressed air and not oxygen owing to the potential of suppressing their "drive to breathe" (see Chapter 8, The Therapeutic Gases: *Oxygen*).

- Large-reservoir air-entrainment nebulizer: To provide continuous oxygen therapy with humidity, a heated (if 100% body humidity is required) large-reservoir air-entrainment jet nebulizer is used. The reservoir capacity is approximately 250 to 400 ml (or up to 1 L in some devices). Sterile water must be used in this device owing to the particulate water produced (aerosol environments are a source for the colonization and spread of pathogenic bacteria).
- Babington nebulizer (Solosphere, Hydronamic): The Babington nebulizer is indicated as an aid in mobilizing secretions and for sputum induction. To hydrate secretions for expectoration, the patient inhales a hypertonic saline solution (or sterile water may be used) for 20 to 30 minutes. Following the treatment, the patient is encouraged to expectorate into a specimen cup. The sputum sample obtained is then sent to the laboratory for analysis.
- Ultrasonic nebulizer (USN): The ultrasonic nebulizer incorporates a piezoelectric transducer that has the ability to change its shape (oscillate) when a current is ap-

plied. The aerosol particles produced are in the 1- to 5-μm range, ideally suited for bronchiolar and alveolar deposition. The USN is indicated to facilitate the mobilization of bronchial secretions. This is accomplished by thinning thick, retained secretions. Treatments are usually given for 20 to 30 minutes t.i.d. or q.i.d.

Because the Babington and ultrasonic nebulizers deliver highly dense aerosol mists, an inherent hazard to their use is the precipitation of bronchospasm, especially for individuals with hyperreactive airways. An alternative to the use of a hypertonic saline solution or sterile water is normal saline or a hypotonic (half-normal) saline solution, which are less irritating to airways (see Chapter 13). However, if bronchoconstriction occurs with the use of these nebulizers, the treatment must be stopped and safer techniques should be employed.

Metered-dose inhalers (MDIs) are pressurized glass, ceramic, or metal canisters containing a drug to be nebulized. A metered-dose aerosol is produced with the use of a propellant and a valve mechanism designed to deliver a specific amount of medication with each activation. The propellant is some physiologically inert gas (usually Freon 11 or some other fluorocarbon) that liquefies under pressure.

When the nozzle of the canister is depressed, a fine aerosol spray is released that consists of the drug enclosed within the propellant. As the propellant evaporates, the drug remains suspended and continues on in the airstream.

Recent advances in MDI administration include the use of mist-confining (extension devices, holding chambers, spacers) and demand (synchronized medication discharge with inspiration) systems. Designed to facilitate application and minimize aerosol waste, these devices may provide a more stable aerosol particle with a deeper **penetration** into the lungs. These MDI adjuncts are especially beneficial for patients who are unable to coordinate proper technique.

Dosage is extremely variable depending on patient technique and compliance. Unfortunately, many patients do not receive an optimal dose or optimal aerosol deposition because of incorrect use of the MDI. Even with an ideal technique, a high percentage of each drug dose commonly gets trapped in the upper airways or is swallowed with only approximately 9 to 11% of the drug being retained within the lungs (Lewis and Fleming 1985, Zainudin et al. 1990). Owing to these factors, it is extremely important for the practitioner to properly instruct the patient regarding MDI use. Proper technique and application include:

- If using both a bronchodilator and corticosteroid, use the bronchodilator first and then the corticosteroid.
- Remove the MDI and shake it vigorously. If the device has not been used in more than 24 hours, charge the inhaler by holding the canister upside down and actuate by depressing the nozzle.
- Exhale to resting level.

- Open the mouth wide and place the canister, nozzle down, about 1 inch from the mouth, making sure the lips and teeth do not obstruct the aerosol flow. If the lips and teeth are closed around the mouthpiece, the aerosol will be deposited mainly in the mouth or hypopharynx. An exception to this is when the MDI is used with a spacer. The patient places his/her mouth around the spacer's mouthpiece.
- Activate the MDI by depressing the nozzle of the canister *after* inspiration has started and maintain a slow deep inspiration.
- Maintain an inspiratory pause of at least 5 to 10 seconds to maximize deposition and distribution of the drug.
- Repeat the procedure in 1 to 3 minutes.
- Rinse the mouth and throat with water after use (this is especially important when using corticosteroids because of the risk, although low, of developing an oral fungal infection such as that caused by *Candida albicans*). Use of a spacer and hyperextending the neck is also recommended to decrease the incidence of fungal infection.

Care of inhalers is also a vital aspect of patient education. The patient should be instructed to rinse the mouthpiece daily and disinfect once a week with a solution containing one-half white vinegar and one-half water for approximately 30 minutes and then rinse with water and allow to air dry.

Each MDI contains approximately 200 puffs when full. A patient can check for the amount of puffs left in his/her MDI by placing the canister in a bowl of water. A full canister will sink and completely submerge itself under the water; a half-full canister will tilt with the nozzle submerged and the flat end of the canister above the surface of the water, whereas an empty canister floats on its side on the surface of the water (Fig. 3.6).

MDIs are a popular form of aerosol drug administration owing to their compactness and ease of operation. Commonly prescribed for self-administration and home use, MDIs may be a considerable source for potential abuse among chronic respiratory patients. The practitioner should assume a primary role with these patients in proper education and application.

Dry-powdered inhalers (DPIs) are another form of delivering medications into the respiratory tract. These devices are small and portable, similar in size to MDIs. Only a few drugs are available that deliver medication via the DPI (e.g., cromolyn sodium [via the *Spinhaler*], albuterol [via the *Rotahaler*], and terbutaline [via the *Turbuhaler*]). Figure 3.7 illustrates these three types of DPIs.

With the Spinhaler and Rotahaler, a gelatin capsule that contains the drug to be inhaled is inserted into the DPI, which opens the capsule to release the powder. A rapid and deep inspiratory effort on the part of the user provides the powering mechanism to deliver the solid drug particles into the respiratory tract. Considerably high inspiratory flow rates (generally >60 L/min) are required for an effective treatment to be administered, which may be a disadvantage in some users.

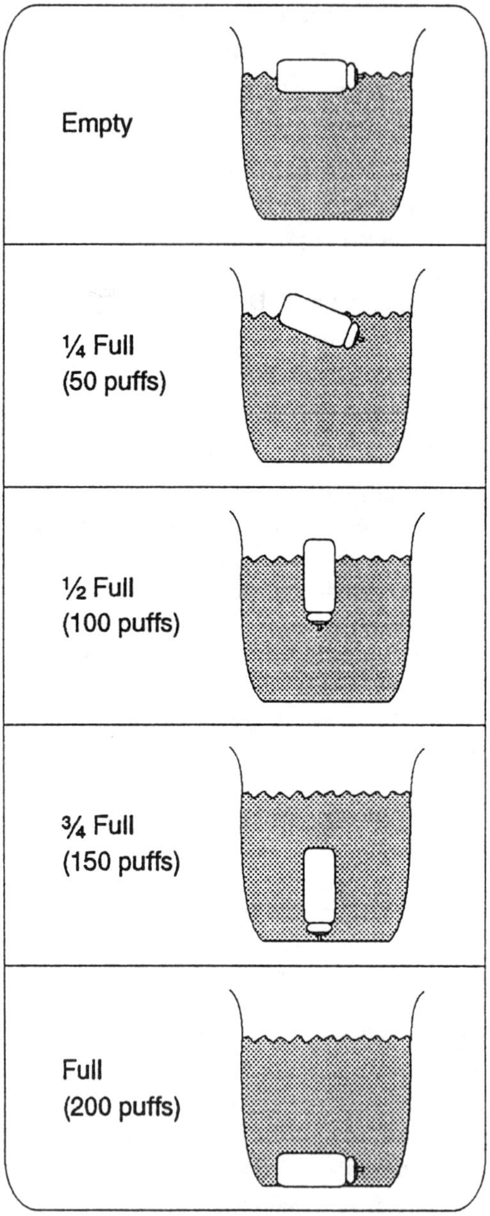

Figure 3.6. Estimating the contents of a metered-dose inhaler. Place the canister in a bowl of water and compare its position to the chart.

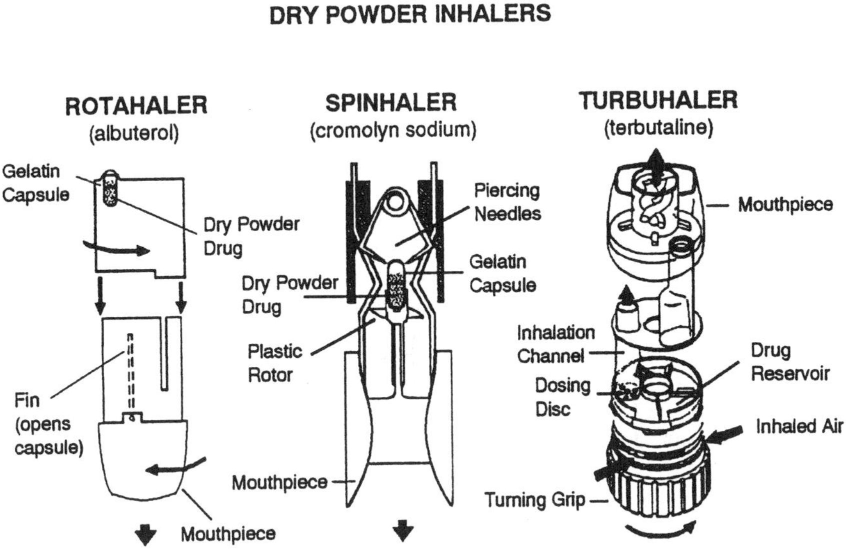

Figure 3.7. Three examples of delivery devices for inhalation of dry-powder aerosols: Rotahaler, Spinhaler, and Turbuhaler. Used with permission from Rau J. Respiratory Care Pharmacology. 4th ed. St. Louis: Mosby-Year Book, Inc., 1994.

The Turbuhaler is a multi-dose DPI that contains approximately 200 doses per inhaler. An advantage to the use of this device over the Spinhaler and Rotahaler is that the Turbuhaler is effective at approximately half the inspiratory flow rates required by the above-mentioned DPIs (Pedersen et al. 1990).

Protocols have been developed by various institutions that aid the practitioner in choosing the appropriate delivery device for administering bronchoactive substances into the respiratory tract.

A small-volume nebulizer is indicated if the patient:

- is unable to cooperate or is disoriented
- is unable to take a deep breath and maintain an inspiratory pause
- is tachypneic (>25 breaths/minute) or exhibits an unstable ventilatory pattern
- needs a drug that is only available in a solution to be nebulized.

A metered-dose inhaler (or a change from SVN to MDI) is indicated if the patient:

- is alert and oriented
- is strong enough to actuate the MDI and able to coordinate inspiration with actuation of the MDI (if a spacer is used, the patient should still be able to demonstrate an effective technique)

- is able to take a slow, deep breath with an inspiratory hold
- is not tachypneic and has a stable ventilatory pattern
- needs a drug that is only available in MDI form.

A dry-powder inhaler is indicated if the patient:

- is sensitive to the fluorocarbon propellant contained in MDIs
- is able to demonstrate high inspiratory flow rates
- uses a drug available in DPI form and has difficulty with MDI actuation or co-ordination.

The most effective method for administering an aerosolized drug to a nonintubated patient is to have the patient use a mouthpiece; however, this is not feasible with infant and pediatric patients as well as unconscious or debilitated patients. For these patients, a face mask is used in conjunction with the SVN or MDI. Several investigators have shown that, even with optimal patient compliance, considerably less than the usual 9 to 11% dosage is being delivered when using a face mask over a mouthpiece (Conner et al. 1989, Kraemer et al. 1991).

Two other adjuncts for aerosol delivery include the small-particle aerosol generator (SPAG) and the intermittent positive pressure breathing machine (IPPB). The SPAG unit is detailed in Chapter 16 under ribavirin. The IPPB machine is a type of lung hyperinflation technique that delivers medication via an in-line SVN during a pressurized breath. The use of this device for medication delivery has declined over the years because it has been demonstrated that the use of the IPPB machine is no more clinically effective over a proper technique employed with the SVN (Dolovich et al. 1977).

Finally, another route of administering medications into the lungs is by direct instillation of the drug through an endotracheal tube. This route is typically reserved for wetting agents (such as lavaging with normal saline when performing endotracheal suctioning), surface-active agents (such as surfactant replacement therapy), and emergent cardiac life support drug management when an intravenous site has not yet been established.

PART II: PHARMACOKINETIC PHASE (MOVEMENT OF DRUGS WITHIN THE BODY)

The processes involved in the movement of a drug after it is administered to the body are collectively known as the *pharmacokinetics* of a drug. The biological processes that constitute the pharmacokinetics of a drug (Fig. 3.8) include absorption (the ability of a drug to gain entrance to the bloodstream), distribution (the movement of the drug throughout the body to various receptor sites), **bio-**

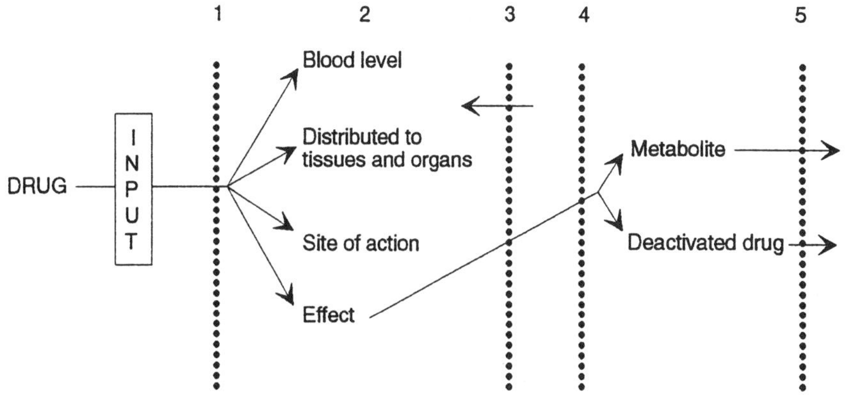

Figure 3.8. *1,* Absorption; *2,* distribution; *3,* redistribution; *4,* biotransformation; *5,* elimination. See text for explanation.

transformation (the chemical alteration of the drug), and elimination (the removal or excretion of the drug).

Drug Absorption

Generally, a drug must first be absorbed (transferred from the site of administration into the bloodstream) before it can gain access to the body's receptor sites. Exceptions are those drugs injected intravascularly, drugs applied topically for their effect on the skin and mucous membranes, drugs injected for a local effect on a specific body area, and drugs administered for their actions within the intestinal lumen. The rate and extent of absorption of a drug into the general circulation, which is defined as bioavailability, is dependent on several factors.

How much of a dose actually gets into the body is the first factor. With intravenous injection, bioavailability of a drug is 100%, owing to the fact that the drug is immediately injected into the bloodstream and bypasses the process of absorption. With other routes of administration, the entire amount of a drug may or may not reach the systemic circulation. With these other routes of administration, the rate and extent at which drug absorption occurs is dependent on types of cellular transport systems, the **physiochemical** properties of the drug (i.e., lipid **solubility, ionization**), blood flow at the site of absorption, the concentration of the drug, and the ambient absorbing surface area.

Transport Mechanisms

As mentioned, intravenous injection enables a drug to be administered directly into the bloodstream, allowing its absorption to be immediate. However, other drug forms must first penetrate one or more cell-membrane barriers from the administration site to reach the circulatory system. These drugs are allowed to reach the circulatory system by one of five transport mechanisms.

Passive diffusion—The most common transport mechanism. A concentration gradient exists from one side of the cell membrane to the other when a drug is introduced into the body. With no energy expended, the drug diffuses across the cell membrane until the drug concentration equalizes on both sides of the cell membrane.

Filtration—Filtration of drugs across cell membranes occurs when the drug molecules are small enough to simply *filter* through the pores of cell membranes.

Facilitated diffusion—Like passive diffusion, facilitated diffusion operates by means of a concentration gradient and also requires no energy expenditure. Drug molecules combine with carrier substances, enabling the drug to penetrate the cell membrane until equal amounts are present on both sides of the cell membrane.

Active transport—This process requires energy because it transfers drug molecules against the concentration gradient. A drug combines with a carrier substance, which takes it from a lower concentrated area to a higher concentrated area.

Pinocytosis—This form of active transport occurs when the cell membrane actually engulfs drug molecules, thereby transporting the drug into the cell. Only a few drug types can be absorbed by this process.

Figure 3.9 presents a graphic representation of these five transport mechanisms.

Physiochemical Properties of Drugs

The physiochemical properties of the drug will also affect the rate of absorption. Lipid-soluble substances diffuse more rapidly across a cell's membrane than non-lipid-soluble substances. This is because of the lipoid nature of the cell membrane. In addition, aqueous solutions are absorbed more rapidly than colloids or suspensions.

Most drugs are weak acids or weak bases, which exist in either the ionized or the nonionized form. Cell membranes are more permeable to the nonionized form of a given drug than to its ionized form. This is because nonionized drugs are more lipid-soluble and readily cross cell membranes. The degree to which a drug exists in either a highly ionized state or a highly nonionized state is determined by the pH of the tissue fluids into which the drug is dissolved in and the **pK_a** of the drug (defined as the pH at which the drug is 50% ionized and 50% nonionized). The concept of pK_a is derived from the Henderson-Hasselbalch equation. For a weak acid:

$$pK_a = pH + Log\ (\text{concentration of nonionized acid} \div \text{concentration of ionized acid})$$

For a weak base:

$$pK_a = pH + Log\ (\text{concentration of ionized base} \div \text{concentration of nonionized base})$$

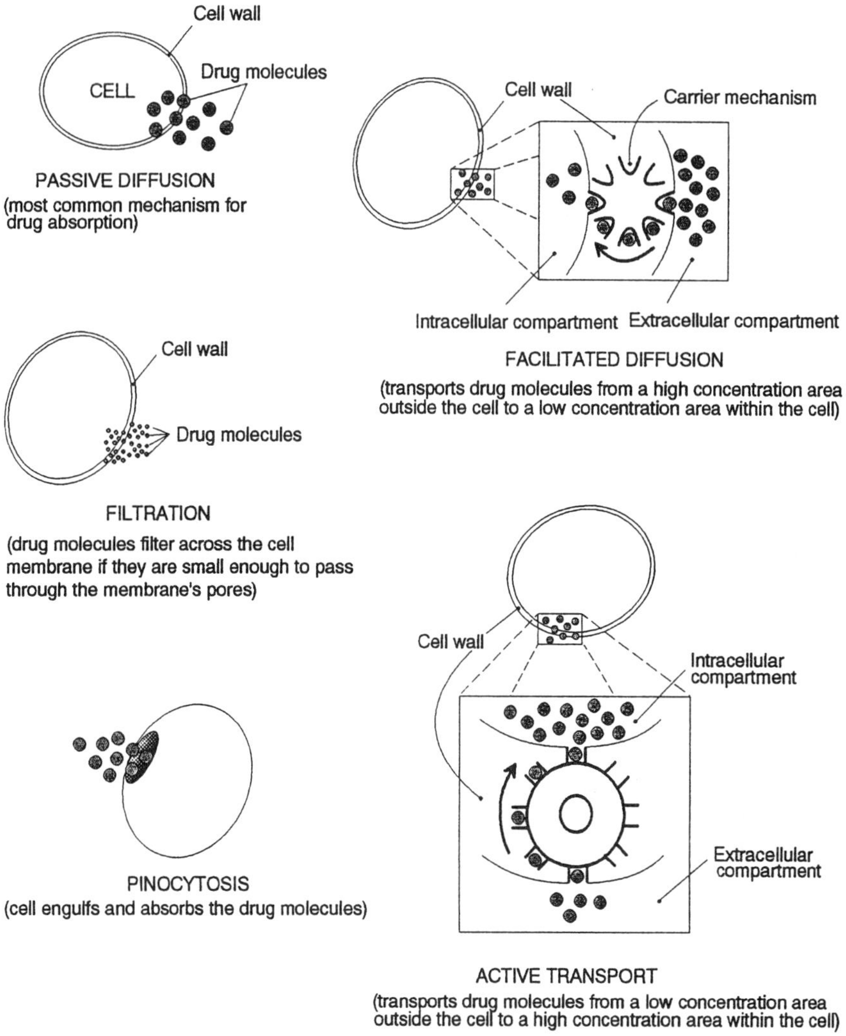
Cell wall
CELL
Drug molecules
PASSIVE DIFFUSION
(most common mechanism for drug absorption)
Cell wall
Carrier mechanism
Intracellular compartment
Extracellular compartment
FACILITATED DIFFUSION
(transports drug molecules from a high concentration area outside the cell to a low concentration area within the cell)
Cell wall
Drug molecules
FILTRATION
(drug molecules filter across the cell membrane if they are small enough to pass through the membrane's pores)
PINOCYTOSIS
(cell engulfs and absorbs the drug molecules)
Cell wall
Intracellular compartment
Extracellular compartment
ACTIVE TRANSPORT
(transports drug molecules from a low concentration area outside the cell to a high concentration area within the cell)

Figure 3.9. Conceptual illustration of the five transport mechanisms: passive diffusion, filtration, facilitated diffusion, active transport, and pinocytosis.

Most drugs have pK_a values between 3 and 11, which means that they exist as partly ionized and partly nonionized over the range of physiologic pH values. The pH in the body varies to its respective location. For example, the pH of plasma is approximately 7.40; the pH of the stomach ranges between 1 and 3; and the pH of urine varies from 4.5 to 8.0.

If the pH that surrounds the drug equals the pK_a of the drug, the drug will be

50% ionized and 50% nonionized. For a weak acid to become more nonionized, and therefore more readily diffusable across the cellular membrane, it would need to be surrounded by a pH that was more acidic (lower) than its pK_a. For a weak **base** to become more nonionized, and therefore more readily diffusable across the cellular membrane, it would need to be surrounded by a more alkaline (higher) pH than its pK_a. Table 3.1 illustrates the comparison between ambient pH and the pK_a of a drug and whether the drug will exist primarily in its nonionized, easily diffusable form.

Blood Flow

Blood flow at the site of absorption is also a vital element when considering the rate of drug absorption. Increased blood flow brought about by massage, fever, or exercise can greatly increase the rate of drug absorption. Decreased blood flow such as that produced by vasoconstrictor agents, shock, or other disease factors can slow the rate of absorption. In addition, absorption of inhaled adrenergic drugs occurs through the lung mucosa and the alveolar capillary membrane. Ventilation-perfusion abnormalities and severe diffusion defects of the lung have the greatest effect of slowing the uptake of the drug.

Drug Concentration and Absorbing Surface

The concentration of a drug also influences the rate of drug absorption. Drugs administered in a highly concentrated state are absorbed more rapidly than drugs of low concentration. The absorbing surface area to which the drug is exposed is an essential consideration in drug absorption rate. Large absorbing surfaces, such as the pulmonary alveolar epithelium and gastrointestinal tract, greatly enhance drug absorption.

In addition to the above-mentioned factors, presystemic metabolism may also affect the rate and extent of absorption. Orally ingested drugs must first pass through the liver prior to entering the systemic circulation. Some drugs may un-

Table 3.1.
The Relationship Between the pK_a of a Drug, Ambient pH, and Drug Nonionization

Weak acid—phenobarbital (pK_a = 7.4)		Weak base—quinine (pK_a = 8.4)	
Ambient pH	% Nonionized	Ambient pH	% Nonionized
6.4	91	7.4	9
7.4	50	8.4	50
8.4	9	9.4	91

If the pH surrounding a drug that is a weak acid is more acidic than the pK_a of the drug, the drug will exist in a more nonionized lipid-soluble stage. If the pH surrounding a drug that is a weak base is more alkalinic than the pK_a of the drug, the drug will exist in a more nonionized lipid-soluble state.

dergo considerable metabolism from the microsomal enzyme system of the liver before entering the bloodstream. This phenomenon is known as *first-pass metabolism.* Sites other than the liver also contain enzymes that can metabolize a drug. The gastric mucosa contains specific enzymes that can chemically alter a drug, thereby potentially inactivating the drug. For this reason, some drugs cannot be given orally. For example, isoproterenol is metabolized and inactivated by a sulfatase enzyme located in the gastric mucosa and is therefore not suited to be administered via the oral route.

Drug Distribution

Through absorption, a drug is made available to the bloodstream. Through distribution, a drug's site of action is attainable by allowing the drug to traverse the body's circulating bloodstream and be exposed to interstitial and cellular fluids and tissues. The rate and pattern of distribution is determined by the physiochemical effects of the drug, by cardiac output, and by circulatory blood flow.

Of major importance in the distribution of a drug is the systemic and pulmonary blood circulation. How soon a drug reaches its target area depends greatly on blood supply. Highly vascular organs (e.g., heart, liver, kidney, brain, and other well perfused areas) receive the drug molecules first, whereas it takes longer for the drug to reach less vascular areas (e.g., muscle, fat, skin). It follows then that impairment of perfusion and circulation may lead to the total dose of the drug not being accessible to receptor sites.

As drugs are absorbed into the circulatory system, one of three actions occurs to the drug molecule: drug molecules may become bound to plasma proteins (usually albumin for acidic drugs and α_1-acid glycoprotein for basic drugs) or red blood cells or may remain free. Both bound and unbound drug molecules traverse the body's circulatory system to reach the fluid compartments and tissues. However, only those drug molecules that remain unbound are able to react with the body's receptor sites and exert a pharmacologic effect.

Plasma protein binding of drug molecules serves as a temporary storage compartment for the drug. As the free drug molecule is metabolized and excreted, the bound drug is gradually released from the plasma protein. This process enables the body to maintain therapeutic drug levels.

When different drug types compete with the same plasma protein, a type of interaction occurs that disturbs the bound/unbound ratio. Either both drugs are not fully bound to the protein or the second drug displaces the first drug. Serious problems occur when a large amount of a bound drug is suddenly displaced from the protein. The patient could suffer the effects of an overdose.

The extent of protein binding depends on the drug's molecular structure and is a highly variable factor with each drug type. For example, 97% of warfarin sodium (Coumadin, an anticoagulant) binds to plasma proteins when administered to the body. Coadministering a drug such as phenylbutazone (an anti-inflammatory agent) will compete with and displace protein-bound warfarin sodium. Freeing just 3% of warfarin from the protein doubles the amount of active drug within the system, which could easily lead to overdose and possible hemorrhage. Eventually, the body may excrete the excess dose.

Other factors that affect the distribution of drugs are tissue solubility, tissue mass, and the blood-brain barrier. Highly lipid-soluble drugs may accumulate in adipose tissue, which then serves as a reservoir for the drug. When circulating concentration of the drug declines, extraction of the drug from these fat reservoirs occurs, thereby extending the duration and therapeutic effect of the drug.

Certain membranes have unique structures that may alter the pattern of drug distribution. For example, many drugs do not reach the central nervous system because of its unique blood-brain barrier. The **blood-brain barrier** is composed of capillary endothelium that is situated between blood vessels and the cerebrospinal fluid (CSF) that cushions the brain. The capillaries of the brain are tightly joined together (there are no pores for a drug to pass through) and covered on the outside by a fatty barrier known as the glial sheath. For a drug to exert a pharmacologic effect on the central nervous system, it must first pass from the plasma, cross the capillary endothelium and then enter the CSF. Once in the CSF, the drug diffuses into brain cells. Highly nonionized lipid-soluble drugs penetrate the fatty layer of the blood-brain interface more readily than their ionized nonlipid-soluble counterparts.

Drug Redistribution

The phenomenon of redistribution may occur when a drug is taken back into the bloodstream after stimulating a receptor and is redistributed to other tissues and sites. For example, thiopental (Pentothal Sodium) is a lipid-soluble drug that readily penetrates all cells and has a high affinity for body fat but does not initially become localized in adipose tissue. When injected intravenously, thiopental will first reach and be deposited in those tissues that have high rates of blood flow (e.g., the brain, liver, kidneys). As the plasma concentration of thiopental declines, the drug will begin to redistribute by diffusing out of these early sites of deposition.

Biotransformation

Biotransformation is a word usually interchangeable with metabolism, which basically means any chemical alterations of a compound (e.g., a drug). A metabolite is the by-product of this alteration. Some drugs may continue to be active until they have undergone metabolism. The ultimate goal of the biotransformation process is to chemically alter the drug so that it can be inactivated or eliminated.

Biotransformation of a drug mainly occurs through the microsomal enzyme system of the liver, but it may also occur in the lungs, kidneys, bloodstream, or intestines. The rate at which biotransformation of a drug occurs is highly variable, depending on an individual's normal metabolic rate, age, any genetic disorders, disease, or drugs in his/her system.

Drug Elimination

A drug may be eliminated from the body chemically unaltered or as a metabolite. The kidneys serve as the most important organ for the excretion of a drug. There are primarily two processes involved in drug excretion by the kidneys: glomerular filtration and tubular secretion. Glomerular filtration is a passive transfer process; the drug simply exits the plasma and enters the tubules by simple filtration. Drugs that are protein bound are poorly filtered and remain in the plasma. Tubular secretion is an active process in which drugs are removed from the plasma by special carriers located within the renal tubules. Even protein-bound drugs can be removed from the plasma by tubular secretion.

Alternating urinary pH by administering acidic or basic drugs is done therapeutically to enhance the excretion of some drugs. For example, amphetamine (a base with a pK_a of 9.8) is ionized and rapidly excreted when the urinary pH is acidic. In an alkaline environment, amphetamine is nonionized and largely reabsorbed.

Excretion of a drug may also occur through perspiration, saliva, tears, or feces. Elimination of a drug by feces is usually unabsorbed orally ingested drugs. Anesthetic gases, paraldehyde, vapors, and aerosols are eliminated through exhalation of the respiratory cycle. Factors hindering drug elimination include interactions with other drugs or impairment of renal, hepatic, or cardiovascular function.

PART III: PHARMACODYNAMIC PHASE (MECHANISM OF ACTION AND EFFECT OF DRUGS)

Pharmacodynamics describe *how* a drug works in the body. This phase of drug therapy involves the biochemical and physiological actions and effects of a drug at the cellular level.

One of the most basic concepts of pharmacology is that drug molecules must attach to specific receptors, either on a cell membrane or within a cell, and thus trigger (or inhibit) a physiologic response. The molecular size, shape, and electrical charge of a drug molecule determines whether it will bind to a specific receptor. Many refer to the drug-receptor complex as a "lock and key" interaction (i.e., the binding is made possible only by a close structural relationship between the drug and the receptor and the drug molecule with the "best fit" to the receptor will elicit the strongest pharmacologic response from the cell; see Fig. 3.1). The matching of a drug to a particular receptor is termed the *structure-activity relationship* (SAR) of the drug.

If a drug binds to and stimulates a response from the receptor, it is known as an *agonist*. However, if a drug binds to a receptor without evoking a response, it is known as an *antagonist*. Both types of drugs (agonists and antagonists) have an *affinity* for the same receptor, but only the agonist will initiate a physiologic response from the receptor. Agonists and antagonists often compete for the same receptor site. For example, both atropine and acetylcholine have an affinity for the muscarinic receptor of the parasympathetic system. If acetylcholine binds to the muscarinic receptor, a series of events will be initiated (i.e., the key that not only fits the lock but also opens the lock). If atropine binds to the muscarinic receptor, no response will be initiated (i.e., the key fits the lock but will not open it). Atropine prevents, or competitively inhibits, acetylcholine from binding to the receptor and thereby exerting any influence on the receptor (Fig. 2.14).

Drug specificity is an important consideration in pharmacodynamics. Many circumstances warrant the use of a very specific agent that will bind to only one type of receptor. For example, the administration of exogenous epinephrine will stimulate all adrenoceptors. If the goal is to relieve bronchospasm (i.e., activate the β_2-adrenoceptor), then epinephrine would not be a good choice owing to its nonselective adrenergic properties. Stimulating the α- and β_1-adrenoceptors could lead to unwanted adverse effects. Selective β_2-adrenoceptor agents, such as albuterol (Proventil, Ventolin) or salmeterol (Serevent), will cause bronchodilation with minimal effects on heart rate (β_1) or blood pressure (α).

Once the actions and effects of a drug can be explained in terms of its interaction with a specific type of receptor, those data will not only be useful in determining a classification scheme for the drug but also as a basis for the development of new drugs. It is not necessary, nor even possible, for the practitioner to learn every new drug marketed; however, it is feasible for the practitioner to learn about the major drug classifications. With this knowledge base, practitioners can acquire a more extensive understanding of the individual drugs commonly used in practice or a specific clinical specialty.

Pharmacokinetics and pharmacodynamics are further detailed in Chapter 4, Factors that Modify Drug Effects.

PHYSIOLOGIC NATURE OF THE LUNGS

Many are aware of the lung's primary function—gas exchange. However, the lung performs several vital nonrespiratory functions as well.

Synthesis

The lung is the major site for the synthesis and release of various autacoids. Histamine synthesis occurs in the lung as well as the arachidonic acid metabolites (prostaglandins, thromboxane, leukotrienes).

Certain cells of the lung (e.g., neutrophils and macrophages) complement the synthesis of **oxygen-derived free radicals** for bactericidal action. Active lung neutrophils and other phagocytes also lead to the release of the proteolytic elastase and trypsin.

The lung contains a unique transport system to rid itself of these dangerous proteases. These enzymes are transported (via the flow of mucus) to the larynx, where the enzymes are conjugated by α_1-antitrypsin. This action forms a detoxified product for elimination through the pulmonary vascular bed and lymph system.

Synthesis of surfactant occurs within the lung by the alveolar (type II) cells. Surfactant has the capacity to reduce alveolar surface tension, enhancing the elasticity of the pulmonary tissue (see Chapter 13). Liberated surfactant is found throughout the alveoli and respiratory air passages.

Filtration

Because of the unique position of the lung between the venous and arterial circulations, the pulmonary vascular bed has the ability to process and filter various substances, thereby protecting the coronary and cerebral circulations. The large surface of the pulmonary vascular bed is ideally suited for this task. This filtration process is why there is a difference in blood levels of a substance between venous and arterial samples.

By active uptake, serotonin and epinephrine are removed from the pulmonary circulation, although histamine is relatively unaffected by the lung's filtration process. Many of the prostaglandins, the leukotrienes, and bradykinin are also removed through the pulmonary circulation. PGE, PGF2α, and bradykinin are removed during a single pass through the pulmonary circulation, making their duration of action very limited.

Metabolism

Among its various activities, the lungs also have the ability to metabolize various vasoactive substances from blood or tissues. Angiotensin I (a decapeptide hormone) is hydrolyzed by a peptidase located within the lung to angiotensin II, a potent vasopressor and stimulator of aldosterone production and secretion.

The pulmonary system contains an abundant source of thromboplastin and plasmin activator. Thromboplastin aids in the conversion of prothrombin to thrombin, which then converts fibrinogen to fibrin. Plasmin activator contributes in the dissolution of formed fibrin clots by initiating the conversion of plasminogen to plasmin.

The lung also contains an active cytochrome P-450 enzyme system (a group of hemoproteins), which gives it the ability to biotransform and detoxify many substances, including drugs.

Elimination

Elimination of a substance may occur through the pulmonary circulation as mentioned above or through exhalation of the respiratory cycle. As mentioned earlier, the various inhaled drugs (anesthetic gases, paraldehyde, vapors, and aerosols) are eliminated through exhalation in the respiratory cycle.

REFERENCES/RECOMMENDED READING

Ariens EJ, Simonis AM. Drug action: target tissue, dose response relationships, and receptors. In: Teorell T, Dedrick RL, Condliffe PG. Pharmacology and Pharmacokinetics. New York: Plenum Press, 1974.

Benet LZ. Effect of route of administration and distribution on drug action. J Pharmacokinet Biopharm 6:559, 1978.

Conner WT, et al. Reliable salbutamol administration in 6- to 36-month-old children by means of a metered dose inhaler and aerochamber with mask. Pediatr Pulmonol 6:263, 1989.

Dipalma JR, DiGregorio GJ. Basic Pharmacology in Medicine. 3rd ed. New York: McGraw-Hill, Inc., 1990.

Dolovich MB, et al. Pulmonary aerosol deposition in chronic bronchitis; intermittent positive pressure breathing versus quiet breathing. Am Rev Respir Dis 115:397, 1977.

Goodman L, Gilman A. The Pharmacologic Basis of Therapeutics. 8th ed. New York: McGraw-Hill, Inc., 1993.

Greenblatt D, Shader RI. Pharmacokinetics in Clinical Practice. Philadelphia: WB Saunders, 1985.

Katzung BG. Basic & Clinical Pharmacology. 6th ed. Norwalk: Appleton & Lange, 1995.

Koch-Weser J. Bioavailability of drugs. N Engl J Med 291:233, 1974.

Kraemer R, et al. Short-term effect of albuterol, delivered via a new auxillary device in wheezy infants. Am Rev Respir Dis 144:347, 1991.

Lewis RA, Fleming JS. Fractional deposition from a jet nebulizer: how it differs from a metered dose inhaler. Br J Dis Chest 79:361, 1985.

Morgan MDL, et al. Terbutaline aerosol given through pear spacer in acute severe asthma. Br Med J Clin Res Ed 285:849, 1982.

Pedersen S, Hansen OR, Fuglsang G. Influence of inspiratory flow rate upon the effect of a Turbuhaler. Arch Dis Child 65:308, 1990.

Prescott LF, Nimmo WS. Drug Absorption. New York: ADIS Press, 1981.

Ridout G, Santus GC, Guy RH. Pharmacokinetic considerations in the use of new transdermal formulations. Clin Pharmacokinet 15:114, 1988.

Tenholder MF, Bryson MJ, Whitlock WL. A model for conversion from small volume nebulizer to metered dose inhaler aerosol therapy. Chest 101:634, 1992.

Zainudin BMZ, et al. Comparison of bronchodilator responses and deposition patterns of salbutamol inhaled from a pressurised metered dose inhaler, as a dry powder, and as a nebulised solution. Thorax 45:469, 1990.

FACTORS THAT MODIFY DRUG EFFECTS 4

The degree to which a drug produces an effect within the body is dependent on several factors and interacting relationships. Before administering a drug, these factors must be taken into account and the dosage must be adjusted to meet the specific requirements of individual patients. The more important factors that modify drug effects are represented in Figure 4.1.

LEARNING OUTCOMES

Upon completion of this chapter, the learner will be able to:

1. Define the terms listed in *Key Terms*.
2. Identify the physiological variables that modify drug effects.
3. Explain how the following disease conditions may alter drug effects:

   Renal failure
   Hepatic failure
   Cardiovascular disorders
   Pulmonary disease

4. Explain the dose-effect relationship. Interrelate how potency, slope, variability, and maximal efficacy affect the dose-effect relation. Define potency, drug efficacy, hyperreactive, hyporeactive, idiosyncrasy, hypersensitivity, supersensitivity, ED_{50}, LD_{50}, TI. Be able to calculate TI when given ED_{50} and LD_{50}.
5. Indicate how compensatory reflex affects the autonomic nervous system.
6. Describe biologic half-life, give an example of and the factors affecting biologic half-life of a drug.

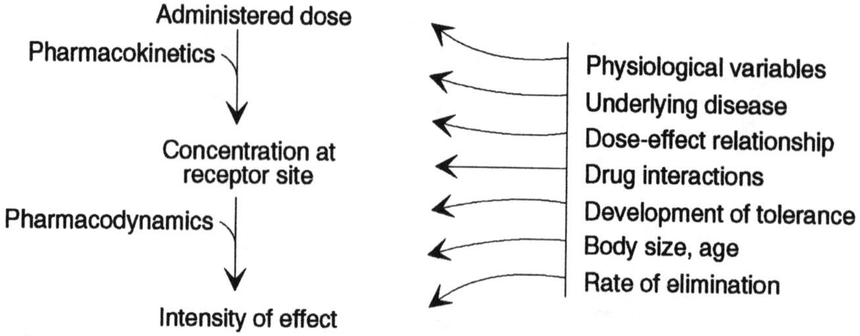

Figure 4.1. Factors that determine the relationship between an administered drug and alterations in expected drug effect.

7. Identify and discuss the pharmacokinetic and pharmacodynamic variables that may alter drug effects. Define and give an example of:

   Additivity
   Synergism
   Potentiation
   Physiologic antagonism
   Chemical antagonism
   Pharmacological antagonism

8. Explain how the following variables may alter the therapeutic outcome of drug therapy:

   Tolerance
   Tachyphylaxis
   Cross-tolerance
   Down-regulation
   Accumulation of drugs
   Age, sex, and weight
   Allergic reactions
   Patient noncompliance
   Pregnancy and lactation
   Hereditary factors
   Environmental factors

9. When given a mean clearance, a target concentration value, and an oral availability factor for a particular drug, be able to calculate the intravenous (IV) dosing rate and oral maintenance dose of a drug.

10. Identify and describe the types of allergic reactions and state an example of each.

KEY TERMS

(The following key terms are highlighted in **bold** when they first occur in the text of this chapter.)

efficacy—A measure of the effectiveness of a drug.

FEV_1—Forced expiratory volume in 1 second. The amount of air that can be exhaled in 1 second starting from a maximal inspiration.

Pharmacogenetics—The study of the hereditary factors that influence the response to drugs.

Potency—Strength of a medicine.

Teratogenic—Causing the development of abnormal structures in an embryo resulting in a severely malformed fetus.

Toxicity—The degree or extent to which a poison exists in the body. The accumulation of a drug or drugs within the body can result in poisonous effects.

Uremia—Retention in the blood of nitrogenous substances normally excreted by the kidney. Results in a toxic condition within the body.

PHYSIOLOGIC VARIABLES

The physical and chemical processes of the body (such as water and electrolyte balance [see Chapter 17], body temperature, acid-base status, and other physiological variatives) may alter drug effects. Of special concern to the practitioner is acid-base status. Acidosis, regardless of etiology, may change the protein binding capability of the cell membrane. This limits a portion of the drug available for diffusion out of the capillary and into tissue. This then may lead to a decreased response to adrenergic drugs in the acidemic patient.

Other physiologic factors that may alter drug effects include disturbances in the hepatic microsomal enzyme system, alterations in body composition (fluid/solid ratio), and a decline in organ function. The neonatal, pediatric, and geriatric populations are especially at high risk for altered drug effects because of their comparative physiologic variances from the normal adult population (see Chapter 7).

PATHOLOGIC FACTORS

A single disease may cause multiple changes in the processes of drug absorption, distribution, metabolism, excretion, and effect. Renal, hepatic, cardiovascular, and pulmonary disease are major pathological factors that may modify drug effects. Drug therapy and dosage should be frequently monitored for clinical response and early indications of **toxicity.**

Renal Disease, Uremia

Renal failure may significantly alter a drug's elimination or clearance from the body. As discussed in Chapter 3, the kidney is the primary organ for drug excretion. In the presence of renal failure, there is a diminished glomerular filtration and tubular secretion of drugs as well as other substances. This then leads to an accumulation of administered drugs within the body, potentially creating life-threatening toxic conditions. Thus, potential toxicity is a major consideration for the uremic patient and requires that special care be taken, not only in regulating the dosage regimen but also in monitoring serum blood levels. The dose of drugs administered to uremic patients must be reduced; the extent of reduction depends on the severity of the renal disease. There are several types of blood tests that test for the presence of renal failure. These include blood urea nitrogen (BUN), creatinine, and uric acid. Appendix B (*VI*) details these blood tests.

Hepatic Disease

Because the liver is the major organ for drug biotransformation and is secondary to the kidney for removal of drugs, it is reasonable to assume that a loss of liver parenchyma or function will lead to a decrease in the capacity of the liver to biotransform or eliminate drugs. In the presence of liver failure, it is best to avoid drugs that must be extensively metabolized by the oxidative enzymes of the liver. Or, as in the case of orally ingested drugs that must first pass through the liver before reaching the systemic circulation, intravenous (IV) or intramuscular (IM) administration should be given priority. Drugs that are inherently toxic to the liver (e.g., ethanol, tetracyclines, dactinomycin, and isoniazid) and drugs that cause a hypersensitivity-like reaction in the liver (e.g., halothane, phenytoin, phenylbutazone) should be avoided, if possible, when impaired liver function is present. It is of utmost importance to frequently measure serum blood levels, as well as clinical effect when administering drugs to patients with liver failure to avoid overt toxic reactions. Appendix B (*VI* and *VII*) details the blood tests available for testing liver function.

Cardiovascular Impairment

Impairment of circulatory blood flow, as with cardiovascular or peripheral vascular disease, has the greatest effect of altering a drug's distribution to its receptor site. In the presence of severe cardiovascular disease, a portion of the blood flow is redistributed to vital organs, leaving other organs with inadequate tissue perfusion. Of special concern are conditions associated with low cardiac output states (congestive heart failure, hypovolemia, shock) in which the liver and kidneys do not receive adequate blood flow and are therefore unable to maintain their bodily functions of biotransformation and elimination of substances. With abnormal tissue blood flow, all routes of drug administration may be ineffective, other than the intravenous or inhalation routes.

Pulmonary Disease

Pulmonary disease has the capability of altering a drug's onset of action and peak effectiveness. Aerosolized drugs are well absorbed by the lung mucosa, and the onset of drug action is rapid if the airway is patent. Lung disease in which there is a large ventilation-perfusion abnormality profoundly affects the absorption of a drug through the alveolocapillary membrane. A quantity of the drug may be lost to the nonperfused, nonventilated areas. Although a quantity of the aerosolized drug may be displaced, it is still an effective means of drug administration, because aerosolized drugs have the advantage of direct utilization to the receptor organ (smooth muscle of the bronchioles).

DOSE-EFFECT RELATIONSHIP

The distribution of a drug throughout the body is not a selective process; however, a drug's ability to stimulate and act upon specific receptor sites is selective. At reduced dosages, a drug may interact with only a few specific receptors, producing a minimum of effects. At higher dosages, a drug may interact with more receptors, initiating and intensifying a variety of effects. The relation between the given amount (dose) of a drug and the intensity of the response elicited is referred to as the dose-effect relation (Fig. 4.2). Each effect and the intensity of the response produced at varying dosage levels may be assimilated into a dose-effect curve. Four pertinent components of the curve include **potency,** slope, variability, and maximal **efficacy.**

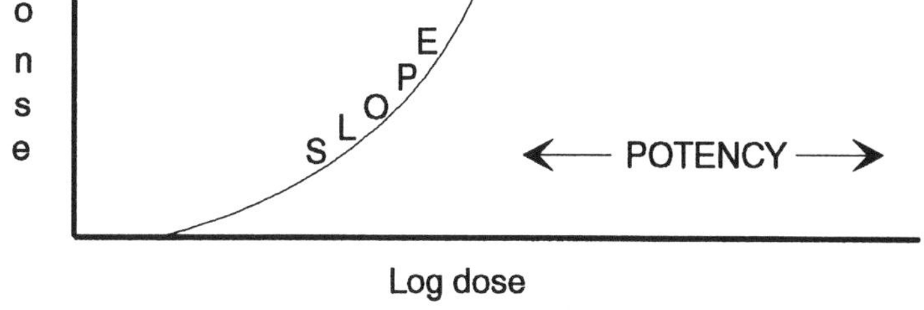

Figure 4.2. The dose-effect relation.

Potency

Potency is a dose-related occurrence that refers to the amount of a drug required to elicit a certain effect. The lower the dose required to elicit a response, the more potent the drug (Fig. 4.3). For a given range of expected responses from a drug, the lowest dose should be administered that will produce the effects desired. Pharmacokinetics, the concentration of the drug, and the drug's intrinsic ability to combine with receptors influence potency. In the case of transdermal absorption, a highly potent drug is mandated owing to the limited capacity of the skin to absorb drugs. For therapeutic purposes, the potency of a drug should be stated in dosage increments and related to the desired therapeutic effect. For example, to treat hypotensive bradycardia, 0.5 mg of atropine may be given, whereas to treat asystole, 1.0 mg of atropine may be administered. Comparatively, potency (located along the dose axis) does not equate with the degree of effectiveness of a drug; therefore, a highly potent drug may not necessarily be the most effective drug (Fig. 4.4).

Slope

The central, more or less linear portion of the curve forms the slope. A sheer upright slope signifies that maximal effects will be achieved with very small increments in dose (Fig. 4.5). It is necessary to be aware of this factor when considering the relative safety of a drug.

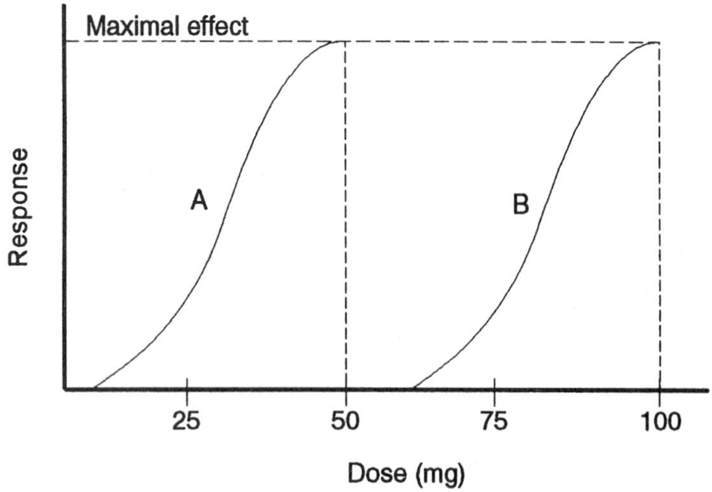

Figure 4.3. Drug A is more potent that drug B because drug A produces its maximal effect at a lower dose.

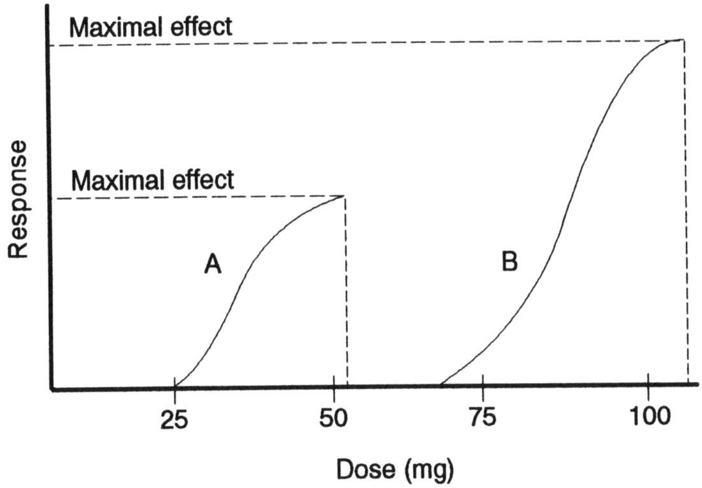

Figure 4.4. Drug A is more potent that drug B because it requires a lower dose to reach maximal efficacy, but drug B is more effective because it possesses a higher drug efficacy.

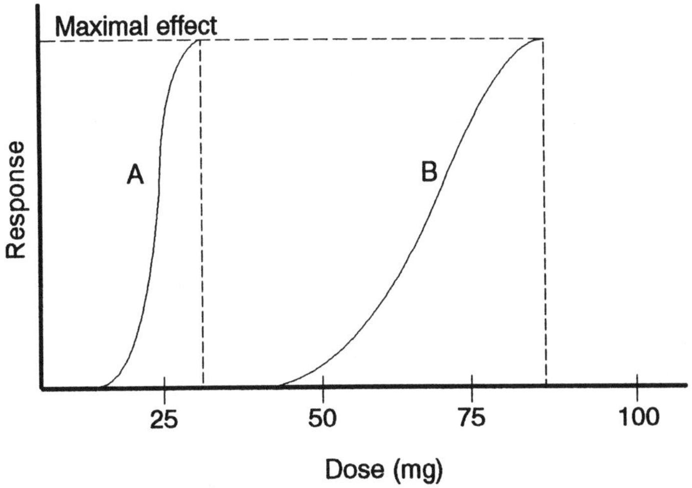

Figure 4.5. Very small increments in dose of drug A (compared to drug B) greatly increases the drug's effect, but both drugs possess the same maximal efficacy.

Maximal Effect

Intrinsic to a drug is its maximal effect, referred to as drug efficacy. Drugs are inherently capable of generating greater effects; however, as undesired effects limit a drug's dosage, its efficacy is also limited. Drug efficacy is sometimes confused with potency; however, the two properties are not related. It is much more important clinically to determine a drug's effectiveness rather than its potency, because a drug may be highly potent but not as effective as a drug lower in potency. This mechanism is illustrated in Figure 4.4. For example, some thiazide diuretics (such as chlorothiazide [Diuril]) have a greater potency than the loop diuretic furosemide (Lasix), but the maximal efficacy of furosemide is considerably greater.

Variability

The final component to be considered in the dose-effect relationship is biological variation. Exact drug response is never identical in all patients; therefore, a drug's dose produces varying effects in each individual. Individuals who obtain the desired response from a lower than normal dose of a drug are said to be *hyperreactive*. As such, individuals who require a higher than average dose to produce the desired response to a drug or who are resistant to the drug's effect are *hyporeactive*. *Tolerance* (as discussed later in this chapter) denotes hyporeactivity that is acquired from repeated, chronic administration of a drug. *Idiosyncrasy* refers to an unusual effect generated from a drug that is not related to the dosage or its intensity; this is usually a result of drug allergy or hereditary factors. Many of the reasons for the above-mentioned variances in drug therapy relate to some type of alteration in the hepatic microsomal enzyme system in which the rate of drug biotransformation is either enhanced or repressed.

The dose of a drug required to elicit the desired response in 50% of the population is designated as the median effective dose (ED_{50}) (Fig. 4.6). If death is the end effect of a drug, then the median lethal dose (LD_{50}) replaces the median effective dose. Therapeutic index (TI) refers to the relative safety of a drug and is calculated by dividing LD_{50} by ED_{50} (Fig. 4.7). As the index approaches zero, the margin of safety of a drug's given amount of dosage is greatly reduced. The therapeutic index changes according to the purpose for which a certain drug is administered. For example, the dose of codeine needed for cough suppression is much less than the dose required for control of pain. Thus, the therapeutic index or margin of safety for codeine's antitussive abilities is much greater than that of its analgesic abilities.

COMPENSATORY REFLEX EFFECTS

Compensatory reflex action of the autonomic nervous system initiates a series of events that leads to a modification in the response to sympathomimetic drugs. Compensatory reflex response determines the sympathetic tone when an α- or β-adrenoceptor is actuated. For example, the compensatory reflex effect in the cardio-

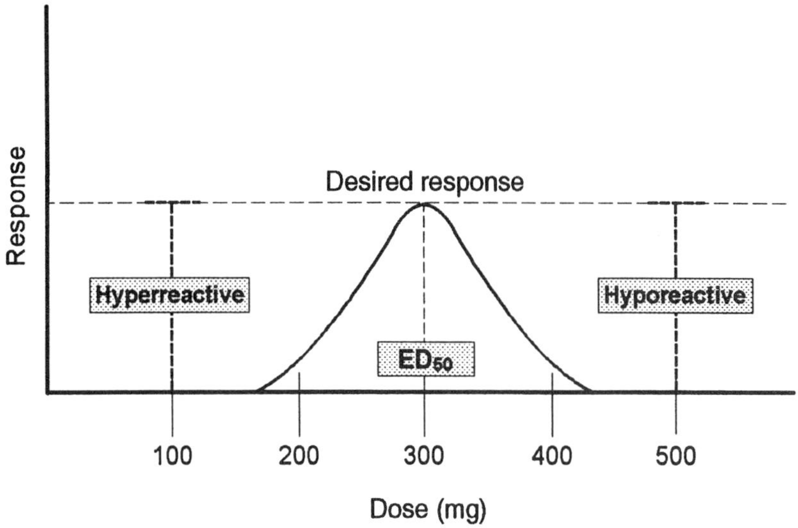

Figure 4.6. Biological variation in susceptibility to a given drug. The median effective dose (ED_{50}) is the dose at which the desired response is produced in 50% of the tested population. Hyperreactive subjects produce the desired response at a lower than normal dose, whereas hyporeactive subjects need a much higher dose to produce the desired response.

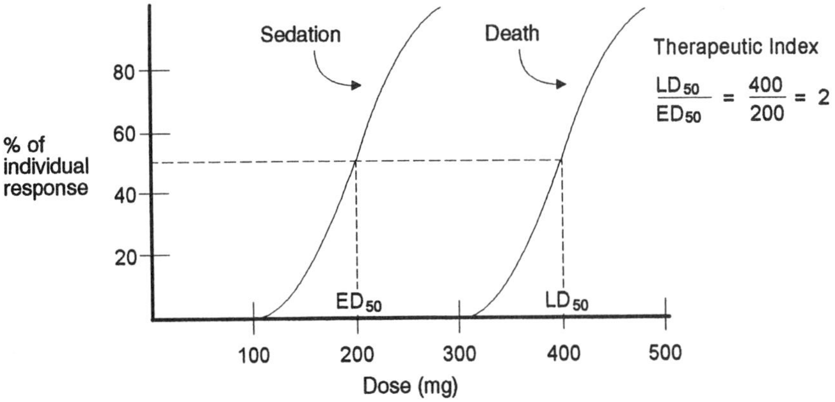

Figure 4.7. Comparison of a drug's dose that produces sedation in 50% of the population versus that dose that causes death in 50% of the population. For a given increase in the amount of a dose, the median lethal dose (LD_{50}) is observed.

vascular system to α_1-adrenoceptor stimulation is a rise in blood pressure through constriction of blood vessels. This results in a diminution of sympathetic tone throughout the system that tends to lessen the intensity of the effects produced by sympathomimetic drugs. β_2-adrenoceptor stimulation produces dilation of skeletal muscle blood vessels with corresponding constriction of other vascular beds through compensatory reflex action to maintain equilibrium of the blood pressure. This enhances overall sympathetic tone and the effectiveness of sympathomimetic drugs.

BIOLOGIC HALF-LIFE

Biologic half-life ($t_{1/2}$) refers to the time in which 50% of an administered drug is eliminated from the body. Biologic half-life establishes dosage frequency for each particular drug. For example, if it takes 4 hours for a drug to be 50% eliminated from the body, then the drug may be given six times per day. Biologic half-life varies with age, body weight, underlying disease, and the presence of other drugs. It is an important factor to be considered in dosing regimens.

DRUG INTERACTIONS

A drug interaction occurs whenever a drug's expected therapeutic effect is restricted, modified, enhanced, or altered in any way by an interactant chemical. The most common interactant is another drug or a combination of drugs (drug-drug interaction). The use of several drugs, administered singly or in combination, is often essential to maintain a desired therapeutic outcome or to treat coexisting diseases. For example, to successfully treat patients with heart failure, the concurrent use of a diuretic and a vasodilator is essential to achieve an adequate cardiac output. The primary goal of multiple drug therapy is to improve drug efficacy.

Drug-drug interactions may alter some aspect of a drug's pharmacokinetic properties (alteration of the absorption, distribution, metabolism, or elimination of one drug by another) or the interaction may involve the pharmacodynamic process (e.g., interactions between agonists and antagonists at drug receptors).

Pharmacokinetic Interactions

Absorption

Some drugs may circumvent absorption by interacting in an IV solution to produce an insoluble precipitate, which may or may not be observable. The rate and sometimes the extent of absorption of orally ingested drugs can be significantly affected by other drugs or conditions that inhibit gastrointestinal absorption. Alterations in gastric pH have the greatest effect of slowing the absorption of orally administered drugs. An acidic environment in the stomach is crucial for the absorption of drugs that are weak acids. Coadministering antacids or sodium bicarbonate (which create an alkaline environment) with orally ingested weak acids (e.g., ketoconazole, tetracyclines) leads to diminished absorption of the weak acid.

Distribution

As mentioned in Chapter 3, many drugs are extensively bound to plasma albumin (acidic drugs) or α-acid glycoprotein (basic drugs). Generally, only unbound drugs are able to exert a biological effect. Thus, when unexpected displacement of a drug from its binding site occurs from the interactions of another drug or substance, the expected result may potentiate the drug's effect and induce an overdose condition.

Metabolism or Biotransformation

Alteration of a drug's metabolism by another is a well-established mechanism for causing either an enhanced drug effect or a repressed drug effect. The cholinergic muscle stimulants are well known for their enzyme-inhibiting action on acetylcholinesterase, which leads to an enhanced effect of acetylcholine, succinylcholine (a depolarizing neuromuscular blocking agent [see Chapter 14]), and some other choline esters. Monoamine oxidase inhibitors have, at times, caused severe hypertensive conditions by preventing the destruction of catecholamines.

Many drugs can induce or inhibit the hepatic microsomal enzyme system, which then leads to alterations in the rate of drug biotransformation. In addition, some drugs alter another drug's metabolism by altering hepatic blood flow. For example, β-adrenoceptor blocking agents have a tendency to diminish hepatic blood flow, which then results in inhibition of another drug's metabolism. By this mechanism, β-adrenoceptor blocking agents raise lidocaine concentrations.

Elimination

Drug interactions that influence the renal tubular secretion of drugs or that alter the pH of urine can greatly affect the clearance of some drugs. Of special concern for patients receiving digoxin therapy are the toxic conditions that result when other drugs inhibit the renal secretion of digoxin. Such drugs include quinidine, amiodarone, verapamil, spironolactone, and cyclosporine.

Pharmacodynamic Interactions

Many pharmacodynamic interactions take place at the receptor level. These interactions may be at the same receptor or at different receptors. The response to receptor interaction may result in either an augmented drug effect by the coadministered drugs or in a reduced effect. In addition, an increase in the incidence of an adverse side effect may be noted with drug-drug interactions.

Augmented drug effects caused by an interactant are composed of three types: additivity, synergism, and potentiation.

Additivity

Additivity occurs whenever the combined effect of two drugs is equal to the sum of their independent effects. Additive effects are usually noted when both drugs act on the same target organ. Additive effects may be beneficial or harmful to the patient. An example of a harmful effect is coadministration of alcohol and chlorpromazine (Thorazine, an antipsychotic agent), the result of which is an additive central nervous system (CNS) depressive effect. Beneficial additive effects include studies that have shown that combination therapy with a β_2-adrenoceptor bronchodilator (e.g., albuterol) and an antimuscarinic bronchodilator (e.g., atropine or ipratropium) result in a rise in the **FEV$_1$** that is greater than the rise in the FEV$_1$ that either agent could produce when administered alone. This phenomenon is especially noted when the antimuscarinic bronchodilator is administered prior to the β_2-adrenoceptor bronchodilator (see Chapter 10). The mathematical expression of drug additivity could be regarded as $1 + 1 = 2$, where *the combined effect of drug A and drug B is equal to the sum of the effect of each agent when given alone.*

Synergism

Synergism occurs whenever the combined effect of two drugs is greater than the sum of their independent effects. Like additive effects, synergistic effects result when both drugs act on the same target organ. For example; combination therapy using a β_2-adrenoceptor bronchodilator (e.g., albuterol) with a xanthine bronchodilator (e.g., theophylline) can produce synergistic activity. The synergistic activity that results when using these two types of bronchodilators may be beneficial to the patient, in that there may be immediate relief of symptoms (e.g., reversal of bronchospasm), or this synergistic activity may be harmful to the patient, in that there may be an increase in the incidence of adverse effects (e.g., toxic effects). The mathematical expression of drug synergism could be regarded as $1 + 1 > 2$, where *the combined effect of drug A and drug B is greater than the sum of the effect of each agent when given alone.*

Potentiation

Potentiation occurs by combining two drugs, one of which has no intrinsic activity on the target organ while the other drug directly acts on the target organ. This mechanism results in an enhanced effect by the drug that directly influences the target organ. For example, administering morphine for its analgesic (pain-relieving) effect in conjunction with chlorpromazine (Thorazine, an antipsychotic agent and not an analgesic) enhances morphine's analgesic abilities. Potentiation can also occur when coadministering one drug that is not inherently toxic to an organ with another drug that is toxic to an organ. The one drug that is not toxic may greatly increase the toxicity of the other drug. For example, isopropanol (used for rubbing alcohol and in some hand lotions) is not itself hepatotoxic, but it can greatly increase the hepatotoxicity of carbon tetrachloride (used as a spot remover and carpet cleaner). Although there are no medicinal reasons for ingesting or inhaling these agents, the interaction between these two agents was highlighted by an industrial accident in which workers exposed to both agents were more susceptible to the hepatotoxic properties of carbon tetrachloride when isopropanol was also present (Folland et al. 1976). The above-mentioned incident brings about the issue of safety in the work place, where individuals are exposed to potentially lethal chemical combinations. The mathematical expression of drug potentiation could be regarded as $1 + 0 > 1$, where *the effect of active drug A and inactive drug B is greater than that effect produced by drug A alone.*

The term used to describe the pharmacological process in which there is a reduction in the effects of one drug by another at the receptor level is antagonism. The following details the various types of antagonism.

Physiologic Antagonism

Physiologic antagonism occurs whenever two drugs act on the same organ through independent receptor activation but produce biological responses in the opposite direction, which may lead to one drug canceling the effect of another. An example of physiologic antagonism is when the β_1-adrenoceptor agonist epinephrine activates the myocardial β_1-adrenoceptors and produces an increase in the heart rate, whereas the M_2-cholinoceptor agonist acetylcholine activates the myocardial M_2-cholinoceptors and produces a decrease in the heart rate. Both agents are agonists, but because of their specific receptor activation, each produces contradictory biologic responses. This process is also known as *functional antagonism.*

Chemical Antagonism

Chemical antagonism occurs when two drugs chemically interact with one another to produce inactive products. This process usually occurs through oxidation or hydrolysis. This mechanism has special significance in toxicology when certain compounds (e.g., chelating agents) are used to inactivate toxic chemicals in the body.

Pharmacological Antagonism

Pharmacological antagonism occurs whenever two drugs having opposing effects compete for the same receptor site. For example, atropine competes with acetylcholine for the muscarinic receptor. When atropine binds to the receptor, it produces a blockade in which acetylcholine cannot bind to the receptor. Atropine is the competitive antagonist to the muscarinic receptor, whereas acetylcholine is the agonist to the muscarinic receptor. Naloxone (Narcan), a competitive antagonist of opioid receptors, is the standard antidote used to reverse the respiratory-depressant effects of opioid agonists such as morphine. The above-mentioned antagonists work via competitive inhibition, which is a common method of therapeutic intervention.

OTHER FACTORS THAT AFFECT THE THERAPEUTIC OUTCOME OF DRUGS

The variation in pharmacokinetic and pharmacodynamic properties of drugs as previously discussed in this chapter account for much of the need to individualize drug therapy. This section presents the factors that can also determine the success or failure of drug therapy. The following topics serve as an introductory knowledge base of likely mechanisms that alter drug effects; some of these topics are also discussed elsewhere in this text.

Tolerance

Prolonged, repeated, or continuous stimulation of receptors with agonists or antagonists generally results in a state of *tolerance* (also referred to as *desensitization* or *refractoriness*). Tolerance is a condition in which there is a progressive diminution in the capacity of receptors to respond to a stimulus. Rapidly developing tolerance is known as *tachyphylaxis*. These phenomena (tolerance and tachyphylaxis) significantly limit the therapeutic efficacy and duration of action of exogenously administered agents. As reduced functional responsiveness occurs, a higher dose will be necessary to maintain the same level of response that was originally obtained by a smaller dose, or a different drug may have to be substituted for the original one; however, when receptors become desensitized by one drug, they may show this effect for all drugs of that class, which is known as *cross-tolerance*. At this point, the practitioner may have to look to a different class of drugs to maintain safe and effective therapy. *Down-regulation* is a term used to describe a type of advanced tolerance in which there is a reduction in the number of receptors following longer periods of contact with a drug.

Although many kinds of receptors undergo tolerance, in most cases, the mechanism is obscure. The only type of receptor in which the molecular mechanism of agonist desensitization that has been worked out in some detail is that of β-adrenoceptors. It appears that after administering a β-agonist, the β-adrenoceptor's capacity to further synthesize cAMP is markedly reduced. As presented in Chapter 2, it is the level of cAMP that is ultimately responsible for the biological response illicited from β-adrenoceptor stimulation. Thus, if there is a significant reduction in circulating cAMP, the resulting biological response will be diminished. There is evidence that multiple factors interact to cause these phenomena (Benovic et al. 1986, Benovic et al. 1988). Three such factors include functional alteration of the receptor itself, decreased efficiency of the G_s protein to activate adenyl cyclase, and a type of negative feedback mechanism from the cAMP-dependent protein kinase that acts to dampen receptor function.

Although receptor tolerance is a primary concern for clinicians, it is not an irreversible event. Withdrawal of the drug for a few days or few weeks can completely restore receptor sensitivity. This effect is depicted in Figure 4.8, which shows increasing tolerance occurring over time, withdrawal of the drug, and then resumption of therapy with the same drug with restoration of full effects. If discontinuance of the drug is not feasible, coadministering certain types of drugs can reduce the risk for developing tolerance. For example, concurrent corticosteroid therapy (oral or inhaled) with β_2-adrenoceptor therapy appears to effectively cause a reduction in the incidence of tolerance that some investigators state accompanies the use of β_2-adrenoceptor therapy (see Chapters 10 and 12).

Accumulation and Maintenance Dosing

Toxic conditions may occur within the body when the rate of elimination of a drug is slower than the rate of administration (e.g., as in renal failure). Appropriate administration/elimination of a drug is a very important concept when designing a regimen for long-term drug administration. In most clinical situations, drugs are administered in such a way as to achieve and maintain a steady state at which "drug in" should equal "drug out." This can be expressed in the following equation:

$$\text{Dosing rate} = \text{Clearance (CL)} \times \text{Target concentration (TC)}$$

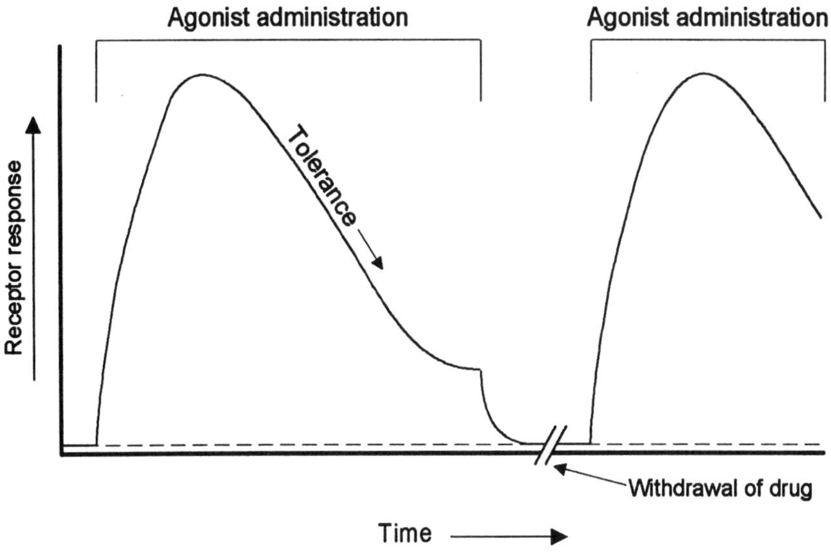

Figure 4.8. Continuous administration of an agonist results in a decreased functional response from a receptor, thereby reducing the efficacy of the agonist. Withdrawal of the agonist restores receptor responsiveness.

The above equation is based on an IV infusion of a drug in which there is 100% bioavailability. Fortunately, mean clearance (CL) for individual drugs of both IV administration and oral administration have been predicted (based on typical population values) and are available to clinicians. If the desired target plasma (or blood) concentration and the mean IV clearance rate of a particular drug are known, the dosing rate for an individual patient can be determined. For example, if one needed to design a dosing regimen for a 70-kg asthmatic patient with acute bronchospasm and were to administer theophylline as the agent to alleviate the patient's bronchospasm, a target plasma theophylline concentration of 10 mg/L would be desired (Holford et al. 1993). If the patient is a nonsmoker and otherwise normal except for asthma, the mean IV clearance for theophylline is 2.8 L/h/70 kg. Factoring in the known parameters would lead to:

$$\begin{aligned} \text{Dosing rate} &= \text{CL} \times \text{TC} \\ &= 2.8\ \text{L/h/70 kg} \times 10\ \text{mg/L} \\ &= 28\ \text{mg/h/70 kg} \end{aligned}$$

Thus, for the above patient, the proper infusion rate is 28 mg/h.

If one wanted to design a dosing regimen for oral theophylline for the above-mentioned patient and also wanted to maintain the 10 mg/L plasma theophylline concentration, the following equation would be used:

$$\text{Maintenance dose} = \text{Dosing rate/F} \times \text{Dosing interval}$$

where Dosing rate is the previously calculated infusion rate, F is the oral availability of theophylline (F_{oral}: in a nonsmoking, otherwise normal patient, F_{oral} for theophylline is 0.96), and Dosing interval is the desired frequency with which theophylline is to be administered in a 24-hour period. Oral theophylline is prepared in immediate release capsules as well as timed-release formulations (8-, 12-, and 24-hour timed-release). In this case, an 8-hour timed-release tablet is desired. Factoring in the known parameters would lead to:

$$\begin{aligned} \text{Maintenance Dose} &= (\text{Dosing rate} \div \text{F}) \times \text{Dosing interval} \\ &= (28\ \text{mg/h} \div 0.96) \times 8\ \text{h} \\ &= 233\ \text{mg} \end{aligned}$$

For this patient, a tablet close to the 233 mg range would be given at 8-hour intervals. If a 12-hour dosing interval were desired, the ideal dose would be 350 mg, and if a 24-hour dosing interval is desired (once a day), the dose would be 700 mg.

Age, Sex, and Weight

Drug dosage is a factor of body weight and surface area. Most standard dosage ranges are for average adults weighing 150 pounds (approximately 70 kg). It follows that drug dosages must be adjusted for infants, children, and the elderly. Chapter 7 details these factors.

Allergic Reactions

An allergic reaction is a response that results from a previous sensitizing exposure to an antigen (or an agent that is structurally similar). The adverse reactions associated with allergic reactions are primarily mediated by the immune system and are of four types:

Type-I reactions are mediated by immunoglobulin E (IgE) antibodies (Ab). This type of allergic reaction is presented in Chapter 2 but will be reviewed again. After exposure to an antigen (Ag), IgE antibodies bind to mast cells and blood basophils. Subsequent exposure to the antigen leads to the Ag-Ab bridge, which then brings about various mediator release (histamine, prostaglandins, leukotrienes). These highly inflammatory mediators precipitate the anaphylactic response (hypotension, edema, bronchoconstriction) that is associated with Type-I reactions. Type-I reactions are also known as *immediate hypersensitivity reactions,* because the anaphylactic response tends to occur quite rapidly after challenge with an antigen with which an individual has been previously sensitized. The primary organs associated with Type-I reactions are the gastrointestinal tract (food allergies), the skin (urticaria and atopic dermatitis), the respiratory tract (rhinitis and asthma), and the vasculature (anaphylactic shock).

Type-II reactions are also known as *cytolytic reactions,* because the primary target tissues are the cells of the circulatory system. Type-II reactions are mediated by both IgG and IgM antibodies. A type of hemolytic anemia ensues from Type-II reactions. The hemolytic anemia can be precipitated from individuals who are allergic to specific drugs such as penicillin and methyldopa. In addition, systemic lupus erythematosus may result in those individuals who are allergic to hydralazine and procainamide. The autoimmune reactions to these drugs usually are abolished within months after removal of the irritating agent.

Type-III reactions, also known as Arthus (from the French bacteriologist, Nicholas Maurice Arthus) reactions, occur in previously sensitized individuals who are injected with an antigen. In the simple form of Type-III reactions, a local necrotic lesion forms as a result of a severe inflammatory reaction at the site of injection. In a more severe form of Type-III reaction, a syndrome known as serum sickness results, the symptoms of which include fever, urticarial skin eruptions, arthritis, and lymphadenopathy. Several types of drugs can induce serum sickness (e.g., sulfonamides, penicillins, some anticonvulsants, iodides). Stevens-Johnson syndrome is a severe form of immune vasculitis mediated by a Type-III reaction from individuals allergic to sulfonamides. Type-III reactions are also the cause of occupational pneumonitis or alveolitis in susceptible individuals. Type-III reactions are mediated by IgG antibodies.

Type-IV reactions are also known as delayed-hypersensitivity reactions, because the symptoms of the adverse reaction to the antigen may not produce a visible change for several hours or even several days. Type-IV reactions result from interactions with sensitized T lymphocytes and macrophages. When these sensitized cells come in contact with an antigen, an inflammatory reaction ensues in which there is a production of lymphokines and an influx of neutrophils and macrophages. An example of a Type-IV reaction is the contact dermatitis caused by poison ivy.

Patient Noncompliance

The desired effects of drug therapy may not be noted if the patient refuses to comply with the dosing regimen. This is an especially difficult area for the clinician who monitors patients that self-administer their drugs.

Pregnancy and Lactation

Administering drugs that cross the placental barrier may be harmful and may cause **teratogenic** effects to the fetus owing to an incomplete and immature enzyme system. Because of this, most drugs carry the warning not recommended for pregnant females. Since the thalidomide episode of 1962 (which generated the passage of the Kefauver-Harris Law of 1962), all drugs are suspected of being capable of causing harmful effects to the fetus. Thalidomine was an antinausea drug administered to pregnant females in the early 1960s that caused malformations in the fetus such as the shortening or loss of limbs. The first trimester of pregnancy is an especially sensitive time for the fetus, and the use of drugs during this time is not recommended unless there is a dire emergency for doing so.

During lactation, most drugs are secreted in the milk. This is especially true of morphine, lithium, and the tricyclic antidepressants. An addicted nursing mother may have an addicted nursing child. If these drugs are necessary, the nursing mother is advised to stop nursing.

Pharmacogenetics

Hereditary factors may greatly influence the dosage of drugs. In most instances, individuals either lack or have an excessive amount of a certain, critical enzyme. The most significant effect hereditary variances have on drug effects is to alter the hepatic microsomal enzyme system, which in turn leads to an unusual rate (either enhanced or repressed) of drug biotransformation. This seems to explain some of the idiosyncratic and hypersensitivity reactions produced from certain individuals, as well as those individuals who are hypo- or hyperreactive to drugs. The goal of pharmacogenetics is not only to identify those individuals at risk for differences in drug effects but also to recognize these differences before the drug is administered to provide an alternative method for these susceptible individuals.

Environmental Factors

The alteration of drug effects in cases of individuals who are exposed to unusual chemicals in the environment is usually mediated by the activity of the hepatic microsomal enzyme system. Agents such as herbicides and pesticides used in agriculture and many organic solvents used in industry are metabolized by the hepatic microsomal enzyme system. These agents can function as both inducers and inhibitors of microsomal enzyme activity.

The many complex chemicals found in tobacco smoke include, in addition to nicotine, nongaseous matter such as hydrocarbons, acids, alcohol, ketones, and tars, and gaseous matter such as carbon monoxide, hydrogen cyanide, nitrous oxide, and nitrogen dioxide. All of these chemicals can affect the hepatic microsomal enzyme system. The chemicals contained in tobacco smoke have a tendency to enhance the activity of microsomal enzymes, which leads to an increased rate of drug biotransformation. For this reason, smokers may exhibit significantly different pharmacologic profiles, and dosage regimens usually need to be adjusted.

REFERENCES/RECOMMENDED READING

Benovic JL, et al. Beta-adrenergic receptor kinase: identification of a noval protein kinase which phosphorylates the agonist-occupied form of the receptor. Proc Natl Acad Sci U S A 83:2797, 1986.

Benovic JL, et al. Regulation of adenylyl cyclase-coupled beta-adrenergic receptors. Annu Rev Cell Biol 4:405, 1988.

Clark DWJ. Genetically determined variability in acetylation and oxidation. Therapeutic implications. Drugs 29:342, 1985.

Folland ED, et al. Carbon tetrachloride toxicity potentiated by isopropyl alcohol. JAMA 236:1853, 1976.

Guyatt G, et al. Determining optimal therapy—randomized trials in individual patients. N Engl J Med 314:889, 1986.

Holford NHG, et al. Theophylline target concentration in severe airways obstruction—10 or 20 mg/L? A randomised concentration-controlled trial. Clin Pharmacokinet 25:495, 1993.

Holford NHG, Sheiner LB. Understanding the dose-effect relationship. Clin Pharmacokinet 6:429, 1981.

Jick H. Adverse drug reactions: the magnitude of the problem. J Allergy Clin Immunol 74: 555, 1984.

Kersten LD. Comprehensive Respiratory Nursing. Philadelphia: WB Saunders, 1989.

Larsson S, Svedmyr N, Thiringer G. Lack of bronchial beta-adrenoceptor resistance in asthmatics during long-term treatment with terbutaline. J Allergy Clin Immunol 59:93, 1977.

McInnes GT, Brodie MJ. Drug interactions that matter: a critical reappraisal. Drugs 36:83, 1988.

Motulsky HJ, Insel PA. Adrenergic receptors in man: direct identification, physiologic regulation, and clinical alterations. N Engl J Med 307:18, 1982.

O' Connor BJ, Aikman SL, Barnes PJ. Tolerance to the nonbronchodilator effects of inhaled $beta_2$-agonists in asthma. N Engl J Med 327:1204, 1992.

Overstreet DH, Yamamurs HI. Receptor alterations and drug tolerance. Life Sci 25:1865, 1979.

Repsher LH, et al. Assessment of tachyphylaxis following prolonged therapy of asthma with inhaled albuterol aerosol. Chest 85:34, 1984.

Rodin SM, Johnson BF. Pharmacokinetic interactions with digoxin. Clin Pharmacokinet 15:227, 1988.

Skorodin MS. Beta-adrenergic agonists: a problem. Chest 103:1587, 1993.

Tatro DS, Olin BR, Hebel SK. Drug Interaction Facts. 2nd ed. Philadelphia: JB Lippincott Co., 1990.

Williams RL, Mamelok RD. Hepatic disease and drug pharmacokinetics. Clin Pharmacokinet 5:528, 1980.

Ziment I. Beta-adrenergic agonist toxicity: less of a problem, more of a perception. Chest 103:1591, 1993.

THERAPEUTIC EVALUATION AND PREPARATION OF MEDICINES 5

Therapeutic maintenance includes supportive care of the patient and the proficient use of pharmacologic agents. The practitioner must have a thorough knowledge of drug action, interaction, and effects before skillfully administering and evaluating these drugs.

LEARNING OUTCOMES

Upon completion of this chapter, the learner will be able to:

1. Define and describe subjective data, objective data, assessment, and plan of action as they pertain to drug evaluation.
2. Interrelate the pharmacologic assessment questions to the type of drug, dosage, administration, etc.
3. List the five rights of drug therapy.
4. Apply the rules for good charting.
5. Identify and discuss the legal factors involved in drug administration.
6. Describe the guidelines that help identify an adverse reaction.
7. List the precautions taken when administering medications.
8. Name the most commonly used medication syringes. List the units in which the syringe scales are calibrated.
9. Compare/contrast the two methods in which medications may be "drawn up" by using syringes.
10. Describe the medicine cup, list the units found on the medicine cup, and identify how the dosage is read.
11. Identify the calibrated dropper and the special precautions observed when using the calibrated dropper.

12. Explain the unit dose method of drug administration and the advantages pertaining to the unit dose.

THE FOUR PARTS OF THERAPEUTIC EVALUATION

Evaluation of drug therapy is the process of determining the effectiveness of drug action. It is an exceedingly important step in identifying the particular needs of a patient. The evaluation is performed purposefully and in an organized way. Four basic methods of collecting data for evaluation must be employed by the practitioner: 1) subjective feelings of the patient, 2) observation and examination of the patient, 3) assessment of the patient and of the data collected, and 4) review of data and reports to determine the course of drug therapy. These methods are collectively termed SOAP or SOAR, which are acronyms for subjective, objective, assessment, and plan (or recommendation).

Subjective

Subjective data are discernible only to the person affected and can only be verified by the person involved. After the administration of respiratory therapeutics, a patient's subjective feeling of comfort, relief of bronchospasm, and well-being are probably the most valuable tools in determining the effectiveness of therapy. Subjective data are known as symptoms.

Objective

Objective data are those that are detectable by the practitioner or can be tested using acceptable standards. The term "overt data" refers to something observed. Before, during, and after the administration of respiratory drugs, the practitioner must note pulse, respirations, auscultatory findings, and the volume of sputum production. Any noticeable improvement of the above may lead to a positive evaluation of the effectiveness of drug action. Objective data are known as signs.

Assessment

Assessment is the systematic collection of data and then the allocation of a meaning to the data. Data may be collected by observation, by interviewing, by physical examination, or by implementing specific tests that act as guidelines to determine the effectiveness of drug therapy. Bedside pulmonary function studies such as vital capacity, peak flow, and FEV_1 are completed before and after bronchodilator therapy to evaluate and document the extent of improvement. Monitoring arterial blood gas parameters and chest x-rays are also useful in assessing the effectiveness of drug action. Basic pharmacological assessment questions (Table 5.1) are also useful in the assessment and evaluation of drug therapy and drug effectiveness.

Table 5.1.
Pharmacological Assessment Questions[a]

Rationale for use	What is the medical diagnosis for which the drug is prescribed? What are the goals of therapy (e.g., relief of hypoxemia, reversal of bronchospasm)?
Dosage	Is the ordered dosage appropriate? Are there any factors that would necessitate a reduced dose (e.g., renal failure, hepatic failure, patient's physical condition)?
Administration	Is the mode of administration appropriate (e.g., intravenous, intramuscular, subcutaneous, oral, inhalation)? Are there factors that will influence administration of the drug and the patient's ability and willingness to take the drug?
Effects	Is the expected therapeutic effect being achieved? Is there observed improvement? Would another drug or dosage be more effective?
Side effects	Is there evidence of adverse effects from previous doses? If so, have they been minimized to a tolerable level? Would another drug produce less adverse effects but promote the same effectiveness?
Patient compliance	Does the patient feel that he/she is benefiting from drug therapy and thereby complying with the regimen?

Modified from Kersten L. Comprehensive Respiratory Nursing. Philadelphia: WB Saunders, 1989.

Plan/Recommendation

All other steps in the evaluation of drug therapy depend on the collection of data, which must be complete, relevant, and carefully recorded. A plan of action is necessary to implement, modify, or alter the course of drug therapy. The practitioner must review, on a daily basis, the course of drug therapy pertaining to a particular patient. After careful review and assessment of the data available, the practitioner may intelligently recommend any modifications that may be necessary for the progress of the patient. In many cases, the physician relies heavily on the information and recommendations relayed to him or her by the practitioner.

Table 5.2 gives an example of a typical drug care plan using the SOAP/SOAR method.

RULES FOR GOOD CHARTING

Most practitioners give medications to patients more often than any other single task. Before administering and charting any drug, make certain the "five rights" are observed: give the *right dose* of the *right medication* to the *right patient* at the *right time* by the *right route*. And add a sixth right—*right technique*. To prevent errors and ensure safe administration, always check the physician's medical orders for date, drug, dosage, route, and frequency. If there are any discrepancies, withhold the drug and check with the doctor or pharmacist.

The primary purpose of charting is to ensure continuity of patient care. Keeping well constructed, accurate, and complete notes not only ensures this continuity of care and protects the patient but also protects the practitioner from any forms of malpractice or negligence litigation if such charges are ever filed. The practitioner's notes serve as a legal document and should thus comply with the following guidelines for good charting:

Table 5.2.
An Example of a Drug Care Plan Using the SOAP/SOAR Method

Patient's Name: Janice Jones Date: 6/4/95

Patient's ID #: E4659862 Diagnosis: Asthma

Weight	Height	Age	Sex
61 kg	5′6″	34	F

Subjective Data	Objective Data	Assessment	Plan/Recommendation
Patient c/o tightness in chest, shortness of breath.	Breath sounds: diminished aeration throughout, bilateral inspiratory and expiratory wheezes. Respiratory rate: 22 breaths/min Heart rate: 116 beats/min Blood pressure: 134/72 mmHg Arterial blood gases: pH 7.46; $PaCO_2$ 32 mmHg; PaO_2 69 mmHg	Patient is having an acute bronchospastic attack. The patient's work of breathing and the work of her heart are abnormally high, most likely because of hypoxemia.	Relief of bronchospasm and inflammation: administer combination therapy with ipratropium (Atrovent) 4 puffs, albuterol (Ventolin) 4 puffs, and triamcinolone (Azmacort) 2 puffs via metered-dose inhaler q 4° and p.r.n. Reevaluate therapy in 24 hours. When patient's respiratory distress and condition improve, use medications p.r.n. Relieve hypoxemia, work of breathing, work of heart: titrate oxygen to achieve an SaO_2 of $\geq$ 95%.

1. Conform to hospital policy regarding notes, and follow up that policy with sound professional judgment. Record only on the proper forms supplied.
2. Enter the date and time before each note. Sign each note with your first initial, last name, and your title (e.g., R.N., C.R.T.T., R.R.T., etc.)
3. Never erase or write between the lines. If a mistake is made, draw a line through it, write "error" and sign your initials.
4. Record on every line in chronological order. Draw a line through any unused or half-used lines before signing your name.
5. Do not let anyone else chart or sign for the care you have given. Do not chart or sign for any care others have given.
6. Do not generalize in your charting; be specific and exclude any bias from your charting.
7. Document any discussions of questionable medical orders and the physician's directives to the order and the actions you took.
8. Record your patient assessment before and after therapy.
9. Above all, maintain accurate records—it is well worth the time and effort.

WHAT THE LAW REQUIRES

As a practitioner's role in medication delivery expands, so do one's legal responsibilities. The best way to protect against liabilities is to deliver quality patient care and to know the rights and responsibilities of medication administration. Along with the rules for good charting presented above, the following tips serve as helpful guidelines that will not only protect the practitioner but will ensure patient safety.

- **Familiarize yourself with the practice act that applies to your profession (e.g., nurse, respiratory care practitioner) from the state or province where you work. In addition, from time to time, review the job description of the position for which you were hired.** If you attempt to perform duties that are outside your realm of practice (or are instructed to do so), you are solely liable for the consequences. In addition, those individuals who are not properly licensed or certified who perform your assigned duties are breaking the law. As a result, both of you can be prosecuted and you may lose your license or certificate. In most states and Canadian provinces, practicing as a licensed profession without a current, valid license is a serious offense—at least a misdemeanor.
- **Be aware of federal and state drug abuse laws.** Chapter 1 details the Controlled Substances Act of 1971, which categorizes drugs by how dangerous they are (some are forbidden for use whereas others have severe restrictions).
- **Know about the drugs you administer.** You are expected to have a sound knowledge base about every drug you give to a patient. This means that you are legally responsible for knowing the drug's safe dosage range, expected therapeutic effects, most common risks and hazards, as well as why the patient is receiving the drug.
- **As mentioned above, make sure that you are giving the right drug to the right patient and that you are doing so with the correct and safe technique.** Do not administer medications that have expired or use accessories (syringes, needles, medicine cups, diluents, nebulizers) that are suspect. Medications must be administered to patients in a sterile or aseptic manner. Do not contaminate medications by using an inappropriate technique.
- **Ask if you are not sure.** If you do not have a clear understanding or if you have a question regarding a drug order, investigate further. There are several resources available to you:

Look up the drug in a standard drug reference book. Many institutions carry the *Physician's Desk Reference* or *Drug Facts and Comparison.*

Ask your hospital's pharmacist.

Check your institution's policy regarding the guidelines that have been established for giving the drug.

Ask the practitioner in charge.
Call the prescribing doctor.
If interacting with a resident or intern and he/she cannot answer your question, ask his/her supervisor.
You may have to call your institution's legal department if no one can satisfactorily answer your question.

- **Seriously think twice before administering a drug if you think the drug may cause harm to the patient.** Under certain circumstances, you may refuse to give a drug. For example, if the prescribed dosage is too high or if the drug is contraindicated owing to previously administered drugs (including alcohol). If you refuse to carry out a drug order, you must notify your immediate supervisor and the physician ordering the drug. Follow through with an incident report documenting why you withheld the drug.
- **Document thoroughly.** Always document drug administration as soon as feasible after giving the drug. Never document before administering a drug. If you have made a medication error, fill out an incident report describing the circumstances surrounding the error as well as the corrective action taken following the error.

IDENTIFYING AN ADVERSE REACTION

Recognizing an adverse reaction is not always easy. The signs and symptoms accompanying the adverse reaction may correspond to the patient's disease state, or the severity of the reaction may be masked by the patient's physical condition and other previously administered drugs. Adverse reactions also vary from person to person. The following guidelines are helpful if a patient is suspected of having an adverse reaction:

- Determine when the change in the patient's condition occurred—before, during, or after therapy.
- Determine whether the presenting symptom is related to the patient's condition or disease.
- Given the patient's age and condition, determine whether the appropriate dose was administered or if the frequency of administration is appropriate.
- Determine whether other previously administered drugs are potentiating the effects and thereby the side effects of the drug.
- Determine whether the patient is allergic to other drugs and, thus, may be allergic to the current drug. Does the patient exhibit adverse symptoms with this drug that he/she has previously experienced from other drugs?
- Determine whether there are any contributing factors, such as liver or renal disease, that could be causing the adverse reaction.

Although some adverse reactions are minor and nonsignificant, severe life-threatening reactions can and do occur. Your immediate assessment of the situation and actions can dictate the outcome to such reactions.

PREPARATION OF MEDICINES

There are several methods to prepare or "draw up" medications. This section focuses on the primary systems.

Syringes

Figure 5.1 shows the three types of syringes most commonly used for medication preparation. The tuberculin syringe (1-cc dosage), the 3-cc syringe, and the 6-cc syringe have double calibrated scales that measure dosages in cc on one side and in minims on the other side.

Two methods are available for drawing up medications with syringes. The *single syringe method* uses one syringe for drug administration. This system is preferred when only one agent is required. However, it may also be used when an active ingredient (e.g., albuterol) and a diluent (e.g., normal saline) are needed. Both the active ingredient and diluent are drawn into the syringe in proper proportions (e.g., 0.5 ml albuterol plus 2.5 ml normal saline). Disadvantages to this system include possible cross-contamination and inaccurate dosage when two agents are mixed in one syringe.

The *double or separate syringe method* uses two syringes for drug administration. The active ingredient is drawn into one syringe while the diluent is drawn into another separate syringe. This allows accuracy of drug dosage while elimi-

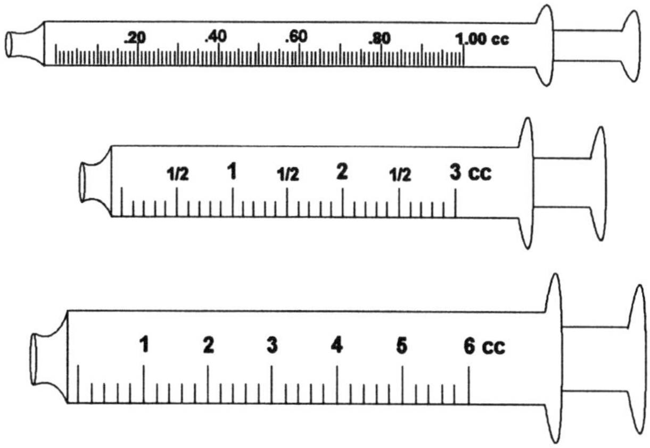

Figure 5.1. Commonly used medication syringes.

nating cross-contamination of the agents used. This is the preferred method when two or more agents are used.

Medicine Cup

The medicine cup is a small, plastic 30-cc cup (Fig. 5.2) that has the following graduations: teaspoons (tsp), tablespoons (tbs), dessert spoons (dssp), ounces (oz), drams, milliliters (ml), cubic centimeters (cc).

Measurements of teaspoons, tablespoons, and dessert spoons are from the household measuring system; measurements of ounces and drams are apothecary measures; and milliliters and cubic centimeters are from the metric system.

The reading of the dose must be made at the lowest point of the meniscus and observed at eye level. If more than one agent is used, careful consideration of dosage dilution and accuracy must be realized. Cross-contamination of vials is prevented if agents are drawn up separately and then added to the measuring cup or if they are poured separately into the cup.

Calibrated Dropper

Certain drugs are supplied with a calibrated dropper (Fig. 5.3). Graduations may be milliliters, cubic centimeters, teaspoons, or ounces. Careful consideration must be given to eliminate air bubbles and excess solution. Drug manufacturers have specific calibration guidelines for a particular drug; therefore, substituting a medicine dropper to use with a drug other than the one recommended may result in inaccurate dosage.

Unit Dose

The unit dose method provides a one-time-use, premeasured dosage placed in a container (usually a vial or ampule). The container may hold the active ingredient alone or the active ingredient mixed with a diluent. Medication errors and

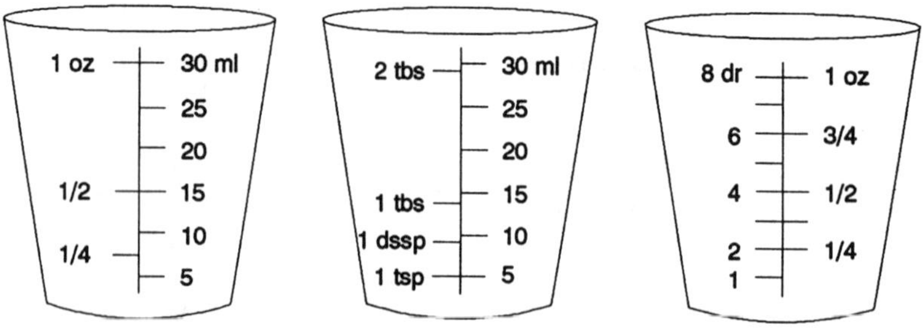

Figure 5.2. Commonly used medicine cups with various graduations.

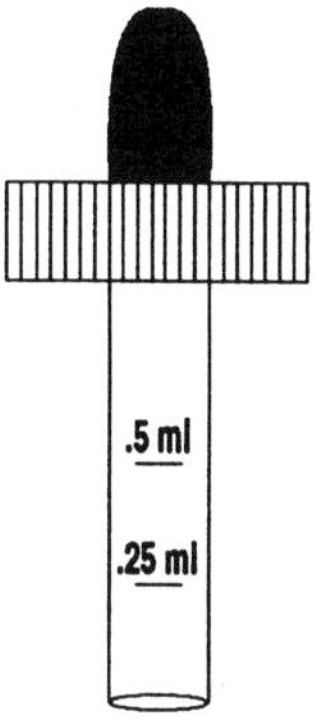

Figure 5.3. The calibrated dropper.

drug waste are eliminated, which results in safe administration and lower costs for the patient.

REFERENCES/RECOMMENDED READING

Deglin JM, Mandell HN. Drug interactions without anguish. Postgrad Med 72:199, 1982.
Govoni L, Hayes J. Drugs and Nursing Implications. 7th ed. Norwalk, CT: Appleton & Lange, 1992.
Kersten LD. Comprehensive Respiratory Nursing. Philadelphia: WB Saunders, 1989.
Nursing Now: Drug Interactions, Springhouse, PA: Springhouse, 1984.
Poirier TI. Factors involved in adverse drug reactions. US Pharmacist 8:33, April 1983.

Mathematics of Drugs and Solutions 6

One of the more difficult areas of drug therapy for practitioners is the mathematics of drugs and solutions. The comprehension and application of mathematical concepts as applied to the administration of drugs and solutions are of utmost importance to the practitioner because calculations must be made and accuracy is essential.

Learning Outcomes

Upon completion of this chapter, the learner will be able to:

1. Name and describe the systems of measurement, their symbols and abbreviations, and any special considerations for use. Apply the conversions of equivalents within and between the metric, the apothecary, the household, and the avoirdupois methods.
2. Convert percentage strength to a ratio and a ratio to percentage strength.
3. Convert a given amount of g:mL to the amount of mg:mL.
4. When given a drug dosage problem, provide an appropriate equation to solve for an unknown variable. The unknown variable may be:

   the percentage strength or ratio
   the solute or the total solution amount
   the desired dosage or desired concentration

5. Calculate and solve the various problems/examples given in this chapter.
6. Calculate the proper dose to administer when given a dosage schedule in mg/kg and the patient's weight.
7. Differentiate between the various rules and equations that apply for the appropriate administration of drugs in infants and children.

8. When given an intravenous (IV) drug, calculate the flow rate and infusion time.

METHODS OF MEASUREMENT

The Metric System

The metric system—also called the decimal system—is a method of weights and measures using multiples and fractions of 10. Denominations may be changed by simply moving the decimal point. The metric system is the most commonly used system of measurement owing to its accuracy and uniformity.

The unit of length in this system is the meter (hence "metric"). The units applied to weight (i.e., the kilogram, the gram, and the milligram) and the units applied to volume (i.e., the liter and the milliliter or the cubic centimeter) are used to measure medications.

Primary Units

METER (m) . . . . .unit of LENGTH
GRAM (g) . . . . .unit of WEIGHT
LITER (L) . . . . .unit of VOLUME

Latin prefixes are designated to express quantities less than a meter, a gram, or a liter.

Unit	Meaning	Written As
nano (n)	10^{-9}	0.000000001
micro (μ)	10^{-6}	0.000001
milli (m)	10^{-3}	0.001
centi (c)	10^{-2}	0.01
deci (d)	10^{-1}	0.1

For all quantities less than 1, decimals are used (i.e., 0.5 g, 0.1 g)

Greek prefixes are designated to express quantities greater than a meter, a gram, or a liter.

Unit	Meaning	Written As
kilo (k)	10^3	1000
hecto (h)	10^2	100
deca (da)	10	10
meter, gram, liter	1	1

Summary

Weight		Volume	
kilogram (kg)	$g \times 10^3$	kiloliter (kL)	$L \times 10^3$
hectogram (hg)	$g \times 10^2$	hectoliter (hL)	$L \times 10^2$
decagram (dag)	$g \times 10$	decaliter (daL)	$L \times 10$
gram (g)	1	liter (L)	1
decigram (dg)	$g \times 10^{-1}$	deciliter (dL)	$L \times 10^{-1}$
centigram (cg)	$g \times 10^{-2}$	centiliter (cL)	$L \times 10^{-2}$
milligram (mg)	$g \times 10^{-3}$	milliliter (mL)	$L \times 10^{-3}$
microgram (μg, mcg)	$g \times 10^{-6}$	microliter (μL, mcL)	$L \times 10^{-6}$
nanogram (ng)	$g \times 10^{-9}$	nanoliter (nL)	$L \times 10^{-9}$

Equivalents within the Metric System

Weight	Volume
1 gram = 1000 mg	1 liter = 1000 mL*
= 100 cg	= 100 cL
= 10 dg	= 10 dL
= 0.1 dag	= 0.1 daL
= 0.01 hg	= 0.01 hL
= 0.001 kg	= 0.001 kL

*mL is frequently written as cc (cubic centimeter). Both terms represent 1/1000 of a liter. For general purposes, 1 mL = 1 cc and weighs 1 g (water at 4°C).

Helpful Hints

1. 10 times 1 unit = the next higher unit
   Example: 10×1 mg = 1 cg
   10×1 cg = 1 dg
   10×1 dg = 1 g
2. Placing the decimal point one place to the right multiplies its value by 10.
   Example: $0.001 \times 10 = 0.01$
3. Placing the decimal point one place to the left divides its value by 10.
   Example: $0.001/10 = 0.0001$

The Apothecary System

The apothecary system is an ancient English method that is being replaced by the metric system. However, some hospitals and physicians still use this system.

Apothecary Weight

The units for weighing solids are (from smallest to largest):

grain (gr)
scruple (℈)
dram (ʒ)
ounce (℥, oz)
pound (lb)

In apothecary weight, 12 ounces equal 1 pound, whereas in avoirdupois weight, 16 ounces equal 1 pound.

Apothecary Volume

The units for measuring volume are (from smallest to largest):

minim (♏)
fluiddram (f ʒ)
fluidounce (f ℥)
pint (pt)
quart (qt)
gallon (gal)

Equivalents within the Apothecary System

Weight	Volume
20 grains = 1 scruple	60 minims* = 1 fluidram
3 scruples = 1 dram	8 fluidrams = 1 fluidounce
8 drams = 1 ounce	16 fluidounces = 1 pint
12 ounces = 1 pound	2 pints = 1 quart
	4 quarts = 1 gallon

*One minim is *almost equal to one drop*. A minim is measured with a minim glass and a drop is measured with a medicine dropper. For accuracy, if a drug is prescribed in minims, it is best to measure it in minims, not drops.

Symbols and Abbreviations

Lower-case Roman numerals and fractions express quantities in the apothecary system. When a symbol or abbreviation of a unit is used, the symbol or abbreviation is expressed first, followed by the quantity, which is written either in Roman numerals or as a fraction.

For example, if the quantity is 1 or greater, Roman numerals are used:

2 drams is ʒii
6 grains is gr vi

If the quantity is less than 1, fractions are used:

¼ ounce is ℥ ¼ or oz ¼
¾ grain is gr ¾

An exception to the rule is the fraction ½, which has its own symbol, $\overline{ss}$. Therefore, an order for ½ grain may be written as gr $\overline{ss}$.

5½ ounces is ℥ v$\overline{ss}$
7½ grains is gr vii$\overline{ss}$

Some Commonly Used Symbols and Lowercase Roman Numerals

$\overline{ss}$ = ½	iii = 3	vi = 6	ix = 9
i = 1	iv = 4	vii = 7	x = 10
ii = 2	v = 5	viii = 8	xv = 15
			xx = 20

Approximate Conversion Equivalents*

	Metric	Apothecary
Weight	60 milligrams	1 grain
	1 gram (1000 mg)	15 grains
Volume	1 mL	15 minims
	30 mL	1 fluidounce
	500 mL	1 pint
	1000 mL	1 quart

*For a complete list of conversion equivalents, refer to Appendix C.

The Household System

The household system of measurement is the least accurate method of weights and measures and contains only approximate equivalents. Therefore, it is not advisable to substitute household equivalents for medication prescribed by physicians. The household system is used only when it is impractical to measure doses by other systems. This system is based on cooking utensils such as the teaspoon and tablespoon and is commonly used in everyday home situations.

Household Measurements

60 drops (gtt) = 1 teaspoon (t)	2 cups = 1 pint (pt)
3 teaspoonfuls = 1 tablespoon (T)	2 pints = 1 quart (qt)
2 tablespoonfuls = 1 fluidounce (oz)	1 quart = 4 cups

8 fluidounces = 1 glassful
16 ounces (dry measure) = 1 pound
4 quarts = 1 gallon (gal)

Approximate Conversion Equivalents

Metric	Apothecary	Household
0.06 mL	1 minim	1 drop
1 mL	15 minims	15 drops
5 mL	1 fluidram	1 teaspoon
15 mL	½ fluidounce	1 tablespoon
30 mL	1 fluidounce	2 tablespoons
240 mL (~250 mL)	8 fluidounces	1 cup
473 mL (~500 mL)	16 fluidounces	1 pint
946 mL (~1000 mL)	32 fluidounces	1 quart
3785 mL	128 fluidounces	1 gallon

The Avoirdupois System

The avoirdupois method is a system of weight only and is mainly used in English-speaking countries. The avoirdupois and the apothecary systems contain the same terms, but the grain is the only term that is an equal amount. The avoirdupois pound contains 16 ounces, whereas the apothecary pound contains 12 ounces.

Avoirdupois Measurements

437.5 grains = 1 ounce
16 ounces = 1 pound
7000 grains = 1 pound

Approximate Conversion Equivalents*

Metric	Avoirdupois
1 g	0.035274 ounce
28.3 g	1 ounce
454 g	1 pound
1 kg	2.2 pounds

*Note: All of the above lists of equivalents are only approximate. Different sets of equivalents can be found in different texts.

CHEMICAL SOLUTIONS: DEFINITIONS AND TERMS

solute—The substance dissolved in a solution: the active ingredient (i.e., the drug). The solute is usually expressed in grams or milligrams.

solvent—The dissolving medium (the component in a solution present in the greatest amount). The solvent, in pharmacology, is usually expressed in ml or cc.

solution—A homogeneous mixture of one or more substances (solute) dissolved in a quantity of a dissolving medium (solvent).
aqueous solution—A solution in which water is the dissolving medium.
strength of a solution—Percentage of solute present in a solution, expressed as parts of solute in 100 parts solution.
normal solution—A solution in which 1 liter contains 1 gram equivalent of the solute.
buffer solution—A solution of a weak acid and its salt, maintains a constant pH.
milliequivalent (mEq)—Concentration of electrolytes in a certain volume (usually 1 liter) of solution.
molar solution—A solution in which 1 mole (Avogadro's number) of the solute is dissolved in 1 liter.
osmolar solution—Concentration of osmotically active particles in solution.
isotonic, hypertonic, hypotonic solutions—See Chapter 13.

DRUG DOSAGE CALCULATIONS

The crucial steps in learning dosage calculations are to first identify the appropriate equation to use and then to set up the equation or proportions in the same sequence of measurement units; otherwise, the problem cannot be solved correctly. For example, grams and milligrams cannot be mixed in an equation or in a proportion. Either convert to grams or convert to milligrams.

Types of Percentage Preparations

Three types of percentage preparations exist:

Weight-to-weight (W/W): the amount (grams of active ingredient) in 100 grams of a mixture.

$$\text{W/W\%} = \frac{\text{grams (solute)}}{\text{100 grams (solution)}} \times 100$$

Example: 1% = (1 g solute/100 g solution) × 100

Weight-to-volume (W/V): the amount (grams of active ingredient) in 100 milliliters of a mixture.

$$\text{W/V\%} = \frac{\text{grams (solute)}}{\text{100 milliliters (solution)}} \times 100$$

Example: 5% = (5 g solute/100 mL solution) × 100

Note: prescription usage favors weight-to-volume percentage solutions. When a ratio or percent is given of a drug strength it is understood to be g:mL unless otherwise stated.

Volume-to-volume (V/V): the amount (milliliters of active ingredient) in 100 milliliters of a mixture.

$$V/V\% = \frac{\text{milliliters (solute)}}{\text{100 milliliters (solution)}} \times 100$$

Example: 0.1% = (0.1 mL solute/100 mL solution) × 100

Solutions In Which Strength Is Expressed in Ratio

A ratio designates the relation between the solute and the total solution (solute plus solvent) and is usually expressed in g:mL. However, "ratio by simple parts" still exists. For example, a physician may order Bronkosol 1:8, which means one part drug to eight parts diluent. This type of drug order does not give the actual dosage amount, although milliliters is assumed. Knowledge of correct dosage when interpreting this type of order is essential. The dosage range for Bronkosol 1% is 0.25 to 0.5 mL diluted with normal saline; therefore, you would not give more than that amount.

Converting a ratio to a percent strength

As mentioned, most drug ratios are expressed as a weight:volume in which, for example, 1:100 is assumed to be 1 g solute (active ingredient) per 100 mL solution. To convert the ratio 1:100 to a percent strength, simply divide 1 by 100 and then multiply by 100. Thus, the percent strength of a drug that is expressed as a 1:100 ratio is 1%.

The equation for converting a ratio to a percent strength is:

$$\text{Percent strength} = \frac{\text{solute (g)}}{\text{solution (mL or cc)}} \times 100$$

Examples:

1. A physician has written orders for your patient to receive Isuprel 1:200. Express this ratio as a percent strength. (Remember, 1:200 is assumed to be 1 g:200 mL).

Answer:

$$\text{Percent strength} = \frac{\text{solute (g)}}{\text{solution (mL)}} \times 100$$

$$= \frac{1\text{ g}}{200\text{ mL}} \times 100$$

$$= 0.5\%$$

2. Epinephrine's cardiopulmonary resuscitative (CPR) strength is 1:10,000. Express this ratio as a percent strength.

Answer:

$$\text{Percent strength} = \frac{\text{solute (g)}}{\text{solution (mL)}} \times 100$$

$$= \frac{1\text{ g}}{10{,}000\text{ mL}} \times 100$$

$$= 0.01\%$$

Converting a Percent Strength to a Ratio

When converting a percent strength to a ratio one must remember two things:

1. The percent strength must be converted to a decimal prior to using it in the equation. This can be done by simply dividing the percent strength by 100. For example, the decimal of 5% is 0.05 (5 ÷ 100 = 0.05).
2. When converting a percent strength to a ratio, the ratio will be a 1 g:? mL, where the solution in mL is the unknown portion of the ratio.

Converting a percent strength to a ratio:

$$X = \frac{1}{\text{percent strength (in decimals)}}$$

Examples:

1. Express 0.3% as a ratio.

Answer:

$$X = \frac{1}{\text{percent strength (in decimals)}}$$

$$X = \frac{1}{0.003}$$

$$= 333$$

Thus, 0.3% expressed as a ratio is 1:333.

2. Convert 0.125% to a ratio.

Answer:

$$X = \frac{1}{\text{percent strength (in decimals)}}$$

$$X = \frac{1}{0.00125}$$

$$= 800$$

Thus, 0.125% expressed as a ratio is 1:800.

Converting g:mL to mg:mL

When converting g:mL to mg:mL, one must remember that 1000 mg = 1 g.

Examples:

1. How many mg are in Isuprel 1:200?

Answer:

a. Recall that Isuprel 1:200 = 1 g:200 mL
b. Convert g to mg: 1 g = 1000 mg
c. Thus, we have a ratio that is 1000 mg:200 mL
d. 10 ~~00~~ mg:2 ~~00~~ mL = 10 mg:2 mL = 5 mg:1 mL (or 5 mg)

There is 5 mg of active ingredient in Isuprel 1:200.

Another method for solving the above problem:

a. Isuprel 1:200 = 0.005 g/mL (1 ÷ 200 = 0.005)
b. There are 1000 mg in 1 g; therefore, 0.005 g/mL × 1000 mg/g = 5 mg/mL (or 5 mg)

In Summary: Isuprel 1:200 has a strength of 0.5% and contains 5 mg (or 0.005 g).

Percentage and Ratios of Solutions (Weight to Volume)

Ratio	Percentage (%)	g/mL	mg/mL
1:1000	0.1	0.001	1
1:500	0.2	0.002	2
1:200	0.5	0.005	5
1:100	1	0.01	10
1:20	5	0.05	50

Ratio	Percentage (%)	g/mL	mg/mL
1:10	10	0.1	100
1:5	20	0.2	200
1:1	100	1	1000

Percentage and Ratio Calculation Problems

The basic equation for solving one drug's solute amount, solution amount, or strength is as follows:

$$\text{Strength (in decimals)} = \frac{\text{solute (g)}}{\text{total solution (mL or cc)}}$$

This equation provides three variables:

a. If solute and solution are known, solve for strength (use the equation above).
b. If solution and strength are given, solve for solute. Rearranging the equation to solve for solute gives:
 Solute (g) = strength (in decimals) × solution (mL or cc)
c. If solute and strength are given, solve for solution. Rearranging the equation to solve for solution gives:

$$\text{Solution (mL or cc)} = \frac{\text{solute (g)}}{\text{strength (in decimals)}}$$

Rules:

1. If a ratio is given as the strength, it must be converted to g/mL (e.g., 1 ÷ 200 = 0.005 g/mL) prior to using it in the equation.
2. If strength is given in percent, it must be converted to decimals prior to using it in the equation (e.g., 5%/100 = 0.05).
3. Solute (if given in milligrams) must be converted to grams prior to using it in the equation (e.g., 5 mg × 1 g/1000 mg = 0.005 g).

Examples:

1a. What is the percentage strength of a solution that contains 5 g of drug to 100 mL of solution (5:100)?

Percent strength - unknown
Solute - 5 g
Total solution = 100 ml

$$\text{Percent strength} = \frac{\text{solute (g)}}{\text{total solution (mL)}} \times 100$$

$$= \frac{5\text{ g}}{100\text{ mL}} \times 100$$

$$= 5\%$$

1b. Express the ratio given in problem 1a in milligrams.

5 g:100 mL = 50 ~~00~~ mg:1 ~~00~~ mL = 50 mg

or

$$5 \div 100 = 0.05\text{ g}$$

$$0.05\text{ g} \times 1000\text{ mg/g} = 50\text{ mg}$$

2. How many milligrams are there in 4 mL 1:100 epinephrine?
   Strength = 1:100 = 0.01 g/mL
   Solute = unknown
   Total solution = 4 mL

$$\text{Solute (g)} = \text{strength (in decimals)} \times \text{solution (mL)}$$

$$= 0.01 \times 4$$

$$= 0.04\text{ g}$$

$$0.04\text{ g} \times 1000\text{ mg/g} = 40\text{ mg}$$

3. A physician orders Isuprel 1:200, 2 mg to be administered to your patient. What is the amount of Isuprel you will give to your patient?
   Strength = 1:200 = 0.005 g/mL
   Total solution = unknown
   Solute = 2 mg = 0.002 g

$$\text{Solution (mL)} = \frac{\text{solute (g)}}{\text{strength (in decimals)}}$$

$$= \frac{0.002\text{ g}}{0.005}$$

$$= 0.4\text{ mL}$$

Dilution Calculations

Another type of dosage equation involves the use of two strengths, where the strength of one drug will need to be diluted. For example, if the physician orders a 6-mL dose of an 8% solution and the only type of preparation on hand is a 20% solution, the more concentrated drug will need to be diluted to obtain an 8% solution. The equation for this is:

$$V_1 \times C_1 = V_2 \times C_2$$

Where:
V_1 is the volume before dilution
C_1 is the concentration before dilution
V_2 is the volume after dilution
C_2 is the concentration after dilution

Example 1: In the above-mentioned scenario in which the physician wants a 6-mL dose of an 8% solution and the stock solution contains 20%, the setup would be as follows:
V_1 = unknown
C_1 = 20%
V_2 = 6 mL
C_2 = 8%

$$\begin{aligned} V_1 \times C_1 &= V_2 \times C_2 \\ (X) \times (20) &= (6) \times (8) \\ X &= \frac{6 \times 8}{20} \\ &= 2.4 \end{aligned}$$

Thus, 2.4 mL of the 20% solution will be needed. To obtain the desired 8% solution, a diluent will be added to the 2.4 mL. In this case, 3.6 mL of a diluent will be added to the 2.4 mL from the 20% solution for a total dose of 6 mL (3.6 + 2.4 = 6) at 8% strength.

Example 2: Mucomyst is prepared in 10% and 20% solutions. You have on hand a 20% Mucomyst solution. The physician orders 8 mL of 10% Mucomyst to be administered by nebulization. How many mL of the 20% solution are needed to prepare a 10% solution?
V_1 = unknown
C_1 = 20%
V_2 = 8 mL
C_2 = 10%

$$V_1 \times C_1 = V_2 \times C_2$$

$$(X) \times 20 = (8) \times (10)$$

$$X = \frac{8 \times 10}{20}$$

$$= 4$$

Thus, 4 mL of the 20% solution will be needed, in addition to 4 mL of a diluent (e.g., normal saline) to deliver an 8-mL dose at 10% strength.

Example 3: Prepare a 3-mL dose of isoetharine 0.2% from a stock solution containing 1% isoetharine.
V_1 = unknown
C_1 = 1%
V_2 = 3 mL
C_2 = 0.2%

$$V_1 \times C_1 = V_2 \times C_2$$

$$(X) \times (1) = (3) \times (0.2)$$

$$X = \frac{3 \times 0.2}{1}$$

$$= 0.6$$

In this case, 0.6 mL of the 1% solution will be added to 2.4 mL of a diluent to administer a 3-mL dose at 0.2%.

Example 4: If you have 15 mL of a 3% atropine solution and add 6 mL of normal saline, what is the new concentration?
V_1 = 15 mL
C_1 = 3%
V_2 = 21 mL (15 + 6 = 21)
C_2 = unknown

$$V_1 \times C_1 = V_2 \times C_2$$

$$(15) \times (3) = (21) \times (X)$$

$$X = \frac{15 \times 3}{21}$$

$$= 2.14\%$$

Example 5: If you have 18 mL of a 5% solution of metaproterenol (Alupent) and you dilute it to a 0.9% solution with normal saline (NS), how much NS did you add? (this one can be tricky!)
V_1 = 18 mL
C_1 = 5%
V_2 = unknown
C_2 = 0.9%

$$V_1 \times C_1 = V_2 \times C_2$$
$$(18) \times (5) = (X) \times (0.9)$$
$$X = \frac{18 \times 5}{0.9}$$
$$= 100$$

At first glance, it would appear that 100 mL is the answer, but the question asked *how much NS did you add?* Because you started with 18 mL (V_1) at 5% strength and the total volume of diluted Alupent is 100 mL (V_2), you added 82 mL of NS ($V_2 - V_1 = 100 - 18 = 82$) to get to 0.9% strength. Therefore, 82 mL is the correct answer.

Example 6: If you have 0.8 mL of a 1:200 solution and add 1.2 mL to this solution, what is the new concentration by ratio?
V_1 = 0.8 mL
C_1 = 1:200 = 0.005
V_2 = 2 mL (0.8 + 1.2 = 2)
C_2 = unknown

Step 1:

$$V_1 \times C_1 = V_2 \times C_2$$
$$(0.8) \times (0.005) = (2) \times (X)$$
$$X = \frac{0.8 \times 0.005}{2}$$
$$= 0.002$$

Converting a decimal to a ratio was presented earlier in this chapter. The setup is as follows:

Step 2:

$$X = 1/0.002$$
$$= 500$$

The new concentration by ratio is 1:500.

Calculating Dosages Using Proportions

Another way to solve dosage problems is to set up proportions or ratios in which:
A : B :: C : D or A/B = C/D

In mathematics:
A and D (the first and fourth terms) are the "extremes."
B and C (the second and third terms) are the "means."
The product of the extremes equals the product of the means:
$A \times D = B \times C$

Example:
2 : 3 :: 4 : 6 or 2/3 = 4/6
2×6 (extremes) = 3×4 (means)

Applying the above concept to solve dosage problems results in the following proportion:

original dose : amount supplied :: desired dose : desired amount

In other words, original dose (in g or mg) per amount supplied (in mL or cc) is equal to desired dose (in g or mg) per amount of desired dose (in mL or cc).

The equation for the above is:

$$\overset{\textit{Known}}{\frac{\text{original dose}}{\text{amount supplied}}} = \overset{\textit{Unknown}}{\frac{\text{desired dose}}{\text{desired amount}}}$$

Example 1: A physician orders 1 g ampicillin to be administered to your patient. You have on hand 250 mg ampicillin capsules. (Because the drug on hand is 250 mg, the 1 g desired dosage will need to be converted to mg: 1 g = 1000 mg.)

Original dose = 250 mg
Amount supplied = 1 capsule
Desired dose = 1000 mg (1 g)
Desired amount = unknown

$$\frac{\text{original dose}}{\text{amount suppled}} = \frac{\text{desired dose}}{\text{desired amount}}$$

$$\frac{250\text{ mg}}{1\text{ capsule}} = \frac{1000\text{ mg}}{X}$$

$$250\,X = 1000 \times 1$$

$$X = \frac{1000 \times 1}{250}$$

$$= 4$$

You will give your patient 4 capsules (250 mg each) for a dose of 1 g.

Example 2: A patient with severe myasthenia gravis is to receive Mestinon syrup 0.36 g. The stock dosage on hand is 60 mg/5 mL. How many milliliters will the patient receive?

Original dose = 60 mg
Amount supplied = 5 mL
Desired dose = 0.36 g, which must be converted to mg: 0.36 g × 1000 mg/g = 360 mg
Desired amount = unknown

$$\frac{\text{original dose}}{\text{amount supplied}} = \frac{\text{desired dose}}{\text{desired amount}}$$

$$\frac{60 \text{ mg}}{5 \text{ mL}} = \frac{360 \text{ mg}}{X}$$

$$60\,X = 360 \times 5$$

$$X = \frac{360 \times 5}{60}$$

$$= 30$$

The patient will receive 30 mL for a dose of 0.36 g (360 mg).

The above examples were given with the dosage calculations given within the same measurement system. If a two measurement system is given, one system must be converted to the other. For example, a physician orders 1.5 grains of a drug to be administered. Stock tablets on hand contain 0.2 g each.

First, convert the amount to be given into a common unit with the amount of the drug on hand. Referring to the table of equivalents (Appendix C): 1 gram = 15 grains.

How many grains are in each tablet?

$$\frac{1 \text{ g}}{15 \text{ grains}} = \frac{0.2 \text{ g}}{X}$$

$$1\,X = 0.2 \times 15$$

$$X = \frac{0.2 \times 15}{1}$$

$$= 3$$

There are 3 grains in each tablet.

Now set up the proportion:

The three known terms are: dose is 1.5 grains (desired dose). There are 3 grains (original dose) per tablet (amount supplied). The unknown term is how many tablets should be given (desired amount).

$$\frac{\text{original dose}}{\text{amount supplied}} = \frac{\text{desired dose}}{\text{desired amount}}$$

$$\frac{3 \text{ grains}}{1 \text{ tablet}} = \frac{1.5 \text{ grains}}{X}$$

$$3X = 1.5 \times 1$$

$$X = \frac{1.5 \times 1}{3}$$

$$= 0.5$$

You will give your patient ½ tablet.

To Give Units

Some drugs are supplied in ampules or vials that contain a specific number of units per cc of solution.

Example: An ampule of Tetanus antitoxin contains "1500 U per cc." How much of the solution would you give if the physician has ordered a total dose of 1000 units?

$$\frac{\text{original dose}}{\text{amount supplied}} = \frac{\text{desired dose}}{\text{desired amount}}$$

$$\frac{1500 \text{ U}}{1 \text{ cc}} = \frac{1000 \text{ U}}{X}$$

$$1500X = 1000 \times 1$$

$$X = \frac{1000 \times 1}{1500}$$

$$= 0.67 \text{ or } \tfrac{2}{3}$$

You will give ⅔ cc of the antitoxin.

Dosage Calculations Based on the Weight of a Patient

Many drug dosages are given based on kilogram weight of a patient. For example, if an adult patient weighs 60 kg and the normal adult drug dose is 5 mg/kg, the patient would receive 300 mg of the drug (5 mg/kg × 60 kg). If a patient's weight is given in pounds instead of kilograms, you must convert to kilograms. For example, because there is 1 kilogram in 2.2 pounds (1 kg/2.2 lb), a 180-pound patient would weigh 81.8 kg (180 lb × 1 kg/2.2 lb). As you can see, converting from pounds to kilogram reduces the number by approximately half.

Normally, an individual older than 12 years of age is given an adult dose. However, some cases may warrant a reduction in the adult dose (e.g., severe emaciation, severe dehydration, or major organ failure). For some, the reduced dose would be proportional to the individual's weight. Considering that a normal adult dose is based on a 150-pound (~70 kg) person and your patient is an individual that weighs 75 pounds who needs a reduced dose, the dose would need to be one-half that of the adult dose.

Example: If the normal adult dose of a drug is 750 mg and your patient is a 90-pound adult frail female, what dose would be appropriate?
Solution:
Because 90 pounds is 60% of 150 pounds (90/150 × 100), the patient's dose would be 60% of 750 mg. The patient's dose would be 450 mg (0.6 × 750 = 450).
Another way to solve this problem is to set up a proportion:

$$\begin{aligned} &\textit{Normal dose} \quad \textit{Patient's dose} \\ \frac{750\text{ mg}}{150\text{ lb}} &= \frac{X}{90\text{ lb}} \\ 150\,X &= 750 \times 90 \\ X &= \frac{750 \times 90}{150} \\ X &= 450\text{ mg} \end{aligned}$$

Setting up the above proportion using kilograms instead of pounds would yield approximately the same result. The normal dose would be 750 mg/70 kg, and the patient's dose would be *X*/41 kg.

A special situation exists in which premature infants are concerned owing to the measurement of their weight in grams. To calculate drug dosages for these patients, the weight must be converted to kilograms. For example, if a premature infant weighs 1600 grams, the kilogram weight would be 1.6. This was calculated by 1600 g × 1 kg/1000 g, which is the same as the following proportion:

$$\frac{1000\text{ g}}{1\text{ kg}} = \frac{1600\text{ g}}{X}$$

$$1000\,X = 1600 \times 1$$

$$X = \frac{1600 \times 1}{1000}$$

$$X = 1.6 \text{ kg}$$

If a newborn's weight is given in pounds instead of grams, the conversion factor is 1 lb/454 g.

Example: a premature infant weighs 3.52 pounds. What is this infant's gram weight? Kilogram weight?

g weight = 3.52 lb × 454 g/1 lb = 1598 g

Which is the same as:

$$\frac{1 \text{ lb}}{454 \text{ g}} = \frac{3.52 \text{ lb}}{X}$$

$$1\,X = 3.52 \times 454$$

$$X = \frac{3.52 \times 454}{1}$$

$$X = 1598 \text{ g}$$

Kg weight = 1598 g × 1 kg/1000 g = 1.59 or (rounded up) 1.6 kg

Suppose the above 1.6-kg patient needs a drug in which the dosing schedule is 75 mg/kg? The appropriate dose is 120 mg (75 mg/kg × 1.6 kg). Taking this concept one step further, suppose the drug is formulated in a 150 mg/5 mL solution. How many milliliters of the drug would you give to administer a dose of 120 mg?

Solution:

$$\frac{\text{original dose}}{\text{amount supplied}} = \frac{\text{desired dose}}{\text{desired amount}}$$

$$\frac{150 \text{ mg}}{5 \text{ mL}} = \frac{120 \text{ mg}}{X}$$

$$150\,X = 120 \times 5$$

$$X = \frac{120 \times 5}{150}$$

$$= 4 \text{ mL}$$

For a 120-mg dose, you would give the patient 4 mL of the drug.

DRUG FORMULAS FOR INFANTS AND CHILDREN

Dosages of drugs for toddlers and infants are reduced proportionately to the age or weight of the child. Various rules apply.

Young's Rule (for children 2–12 years of age)

$$\text{Child's dose} = \frac{\text{age in years}}{\text{age in years} + 12} \times \text{adult dose}$$

Clark's Rule

$$\text{Child's dose} = \frac{\text{weight in pounds}}{150\ \text{(adult weight)}} \times \text{adult dose}$$

Fried's Rule (children younger than 2 years of age)

$$\text{Child's dose} = \frac{\text{age in months}}{150} \times \text{adult dose}$$

BSA (body surface area) Formula

$$\text{Child's dose} = \frac{\text{BSA of child in M}^2}{1.7\ \text{(av adult BSA)}} \times \text{adult dose}$$

The BSA formula is the most accurate of all the formulas for calculating drug dosages in children. This is because it is a much more individualized calculation in that it takes into account *both* the height and weight of the child. The BSA of a child is determined using a graph of normal or average values for the child's height and weight, called the West nomogram.

Note: These rules are intended to serve as an approximate guide only. Other factors such as physiologic and pathologic conditions may also regulate the dose of a drug.

INTRAVENOUS CALCULATIONS

Initiating and maintaining proper IV flow rates and infusion times are an essential part of managing a critically ill patient. This section details the equations necessary for such calculations.

Calculation of IV Flow Rates

IV solutions are generally ordered in either mL/hr or mL/min. The IV flow rate controls the administered volume, which is calculated in drops per minute (gtt/min).

Because IV flow rates are regulated in drops/minute, the type of IV set used plays an integral role in determining how many drops there are per mL. Normally, there are 15 gtt/mL, but the drops from various IV tubing may range from 10 gtt/mL to as high as 60 gtt/mL. A standard macrodrip administration ranges from

10, 15, or 20 gtt/mL, whereas a microdrip administration will give 60 gtt/mL. The calibration for gtt/mL (known as the drip factor) is printed on each IV package and must be adhered to when setting up infusion rates.

The formula for calculating flow rates is:

$$\text{Flow rate} = \frac{\text{Volume} \times \text{Calibration}}{\text{Time (min)}}$$

Example 1: The physician orders an IV drug to infuse at 150 mL/hr. Calculate the flow rate required using an IV set calibrated at 20 gtt/mL.

$$\text{Flow rate} = \frac{\text{Volume} \times \text{Calibration}}{\text{Time (min)}}$$

$$= \frac{150 \text{ mL} \times 20 \text{ gtt/mL}}{60 \text{ min}}$$

$$= 50 \text{ gtt/min}$$

The IV would be set up to deliver 50 gtt/min.

Example 2: You need to administer 120 mL of an IV drug in 30 minutes. You are using an IV set calibrated at 15 gtt/mL.

$$\text{Flow rate} = \frac{\text{Volume} \times \text{Calibration}}{\text{Time (min)}}$$

$$= \frac{120 \text{ mL} \times 15 \text{ gtt/mL}}{30 \text{ min}}$$

$$= 60 \text{ gtt/min}$$

You would set the IV flow rate to deliver 60 gtt/min.

An IV flow rate should be checked every hour by actually counting the number of drops administered in a minute's time and adjusting the flow rate accordingly. In the acutely critically ill patient, for whom extreme accuracy of flow rates is necessary, electronic flow rate monitors such as the volumetric pump are used.

Calculating IV Infusion Times

Calculating IV infusion times is necessary to determine when to change the IV solution or when to discontinue the drug. The one-step formula for calculating IV infusion times is:

$$\text{Infusion time} = \frac{\text{total volume to infuse}}{\text{mL/hr being infused}}$$

Example 1: 1000 mL Ringer's Lactate is ordered to infuse at a rate of 60 mL/hr. What is the infusion time?

$$\text{Infusion time} = \frac{\text{total volume to infuse}}{\text{mL/hr being infused}}$$

$$= \frac{1000 \text{ mL}}{60 \text{ mL/hr}}$$

$$= 16.67$$

= 16 hours and 40 minutes
(the 40 minutes was obtained by multiplying 0.67 by 60 min)

If the mL/hr infusion rate is not known, then several steps are needed to determine infusion time. If the total volume to infuse is known, as well as the flow rate and the set calibration, then a proportion must be set up. For example, if the volume to infuse is 750 mL, the flow rate is 30 gtt/min, and the set calibration is 10 gtt/mL the proportion would be as follows:

Step 1: Determine the mL/min infusing.

$$\frac{10 \text{ gtt}}{1 \text{ mL}} = \frac{30 \text{ gtt}}{X \text{ mL}}$$

$$10\,X = 30 \times 1$$

$$X = \frac{30 \times 1}{10}$$

$$X = 3 \text{ mL/min}$$

Step 2: Convert mL/min to mL/hr.

$$3 \text{ mL/min} \times 60 \text{ min} = 180 \text{ mL/hr}$$

Step 3: Calculate the infusion time.

$$\text{Infusion time} = \frac{\text{total volume to infuse}}{\text{mL/hr being infused}}$$

$$= \frac{750 \text{ mL}}{180 \text{ mL/hr}}$$

$$= 4.17$$

= 4 hours and 10 minutes

Table 6.1
Mathematics of Drugs and Solutions

1. Conversion of g to mg: mg = number of grams × 1000 mg/1 g
2. Conversion of mg to g: g = number of mg × 1 g/1000 mg
3. Conversion of kg to lb: lb = number of kg × 2.2 lb/1 kg
4. Conversion of lb to kg: kg = number of lb × 1 kg/2.2 lb
5. Conversion of g to lb: lb = number of g × 1 lb/454 g
6. Conversion of lb to g: g = number of lb × 454 g/1 lb
7. Conversion of a ratio to a percent: Percent strength = [solute (g) ÷ solution (mL, cc)] × 100
8. Conversion of a percent strength to a ratio: $X = 1 \div$ percent strength (in decimals) (The ratio will take the form of 1:*X*.)
9. Calculation of how many g/mL are in a dosage strength: g/mL = strength (in decimals) or solute (g) ÷ solution (mL)
10. Solving for one drug's strength, solute amount, or solution amount:
    a. Strength (in decimals) = solute (g) ÷ solution (mL or cc)
    b. Solute (g) = strength (in decimals) × solution (mL or cc)
    c. Solution (mL or cc) = solute (g) ÷ strength (in decimals)
11. Dilution calculation: $V_1 \times C_1 = V_2 \times C_2$
12. Proportion calculation: original dose/amount supplied = desired dose/desired amount
13. Calculation of a patient's dose when a drug is given in a mg/kg form: patient's weight in kg × dose (number of mg/kg)
14. Calculation of a reduced dose based on a patient's weight in lb: patient's dose = (number of mg in normal dose ÷ 150 lb) × patient's weight in lb
15. Calculation of a reduced dose based on a patient's weight in kg: patient's dose = (number of mg in normal dose ÷ 70 kg) × patient's weight in kg
16. Young's rule for a child's dose: child's dose = (age in years ÷ age in years + 12) × adult dose
17. Clark's rule for a child's dose: child's dose = (weight in lb ÷ 150) × adult dose
18. Fried's rule for a child's dose: child's dose = (age in months ÷ 150) × adult dose
19. Body surface area formula for a child's dose: (BSA of child in M^2 ÷ 1.7) × adult dose
20. Calculation of IV flow rate: flow rate = (volume × calibration) ÷ time (min)
21. Calculation of infusion time: infusion time = total volume to infuse ÷ mL/hr being infused
22. Conversion a decimal portion of an hour to minutes: decimal portion of hour × 60 min

SUMMARY

Understanding and applying the mathematics of drugs and solutions are vital aspects of drug therapy. Familiarity with the equations presented in this chapter will help the practitioner in administering accurate dosages. Table 6.1 lists the various equations that were presented in this chapter. Additional dosage calculations for this chapter can be found in the software program accompanying this textbook.

REFERENCES/RECOMMENDED READING

Carr JJ, McElroy NL, Carr BL. How to solve dosage problems in one easy lesson. Am J Nurs 76:1934, 1976.

Curren AM, Munday LD. Math for Meds: A Programmed Text of Dosages and Solutions. 5th ed. San Diego: Wallcur Inc., 1986.

Frey AM. Pediatric dosage calculations. NITA 8:373, 1985.
Glasper A, Oliver RW. A simple guide to infant drug calculations. Nursing—Oxford 2:649, 1984.
Govoni L, Hayes J. Drugs and Nursing Implications. 7th ed. Norwalk, CT: Appleton & Lange, 1992.
Kacmarek RM, Mack CW, Dimas S. The Essentials of Respiratory Care. 3rd ed. St. Louis: Mosby-Year Book, Inc., 1990.
Neu J, et al. Calculator assisted determination of dilutions for continuous infusion ICU medications. Crit Care Med 10:610, 1982.
Zenk KE. Dosage calculations for drugs administered by infusion. Am J Hosp Pharm 37:1304, 1980.

SPECIAL ASPECTS OF NEONATAL, PEDIATRIC, AND GERIATRIC DRUG THERAPY 7

Providing drug therapy to the neonate, pediatric, and elderly patient presents the practitioner with a unique set of challenges. Because drug effects are often less predictable in these patients, careful monitoring after administration of drugs is necessary to ensure safe and effective therapy.

LEARNING OUTCOMES

Upon completion of this chapter, the learner will be able to:

1. Identify and discuss the physiologic factors that alter drug absorption, distribution, metabolism, and elimination in the neonate and pediatric patient.
2. Identify and discuss the physiologic factors that alter drug absorption, distribution, metabolism, and elimination in the geriatric patient.

DRUG THERAPY IN THE NEONATAL AND PEDIATRIC PATIENT

In a newborn, infant, and child, a drug undergoes the same pharmacokinetic processes as in an adult. However, the physiologic contexts in which the pharmacokinetic processes occur are different in these smaller patients owing to the growth and development of organ systems and changes in body composition. The changing body size and metabolic rate changes associated with infancy and childhood can significantly alter the absorption, distribution, metabolism, and elimination of drugs.

Variances in Pharmacokinetic Processes

Drug Absorption

Various factors influence the rate and completeness of absorption in neonatal and pediatric patients. Most importantly, the route of administration is a primary concern.

- *Oral administration:* Several physiologic variables may inhibit or accelerate the absorption of orally ingested medications. For example, neonatal and pediatric patients generally exhibit a slower gastrointestinal (GI) tract motility, an underdeveloped drug transport mechanism, and low gastric acidity as compared to the adult. A neonate generally has an erratic and prolonged gastric emptying time, which can enhance drug absorption. On the other hand, a child's more rapid gastric emptying time can decrease drug absorption. Low gastric acidity is a primary issue in children younger than 3 years of age. Administration of drugs that are weak acids may not be fully absorbed owing to the increase in the ionized form of the drug.
- *Topical administration:* Unlike orally ingested drugs, topically administered drugs are generally absorbed much faster and more completely in a neonate and child than in an adult. This is because neonates, infants, and children usually have thinner epithelial layers, which enhance the delivery of the drug across skin and mucous membranes.
- *Intramuscular administration:* Because neonatal and pediatric patients have relatively low skeletal muscle mass (this is especially true of neonates and very young infants), intramuscularly administered drugs may have erratic, unpredictable patterns of absorption. In addition, blood flow to muscle tissue may fluctuate, which makes it difficult to determine absorption rates.

Drug Distribution

Drug distribution in the neonate, infant, and child, as in the adult, is influenced by protein binding, membrane permeability, and body composition. Because neonates and pediatric patients have a lower number of plasma proteins (and therefore fewer protein binding sites), more free or active drug is distributed to receptor sites. This could cause an exaggerated response from drugs and would necessitate a lower dose to avoid toxicity.

The comparative immaturity of the blood-brain barrier system of the neonatal patient could possibly cause central nervous system toxicity owing to the drug's ability, especially lipid-soluble drugs, to readily penetrate the central nervous system.

One other physiologic factor affecting drug distribution relates to the developmental changes in body composition that occurs during childhood. In the normal adult, body fluids account for approximately 50% of total body weight, whereas in the neonatal patient, the fluid body weight may be as high as 70% to 80% (especially in premature infants). Because of the neonate's higher ratio of fluid to solid body weight, water-soluble drugs are distributed faster, whereas lipid-soluble drugs are distributed more slowly.

Drug Metabolism

Because a neonate's liver is immature and the hepatic microsomal enzyme system is not fully developed, drugs are metabolized slower, which could lead to toxic conditions. On the other hand, older infants and children (6 months to 9 years of age) metabolize some drugs (for example, theophylline) at a faster rate than normal. Therefore, they require a higher drug dosage than recommended for adults. The ability of the practitioner to recognize these differences in neonatal and pediatric patients is crucial in determining the success of drug therapy.

Elimination

The kidneys of a neonate or infant younger than 1 year of age have yet to fully develop their capacity to effectively filter and secrete drugs. In fact, during the first month of life, the ability of the kidney to filter drugs may be as low as 5% of that of an adult kidney. Dehydration, as sometimes occurs in severely ill infants, can also greatly decrease filtration. The above-mentioned physiologic factors can greatly diminish the response of those drugs that have a high glomerular filtration rate (GFR), such as thiazide diuretics. Either a higher dose or substitution of a drug that is less dependent on GFR, such as furosemide, will be necessary.

Pediatric Drug Dosage

Chapter 6 listed the various formulas used to calculate a child's dose. Because formulas based on age or weight (e.g., Clark's, Young's, or Fried's rules) are conservative, they tend to underestimate the required dose. Most drugs approved for use in neonates, infants, and children have recommended doses, generally stated as mg/kg or per pound. Because of differences in pharmacokinetics in neonates, infants, and children, simple proportional reductions in the adult dose may not be adequate to determine safe and effective dosage.

The most accurate and commonly used pediatric drug dose formula is the body surface area (BSA) formula. This is because calculating required doses using total body surface area is a much more individualized and exact parameter than just using age, height, or body weight.

DRUG THERAPY IN THE GERIATRIC PATIENT

Geriatric patients are the population older than 65 years of age. Concurrent with the external physical signs of aging are internal physiologic changes that can significantly alter the absorption, distribution, metabolism, and elimination of drugs in the elderly.

Variances in Pharmacokinetic Processes

Drug Absorption

Some studies suggest that aging reduces the absorption rate in an elderly patient. There are several reasons for this. The low gastric acidity that accompanies the decreased hydrochloric acid secretion noted with aging is one such reason. As a result, orally ingested drugs that require an acid environment are absorbed more slowly or not at all. Another critical factor is intestinal blood perfusion, which may decrease as much as 50% in elderly patients.

Drug Distribution

As in the neonate and infant, the elderly patient demonstrates altered drug disposition due to low plasma protein levels (particularly albumin), a less efficient passive and active transport system, and changes in body composition.

Water volume and lean tissue diminish with age, whereas adipose tissue increases with age. Water volume and lean tissue loss results in a reduced volume distribution of water-soluble drugs because these drugs normally distribute to body fluids and lean tissue. Because of this, a higher blood concentration of these drugs is noted. Comparatively, because the proportion of fatty tissue increases with age, lipid-soluble drugs distribute more readily, are retained within the body for longer periods of time, and exhibit prolonged action and effects.

Drug Metabolism

Cardiac output declines approximately 1% per year beginning at 19 years of age. Consequently, with age, a decreased proportion of this output is distributed to the liver and kidneys. The net effect of reduced blood flow to these organs is a decreased capacity to function. Therefore, drugs remain active for longer periods of time in elderly patients. Smaller liver size and a reduced production of enzymes that function to deactivate drugs also contribute to alterations in drug metabolism. These metabolic changes can be further aggravated by medical conditions such as hepatic failure or congestive heart failure.

Elimination

Because renal blood flow has a tendency to diminish with age, the kidney's ability to filter and excrete drugs is reduced, resulting in an accumulation of drugs. In addition, as the aging process progresses, the overall performance of the renal tubules declines owing to a loss of functioning renal tubules. As a result, glomerular filtration, tubular reabsorption, and active tubular secretion occur much more slowly.

The combined effect of the above-mentioned age-related changes brings about a longer half-life for most drugs which, in turn, can result in drug toxicity in the elderly patient. In addition, because elderly patients are predisposed to chronic diseases—especially renal, hepatic, and cardiovascular disorders—the incidence of adverse drug reactions is more prevalent. Thus, practitioners should realize that drug dosages may need modification in elderly patients.

REFERENCES/RECOMMENDED READING

Beers MH, Ouslander JG. Risk factors in geriatric drug prescribing: a practical guide to avoiding problems. Drugs 37:105, 1989.

Bender AD, et al. Plasma protein binding of drugs as a function of age in adult human subjects. J Pharm Sci 64:1711, 1975.

Besunder JB, Reed MD, Blumer JL. Principles of drug biodisposition in the neonate: a critical evaluation of the pharmacokinetic-pharmacodynamic interface. Clin Pharmacokinet 14:189, 1988.

Everitt DE, Avorn J. Drug prescribing for the elderly. Arch Intern Med 146:2393, 1986.

Gilman JT. Therapeutic drug monitoring in the neonate and paediatric age group: problems and clinical pharmacokinetic implications. Clin Pharmacokinet 19:1, 1990.

Gorrod JW. Absorption, metabolism and excretion of drugs in geriatric subjects. Gerontol Clin 16:30, 1974.

Greenblatt DJ, Sellers EM, Shader RI. Drug disposition in old age. N Engl J Med 306:1081, 1982.

Morselli PL. Clinical pharmacology of the perinatal period and early infancy. Clin Pharmacokinet 17(Suppl 1):13, 1989.

Prandota J. Clinical pharmacokinetics of changes in drug elimination in children. Dev Pharmacol Ther 8:311, 1985.

Individual Pharmacologic Agents

I

Chapters 8 through 19 present the specific pharmacologic agents. For consistency, Chapters 9 through 19 are organized in a similar fashion. The learning outcomes for Chapters 9 through 19 are summarized as follows (Chapter 8 has its own specific outcomes):

1. If included in the chapter, define the terms listed under *Key Terms*.
2. If a preparatory review is included in the chapter, briefly discuss the physiology of the organ system involved and how the individual classes of drugs in the chapter affect that particular organ system.
3. State the primary mechanism of action, indications for use, contraindications, precautions, adverse reactions, and symptoms and treatment of overdose for each class of drugs listed in the chapter.
4. Identify, if applicable, the prototypic drug for a particular class of drugs.
5. Although it is virtually impossible, and not expected, for the practitioner to memorize all drug dosages contained in this book, the cardiopulmonary practitioner (especially respiratory care practitioners) should know the correct dosages for the following pharmacologic agents:

- All respiratory drug dosages, including:

  The therapeutic gases oxygen, carbon dioxide, and helium
  The inhalational sympathomimetic bronchodilators
  The inhalational anticholinergic (antimuscarinic) bronchodilators
  The inhalational prophylactic antiasthmatic agents (cromolyn and nedocromil)
  The inhalational anti-inflammatory agents
  The inhalational mucokinetic agents and surface-active agents

- All cardiopulmonary resuscitative (CPR) drug dosages
- Additionally, the practitioner should be familiar with the dosages of the more commonly delivered cardiovascular drugs and others such as morphine, pan-

curonium (Pavulon), and lidocaine (Xylocaine). Your instructor or institution will advise which drugs and drug dosages should be known.

Note: All drug dosages presented in the following chapters are to be used as a general guideline only, not as absolute. Many factors play a vital role in determining the proper dosage for a certain patient. Chapters 2, 3, 4, and 7 presented the various mechanisms that can alter or modify a drug's action and final effect. These same mechanisms also apply to a drug's dosage.

8 THE THERAPEUTIC GASES

This chapter focuses on various aspects that pertain to the safe and effective administration of the inhaled therapeutic gases—oxygen, carbon dioxide, helium, and nitric oxide. The inhaled general anesthetic gases are presented in Chapter 15. The therapeutic gases presented in this chapter are drugs and should be treated as any pharmacologic agent. One should apply the lowest dose that produces the desired outcome in addition to monitoring responses and implementing changes in the dose to meet predetermined goals.

LEARNING OUTCOMES

Upon completion of this chapter, the learner will be able to:

Oxygen:

1. Identify the four main organ systems that are involved in the transport of oxygen from the atmosphere to the cells of the body.
2. Using the appropriate formula, calculate the following:

   Oxygen dissolved in plasma
   Oxygen chemically combined with hemoglobin
   Systemic oxygen transport
   Oxygen consumption ($\dot{V}O_2$)

3. List the normal values and the significance of an abnormal value for the following:

   SaO_2 $C(a\text{-}v)O_2$
   SvO_2 Systemic oxygen transport

CaO_2 Oxygen consumption
CvO_2 P50

4. Identify the factors that will shift the oxyhemoglobin curve to the left and to the right and the significance of a left-shifted curve and right-shifted curve.
5. State the expected PO_2 for an SO_2 of 50%, 75%, and 90% when the oxyhemoglobin curve is in its normal position.
6. Define hypoxemia and differentiate between mild hypoxemia, moderate hypoxemia, and severe hypoxemia.
7. Establish a normal PaO_2 range for an adult individual based on age.
8. List and describe the four mechanisms that cause hypoxemia.
9. Define hypoxia and list the causes for:

   hypoxic hypoxia (hypoxemic hypoxia)
   anemic hypoxia
   circulatory hypoxia (stagnant hypoxia)
   histotoxic hypoxia

10. In the above hypoxias, state the specific organ system that is involved with the type of hypoxia.
11. Describe the body's natural acute compensatory mechanism that activates in response to hypoxia.
12. Describe the body's natural compensatory mechanism that activates in response to chronic, longstanding hypoxia.
13. Identify the signs and symptoms that accompany the hypoxic patient.
14. State how oxygen is commercially packaged, identify its cylinder color code, and state the percentage of purity that is mandated by the Food and Drug Administration (FDA).
15. Name and describe the four most commonly used adult oxygen delivery systems and any special precautions for use.
16. Discuss the four primary indications for administering supplemental oxygen. State the three goals of oxygen therapy for the hypoxemic patient.
17. List and explain the four primary hazards of oxygen therapy.
18. Identify the conditions or situations in which 100% oxygen is required.
19. Discuss the factors that apply in monitoring and evaluating the patient receiving supplemental oxygen.

Carbon dioxide:

20. State the three compartments that carbon dioxide is transported in the blood and identify the normal value for carbon dioxide production and elimination, at rest.

21. Identify the normal value for $PvCO_2$ and $PaCO_2$.
22. Define respiratory acidosis and respiratory alkalosis.
23. Describe the physiologic alterations that occur on respiration, circulation, and the CNS when there is an abnormal amount of carbon dioxide in the blood.
24. State how carbon dioxide is commercially packaged, identify its cylinder color code, and state the percentage of purity that is mandated by the FDA.
25. Identify the percent combinations of carbon dioxide-oxygen mixtures.
26. Describe the procedure for administering carbon dioxide therapy.
27. Identify the specific, therapeutic indications for administering carbon dioxide therapy.
28. List the potential hazards and side effects that may occur when administering carbon dioxide therapy.
29. Discuss the factors that apply in monitoring and evaluating the patient receiving carbon dioxide therapy.

Helium:

30. Identify helium's inherent properties that make it a useful therapeutic gas.
31. State how helium is commercially packaged, identify its cylinder color code, and state the percentage of purity that is mandated by the FDA.
32. Identify the percent combinations of helium-oxygen mixtures.
33. State the appropriate delivery device to use when administering helium-oxygen mixtures as well as the special precautions that apply when using an oxygen flowmeter. Be able to correctly calculate the actual flow rate delivered when using an oxygen flowmeter to administer a helium-oxygen mixture.
34. Identify and describe the specific indications for administering helium therapy.
35. List the hazards and side effects that pertain to the administration of helium therapy.

Nitric oxide:

36. Explain the therapeutic usefulness and physiologic responses elicited from the administration of inhaled nitric oxide.
37. Briefly describe how nitric oxide is supplied.
38. Identify the dosage and criteria that define the lowest effective dose of nitric oxide.
39. Explain the overall purpose for administering nitric oxide and the types of conditions or disease states that would benefit.
40. List the potential hazards and side effects of nitric oxide administration.

OXYGEN

As one of the most plentiful chemical elements on earth, oxygen constitutes approximately 21% of inspired air. Oxygen is a colorless, odorless, tasteless, combustible gas that is essential to life; without oxygen, irreparable tissue damage and cell death ensue.

Inhalational oxygen therapy emerged soon after Priestley's discovery of oxygen in 1772. Just before the turn of the 18th century, Beddoes and colleagues used oxygen to treat all kinds of diseases, including leprosy and paralysis. Naturally, such inappropriate use of oxygen led to many failures and it was not until the pioneering works of Haldane, Hill, Barcroft, Krogh, L.J. Henderson, and Y. Henderson (Sackner 1974) that the physiologic effects and therapeutic usefulness of oxygen was realized.

Oxygen Transport—An Overview

Oxygen gains entrance to the body by way of the gas-exchange units (alveoli) of the lungs. The movement of oxygen through the alveoli and into the pulmonary blood capillary system occurs through simple diffusion (Fig. 8.1). Once in the blood, oxygen is carried by the circulation to the tissues, where it is used by the cells of the tissues (specifically, the mitochondria) during aerobic metabolism. Thus, four body systems are ultimately responsible for the delivery of atmospheric oxygen to the mitochondria: lungs, blood, circulation, and tissues. An abnormality or malfunction in any one of these four body systems can lead to a lack of oxygen for cellular metabolism resulting in anaerobic metabolism and the production of lactic acid.

The blood carries oxygen in two distinct compartments: physically dissolved in plasma and chemically combined to hemoglobin (Hb) molecules.

Physically Dissolved in Plasma

The amount of dissolved oxygen in plasma can be calculated by:

$$PO_2 \times 0.003$$

where:

PO_2 = the partial pressure of oxygen. If the partial pressure of oxygen in arterial blood is known, the designation is PaO_2, whereas partial pressure of oxygen in venous blood is designated as PvO_2. Normally, the PO_2 of arterial blood (PaO_2) is 80 to 100 mmHg, whereas that of venous blood (PvO_2) is approximately 40 mmHg.

0.003 = a constant that is equivalent to the milliliters of oxygen per deciliter (100 mL) physically dissolved for each mmHg PO_2. The unit for this factor is mL

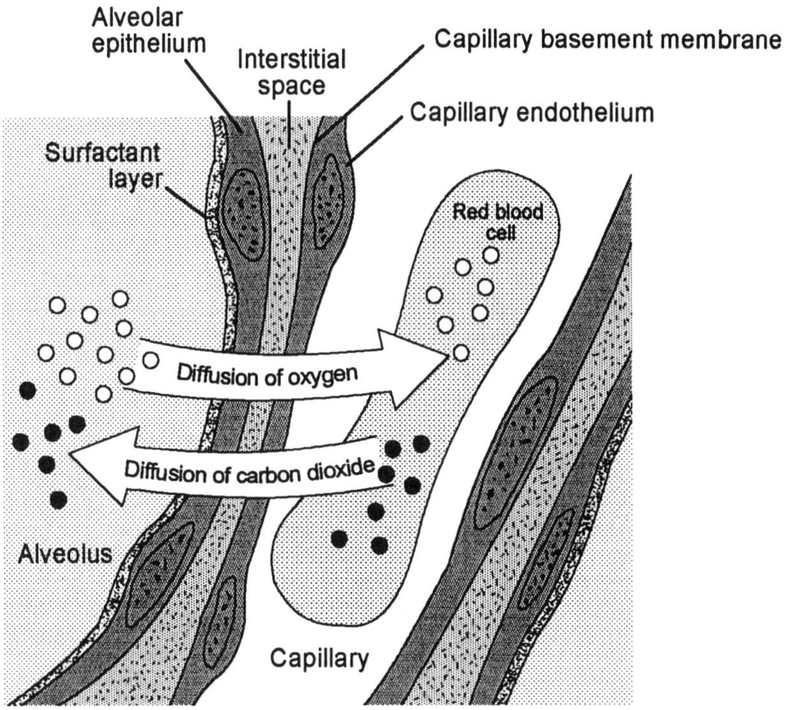

Figure 8.1. The alveolar-capillary membrane displaying the structures through which oxygen and carbon dioxide must diffuse.

O_2/dL/mmHg PO_2. However, the older term "volume%" (or vol%) is still commonly used. Volume% is equivalent to mL/dL, which means number of mL of a substance per 100 mL of plasma.

Multiplying the PO_2 by 0.003 yields the amount of oxygen physically dissolved in plasma, which accounts for less than 2% of the oxygen contained in a given volume of blood.

Example: If the PaO_2 measured by arterial blood gas analysis is 67 mmHg, what is the amount of dissolved oxygen in the blood?

67 mmHg $\times$ 0.003 mL O_2/dL/mmHg PO_2 = 0.201 mL O_2/dL *(another way of expressing this is 0.201 vol%)*

Chemically Attached to Hemoglobin

The greatest part (approximately 97% to 98%) of oxygen is carried chemically bound to hemoglobin. Arterial blood saturation of hemoglobin with oxygen is normally $\geq$97% (designated as SaO_2), whereas venous blood saturation of hemoglobin with oxygen is normally 75% (SvO_2—range of 60% to 80%). At 100% saturation, each gram of hemoglobin can maximally bind with 1.34 mL of oxygen. This factor, 1.34 mL O_2/g Hb, is calculated at standard temperature and pressure (STP). Some authors use the factor 1.39 mL O_2/g Hb, which is derived from converting 1.34 mL O_2/g Hb at STP to its volume at body temperature and pressure, saturated (BTPS). Although the factor 1.39 mL O_2/g Hb is a more accurate measure, for purposes of standard use, 1.34 mL O_2/g Hb will be used throughout this book.

The total amount of oxygen carried in the blood chemically bound with hemoglobin is a function of three variables:

- hemoglobin
- the amount of oxygen that can attach to each gram of hemoglobin (1.34)
- the saturation of hemoglobin with oxygen (SO_2).

By multiplying these variables, one can determine the total volume of oxygen chemically attached to hemoglobin:

$$\text{Hb content} \times 1.34 \text{ mL } O_2/\text{g Hb} \times SO_2 \text{ (in decimals)}$$

For example, given a patient with a hemoglobin of 14 g/dL and an arterial oxygen saturation of 92%, the quantity of oxygen chemically attached to hemoglobin would be:

$$14 \text{ g Hb/dL} \times 1.34 \text{ mL } O_2/\text{g Hb} \times 0.92 = 17.26 \text{ mL } O_2/\text{dL}$$

(another way to express this is 17.26 vol%)

Hemoglobin plays a vital role in transporting the bulk of oxygen to the tissues. If the amount of hemoglobin would significantly drop, such as that which occurs in patients with anemia or hemorrhage, the tissues could suffer irreversible damage because of the lack of sufficient circulating oxygen:

$$7 \text{ g Hb/dL} \times 1.34 \text{ mL } O_2/\text{g Hb} \times 0.92 = 8.64 \text{ mL } O_2/\text{dL}$$

It is of utmost importance to administer whole blood or packed red blood cells under these circumstances. Appendix B, IV details the activity as well as the types of red blood cells and hemoglobin normally found in the body.

Total Oxygen Content

The total content of oxygen in the blood is the sum of the amount of physically dissolved oxygen and the amount chemically bound to hemoglobin. The mathematical equation for calculating the oxygen content of arterial blood (CaO_2) is expressed as:

$$CaO_2 = (Hb \times 1.34 \times SaO_2) + (PaO_2 \times 0.003)$$

The total content of oxygen in venous blood is:

$$CvO_2 = (Hb \times 1.34 \times SvO_2) + (PvO_2 \times 0.003)$$

The normal value for CaO_2 is 20 mL O_2/dL, whereas the normal value for CvO_2 is 15 mL O_2/dL. Thus, the difference between CaO_2 and CvO_2 ($avDO_2$ or $C[a\text{-}v]O_2$) is normally 5 mL O_2/dL.

Oxygen Transport

The rate at which oxygen is delivered to the tissues (cardiac output [CO], normally about 5 L/min) and the arterial oxygen content (CaO_2) determine the total quantity of oxygen that is transported and therefore available for tissue use:

$$\begin{aligned} O_2 \text{ transport} &= CO \times CaO_2 \times 10 \\ &= 5 \times 20 \times 10 \\ &= 1000 \text{ mL } O_2/\text{min} \end{aligned}$$

Oxygen Consumption

As can be seen from above, the normal amount of oxygen transported to the tissues is approximately 1000 mL O_2/min. Of this amount, the body's tissues normally extract approximately 250 mL O_2/min. This leaves a venous reserve of 750 mL, or 75% (normal saturation of venous blood).

The extraction of oxygen from the blood by the tissues is known as oxygen consumption ($\dot{V}O_2$). Factors that can alter $\dot{V}O_2$ include the level of physical activity (metabolic rate), physiologic stress, body temperature, and alterations in peripheral perfusion.

The amount of oxygen extracted by the tissues is a reflection of the cardiac output and the difference between arterial oxygen content and venous oxygen content:

$$\begin{aligned} \dot{V}O_2 &= CO \times (CaO_2 - CvO_2) \times 10 \\ &= 5 \times (20 - 5) \times 10 \\ &= 250 \text{ mL } O_2/\text{min} \end{aligned}$$

A helpful feature of knowing the arterial to venous oxygen content difference ($avDO_2$ or $C[a\text{-}v]O_2$) is that it can estimate whether the cardiac output is high or low. For example, if the $C(a\text{-}v)O_2$ is greater than 5 mL O_2/dL, then it can be assumed that cardiac output is reduced, whereas a $C(a\text{-}v)O_2$ gradient less than 5 mL O_2/dL usually means that the cardiac output is increased or that there is an inability of the cells to use the oxygen brought to them (sepsis, cyanide, or ethanol toxicity). If, in fact, $CaO_2 = CvO_2$, anaerobic metabolism is occurring and death soon follows.

Oxyhemoglobin Dissociation Curve

The oxyhemoglobin (HbO_2) dissociation curve (Fig. 8.2) compares the relationship between the percentage of hemoglobin bound with oxygen (SO_2) with the PO_2 in blood. As can be seen in Figure 8.2, when all factors are equal (normal body temperature, normal pH and $PaCO_2$, normal 2,3-diphosphoglycerate [DPG]), for any given PO_2, there is a correlating SO_2.

Illustrated in the *sigmoid* shape of the dissociation curve, one can see a notable and significant rise in SO_2 for a given increase in PO_2 at the lower end of PO_2 ranges, whereas there are very small increments in saturation as the PO_2 levels rise to higher than 90 mmHg. A rule for the practitioner to remember is that for an oxyhemoglobin saturation of 90%, one can expect a PO_2 of 60 mmHg, whereas an oxyhemoglobin saturation of 75% correlates with a PO_2 of 40 mmHg. This guideline is helpful when measuring oxygen saturations via pulse oximetry. The term P50 designates that PO_2 level at which there is an oxygen saturation of 50%. The normal P50 is 27 mmHg.

Changes in body temperature, pH and $PaCO_2$, 2,3-DPG (a substance in the red blood cell that affects the affinity of the hemoglobin molecule for oxygen), and the presence of carbon monoxide in the blood will change the position of the curve. What this means to the practitioner is that for any given oxyhemoglobin saturation, the PO_2 will not be as expected.

Those factors that shift the curve to the left are hypothermia, decreased levels of 2,3-DPG, carbon monoxide poisoning, and alkalemia (increased pH, decreased $PaCO_2$). As can be seen in Figure 8.2, with a left-shifted curve, the P50 decreases and the PO_2 is less than expected for any given oxyhemoglobin saturation. A left-shifted curve can be life-threatening because the hemoglobin molecule has a tendency to cling to its oxygen, a condition known as an increased affinity of hemoglobin for oxygen. By this mechanism, a severe shift of the curve to the left may result in anaerobic metabolism.

The factors that shift the curve to the right are hyperthermia, acidemia (decreased pH, increased $PaCO_2$), and increased 2,3-DPG. In this instance, the P50 will be increased and the PO_2 is greater than expected for any given oxyhemo-

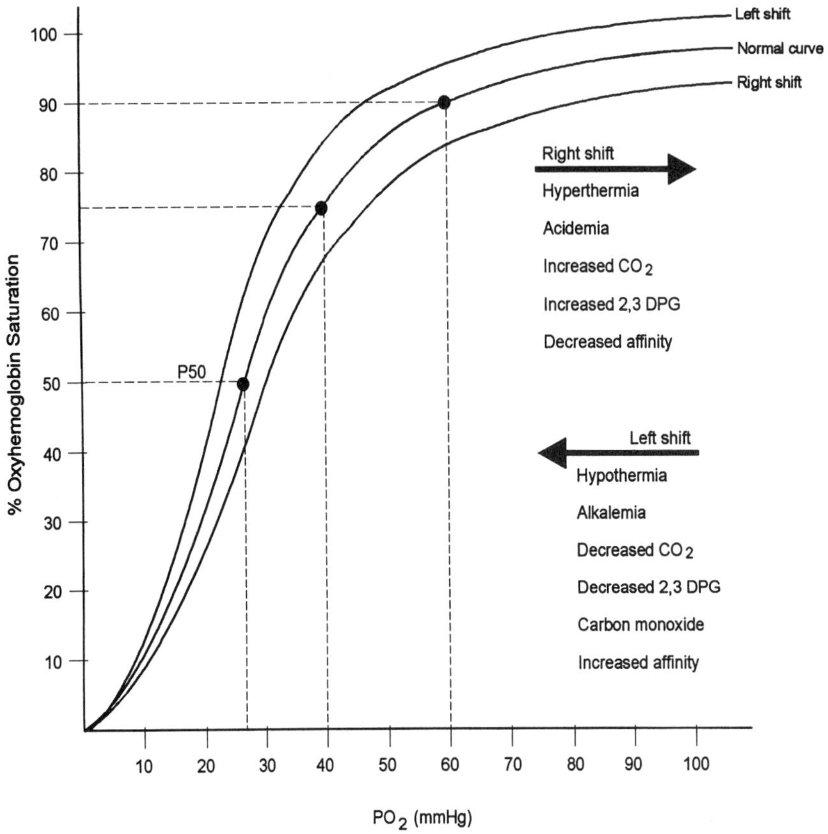

Figure 8.2. The oxyhemoglobin dissociation curve. Illustrated are the factors that will shift the curve to the right and to the left. There is a decreased affinity of hemoglobin for oxygen when the curve is shifted to the right, whereas there is an increased affinity of hemoglobin for oxygen when the curve shifts to the left. P50 is that PO_2 in which the oxyhemoglobin saturation is 50%.

globin saturation. In addition, the affinity of hemoglobin for oxygen is reduced, thus facilitating the unloading of oxygen for increased uptake and utilization by the cells.

Oxygen Deprivation

Hypoxemia is a term used to designate that there is an inadequate amount of oxygen in the blood (i.e., a PaO_2 <80 mmHg). *Mild hypoxemia* exists when the PaO_2 ranges between 60 and 79 mmHg, *moderate hypoxemia* describes a PaO_2 that is between 40 and 59 mmHg, whereas *severe hypoxemia* is a PaO_2 that is less than 40 mmHg.

As an individual ages, the lungs become less efficient in oxygenation capabilities; therefore, the normal limits of PaO_2 for these individuals are lowered in an amount that is proportional to their age. The general guidelines are that for every year over 60 years of age, the lower limit of normal PaO_2 decreases 1 mmHg. For example, a normal PaO_2 for a 70-year-old individual can be 70 mmHg and this would be considered a normal PaO_2 and not hypoxemia. Table 8.1 delineates the normal PaO_2 ranges for individuals 60 years of age and older.

There are four primary reasons for the existence of hypoxemia:

1. Low inspired oxygen tension: This can be caused by high altitude, or the patient is not receiving the appropriate level of supplemental oxygen.
2. Alveolar hypoventilation: This can be brought on by drug overdose (especially narcotic overdose), sleep apnea, or severe chronic obstructive pulmonary disease (COPD).
3. Ventilation to perfusion mismatching (V/Q mismatch): V/Q mismatch is usually caused by some form of pulmonary disease, such as COPD, asthma, and interstitial pulmonary fibrosis.
4. Right-to-left shunt: This occurs when the blood exiting the right heart bypasses a portion of the pulmonary circulation and thus enters the left heart unoxygenated. Right-to-left shunting occurs in conditions such as cardiogenic pulmonary edema, adult respiratory distress syndrome (ARDS), lobar pneumonia, and atelectasis.

Hypoxemia caused from factors 1 through 3 can usually be corrected by applying supplemental oxygen, whereas factor 4, right-to-left shunt, requires, in addition to oxygen therapy, positive end-expiratory pressure (PEEP) or continuous positive airway pressure (CPAP) to overcome the loss of ventilating units.

Hypoxia is a term that denotes a lack of oxygen at the tissue level. As mentioned previously, there are four body systems that conduct atmospheric oxygen

Table 8.1.
Normal PaO_2 Ranges for Elderly Individuals

Age	Normal PaO_2
60	≥80 mmHg
65	≥75 mmHg
70	≥70 mmHg
75	≥65 mmHg
≥80	≥60 mmHg

Note: a PaO_2 lower than 60 mmHg is always considered hypoxemia, regardless of age or disease.

to cells—the lungs, blood, circulatory system, and tissues. Therefore, normal functioning of these processes is necessary for proper tissue oxygenation and any pathophysiologic problems along the circuit may lead to hypoxia. Hypoxia caused from gas exchange abnormalities at the lung level is termed *hypoxic hypoxia* or *hypoxemic hypoxia;* hypoxia caused by inadequate oxygen-carrying capacity is *anemic hypoxia;* hypoxia resulting from inadequate circulatory transport is *stagnant* or *circulatory hypoxia;* and hypoxia resulting from the inability of the tissues to use the oxygen brought to them is termed *histotoxic hypoxia.*

Causes for hypoxic hypoxia are those listed previously for hypoxemia. Anemic hypoxia is caused by either a lower than normal hemoglobin content in the blood or the inability of hemoglobin to combine with oxygen such as that which occurs with carbon monoxide poisoning. Any factors that reduce the cardiac output (e.g., cardiogenic shock, left heart failure, hypovolemia) may cause stagnant or circulatory hypoxia. Histotoxic hypoxia is a life-threatening condition caused from cyanide poisoning, in which the tissues are unable to use the oxygen brought to them.

The body has excellent adaptive mechanisms designed to protect the cells from hypoxia. The compensatory mechanism that initiates in response to hypoxemia or hypoxia are such that the work of the heart (heart rate and/or blood pressure) increase, the work of breathing increases, and the pulmonary vascular bed constricts while other vital organ vascular systems dilate to supply life-sustaining oxygen to them.

A final response is for the body to increase the production of hemoglobin. However, this is not an acute response. With longstanding, chronic hypoxemia as seen with COPD, severe anemias, individuals living at high altitudes, and individuals with heart failure, hemoglobin and red blood cell mass increase to maintain oxygen transport and aerobic metabolism. The mechanism by which this occurs is depicted in Figure 8.3. Diaphoresis and pallor often accompany the hypoxemic patient, as well as restlessness, agitation, and confusion.

Preparations and Methods of Administration

Oxygen is available in compressed gaseous form in steel cylinders with a purity of 99%, as regulated by the FDA. Most hospitals contain a bulk liquid oxygen system in which the stored liquid oxygen is converted to gaseous oxygen and piped into patient areas. All oxygen cylinders and oxygen piping systems are color coded (green in the USA, white internationally) and have a specific indexing system that prevents inadvertent attachment of other gases.

There are various types of oxygen administration devices that enable the practitioner to select a device that would best meet the clinical objectives of oxygen therapy and the patient's particular needs. Figure 8.4 illustrates the most commonly used adult oxygen administration devices; Table 8.2 summarizes the oxygen concentrations and precautions for use that pertain to these devices.

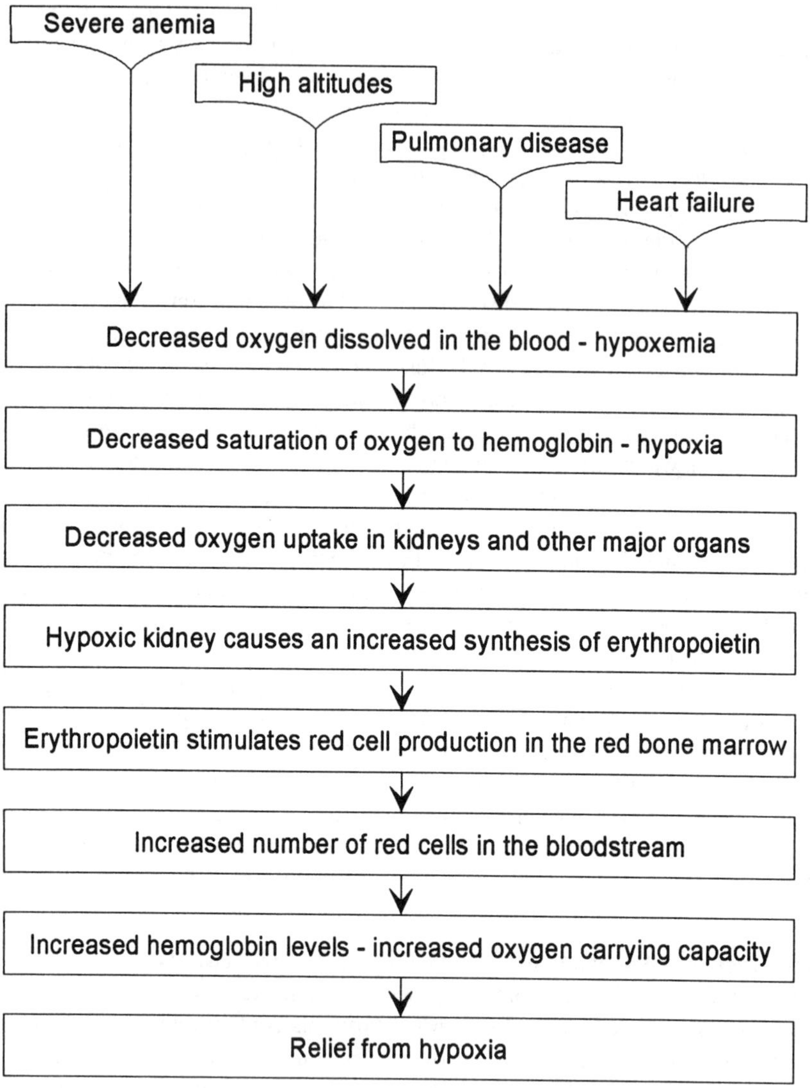
Severe anemia
High altitudes
Pulmonary disease
Heart failure
Decreased oxygen dissolved in the blood - hypoxemia
Decreased saturation of oxygen to hemoglobin - hypoxia
Decreased oxygen uptake in kidneys and other major organs
Hypoxic kidney causes an increased synthesis of erythropoietin
Erythropoietin stimulates red cell production in the red bone marrow
Increased number of red cells in the bloodstream
Increased hemoglobin levels - increased oxygen carrying capacity
Relief from hypoxia

Figure 8.3. Red blood cell production in response to hypoxia.

Therapeutic Indications for Oxygen Therapy

Therapy for hypoxia is always aimed at correcting the underlying cause of the hypoxia. For general purposes, oxygen therapy is only useful in reversing or preventing tissue hypoxia when the problem is caused by hypoxemia. However, oxygen therapy should not be withheld when hypoxia is caused by low cardiac output states, anemia, carbon monoxide poisoning, or cyanide poisoning, because this could fur-

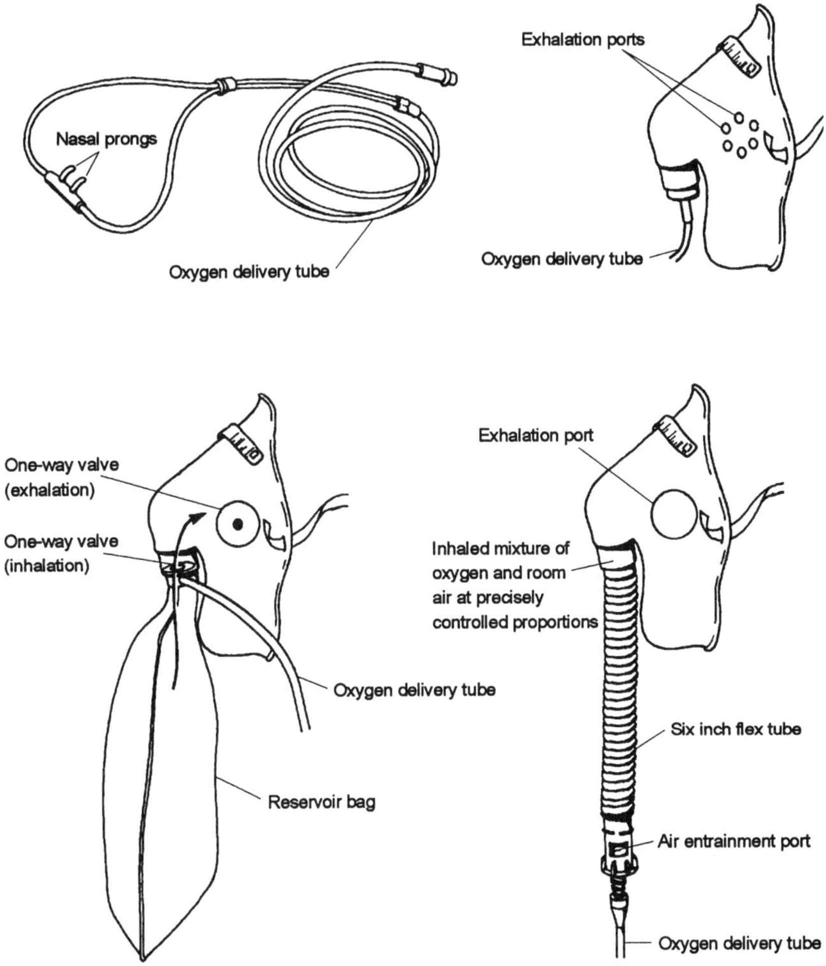

Figure 8.4. Common oxygen delivery devices. *Top left,* nasal cannula; *top right,* simple oxygen mask; *bottom left,* nonrebreathing mask (NRB); *bottom right,* venturi mask.

ther compromise the patient. There are four primary therapeutic uses for oxygen therapy:

- Correction of hypoxemia and/or hypoxia is the mainstay of oxygen therapy. Because hypoxia is most commonly associated with an underlying disease, the administration of supplemental oxygen is primarily for symptomatic and temporary purposes. When administering oxygen therapy to relieve hypoxemia,

Table 8.2
Commonly Used Oxygen Delivery Systems

Delivery Device	Approximate Oxygen Concentration	Comments
Nasal cannula	~24% @ 1 L/min ~28% @ 2 L/min ~32% @ 3 L/min ~36% @ 4 L/min ~40% @ 5 L/min ~44% @ 6 L/min	Oxygen concentration varies widely with patient's ventilatory pattern; not indicated for high oxygen concentrations or for the severely hypoxemic patient. Flowmeter setting should not be set above 6 L/min because there will be no appreciable gain in oxygen concentration and nasal mucosal drying and irritation may occur. Ideal device for patients who are mildly hypoxemic and for patients who are chronic CO_2 retainers.
Simple oxygen mask	~40% to 60% @ 5 to 8 L/min	Oxygen concentration varies widely with patient's ventilatory pattern. The flowmeter setting should never be set less than 5 L/min because exhaled gases, most notably CO_2, will accumulate in the face mask, resulting in rebreathing of CO_2.
Mask with reservoir bag	~60% to 100% @ 10 to 15 L/min	Oxygen concentration varies widely with patient's ventilatory pattern. Flowmeter setting must be set high enough so that the reservoir bag never collapses during inspiration. A system without any one-way valves is known as a partial rebreathing mask; a portion of exhaled gases are rebreathed. A system with one-way valves placed at the exhalation ports and between the mask and reservoir bag is known as a nonrebreathing mask (Fig. 8.4); no portion of exhaled gases are rebreathed. Ideally suited for short-term oxygen therapy for the severely hypoxemic patient.
Venturi mask	Delivers a specific oxygen concentration (up to 50%) at variable flow rates	Delivers very precise oxygen concentrations; the patient's ventilatory pattern does not affect oxygen delivery. Ideally suited for patients who are mildly or moderately hypoxemic who exhibit an unstable ventilatory pattern. The flowmeter setting must be set high enough to meet the patient's inspiratory flow requirements or additional room air will be entrained through the exhalation ports of the face mask, thus diluting the oxygen concentration. Never allow the air entrainment port to become occluded with blankets or sheets or the delivered oxygen concentrations will be higher than desired.

there are three goals the practitioner should meet: 1) elevate the PaO_2, 2) reduce the work of the heart, and 3) reduce the work of breathing.

- Reduction of the partial pressure of an inert gas, most notably nitrogen, is another reason for administering supplemental oxygen to a patient. High inspired oxygen concentrations lower the total body partial pressure of nitrogen, which then enhances the removal of nitrogen from the body's gas spaces. Such gas-filled spaces result from air gas embolism, pneumothorax, and intestinal obstruction or ileus.
- Oxygen is commonly combined with other inhaled vapors and gases, in which it is then used as a carrier gas or a diluting agent. Oxygen is commonly used in combination with anesthetic gases, carbon dioxide, and helium.

- Hyperbaric oxygen therapy is a method of administering oxygen to the body at above atmospheric pressures. The procedure is to place the patient in an air-tight chamber, apply 100% oxygen, and slowly increase the atmospheric pressure from 1 up to 3 atmospheres. The treatment time is usually 1 to 2 hours at full pressure. While breathing 100% oxygen at 3 atmospheres, the patient's PaO_2 may rise to as high as 1900 mmHg. The physiologic effects of such treatment include arteriolar constriction, new capillary bed formation, reduction in the size of nitrogen bubbles dissolved within the blood and other tissue cavities, and alterations in the metabolism of both aerobic and anaerobic organisms. Hyperbaric oxygen therapy is especially suited for patients with deficient tissue oxygenation such as that which occurs in carbon monoxide poisoning, cyanide poisoning, thermal burns, and anaerobic bacterial infections (e.g., gas gangrene). Hyperbaric oxygen therapy is also indicated for the gas-lesion diseases, decompression sickness (the "bends"), and air embolism.

Hazards of Oxygen Therapy

High oxygen concentrations (higher than 40%) used for an extended time period (more than 3 days) may result in adverse effects. Four such effects include:

1. Retinopathy of prematurity (ROP), also known as retrolental fibroplasia (RLF): This condition occurs when supplemental oxygen therapy elevates the PaO_2 to higher than 80 mmHg in the premature infant. Hyperoxia causes vasoconstriction of the retinal blood vessels, which may lead to irreversible blindness in the premature infant.
2. Absorption atelectasis: Nitrogen constitutes approximately 80% of alveolar gas which is essential in maintaining alveolar stability. Replacement of nitrogen with high inspired oxygen concentrations (more than 70%) will wash out nitrogen from the alveoli resulting in alveolar collapse and atelectasis.
3. Oxygen toxicity: High inspired oxygen concentrations over a given time period result in pathophysiologic changes in lung tissue. In as little as 6 to 8 hours, there is a noticeable decrease in the velocity of tracheal mucous; tracheobronchial irritation and chest tightness may occur within 12 hours of inspiring 100% oxygen; increased alveolar permeability and inflammation occur after 17 hours; and decreased pulmonary function ensues after 10 to 24 hours of inspiring 100% oxygen. Clinical manifestations of oxygen toxicity include substernal pain, cough, nausea and vomiting, refractory hypoxemia (hypoxemia that does not respond to oxygen therapy), diffuse patchy bilateral infiltrates, anorexia, alveolar atelectasis, and parasthesia.
4. Oxygen-induced hypoventilation: A high inspired oxygen concentration, leading to an elevated PaO_2, causes respiratory depression in patients who are chronic retainers of CO_2. Two chemoreceptor mechanisms exist that monitor

blood pH (central chemoreceptors) and arterial PO_2 (peripheral chemoreceptors). The response elicited from either chemoreceptor is to stimulate ventilation. Chronic CO_2 retention, leading to a normalized pH, desensitizes the central chemoreceptors. Thus, the only mechanism that stimulates ventilation in chronic CO_2 retainers is the continual activation of the peripheral chemoreceptors caused by the mild hypoxemic state in which these patients normally live. Abolishment of this hypoxic drive to breathe (i.e., inactivation of the peripheral chemoreceptors) by allowing these patients to inspire a high oxygen concentration, thus elevating the PaO_2 to a normal level, leads to hypoventilation, which can ultimately result in respiratory failure. For this reason, for patients with chronically elevated levels of CO_2, supplemental oxygen therapy should be carefully monitored so that the PaO_2 remains approximately 60 mmHg.

Despite the above-mentioned possibilities, 100% oxygen should never be withheld in conditions in which the patient is at risk for developing tissue hypoxia. Such conditions include cardiopulmonary arrest (see Chapter 19), acute cardiopulmonary instability, and carbon monoxide poisoning.

Monitoring and Assessment of Oxygen Therapy

Owing to the risk factors involved with the administration of oxygen therapy, the dose of oxygen should always be titrated to deliver just that amount needed to obtain the desired PaO_2. This can be done through arterial blood gas analysis or pulse oximetry. In addition, it is important to evaluate the work of breathing and the work of the myocardium to determine the overall effectiveness of oxygen therapy.

CARBON DIOXIDE

At normal atmospheric temperatures and pressures, carbon dioxide is a colorless, odorless gas that is approximately 1.5 times heavier than air. Carbon dioxide does not support combustion or maintain life. Carbon dioxide plays a vital role in regulating many bodily functions. At rest, approximately 200 mL of CO_2 per minute is produced from cellular metabolism. The gas is then transferred to the bloodstream, where it is carried partly as bicarbonate ion, partly in chemical combination with hemoglobin and plasma proteins, and partly dissolved in plasma at a partial pressure of approximately 45 mmHg in mixed venous blood. Carbon dioxide is transported to the lung by the circulatory system, where it is exhaled at the same rate at which it is produced.

Normal arterial PCO_2 ranges between 35 and 45 mmHg. Alveolar hypoventilation results in a rise in arterial PCO_2 with a corresponding fall in blood pH. This condition is known as respiratory acidosis. Alveolar hyperventilation results in an arterial PCO_2 that is less than normal with a pH that is greater than normal. This mechanism is termed respiratory alkalosis.

Physiologic Effects of Carbon Dioxide

Small changes in blood PCO_2 and pH induce widespread physiologic alterations on respiration, circulation, and the CNS.

Respiratory Response

Carbon dioxide is a potent respiratory stimulant that produces, within minutes of inhalation, a marked increase in both the rate and depth of ventilation. Activation of the medullary chemoreceptors, which monitor blood PCO_2 and pH, are primarily responsible for the noticeable change in alveolar ventilation.

Circulatory Response

The major circulatory effects induced by inhalation of carbon dioxide include marked cerebral vasodilation, coronary vasodilation, an increase in cardiac output and heart rate, elevation of the arterial blood pressure, and an increase in pulse pressure. Vasodilation is considered a local tissue effect, whereas stimulation of the myocardium results from carbon dioxide's ability to activate the cardiovascular brain centers and the sympathetic nervous system.

CNS Response

High concentrations of carbon dioxide depress cerebral activity, resulting in CNS depression. Inhalation of as little as 5% carbon dioxide may produce mental confusion, whereas inhaling 10% carbon dioxide may lead to unconsciousness.

Preparations and Methods of Administration

Because carbon dioxide does not support life, it is commonly marketed in metal cylinders in combination with oxygen (gray/green cylinders). The FDA purity standard for carbon dioxide is 99.9%. The CO_2/O_2 mixture consists of either 5% CO_2 and 95% O_2 or 10% CO_2 and 90% O_2. The procedure for administering carbon dioxide therapy is to have the patient breathe the CO_2/O_2 mixture through a well-fitting nonrebreathing mask for a duration of 6 to 10 minutes. The therapy should be stopped immediately if adverse effects are noted (see below). For patients with artificial airways, carbon dioxide therapy is administered through the endotracheal or tracheostomy tube.

Another form of administering carbon dioxide is to allow the patient to rebreathe his/her own exhaled CO_2. This can be done simply by having the patient breathe from a paper bag or by removing the soda lime canister from a patient breathing circuit. Patients with artificial airways who also are receiving mechanical ventilation can rebreathe his/her own exhaled CO_2 by placing mechanical dead space (wide bore flex tubing) between the patient's artificial airway and the Y of the breathing circuit.

Therapeutic Indications for Carbon Dioxide Therapy

The overall purpose of administering carbon dioxide therapy is to elevate the arterial PCO_2. Carbon dioxide therapy has very limited uses because other, safer methods of therapy with fewer adverse effects are available. The current therapeutic indications for carbon dioxide therapy include the following:

- Reversal of the CNS and respiratory depressive effects caused by inhalation of anesthetic gases: This is brought about by carbon dioxide's ability to stimulate ventilation and improve cerebral blood flow.
- Abolish hiccups (singulation): Hiccups occur when an irritated phrenic nerve sends erratic impulses to the diaphragm, the result of which causes the diaphragm to spasmodically contract. Inhalation of low concentrations of carbon dioxide stimulates the respiratory center, which initiates a series of events that override the spasmodic impulses to the diaphragm, thereby restoring normal breathing.
- Improve cerebral blood flow: Because carbon dioxide is a potent cerebrovasodilator, it has a long history of use in overcoming the cerebral vasospasm that is associated with certain types of cerebral vascular disease. However, studies using hypercapnic cerebrovasodilation have demonstrated mixed results in which hypercapnic cerebrovasodilation was beneficial in some and deleterious in others (Klassen et al. 1979).
- Improve retinal blood flow: Some ophthalmologists use carbon dioxide therapy to vasodilate the vessels supplying the retina of the eye to restore blood flow when thromboses have hindered circulation.

Hazards of Carbon Dioxide Therapy

Carbon dioxide produces toxic effects when given in excessive amounts. Such effects include nausea, vomiting, dizziness, headaches (due from cerebral vasodilation), palpitations, muscle tremors, and mental confusion. In addition, the blood pressure may rise to dangerous levels that can lead to convulsions and cardiac or respiratory failure. Carbon dioxide therapy is contraindicated for patients who are chronic retainers of CO_2 because these patients are already hypercapnic, and additional carbon dioxide will further aggravate their condition.

Monitoring and Assessment of Carbon Dioxide Therapy

It is vital that the practitioner remain in constant attendance and continuously monitor the patient for signs of adverse reactions while administering carbon dioxide therapy. Therapy should be discontinued immediately if any of the above adverse effects occur.

HELIUM

Helium is an odorless and tasteless gas that is both chemically and physiologically inert as well as a good conductor of heat, sound, and electricity. Helium is poorly soluble in water and the lightest of gases, second only to hydrogen. Helium's therapeutic usefulness is based on its inherent properties: it is an inert gas that has low solubility, low density, and high thermal conductivity.

Preparations and Methods of Administration

Because helium, like carbon dioxide, does not support life, it is available for therapeutic use only in combination with oxygen. The helium-oxygen mixture is marketed in compressed form in steel cylinders color-coded brown (helium) and green (oxygen) with a percentage combination of either 80% He and 20% O_2 or 70% He and 30% O_2. The purity standards mandated by the FDA for helium is 95%.

Helium-oxygen is administered via a well-fitting nonrebreathing mask or, for patients with artificial airways, through an endotracheal or tracheostomy tube. A special flowmeter, calibrated for the helium-oxygen mixture, may be used or an oxygen flowmeter may be used to deliver the helium-oxygen mixture. However, because oxygen flowmeters are calibrated for the density of oxygen, the actual flow rate delivered by the lighter helium-oxygen mixture will be different from the indicated flow rate when using an oxygen flowmeter. To determine the actual flow rate being delivered, multiply the indicated flow rate by 1.8 for an 80% He and 20% O_2 mixture or by 1.6 for a 70% He and 30% O_2 mixture. For example, if the oxygen flowmeter were set at 10 L/min when delivering a 70% He and 30% O_2 mixture, the actual flow rate is 16 L/min ($10 \times 1.6 = 16$).

Calculating the actual flow rate when using an oxygen flowmeter and a 70% He/30% O_2 mixture:

$$\text{Actual flow rate} = \text{Indicated flow rate} \times 1.6$$

Calculating the actual flow rate when using an oxygen flowmeter and an 80% He/20% O_2 mixture:

$$\text{Actual flow rate} = \text{Indicated flow rate} \times 1.8$$

Therapeutic Indications for Helium Therapy

Currently, helium's medical use is limited to the following:

- Treatment of patients with airflow obstruction
- Certain pulmonary function testing

- Laser airway surgery
- Selected hyperbaric applications

Airflow Obstruction

Inhaling a mixture of helium and oxygen has been demonstrated to significantly reduce the work of breathing in patients with airflow obstruction. This is because substituting a lower-density helium-oxygen mixture for higher-density oxygen or air enhances a smooth and even laminar flow throughout the airways, especially in the larger airways where more rough and tumbling turbulent flow is likely to occur during airflow obstruction. Because laminar flow patterns move gases at a lower pressure than turbulent flow patterns and because breathing mixtures of helium and oxygen encourages laminar flow, the work of breathing decreases.

Pulmonary Function Testing

Functional residual capacity (FRC) and residual volume (RV) are obtained by having a patient inhale a known percentage of helium and then collecting the mixed exhaled gas for analysis. The procedure is known as the helium dilution technique or closed circuit test. Because helium is highly inert and poorly soluble (meaning that it does not react with other substances or leave the lung) it is an ideal gas in measuring its concentration in exhaled gas in dilution with the other gases in the lung.

Laser Airway Surgery

Helium's high thermal conductivity makes it useful in deflecting the heat generated from the point of contact of the laser beam, thus decreasing the likelihood of surrounding tissue damage within the airway during laser surgery. In addition, helium improves flow rate throughout the airways by encouraging laminar flow through the small endotracheal tubes commonly used during laser airway surgery.

Hyperbaric Applications

Breathing helium-oxygen mixtures, instead of pure oxygen, for diving activity minimizes the risk of oxygen toxicity, inert gas narcosis, and decompression sickness (commonly known as the "bends"). In addition, breathing helium-oxygen mixtures instead of pure oxygen reduces the work of breathing associated with hyperbaric conditions.

Hazards of Helium-Oxygen Therapy

The most common adverse effect of breathing helium is voice distortion. In the intubated patient, this is not a problem; however, the nonintubated patient should be told to expect a badly distorted voice and be reassured that it will disappear within a few minutes after the completion of therapy.

Breathing helium-oxygen mixtures may affect the cough mechanism. Because an effective cough requires turbulent flow in the larger airways to generate the explosive pressure required to expel airway content, the patient's cough may be somewhat diminished because of the laminar flow within the large airways, which results from breathing helium. For this reason, the clearance of secretions may be impaired. Whereas this is a consideration in the application of helium therapy, the cough should return to normal after washing the helium from the airways.

NITRIC OXIDE

In the early 1980s, it was discovered that the endothelium, a one-cell-thick layer that lines the entire inner luminal surface of the circulatory system, actively produces a chemical substance that is a very potent vasodilator. Subsequently, this chemical was termed endothelium-derived relaxing factor (EDRF). After an intense search to find the chemical identity of EDRF, it was discovered in 1987 that EDRF may possibly be nitric oxide. Of interest, is that nitric oxide is the active metabolite of a group of vasodilators now known as *nitrovasodilators* because they mimic the endothelial cells and produce nitric oxide. Such drugs include sodium nitroprusside, nitroglycerin, isosorbide dinitrate and mononitrate, and amyl nitrite (see Chapter 18, Cardiovascular Agents).

Molecular Basis of Nitric Oxide Function

Nitric oxide binds to the enzyme guanyl cyclase, which as discussed in Chapter 2, catalyzes the conversion of guanosine triphosphate (GTP) to 3,5-guanosine monophosphate (cGMP). It is the rise in intracellular levels of cGMP that produces relaxation of vascular smooth muscle. Without nitric oxide, guanyl cyclase produces cGMP very slowly and because cGMP is rapidly metabolized by cells, the levels stay low. With nitric oxide bound to it, guanyl cyclase produces cGMP quite rapidly and the levels rise significantly, causing marked vasodilation.

The primary problem with using nitric oxide as a drug is that it is rapidly metabolized on contact with blood: nitric oxide readily penetrates the red cell membrane where it then reacts with hemoglobin to form methemoglobin. The advantage of administering *inhaled* nitric oxide is that it is applied topically to the pulmonary vessel wall after it diffuses across the alveolus. By this mechanism, nitric oxide selectively dilates the pulmonary arterioles. Any nitric oxide that diffuses further into the vessel comes in contact with blood, where it is instantly destroyed by circulating hemoglobin. As a result, there is no circulating nitric oxide, no vasodilation of blood vessels downstream of the alveoli, and no systemic vasodilation. Inhaled nitric oxide is a selective pulmonary vasodilator because it only reaches the pulmonary vasculature.

Physiologic Effects of Inhaled Nitric Oxide

Nitric oxide, not to be confused with the anesthetic nitrous oxide, is a gas that has very potent vasodilating properties. Inhalation of nitric oxide produces local vasodilation of well-ventilated lung units. By this mechanism, nitric oxide:

- Lowers pulmonary hypertension
- Reduces pulmonary vascular resistance
- Increases right heart ejection fraction
- Improves arterial oxygenation by redistributing blood flow away from areas with intrapulmonary shunts to areas with a normal ventilation/perfusion ratio

The distinct advantage that inhaled nitric oxide has over systemically infused vasodilators is that inhaled low-dose nitric oxide selectively vasodilates the pulmonary vasculature. Systemic vasodilation does not occur because of the rapid inactivation of nitric oxide by hemoglobin. Inhaled nitric oxide has also been shown to exert a weak bronchodilatory effect in bronchial asthma.

Preparations and Methods of Administration

Nitric oxide is supplied in compressed gas cylinders containing nitric oxide in combination with nitrogen. Nitric oxide must be stored in nitrogen owing to its rapid oxidation in the presence of oxygen. The mechanics of how nitric oxide from the cylinder is added to the inhaled gases is, at present, costly and difficult to use. One major limitation is the problem of measuring the concentration of nitric oxide delivered. The current trend is to find a safe, portable, accurate, and adaptable system to deliver nitric oxide.

Dosage

Many studies have demonstrated that inhaled nitric oxide seems to be relatively effective and safe at doses between 2 and 80 parts per million (ppm). Some investigators define the lowest effective inspiratory nitric oxide dose as that which achieves at least a 30% improvement in the PaO_2/FIO_2 ratio (Gerlach et al. 1993).

Therapeutic Indications for Inhalation of Nitric Oxide

Although not yet approved by the FDA, inhalation of low concentrations (2 to 80 ppm) of nitric oxide is a relatively innovative investigational therapy that benefits patients who exhibit increased pulmonary vascular resistance secondary to severe pulmonary hypertension. Inhalation of nitric oxide has proven beneficial for the following conditions:

- Adult respiratory distress syndrome (ARDS) (Bigatello et al. 1994, Ricou et al. 1994, Gerlach et al. 1993). In addition, inhalation of nitric oxide has been beneficial for patients with ARDS who are being ventilated via permissive hypercapnia. Combining permissive hypercapnia and inhaled nitric oxide seems to decrease the potentially deleterious effects that permissive hypercapnia alone exhibits on lung parenchyma and pulmonary circulation (Puybasset et al. 1994).

- Infant respiratory distress syndrome (Abman et al. 1993).
- Pulmonary hypertension secondary to congenital heart defects (Miller et al. 1994, Journois et al. 1994, Winberg et al. 1994).
- Acute hypoxemic respiratory failure (Watkins et al. 1993).
- Persistent pulmonary hypertension of the neonate (Kinsella et al. 1993).
- Heart transplant candidates with elevated pulmonary vascular resistance (Kieler-Jensen et al. 1994).
- Newborns with right-to-left extrapulmonary shunts (Roze et al. 1994).
- Chronic obstructive pulmonary disease (Moinard et al. 1994).
- Interstitial pulmonary fibrosis and cor pulmonale (Channick et al. 1994).
- Cardiac surgery (e.g., coronary artery bypass grafting and mitral valve replacement) in which there is postoperative pulmonary hypertension (Lindberg et al. 1994, Rich et al. 1994, Wessel et al. 1993, Snow et al. 1994).
- Pulmonary hypertension secondary to postsurgical repair of congenital diaphragmatic hernia (Frostell et al. 1993).
- Bronchopulmonary dysplasia (Abman et al. 1994).
- Acute pneumonitis caused by the respiratory syncytial virus (Abman et al. 1994).
- Asthma (Hogman et al. 1993).

Hazards of Nitric Oxide Therapy

Although many investigators have suggested that short-term, low-dose inhalation of nitric oxide is a relatively safe procedure without important side effects, special precautions still apply. The formation of the toxic metabolites of nitric oxide, such as NO_2, NO_3, should be carefully monitored as well as an increase in methemoglobin concentrations. What remains to be seen is whether inhalational nitric oxide therapy can reduce morbidity or improve survival rates. The safety and efficacy of inhaled nitric oxide therapy is currently being examined in multicenter trials.

REFERENCES/RECOMMENDED READING

Abman SH, et al. Inhaled nitric oxide in the management of a premature newborn with severe respiratory distress and pulmonary hypertension. Pediatrics 92(4):606, 1993.

Abman SH, et al. Acute effects of inhaled nitric oxide in children with severe hypoxemic respiratory failure. J Pediatr 124(6):881, 1994.

Bigatello LM, et al. Prolonged inhalation of low concentrations of nitric oxide in patients with severe adult respiratory distress syndrome. Effects on pulmonary hemodynamics and oxygenation. Anesthesiology 80(4):761, 1994.
Channick RN, et al. Improvement in pulmonary hypertension and hypoxemia during nitric oxide inhalation in a patient with end-stage pulmonary fibrosis. Am J Respir Crit Care Med 149(3 Pt 1):811, 1994.
Clark JM. Pulmonary limits of oxygen tolerance in man. Exp Lung Res 14:897, 1988.
Coursin DB, et al. Adaptation to chronic hyperoxia: biochemical effects and the response to subsequent lethal hyperoxia. Am Rev Respir Dis 135:1002, 1987.
Fahey PJ, Hyde RW. "Won't breathe" vs "can't breathe." Detection of depressed ventilatory drive in patients with obstructive pulmonary disease. Chest 84(1):19, 1983.
Frostell CG, et al. Near fatal pulmonary hypertension after surgical repair of congenital diaphragmatic hernia. Successful use of inhaled nitric oxide. Anaesthesia 48(8):679, 1993.
Gerlach H, et al. Long-term inhalation with evaluated low doses of nitric oxide for selective improvement of oxygenation in patients with adult respiratory distress syndrome. Intensive Care Med 19(8):443, 1993.
Hogman M, et al. Inhalation of nitric oxide modulates adult human bronchial tone. Am Rev Respir Dis 148(6 Pt 1):1474, 1993.
Jacobi MS, et al. Ventilatory responses to inhaled carbon dioxide at rest and during exercise in man. Clin Sci 73(2):177, 1987.
Journois D, et al. Inhaled nitric oxide as a therapy for pulmonary hypertension after operations for congenital heart defects. J Thorac Cardiovasc Surg 107(4):1129, 1994.
Kieler-Jensen N, et al. Inhaled nitric oxide in the evaluation of heart transplant candidates with elevated pulmonary vascular resistance. J Heart Lung Transplant 13(3):366, 1994.
Kinsella JP, et al. Clinical response to prolonged treatment of persistent pulmonary hypertension of the newborn with low doses of inhaled nitric oxide. J Pediatr 123(1):103, 1993.
Klassen AC, et al. Hypercapnic alteration of visual evoked responses in acute cerebral infarction. Arch Neurol 36(10):627, 1979.
Lahari S, et al. Comparison of aortic and carotid chemoreceptor responses to hypercapnia and hypoxia. J Appl Physiol 51:55, 1981.
Lindberg L, et al. Nitric oxide gives maximal response after coronary artery bypass surgery. J Cardiothorac Vasc Anesth 8(2):182, 1994.
Lourenco RV. Clinical methods for the study of regulation of ventilation. Chest 70:109, 1976.
Mathewson HS. Helium—who needs it? Respir Care 27:1400, 1982.
Miller OI, et al. Very-low-dose inhaled nitric oxide: a selective pulmonary vasodilator after operations for congenital heart disease. J Thorac Cardiovasc Surg 108(3): 487, 1994.
Moinard J, et al. Effect of inhaled nitric oxide on hemodynamics and VA/Q inequalities in patients with chronic obstructive pulmonary disease. Am J Respir Crit Care Med 149(6):1482, 1994.
Nunn JF. Carbon dioxide. In: Applied Respiratory Physiology. 3rd ed. London: Butterworths, 1987.
Puybasset L, et al. Inhaled nitric oxide reverses the increase in pulmonary vascular resistance induced by permissive hypercapnia in patients with acute respiratory distress syndrome. Anesthesiology 80(6):1254, 1994.
Redding JS, McAfee DD, Parham AM. Oxygen concentrations received from commonly used delivery systems. South Med J 71:169, 1978.
Rich GF, et al. Inhaled nitric oxide selectively decreases pulmonary vascular resistance without impairing oxygenation during one-lung ventilation in patients undergoing cardiac surgery. Anesthesiology 80(1):57, 1994.

Ricou B, et al. [Nitrous oxide (NO) in the treatment of adult respiratory distress syndrome] [French]. Schweiz Med Wochenschr 124(14):583, 1994.
Rimer S, Gillis CN. Selective pulmonary vasodilation by inhaled nitric oxide is due to hemoglobin inactivation. Circulation 88(6):2884, 1993.
Roze JC, et al. Echocardiographic investigation of inhaled nitric oxide in newborn babies with severe hypoxaemia. Lancet 344(8918):303, 1994.
Sackner MA. A history of oxygen usage in chronic obstructive pulmonary disease. Am Rev Respir Dis 110(Suppl):25, 1974.
Schacter EW, et al. Monitoring of oxygen delivery systems in clinical practice. Crit Care Med 8:405, 1980.
Snow DJ, et al. Inhaled nitric oxide in patients with normal and increased pulmonary vascular resistance after cardiac surgery. Br J Anaesth 72(2):185, 1994.
Snyder JV, Pinsky MR. Oxygen Transport in the Critically Ill. Chicago: Year Book Medical Publishers, 1987.
Sobini CA, Grassi V, Solinas E. Arterial oxygen tension in relation to age in healthy subjects. Respiration 25:3, 1968.
Thom SR. Hyperbaric oxygen therapy. J Intensive Care Med 4:58, 1989.
Viljanen AA, Viljanen B, Mattila S. The effect of inhaled carbon dioxide and hypoxia mixtures on the electrical and mechanical activities of respiratory muscles in dogs. Acta Physiol Scand 128(2):231, 1986.
Watkins DN, et al. Inhaled nitric oxide in severe acute respiratory failure—its use in intensive care and description of a delivery system. Anaesth Intensive Care 21(6):861, 1993.
Wessel DL, et al. Use of inhaled nitric oxide and acetylcholine in the evaluation of pulmonary hypertension and endothelial function after cardiopulmonary bypass. Circulation 88(5 Pt 1):2128, 1993.
Wessel DL, et al. Delivery and monitoring of inhaled nitric oxide in patients with pulmonary hypertension. Crit Care Med 22(6):930, 1994.
Winberg P, Lundell BP, Gustafsson LE. Effect of inhaled nitric oxide on raised pulmonary vascular resistance in children with congenital heart disease. Br Heart J 71(3):282, 1994.

COUGH AND COLD PREPARATIONS 9

The various cough and cold remedies, available either over the counter or by prescription, do not cure the cold nor lessen its duration but only serve to modify or relieve the symptoms (nasal congestion, headache, fever, general malaise, cough, rhinorrhea). This chapter focuses on the four classes of drugs that work, either singly or in combination, to lessen the severity of the cough, cold, or allergy symptoms:

- Nasal decongestants (relieve nasal congestion)
- Antihistamines (dry secretions, symptomatic relief of symptoms associated with various allergic reactions)
- Antitussives (suppress cough)
- Expectorants (increase clearance of secretions)

The efficacy of some of these agents is questionable owing to the lack of objective studies. Many over-the-counter cold and cough remedies are used indiscriminately; therefore, the potential for abuse is high. Of utmost importance is the need to first treat the underlying cause of the cough or allergy.

The addition of other chemicals such as analgesics, anticholinergic agents, preservatives, caffeine, and alcohol is a common but questionable practice. Anticholinergics (such as atropine or methscopolamine) are included for their drying effects on mucosal secretions; however, this may lead to mucus plugging or airway obstruction. Caffeine is included in some preparations for central nervous system (CNS) stimulation to counteract the effects of antihistamine depression. Analgesics (acetaminophen, aspirin, sodium salicylate) are added for symptoms of headache, fever, muscle aches, and pain. Some preparations contain considerable levels of alcohol. When using these combinations, it is necessary to consider whether each ingredient is applicable to the symptoms or condition or whether a particular ingredient is even beneficial. Because various cough and cold preparations are available, one may be very selective.

NASAL DECONGESTANTS

Mechanism of Action and Indications for Use

Decongestants are sympathomimetic amines with primary α-adrenoceptor action. Activation of the α-adrenoceptor sites elicits marked local vasoconstriction to swollen, dilated arterioles when applied directly to the nasal mucosa, which in turn causes shrinkage of the nasal mucosa, thus relieving the stuffy feeling that results from membrane congestion. As a result of this action, promotion of drainage and improved ventilation through the nose occur.

Decongestants administered topically (via nasal sprays, drops, jellies, inhalers) to swollen mucosal membranes or systemically via the oral route (via capsules, tablets, liquids) are useful in the treatment of mucosal congestion that typically accompanies hay fever, allergic rhinitis, vasomotor rhinitis, sinusitis, the common cold, and other upper respiratory allergies. Topical agents are generally more immediately effective than oral agents, but oral agents have a sustained duration of action, cause less local mucosal irritation, and are not associated with the phenomenon of rebound congestion that results from repeated, excessive use of topical agents.

Contraindications

Contraindications to the use of nasal decongestants include monoamine oxidase inhibitor (MAO) therapy, hypersensitivity to sympathomimetic amines, severe hypertension, coronary artery disease, nursing mothers, and narrow-angle glaucoma.

Precautions

1. Excessive use of topical decongestants may result in systemic effects resulting in nervousness, dizziness, or sleeplessness.
2. Rebound congestion (hyperemia, edema of mucosa) may occur following topical administration once the vasoconstrictive effects recede. This is especially noted with excessive, repeated dosing.
3. Use topical administration of decongestants only in acute states, only when needed, and no longer than 3 to 5 days. Significant side effects are associated in patients with allergic rhinitis who use topical nasal decongestants for a prolonged period of time. Patients should be instructed not to exceed recommended dose.
4. Use cautiously in patients with hyperthyroidism, hypertension, diabetes mellitus, increased intraocular pressure, prostatic hypertrophy, or ischemic cardiac disease, because systemic absorption may occur, leading to CNS stimulation, convulsions, or cardiovascular collapse.

5. Some decongestants contain sulfites, which may precipitate an allergic response (hives, itching, wheezing) in sulfite-sensitive individuals.

Adverse Reactions

Cardiovascular: Palpitations, tachycardia, arrhythmias, cardiovascular collapse.
CNS: Fear, anxiety, headache, restlessness, lightheadedness, dizziness, drowsiness, tremor, insomnia, hallucinations, convulsions, CNS depression.
Gastrointestinal (GI): Nausea, vomiting, anorexia.
Genitourinary (GU): Urinary retention, dysuria.
Topical administration: Burning, stinging, sneezing, dryness, mucosal irritation, rebound congestion.
Miscellaneous: Respiratory difficulties, sweating, pallor.

Overdosage

CNS depression (somnolence, sedation, or deep coma) accompanied by hypertension, bradycardia, and rebound hypotension. Treatment consists of supportive care and early intervention with gastric lavage following oral overdose.

Dosage and Administration

Table 9.1 lists the nasal decongestants.

ANTIHISTAMINES

Review of Histamine Action and Effects (see Chapters 2 and 11)

Histamine is a vasoactive substance found in most body tissues (the highest concentration is in the lungs, skin, and stomach) and exists in bound form within subcellular granules of the mast cell. High concentrations of histamine are also located within the basophil blood cell. Various physical and chemical stimuli (including drugs and antigen-antibody reactions) mediate the release of histamine from the mast cell. Once histamine is released from the mast cell, a series of inflammatory reactions are triggered that range from mild itching to shock and death.

Mechanism of Action and Indications for Use

The antihistamines presented in this chapter competitively antagonize histamine at the H_1 receptor but do not bind to histamine to deactivate it. Recall from Chapter 2 that activation of H_1 receptors causes increased capillary permeability and formation of edema and wheal with itching and pain. In addition, histamine induces contraction of bronchiolar and gastrointestinal smooth muscle. Thus, antihistamines countereffect, to varying degrees, most of the pharmacological actions

Table 9.1. The Nasal Decongestants

Decongestant	Dosage Form[a]	Dosage[b]
Ephedrine HCI (Efedron Nasal Jelly)	*Nasal jelly:* 0.5%	Apply a small amount of jelly to nasal mucosa no more than q 4 hr
Ephedrine Sulfate (Vicks Vatronol, Kondon's Nasal, Pretz-D)	*Nasal spray:* 0.25% (Pretz-D) *Nasal drops:* 0.5% (Vicks Vatronol) *Nasal jelly:* 1% (Kondon's Nasal)	Refer to package brochure; dosage is product-specific
Epinephrine HCl (Adrenalin Chloride)	*Nasal solution:* 0.1%	Apply nasally as needed; do not use in children <6 years old unless under the direction of a physician
1-desoxyephedrine (Vicks Inhaler)	*Nasal inhaler:* 50 mg	1 to 2 inhalations each nostril (while occluding the other nostril) not more than q 2 hr; do not use for more than 7 days; not recommended for children <6 years old
Naphazoline HCl (Privine)	*Nasal solution:* 0.05%	1 to 2 drops or sprays each nostril as needed; do not use the spray more than q 6 hr; do not use in children <12 years old unless under the direction of a physician
Oxymetazoline HCl (Afrin, Allerest 12 Hour Nasal, Cheracol Nasal, Chlorphed-LA, Duramist Plus, Duration, Dristan, Genasal, Nasal Relief, Neo-Synephrine 12 Hour, Nōstrilla, NTZ Long Acting Nasal, 12 Hour Sinarest, Sinex Long-Acting, Twice-A-Day, 12 Hour Nasal)	*Nasal solution:* 0.025% (Afrin Children's Nose Drops), 0.05%	2 to 3 sprays or drops each nostril b.i.d.; once in the morning and once in the evening. Children 2 to 5 years: 2 to 3 drops (0.025%) each nostril b.i.d.
Phenylephrine HCl (Neo-Synephrine, Alconefrin, Rhinall, Nōstril, Sinex)	*Nasal solution:* 0.125%, 0.16%, 0.25%, 0.5%, 1%	0.125% to 0.5% solution: 2 to 3 sprays or drops each nostril q 3 to 4 hr 1% solution: 2 to 3 sprays or drops each nostril q 4 hr. Children 6 to 11 years: 2 to 3 sprays or drops (0.25%) each nostril q 3 to 4 hr. Infants >6 months: 1 to 2 drops (0.16%) each nostril q 3 hr
Phenylpropanolamine HCl (Propagest, Rhindecon)	*Tablets:* 25, 50 mg *TR capsules:* 75 mg	25 mg q 4 hr or 75 mg SR q 12 hr (do not exceed 150 mg/24 hr). Children 6 to 12 years: 12.5 mg q 4 hr (do not exceed 75 mg/24 hr) Children 2 to 6 years: 6.25 mg q 4 hr
Propylhexedrine (Benzedrex)	*Nasal inhaler:* 250 mg	1 to 2 inhalations each nostril (while occluding the other nostril) not more than q 2 hr; do not use for more than 3 days; not recommended for children <6 years old

Table 9.1.—*continued*

Decongestant	Dosage Form[a]	Dosage[b]
Pseudoephedrine HCl (Congestion Relief, Dorcol Children's Decongestant, Genaphed, Halofed, Sudafed, Pseudo-Gest, Seudotabs, DeFed-60, Efidac/24, Allermed, Sinustop Pro, Triaminic AM Decongestant Formula, Decofed Syrup, Cenafed Syrup, Novafed)	*Tablets:* 30, 60, 240 mg *Capsultes:* 60 mg *ER tablets:* 120 mg *TR capsules:* 120 mg *Liquid:* 15 mg/5 ml, 30 mg/5 ml *Drops:* 7.5 mg/0.8 ml (PediaCare Infant's Decongestant)	60 mg q 4 to 6 hr or 120 mg SR q 12 hr (do not exceed 240 mg/24 hr). Children 6 to 12 years: 30 mg q 4 to 6 hr (do not exceed 120 mg/24 hr). Children 2 to 5 years: 15 mg q 4 to 6 hr (do not exceed 60 mg/24 hr). Children 1 to 2 years: 7 drops (0.2 ml)/kg q 4 to 6 hr up to 4 doses/24 hr. Infants 3 to 12 months: 3 drops/kg q 4 to 6 hr up to 4 doses/24 hr
Pseudoephedrine Sulfate (Afrin, Drixoral Non-Drowsy Formula)	*ER tablets:* 120 mg (60 mg immediate release/60 mg delayed release)	120 mg SR q 12 hr (do not crush or chew sustained-release tablets)
Tetrahydrozoline HCl (Tyzine)	*Nasal solution:* 0.05%, 0.1%	2 to 4 drops each nostril q 3 to 4 hr as needed; or 3 to 4 sprays each nostril q 4 hr as needed. Children 2 to 6 years: 2 to 3 drops (0.05%) each nostril q 4 to 6 hr. Do not use the 0.1% nasal solution in children < 6 years old
Xylometazoline HCl (Otrivin)	*Nasal solution:* 0.05%, 0.1%	2 to 3 drops or sprays each nostril q 8 to 10 hr. Children 2 to 12 years: 2 to 3 drops (0.05%) each nostril q 8 to 10 hr

[a]TR, timed release; ER, extended release; SR, sustained release.
[b]Usual adult dose unless otherwise stated.

of histamine. These agents have negligible influence on H_2 receptors. The ability of antihistamines to block histamine action depends on both the concentration of histamine present and the concentration of the drug present. Most antihistamines also exhibit anticholinergic (drying), antipruritic, sedative, and antiemetic effects.

The first-generation histamine H_1 receptor antagonists, such as diphenhydramine, tripolidine, and chlorpheniramine, frequently cause somnolence and other CNS effects, whereas the newer, second-generation antihistamines, such as terfenadine, astemizole, and loratadine, represent an advance in therapeutics in which they not only do not produce any significant CNS side effects but also seem to have the ability to inhibit histamine release from human basophils. By this action, these second-generation antihistamines have a more favorable benefit/risk ratio with regard to lack of CNS effects, in addition to their increased effectiveness owing to their antiallergic as well as anti-inflammatory activities. Owing to these recent advances, the emerging evidence suggests that these newer, novel antihistamines may be useful and not necessarily contraindicated for patients who have both asthma and allergic rhinitis.

Antihistamines are indicated for use in the relief of symptoms accompanying allergic rhinitis; vasomotor rhinitis; allergic conjunctivitis; temporary relief of runny nose, watery eyes, and sneezing due to the common cold; angioedema; uncomplicated urticaria; and allergic reactions to blood or plasma. They are also indicated as an adjunctive therapy in anaphylactic reactions. Antihistamines with potent sedative effects are also used as nonprescription sleep aids, and those with antiemetic effects are used to treat nausea, vomiting, and motion sickness.

Contraindications

Contraindications to the use of antihistamines include antihistamine hypersensitivity, patients receiving MAO therapy, narrow-angle glaucoma, stenosing peptic ulcer. Antihistamines are not to be used for newborns, premature infants, or nursing mothers. The newer, second-generation agents are contraindicated for patients receiving erythromycin, ketoconazole, or itraconazole and for patients with significant hepatic dysfunction owing to the occurrence of severe cardiovascular disturbances (see below).

Precautions

1. Antihistamines are generally not indicated to treat lower respiratory tract symptoms owing to the anticholinergic (drying) effect, which may precipitate thickening of mucus secretions and hinder expectoration.
2. Patients must observe caution when driving or operating machinery, because antihistamines may affect alertness.
3. Use phenothiazines with caution for patients with cardiovascular disease, liver impairment, or ulcer disease (owing to cholestasia) and for children with history of sleep apnea, Reye's syndrome, or family history of sudden infant death syndrome (SIDS) (owing to diminished mental alertness).
4. Use with caution in the elderly—may cause dizziness, sedation, syncope, hypotension, or confusion.
5. Usage in pregnancy—use only if acutely indicated (antihistamines may cause harm to the fetus.) Especially not to be used during the third trimester.
6. Do not use with alcohol and other CNS depressants—additive effects are noted.
7. May cause gastrointestinal (GI) upset—antihistamines should be taken with food.
8. Some antihistamines contain sulfites, which may precipitate an allergic response (hives, itching, wheezing) in sulfite-sensitive individuals.

Adverse Reactions

Cardiovascular: Arrhythmias, hypertension, hypotension (elderly), palpitations, tachycardia.

CNS: Most frequent: drowsiness, sedation, dizziness, disturbed coordination, headache.

GI: Epigastric distress, nausea, vomiting, diarrhea, constipation, anorexia.

GU: Urinary frequency, dysuria, urinary retention, impotence.

Hematologic: Hemolytic anemia, hypoplastic anemia, aplastic anemia, thrombocytopenia, leukopenia, pancytopenia, agranulocytosis.

Pulmonary: Thickening of bronchial secretions, chest tightness, nasal congestion, wheezing, respiratory depression, sore throat, dry mouth.

Miscellaneous: Tingling, heaviness and weakness of the hands, urticaria, rash, anaphylactic shock.

Overdosage

Effects vary from CNS depression to CNS stimulation, coma, unconsciousness, cardiovascular collapse, and death. These effects are especially prevalent in very young and elderly individuals. Toxic responses may occur within 30 minutes and include drowsiness, dizziness, ataxia, tinnitus, blurred vision, and hypotension. Treatment consists of supportive measures and early intervention with gastric lavage or the induction of vomiting. To minimize absorption, administer activated charcoal following lavage.

Dosage and Administration

There are six specific groups of compounds that constitute the antihistamines:

Alkylamines: Useful and effective at low doses and practical for daytime use. This group of antihistamines may cause either CNS stimulation (excitation) or CNS depression (sedation).

Ethanolamines: Gastrointestinal effects are minimal; however, ethanolamines have the highest incidence of drowsiness. Most of these agents are available by prescription only.

Ethylenediamines: Pyrilamine—high incidence of GI upset; may cause either moderate drowsiness or excitability and hyperirritability. Tripelennamine—low incidence of side effects; most frequent are drowsiness and dry mouth.

Phenothiazines: Strong CNS depressant effects; may suppress the cough reflex and obscure symptoms of intestinal obstruction, brain tumor, overdosage of toxic drugs.

Piperidines: Available by prescription only; may cause drowsiness and dryness of mouth.

Second-Generation: These agents have a relatively long duration of activity (12 to 24 hours) with minimal CNS effects when used in prescribed doses. Significant abnormal ECG changes (QT interval prolongation, ventricular arrhythmias) have been noted in patients who receive astemizole or terfenadine and who have the following conditions:

- Hepatic dysfunction
- Concomitant administration of erythromycin, ketoconazole, or itraconazole

In some situations, syncope preceded the onset of severe arrhythmias; therefore, if a patient receiving these drugs experiences fainting spells, the drug should be immediately withheld and a full evaluation of potential arrhythmias should be closely assessed.

Table 9.2 lists the antihistamines.

ANTITUSSIVES

Mechanism of Action and Indications for Use

The cough is a protective action by which irritants (dust, liquids, foreign material, etc.) and secretions are cleared from the respiratory tract. Complete cough suppression is detrimental and should be avoided. However, when the cough is disturbing, nonproductive, or potentially exhausting, agents such as antitussives are indicated. They are frequently used to relieve chronic irritation of the airways, either from the common cold or other acute upper airway infections. As with expectorants, antitussives are purely symptomatic medications that relieve the cough, but treating the cause of the cough should be given first priority.

Two classes of antitussives are available: narcotic (primarily codeine, see also Chapter 15) and nonnarcotic. Both classes are generally central acting, suppressing the cough reflex located at the medullary cough center. There are a few nonnarcotic antitussives that act to suppress the cough reflex at its source—the stretch receptors in the respiratory passages (lungs and pleura).

Contraindications

Contraindications to the use of antitussives include hypersensitivity to any component. Use with extreme caution for patients with chronic obstructive pulmonary disease or cor pulmonale, for patients having an acute asthmatic attack, and for patients with decreased respiratory drive.

Precautions

1. The narcotic antitussives are effective cough suppressants at doses below those necessary to achieve analgesia; however, they may still exhibit respiratory depressant effects (see Chapter 15). Normal doses of these agents (especially codeine) may decrease the respiratory drive to the point of apnea. Codeine's drying action on the respiratory mucosa may thicken secretions, precipitating mucous plugging.

Table 9.2.
The Antihistamines[a]

Antihistamine	Dosage Form[b]	Dosage[c]
ALKYLAMINES		
Chlorpheniramine maleate (Chlo-Amine, Chlor-Trimeton, Chlorspan-12, Phenetron, Telachlor, Teldrin, Aller-Chlor, Pedia Care Allergy Formula, Chlor-Pro, Chlor-100, Chlortab-8, Pfeiffer's Allergy, Gen-Allerate, Chlorate, Chlortab-4, Allergy)	*Tablets:* 2, 4, 8, 12 mg *TR tablets:* 8, 12 mg *Capsules:* 12 mg *TR capsules:* 8, 12 mg *Liquid:* 1 mg/5 ml *Syrup:* 2 mg/5 ml *Injection:* 10 mg/ml, 100 mg/ml	*Injection:* 10 to 20 mg, single dose (up to 40 mg/24 hr). *PO:* 4 mg q 4 to 6 hr, or 8 to 12 mg q 8 to 12 hr (SR). Children 6 to 12 years: 2 mg q 4 to 6 hr. Children 2 to 6 years: 1 mg q 4 to 6 hr.
Dexchlorpheniramine maleate (Polaramine, Poladex, Polargen, Dexchlor)	*Tablets:* 2 mg *TR tablets:* 4, 6 mg *Syrup:* 2 mg/5 ml	2 mg q 4 to 6 hr, or 4 to 6 mg bid (SR). Children 6 to 11 years: 1 mg q 4 to 6 hr or 4 mg SR at bedtime. Children 2 to 5 years: 0.5 mg q 4 to 6 hr (do not use SR form)
Brompheniramine maleate (Dimetane, Veltane, Bromphen, Codimal-A, Cophene-B, Dehist, Histaject, Nasahist B, ND Stat, Oraminic II, Sinusol-B, Diamine T.D.)	*Tablets:* 4, 8, 12 mg *TR tablets:* 8, 12 mg *Elixir:* 2 mg/5 ml *Injection:* 10 mg/ml	*Injection:* 5 to 20 mg/dose (up to 40 mg/24 hr). Children <12 years: 0.5 mg/kg/day in 3 or 4 divided doses. *PO:* 4 mg q 4 to 6 hr, or 8 to 12 mg q 8 to 12 hr (SR)
Triprolidine HCl (Actidil, Myidil)	*Tablets:* 2.5 mg *Syrup:* 1.25 mg/5 ml	2.5 mg q 4 to 6 hr. Children 6 to 12 years: 1.25 mg q 4 to 6 hr
ETHANOLAMINES		
Diphenhydramine HCl[d] (Benadryl, Benoject-50, Banophen, Bydramine Cough, Dihydrex, Diphen Cough, Diphenhist, Gen-D-phen, Hyrexin-50, Nidryl, Nordryl, Hydramine, AllerMax, Phendry, Belix, Dormarex 2, Genahist, Scot-Tussin Allergy Relief Formula, Tusstat, Wehdryl)	*Capsules:* 25, 50 mg *Tablets:* 25, 50 mg *Liquid:* 12.5 mg/5 ml *Elixir:* 12.5 mg/5 ml *Syrup:* 12.5 mg/5 ml *Injection:* 10 mg/ml, 50 mg/ml	*Injection:* 10 to 50 mg (up to 100 mg if required, do not exceed 400 mg/24 hr). Children: 5 mg/kg/day (do not exceed 300 mg/24 hr) *PO:* 25 to 50 mg q 6 to 8 hr. Children >10 kg: 12.5 mg to 25 mg q 4 to 6 hr or 5 mg/kg/24 hr
Clemastine fumarate[d] (Tavist, Tavist-1)	*Tablets:* 1.34 mg, 2.68 mg *Syrup:* 0.67 mg/5 ml	1.34 to 2.68 mg q 8 to 12 hr
ETHYLENEDIAMINES		
Tripelennamine HCl (Pelamine, PBZ)	*Tablets:* 25, 50 mg *SR tablets:* 100 mg *Elixir:* 37.5 mg/5 ml	25 to 50 mg q 4 to 6 hr, or 100 mg q 12 hr (SR)
Pyrilamine maleate (Nisaval)	*Tablets:* 25 mg	25 to 50 mg q 6 to 8 hr
PHENOTHIAZINES		
Prometazine HCl[d] (Phenergan, Phenameth, Anergan, Prothazine, K-Phen, Phenazine, Prorex, Phencen, Pro-50, Prometh-50, Pentazine, V-Gan 50)	*Tablets:* 12.5, 25, 50 mg *Syrup:* 6.25 mg/5 ml, 25 mg/5 ml *Suppositories:* 12.5, 25, 50 mg *Injection:* 25 mg/ml, 50 mg/ml (IM use only)	*Injection:* Allergy—25 mg (repeated in 2 hr if necessary); Nausea and vomiting—12.5 to 25 mg not given more than q 4 hr; Sedation—25 to 50 mg. Children <12 years: do not exceed one-half the adult dose *PO:* Allergy—12.5 to 25 mg q 6 to 24 hr; Nausea and vomiting—25 mg q 4 to 6 hr if necessary; Sedation—25 to 50 mg; Motion sickness—25 mg b.i.d.

Table 9.2.—*continued*

Antihistamine	Dosage Form[b]	Dosage[c]
Trimeprazine[d] (Temaril)	*Tablets:* 2.5 mg *SR capsules:* 5 mg *Syrup:* 2.5 mg/5 ml	2.5 mg t.i.d. or 5 mg q 12 hr (SR). Children >3 years: 2.5 mg at bedtime or t.i.d., if necessary Children 6 months to 3 years: 1.25 mg at bedtime or t.i.d. if necessary
Methdilazine HC1[d] (Tacaryl)	*Tablets:* 4, 8 mg *Syrup:* 4 mg/5 ml	8 mg b.i.d. or d.i.d. Children >3 years: 4 mg b.i.d. or q.i.d.
PIPERIDINES		
Cyproheptadine HC1 (Periactin)	*Tablets:* 4 mg *Syrup:* 2 mg/5 ml	Initially, 4 mg t.i.d. (then 4 to 20 mg/24 hr). Children 7 to 14 years; 4 mg b.i.d., t.i.d. Children 2 to 7 years: 2 mg b.i.d. t.i.d.
Azatadine maleate (Optimine)	*Tablets:* 1 mg	1 to 2 mg b.i.d.
Phenindamine tartrate (Nolahist)	*Tablets:* 25 mg	25 mg q 4 to 6 hr. Children 6 to 11 years: 12.5 mg q 4 to 6 hr
SECOND-GENERATION ANTIHISTAMINES: LONG-ACTING, NONSEDATING		
Terfenadine (Seldane)	*Tablets:* 60 mg	60 mg q 12 hr. Children 6 to 12 years: 30 to 60 mg q 12 hr. Children 3 to 6 years: 15 mg q 12 hr
Astemizole (Hismanal)	*Tablets:* 10 mg	10 mg daily
Loratadine (Claritin)	*Tablets:* 10 mg	10 mg daily

[a]Most antihistamines have some degree of anticholinergic activity and sedative effects; however, the newer second-generation antihistamines (long-acting, nonsedating) have very minimal, if any, anticholinergic and sedative effects.
[b]TR, timed release; ER, extended release; SR, sustained release.
[c]Usual adult dose unless otherwise stated.
[d]Antiemetic effects.

2. Use with caution when giving to pregnant women—these agents may cross the placental barrier.
3. Use with caution for patients with head injuries and patients with increased intracranial pressure—narcotic antitussives have the capacity to elevate cerebrospinal fluid pressure.
4. Antitussives are not indicated for chronic cough due to smoking, asthma, or emphysema, or when excessive secretion is present.
5. Medical supervision is highly recommended when using these agents for patients with persistent headache, high fever, rash, nausea, or vomiting.
6. Avoid alcohol use (additive depressant effects) when taking narcotic antitussives.
7. May affect alertness; use with caution when driving or operating machinery.
8. May be addictive; use for only short periods of time.
9. These agents may cause GI upset; take with food or milk.

Adverse Reactions

Narcotic antitussives: Minimal side effects are noted when taking the usual oral dose; the most common are nausea, vomiting, sedation, dizziness, and constipation.

Nonnarcotic antitussives: Sedation, headache, dizziness, constipation, nausea, nasal congestion, hypersensitivity, GI upset.

Overdosage

Narcotic antitussives: CNS depression, respiratory depression, respiratory or cardiac arrest (noted with rapid intravenous administration). 0.5 to 1 g is the lethal oral dose for codeine.

Nonnarcotic antitussives: CNS stimulation (restlessness, tremors), clonic convulsions, followed by CNS depression.

Dosage and Administration

Table 9.3 lists the antitussives.

EXPECTORANTS

Mechanism of Action and Indications for Use

Expectorants increase the amount of fluid in the respiratory tract, resulting in nonproductive coughs becoming productive. Some expectorants stimulate the vagal pathway, innervating the respiratory secretory glands, whereas others absorb into

Table 9.3.
The Antitussives[a]

Antitussive	Dosage Form[b]	Dosage[c]
Codeine	*Tablets:* 15, 30, 60 mg	10 to 20 mg q 4 to 6 hr. Children 6–12 years; 5 to 10 mg q 4 to 6 hr. Children 2–6 years: 2.5 to 5 mg q 4 to 6 hr
Dextromethorphan HBr (Benylin DM, Delsym, Pertussin, Vicks Formula 44, Sucrets Cough Control, St. Joseph Cough Suppressant, Drixoral Cough Liquid Caps, Scot-Tussin DM Cough Chasers, Hold DM, Children's Hold, Robitussin Cough Calmers, Trocal, Suppress, Creo-Terpin, Robitussin Pediatric)	*Capsules:* 30 mg *Lozenges:* 2.5, 5, 7.5 mg *Liquid:* 10 mg/15 ml, 3.5 mg/5 ml, 7.5 mg/5 ml, 15 mg/5 ml *Liquid SA:* 30 mg/5 ml *Syrup:* 15 mg/15 ml, 10 mg/5 ml	10 to 30 mg q 4 to 8 hr or 60 mg q 12 hr (SA). Children 6–12 years: 5 to 10 mg q 4 hr or 15 mg q 6 to 8 hr or 30 mg q 12 hr (SA). Children 2–6 years: 2.5 to 7.5 mg q 4 to 8 hr or 15 mg q 12 hr (SA)
Diphenhydramine HCl (Benylin Cough, Bydramine, Tusstat, Diphen Cough, Silphen Cough, Uni-Bent Cough)	*Syrup:* 12.5 mg/5 ml	25 mg q 4 hr. Children 6–12 years: 12.5 mg q 4 hr. Children 2–6 years: 6.25 mg q 4 hr
Benzonatate (Tessalon Perles)	*Capsules:* 100 mg	100 mg t.i.d.

[a]For a further list of narcotics that have antitussive effects, see Chapter 15.
[b]TR, timed release; ER, extended release; SR, sustained release.
[c]Usual adult oral dose unless otherwise stated.

the respiratory secretory glands. The overall effect of stimulating the respiratory secretory glands is an increase in the production of mucus, thereby liquefying secretions and promoting ciliary activity, making the cough less frequent and more productive. The efficacy of many of these agents is not well documented because of a lack of convincing studies.

Expectorants are used for the relief of dry, nonproductive coughs and when mucus is present in the respiratory tract. These agents are used in the treatment of asthma, chronic bronchitis, bronchiectasis, cystic fibrosis, and emphysema, in which tenacious secretions may complicate the condition.

The expectorants in which guaifenesin is the base are generally considered safe and effective expectorants. Guaifenesin enhances the output of fluid from the respiratory tract by reducing the adhesiveness and surface tension of mucus, which then makes mucus less viscous and more easily expectorated.

The history of using iodides as expectorants dates back to 1939, when they were used for patients with asthma and chronic bronchitis. In addition, these agents have been used as adjunctive therapy for patients with cystic fibrosis, chronic sinusitis, and postoperative surgical patients to help prevent atelectasis. However, owing to the potential adverse effects (thyroid dysfunction [especially noted with iodinated glycerol], pulmonary edema, hypersensitivity reaction to iodide), other expectorating agents are usually preferred.

Contraindications

Contraindications to the use of expectorants includes hypersensitivity to any component. Potassium iodide is contraindicated for patients with acute bronchitis, hyperthyroidism, Addison's disease, renal disease (acute or chronic), acute dehydration, hyperkalemia, iodism, and tuberculosis. Iodinated glycerol is contraindicated for pregnant women, newborns, and nursing mothers.

Precautions

1. These agents should not be used for patients with chronic or persistent coughs without first documenting the underlying condition causing the cough. Persistent coughs usually indicate a serious condition. Medical supervision is recommended for coughs that last for more than 1 week, are recurrent, and are accompanied by fever, headache, or rash.
2. The best pharmacologic agent for persistent, nonproductive coughs is water. Patients should increase their daily intake of fluids and breathe humidified air. Expectorants, to be effective, should be taken with a full glass of water.
3. These agents are not indicated for persistent coughs that occur as a result of smoking or when there is an excessive production of secretions.
4. For some patients, chronic and repeated use of iodides may lead to hypothyroidism. Use with extreme caution, if at all, for patients with thyroid disease history. Thyroid function tests may be altered by iodide.
5. Use of an iodide preparation may cause a flare-up of adolescent acne.

Adverse Reactions

Most common: GI upset, nausea, drowsiness, dizziness, headache, rash.

Iodides: thyroid adenoma, goiter, myxedema, angioneurotic edema (hypersensitivity reaction), cutaneous and mucosal hemorrhages, serum sickness-like symptoms (fever, eosinophilia, arthralgia, lymph node enlargement). In addition, GI bleeding, confusion, arrhythmias, numbness, tingling, fatigue, weakness. Chronic iodide poisoning may occur with prolonged therapy. Manifestations include metallic taste, burning of mouth or throat, sore mouth, ulceration of mucous membranes, sneezing, swelling of the eyelids. Pulmonary edema has also resulted from the use of iodides.

Overdosage

Overdosage of expectorants is not a common problem; however, intensification of the effects listed under *Adverse Reactions* is noted. A large quantity of fluid and salt intake will help eliminate iodide.

Dosage and Administration

Table 9.4 lists the expectorants.

Table 9.4.
The Expectorants

Expectorant	Dosage Form[a]	Dosage[b]
Guaifenesin (Glyceryl Guiaiacolate) (Glycotuss, Hytuss, Gee-Gee, Breonesin, Amonidrin, Glyate, Halotussin, Malotuss, Robitussin, Scot-tussin, Humibid LA, Humibid Sprinkle, GG-Cen, Naldecon Senior EX, Guiatuss, Anti-Tuss, Genatuss, Mytussin, Uni-tussin, Diabetic Tussin EX, Hytuss 2X, Fenesin, Liquibid, Pneumomist, Respa-GF, Sinumist-SR Capsules, Touro Ex)	*Tablets:* 100, 200 mg *SR tablets:* 600 mg *Capsules:* 200 mg *SR capsules:* 300 mg *Syrup:* 100 mg/5 ml *Liquid:* 100 mg/5 ml, 200 mg/5 ml	100 to 400 mg q 4 hr. Children 6–12 years: 100 to 200 mg q 4 hr. Children 2–6 years: 50 to 100 mg q 4 hr
Iodine products (Potassium Iodide, SSKI, Pima, Iodo-Niacin)	*CA tablets:* 135 mg *Syrup:* 325 mg/5 ml *Solution:* 1 g/ml	Initially, 300 to 1000 mg after meals, t.i.d. Then, if tolerated, 1 to 1.5 g t.i.d. Children: one-half the adult dose
Iodinated glycerol (Iophen, R-Gen [21.75% alcohol], Organidin [elixir 21.75% alcohol], Par Glycerol [21.75% alcohol]	*Tablets:* 30 mg *Elixir:* 60 mg/5 ml *Solution:* 50 mg/ml	60 mg qid. Children: up to one-half the adult dose, based on weight
Terpin Hydrate (contains 42% alcohol)	*Elixir:* 85 mg/5 ml	85 to 170 mg t.i.d. or q.i.d.

[a]TR, timed release; ER, extended release; SR, sustained release; CA, controlled action.
[b]Usual adult dose unless otherwise stated.

COUGH AND COLD COMBINATIONS

Table 9.5 lists some of the more commonly used and recognized over-the-counter cough and cold preparations. Refer to package brochures for specific types and amounts of decongestant, antihistamine, expectorant, antitussive, acetaminophen, aspirin, anticholinergic, alcohol, and preservatives contained within the formula.

Table 9.5.
Common Cough and Cold Combinations

Trade Name	Dosage
Some Common Adult Cough and Cold Preparations:	
Sine-Aid Extra Strength Caplets (decongestant + acetaminophen)	2 caplets q 4 to 6 hr
Tylenol Maximum Strength Sinus Tablets and Caplets (decongestant + acetaminophen)	2 tablets q 4 to 6 hr
Actifed Syrup (decongestant + antihistamine)	10 ml q 4 to 6 hr
Allerest 12 Hour Caplets (decongestant + antihistamine)	1 capsule q 12 hr
Contac Maximum Strength 12 Hour Caplets (decongestant + antihistamine)	1 capsule q 12 hr
Dimetapp Extentabs (decongestant + antihistamine)	1 tablet q 12 hr
Sudafed Plus Tablets (decongestant + antihistamine)	1 tablet q 4 to 6 hr
Triaminic Allergy Tablets (decongestant + antihistamine)	1 tablet q 4 hr
Comtrex Liqui-Gels (decongestant + antihistamine + antitussive + acetaminophen)	2 capsules q 4 hr
Dimetapp DM Elixir (decongestant + antihistamine + antitussive)	10 ml q 4 hr
Alka-Seltzer Plus Night-Time Cold Tablets (decongestant + antihistamine + antitussive, aspirin)	2 tablets q 4 hr
CoTylenol Cold Tablets (decongestant + antihistamine + anititussive + acetaminophen)	2 tablets q 6 hr
Contac Severe Cold & Flu Nighttime Liquid (decongestant + antihistamine + anititussive + acetaminophen, 18.5% alcohol)	30 ml q 6 hr or 30 ml hs
NyQuil Nighttime Cold/Flue Medicine Liquid (decongestant + antihistamine + anititussive + acetaminophen, 25% alcohol)	30 ml q 6 hr or 30 ml hs
Robitussin Night Relief Liquid (decongestant + antihistamine + anititussive + acetaminophen)	30 ml hs or 30 ml q 6 hr
Robitussin-PE Syrup (decongestant + expectorant)	10 ml q 4 hr
Robitussin DAC Syrup (decongestant + antitussive + expectorant, 1.4 % alcohol)	10 ml q 4 hr
Robitussin-CF Liquid (decongestant + antitussive + expectorant, 4.75% alcohol)	10 ml q 4 hr
Vicks DayQuil Liquid (decongestant + antitussive + expectorant)	30 ml q 4 hr
Triaminic Expectorant DH Liquid (decongestant + antihistamine + antitussive + expectorant, 5% alcohol)	10 ml q 4 hr
Phanadex Cough Syrup (decongestant + antihistamine + antitussive + expectorant)	10 ml q 4 to 6 hr
Father John's Medicine Plus Liquid (decongestant + antihistamine + antitussive + expectorant)	5 to 10 ml q 3 to 4 hr
Extra Action Cough Syrup (antitussive + expectorant, 1.4% alcohol)	10 ml q 6 to 8 hr
Robitussin-DM Liquid (antitussive + expectorant)	10 ml q 4 hr
Some Common Pediatric Cough and Cold Preparations:	
Children's Allerest Tablets (decongestant + antihistamine)	2 tablets q 4 hr
Triaminic Syrup (decongestant + antihistamine)	10 ml q 4 hr
Pedia Care Cough-Cold Liquid (decongestant + antihistamine + antitussive)	10 ml q 4 to 6 hr
Vicks Children's NyQuil Nighttime Cold/Cough Liquid (decongestant + antihistamine + antitussive)	15 ml q 6 hr
Naldecon-DX Children's Syrup (decongestant + antitussive + expectorant)	5 to 10 ml q.i.d.
Dorcol Children's Cough Syrup (decongestant + antitussive + expectorant)	5 to 10 ml q 4 hr
Pediacof Syrup (decongestant + antihistamine + antitussive + expectorant)	1.25 to 10 ml q 4 to 6 hr
Children's Formula Cough Syrup (antitussive + expectorant)	5 to 10 ml q 6 hr
Vicks Pediatric Formula 44E Liquid (antitussive + expectorant)	7.5 to 15 ml q 4 hr

When using these combination products, carefully consider which symptoms are present and buy accordingly.

REFERENCES/RECOMMENDED READING

Alstead S. Potassium iodide and ipecacuanha as expectorants. Lancet 2:932, 1939.

Becker CB, Gordon JM. Iodinated glycerol and thyroid function. Four cases and a review of the literature. Chest 103:188, 1993.

Busse WW. Role of antihistamines in allergic disease. Ann Allergy 72:371, 1994.

Drug facts and comparisons. 49th ed. St. Louis: Facts and Comparisons, 1995.

Geurian K, Branam C. Iodine poisoning secondary to long-term iodinated glycerol. Arch Intern Med 154:1153, 1994.

Heyman SN, Mevorach D, Ghanem J. Hypertensive crisis from chronic intoxication with nasal decongestant and cough medications. DICP 25:1068, 1991.

Huang T, Peterson GH. Pulmonary edema and iododerma induced by potassium iodide in the treatment of asthma. Ann Allergy 46:264, 1981.

Huseby JS, Bennett SW, Hagensee ME. Hyperthyroidism induced by iodinated glycerol. Am Rev Respir Dis 144:1403, 1991.

Irwin RS, Curley FJ, Bennett FM. Appropriate use of antitussives and protussives. A practical review. Drugs 46:80, 1993.

Kobayashi RH, et al. Topical nasal sprays: treatment of allergic rhinitis. Am Fam Physician 50:151, 1994.

Lurie A, et al. Methods for clinical assessment of expectorants: a critical review. Int J Clin Pharmacol Res 12:47, 1992.

Miadonna A, et al. Inhibitory effect of the H1 antagonist loratadine on histamine release from human basophils. Int Arch Allergy Immunol 105:12, 1994.

Physicians Desk Reference. 49th ed. Montvale, NJ: Medical Economics, 1995.

Simons FE. H1-receptor antagonists. Comparative tolerability and safety. Drug Saf 10:350, 1994.

Zervanos NJ, Shute KM. Acute, disruptive cough. Symptomatic therapy for a nagging problem. Postgrad Med 95:153, 1994.

BRONCHODILATORS 10

Airway smooth muscle tone is regulated by the autonomic nervous system (ANS). Specifically, the sympathetic (adrenergic), the parasympathetic (cholinergic), and the nonadrenergic noncholinergic (NANC) nervous systems. In addition to regulating airway smooth muscle tone, the component nervous systems of the ANS influence secretion of mucus from submucosal glands, vascular permeability and blood flow, fluid transport across airway epithelium, and release of mediators from mast cells that participate in the inflammatory response. Bronchodilators work, in one way or another, to relax and dilate bronchial smooth muscle, inhibit antigen-induced release of mast cell mediators, reduce vascular permeability, and enhance the mucociliary transport of respiratory secretions.

Three primary drug categories comprise the class of drugs known as bronchodilators, which are administered to patients with airflow obstruction:

- Sympathomimetic (β_2-adrenoceptor) bronchodilators
- Anticholinergic (antimuscarinic) bronchodilators
- Xanthine bronchodilators

This chapter focuses on these three classes of bronchodilators, as well as the clinical application of these agents and the factors that precipitate bronchospasm.

SYMPATHOMIMETIC (β_2-ADRENOCEPTOR) BRONCHODILATORS

Sympathomimetic drugs have been used since the days of antiquity to relieve a variety of respiratory and cardiovascular disorders. For more than 5000 years, the Chinese used *Ma Huang,* an ancient oriental remedy, which was derived from the plant *Ephedra equisetina*. In the late 1800s, ephedrine (an epinephrine-like agent) was isolated as the active ingredient, and in 1927, ephedrine became available for use in the USA to treat bronchospastic disorders such as asthma.

The use of the catecholamine epinephrine as a bronchodilator dates back to the turn of the century, when Solis-Cohen used desiccated adrenal glands to treat asthma. Epinephrine, the natural adrenal gland hormone and neurotransmitter, is the prototype drug of all β_2-adrenoceptor bronchodilators. In 1940, isoproterenol, a potent nonselective β-agonist, gained wide acceptance as a bronchodilator. The next bronchodilator to appear, isoetharine, was the first preferentially selective β_2-agonist.

Since the mid-1960s, the direction of development of sympathomimetic bronchodilators has been toward safe, very β_2-specific, longer-acting agents. Distinctions between the various β_2-adrenoceptor agonists are based on differences in chemistry and on selectivity for the β_2-adrenoceptor over the β_1-adrenoceptor. Modification of the primary catechol nucleus has resulted in the very β_2-specific resorcinol and saligenin groups of sympathomimetic bronchodilators. The β_2-adrenoceptor bronchodilators are widely regarded as the mainstay of therapy in treating patients with airflow obstruction.

Mechanism of Action and Indications for Use

Autoradiographic studies have shown that the airways are well populated with β_2-adrenoceptors; high densities of these receptors are found in the smaller, peripheral airways. β-adrenoceptors have also been localized to airway epithelium, alveolar walls, vascular smooth muscle, and submucosal glands. Endogenous catecholamines (the presynaptic neurotransmitter norepinephrine or epinephrine secreted by the adrenal medulla) or exogenous β_2-adrenoceptor agonists (drugs) have the ability to stimulate and activate the β_2-adrenoceptors. The sequence of events that occurs when β_2-adrenoceptors are stimulated leads to the activation of adenyl cyclase, which then catalyzes the conversion of adenosine triphosphate (ATP) to cyclic 3′,5′-adenosine monophosphate (cAMP). It is the level of intracellular cAMP that is responsible for the relaxation of airway smooth muscle (Fig. 10.1).

β_2-adrenoceptor agonists are potent bronchodilators, and this bronchodilation represents the main therapeutic effect of β_2-adrenoceptor drugs. Secondary beneficial actions are also noted with these agents; they inhibit antigen-induced release of mast cell mediators, reduce vascular permeability, and enhance the mucociliary transport of respiratory secretions.

β_2-adrenoceptor bronchodilators are indicated for the relief of acute or chronic bronchospasm such as that which occurs in asthma, bronchitis, emphysema, bronchiectasis, pneumonia, cystic fibrosis, and other respiratory infections. These agents are also beneficial in the prevention of exercise-induced bronchospasm.

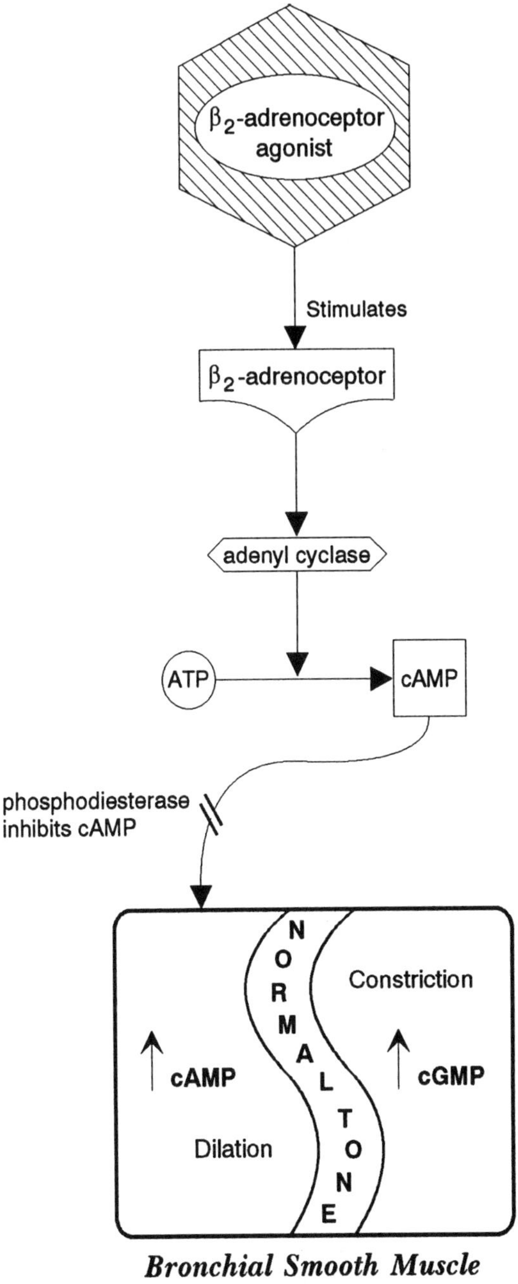

Figure 10.1. Pharmacologic control of bronchomotor tone with β_2-adrenergic agonists.

Classification of the β_2-Adrenoceptor Bronchodilators

Most β_2-adrenoceptor bronchodilators are either catecholamines or catecholamine derivatives. The basic catecholamine structure is depicted in Figure 10.2. Catecholamines contain a benzene ring with hydroxyl groups attached at the third and fourth carbon sites (the catechol nucleus), as well as an amine side chain fixed to the first carbon position.

The exception to the above, in that most β_2-adrenoceptor bronchodilators are either catecholamines or catecholamine derivatives, is ephedrine. Ephedrine is a noncatecholamine; its main advantage is its activity after oral administration. Catecholamines cannot be taken orally owing to their conjugation with sulfate or glucuronide in the gastrointestinal (GI) system. Lacking hydroxyl groups on the benzene ring (see Fig. 10.3), ephedrine is not subject to degradation by sulfate and glucuronide in the GI system and liver or by catechol-O-methyltransferase (COMT). However, ephedrine has two serious disadvantages. First, ephedrine is a weak bronchodilator, the effects of which result primarily from its ability to release endogenous catecholamines, and thus has no receptor selectivity. Second, ephedrine readily crosses the blood-brain barrier because it lacks the hydrophilic hydroxyl groups on the benzene ring. By this mechanism, ephedrine exerts central nervous system (CNS) effects similar to those of amphetamines. Insomnia is

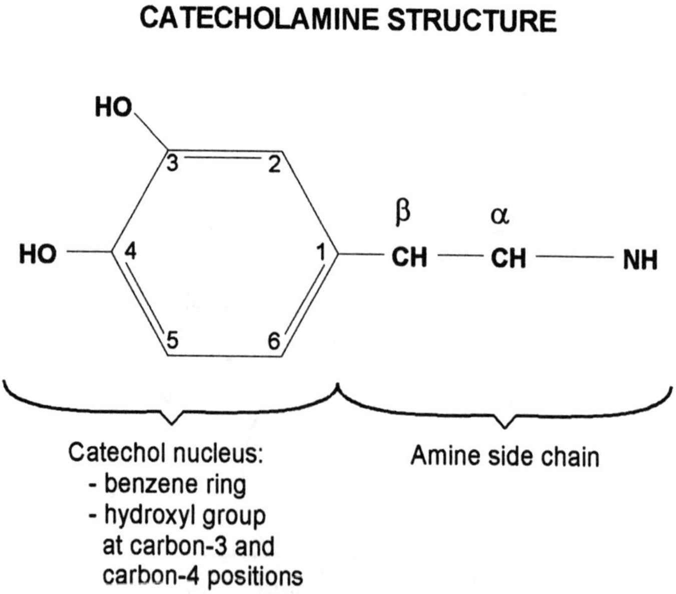

Figure 10.2. The basic catecholamine structure.

EPHEDRINE

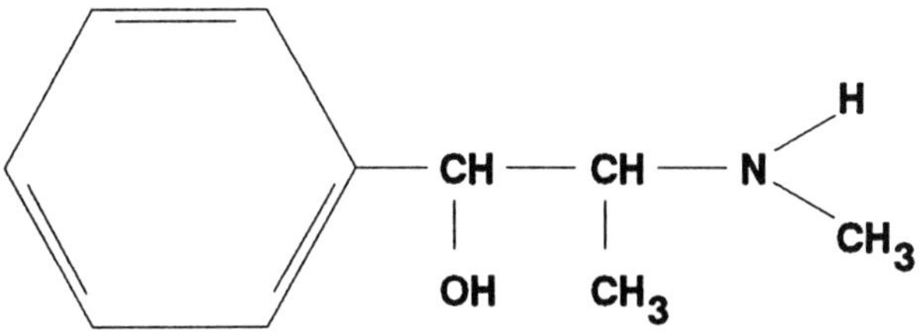

Figure 10.3. Ephedrine's chemical structure. Notice that it lacks the two hydroxyl groups attached to the benzene ring.

a common side effect. Because of ephedrine's properties, it has therapeutic usefulness as a decongestant (see Chapter 9).

Currently, three primary classes of β_2-adrenoceptor bronchodilators are available for use: the catecholamines (first generation) and their synthetic analogues, the resorcinols (second generation), and the saligenins (third generation).

First-Generation β_2-Adrenoceptor Bronchodilators—The Catecholamines

The catecholamine class of bronchodilators includes epinephrine and the synthetic derivatives: isoproterenol, isoetharine, rimiterol, and hexoprenaline. Rimiterol and hexoprenaline are currently available abroad as Pulmadil and Ipradol, respectively. Epinephrine, isoproterenol, and isoetharine were the only approved, most commonly used β_2-adrenoceptor aerosol bronchodilators for many years until several analogues (catecholamine derivatives) became available and were approved for use in the USA.

Figure 10.4 identifies the chemical structures of epinephrine, isoproterenol, and isoetharine. These catecholamines, by their nature, contain a benzene ring with hydroxyl groups attached at the third and fourth carbon sites (the catechol nucleus) as well as an amine side chain fixed to the first carbon position. The shift from an agent that has primary α activity toward one with both potent α and β effects results when the bulk of the amine side chain attached to the catechol base becomes larger and more complex with the addition of a methyl group. For example, the substitution of a methyl group for hydrogen to norepinephrine's side chain (see Chapter 2, Fig. 2.8) creates epinephrine and converts a compound with primary α activity (norepinephrine) to an agent that has both α and β effects (epinephrine). Thus, by its chemical structure, epinephrine is a highly potent stimulator of both α- and β-adrenoceptors.

The addition of a second methyl group in the terminal portion of the side chain

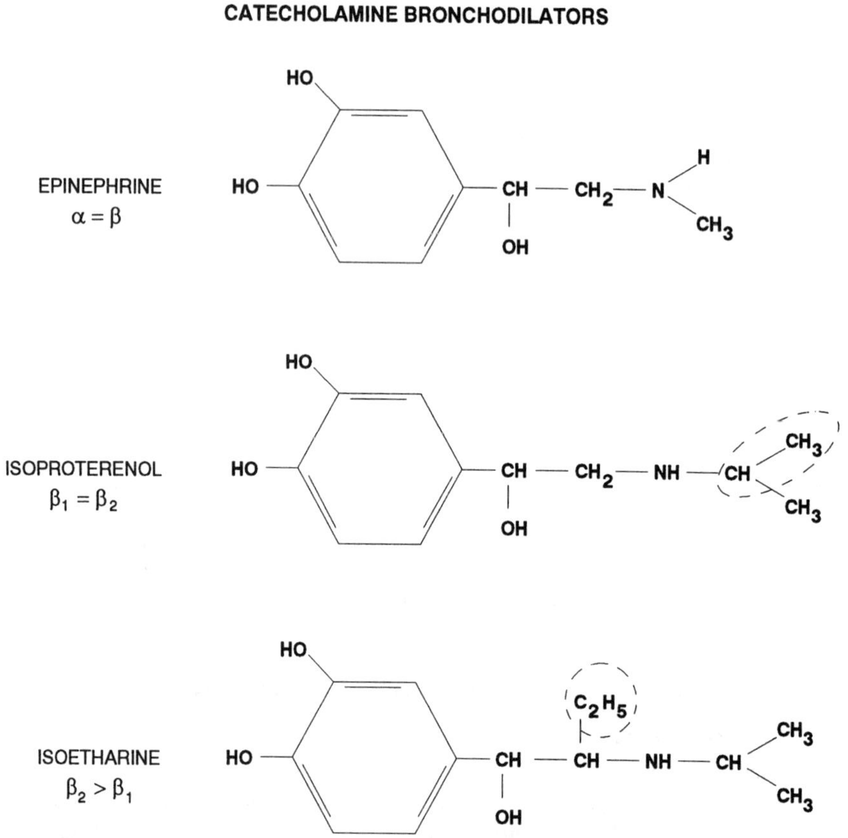

Figure 10.4. The chemical structures of epinephrine, isproterenol, and isoetharine. The shift toward β_2 specificity is through the modification of the amine side chain. The dashed circles represent the modification in the side chain from the previous structure.

diminishes α effects and gives rise to an agent that has mostly β effects. Isoproterenol is such an agent, which is an equal potent stimulator on both β subtypes with little to no α activity. Isoetharine differs from isoproterenol in that an ethyl group has been added in the α carbon of the side chain. This further modification and increase in the side chain produces an agent that has β_2 selectivity over β_1, as well as minimal α activity. Although isoetharine has preferential β_2 selectivity over isoproterenol with less β_1 (cardiostimulation) activity, its bronchodilator activity is not as great as isoproterenol. Thus, an agent may have β_2 preferential activity yet not be the most effective bronchodilator.

Overall, as the bulk of the amine side chain increases, a "better fit" to the β_2-adrenoceptor is realized. This phenomenon is known as the *keyhole theory* of β-adrenoceptors (i.e., the lock and key mechanism referred to in Chapter 3). Extensive investigation into the structure-activity relationships (SAR) of drugs and receptors has led to the development of highly efficacious analogues that have great therapeutic value as bronchodilators. This is especially noted with the resorcinol and saligenin groups of bronchodilators, as discussed later in this chapter.

Although effective and potent (isoproterenol is ranked highest in potency as both a β_1 and β_2 stimulant), the catecholamine class of bronchodilators has two primary disadvantages for use in patients with airflow obstruction. First, the catecholamines are severely limited in their duration of effectiveness, which is 1 to 3 hours at most (rapidly metabolized by the cytoplasmic enzyme COMT). Epinephrine is rapidly degraded to metanephrine (see Chapter 2, Fig. 2.9), whereas isoproterenol is metabolized by COMT to 3-methoxy isoproterenol, a weak β-blocker. Agents that have a longer duration of activity are preferred, especially in those patients who experience nocturnal asthma. In addition, catecholamines are inactivated in the GI tract and liver by sulfate or glucuronide; therefore, they are unsuitable for oral administration.

Second, the catecholamines elicit undesired side effects (dose dependent) owing to their nonselective ability to also stimulate the α- and/or β_1-adrenoceptors (especially noted with epinephrine and isoproterenol). Adverse reactions noted with these drugs include palpitations, tachycardia, increased blood pressure, skeletal muscle tremor (from stimulating the β_2-adrenoceptors of skeletal muscle), headache, dizziness, irritability, anxiety, insomnia, nausea, and worsening of the V/Q ratio (decrease in PaO_2—noted with isoproterenol administration). The reason for the reduced V/Q ratio seems to result from isoproterenol's ability to improve pulmonary blood flow without a concomitant improvement in ventilation (especially in poorly ventilated lung units).

Metabolic derangements such as hypokalemia have also been noted with these agents, as well as with the newer β_2-selective agonists. The decrease in serum potassium level is believed to be a result of intracellular movement of potassium secondary to insulin release from stimulation of pancreatic β_2-adrenoceptors. A primary concern with this reaction is hypokalemic induced arrhythmias. In addition, the practitioner should be aware that the diabetic patient may exhibit unusual reactions to β_2 sympathomimetics owing to the increase in blood glucose and insulin levels that result from the stimulation of pancreatic β_2-adrenoceptors. Occasionally, a diabetic patient may require adjustment of his/her insulin dose when β_2-adrenoceptor therapy is initiated.

All catecholamines are stored in amber containers because they are readily inactivated to inert adrenochromes when exposed to heat, light, or air. The resulting pinkish residue after a nebulizer treatment, as well as a pink tinge to a patient's sputum, occurs from this oxidation of catecholamines.

Bitolterol, a sympathomimetic bronchodilator approved for clinical application in the USA, differs from the previous agents mentioned in that it is a pro-drug that is converted to its parent active catecholamine compound, colterol, by esterase enzymes (Fig. 10.5). The process of hydrolysis is slow, gradually releasing the active catecholamine. By this mechanism, a sustained duration (up to 8 hours) results. Once fully activated, colterol may be metabolized by COMT. Bitolterol is noted to have less cardiovascular side effects when compared with the other sympathomimetics of the catecholamine class.

Racemic epinephrine is yet another catecholamine that is a synthetic mixture of two *stereoisomers* of epinephrine (*l*-epinephrine [active component] and *d*-epinephrine [inactive component]) primarily utilized, not for its β_2-bronchodilator activity, but for its α action. Racemic epinephrine has approximately one-half the vasopressor effects of epinephrine and has been recommended for upper airway edema, such as that which occurs in laryngotracheobronchitis and post-extubation stridor.

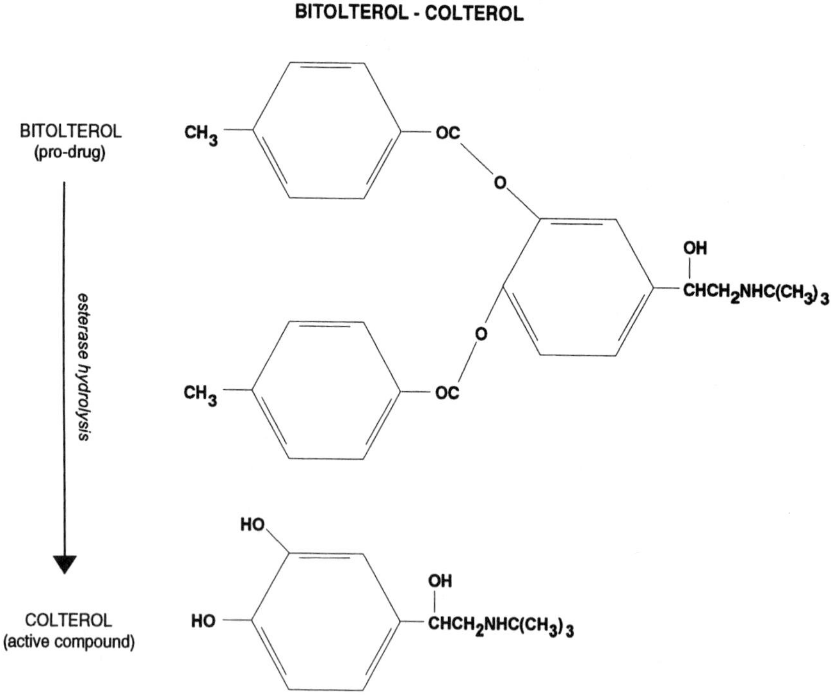

Figure 10.5. The pro-drug, bitolterol, is converted to its active parent compound, colterol (a catecholamine), by esterase enzymes.

Second-Generation β_2-Adrenoceptor Bronchodilators—The Resorcinols

The basic rearrangement of the catechol nucleus by shifting the hydroxyl attachment at the carbon-4 site to the carbon-5 site produces the resorcinol nucleus (Fig. 10.6). Because of this arrangement, the resorcinols are resistant to metabolism by COMT and thus have a relatively longer duration of action (3 to 6 hours) than the catecholamines. In addition, the resorcinols can be taken orally because they are not inactivated in the GI tract and liver by sulfatase enzymes.

The resorcinol class of sympathomimetic bronchodilators includes metaproterenol, terbutaline, and fenoterol. Metaproterenol, reported for the treatment of asthma in the early 1960s, was the first derivative marketed. Terbutaline and fenoterol then followed. Fenoterol is not commercially available in the USA, but metaproterenol and terbutaline are. It is not clear whether fenoterol will be approved for use in the USA owing to concerns regarding fenoterol's margin of safety. Recent studies have linked the regular and long-term use of fenoterol with an increased risk of death or near death in asthmatic patients (Spitzer et al. 1992, Sears et al. 1990). In addition, fenoterol caused more adverse cardiac effects and a greater reduction in plasma potassium concentration than albuterol, terbutaline, or isoproterenol.

Terbutaline is more highly β_2-selective, has less β_1 effects, and has a longer duration of activity than metaproterenol. This fact is illustrated in Figure 10.7. The addition of a tertiary butyl group to terbutaline's terminal portion of the side chain leads to increased β_2-specificity with minimal to no β_1 activity.

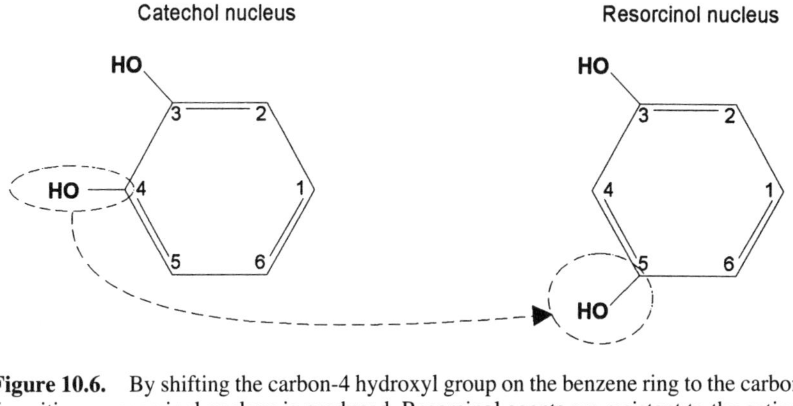

Figure 10.6. By shifting the carbon-4 hydroxyl group on the benzene ring to the carbon-5 position, a resorcinol nucleus is produced. Resorcinol agents are resistant to the actions of catechol-O-methyltransferase (COMT) and to the sulfatases; therefore, they not only have a longer duration of activity than catecholamines but may be taken orally.

RESORCINOL BRONCHODILATORS

METAPROTERENOL

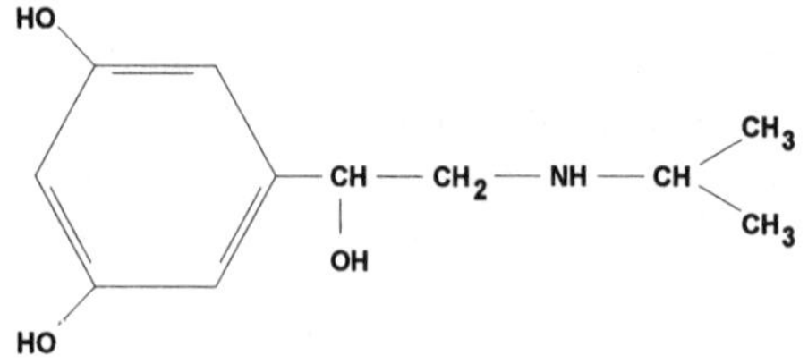

TERBUTALINE

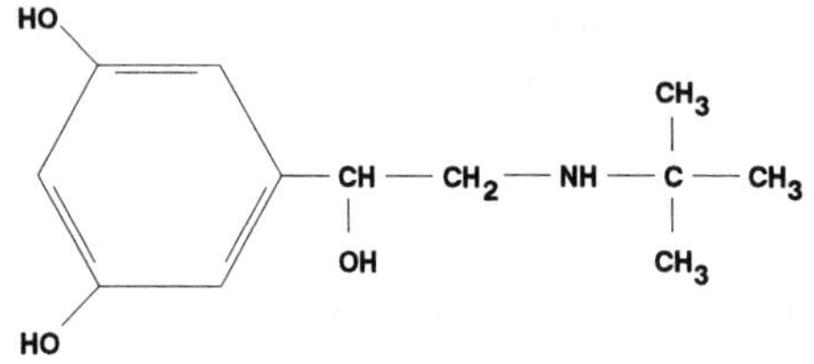

FENOTEROL

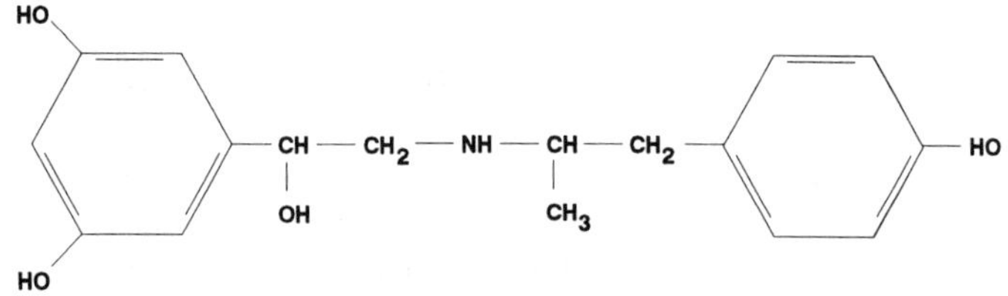

Figure 10.7. The chemical structures of the resorcinol bronchodilators. Terbutaline has greater β_2-receptor selectivity than metaproterenol owing to the addition of a tertiary butyl group. Terbutaline and fenoterol have approximately equal potency.

Third-Generation β_2-Adrenoceptor Bronchodilators—The Saligenins

Substitution of a saligenin for the 3-hydroxyl group on the benzene ring produces the saligenin nucleus (Fig. 10.8). The saligenin group of bronchodilators are not metabolized by COMT or readily conjugated and, thus, are active orally and have a duration of action of several hours.

Albuterol (salbutamol in Europe), pirbuterol, carbuterol, and salmeterol are sympathomimetic bronchodilators of the saligenin class. β_2-specificity, minimal cardiac effects, and a long duration of activity are noted features of this class of drugs. The chemical structures of these agents are detailed in Figure 10.9.

Albuterol has gained tremendous popularity within the last decade as an effective and safe bronchodilator. In addition to its use as a bronchodilator, albuterol may have some unusual clinical values. Intravenous administration of albuterol (as

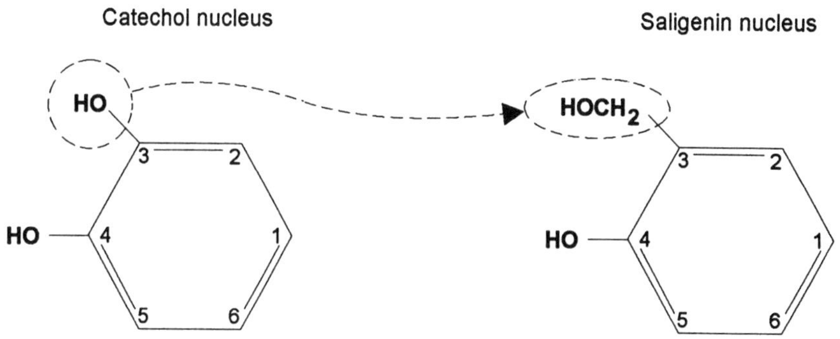

Figure 10.8. Substitution of a saligenin for the 3-hydroxyl group on the benzene ring produces the saligenin nucleus.

well as terbutaline) inhibits premature labor, and nebulized albuterol therapy (10 to 20 mg) has been used as an adjunct in treating serious acute hyperkalemia.

Pirbuterol is structurally similar to albuterol with similar pharmacological effects, although it is slightly less potent. Pirbuterol's difference from albuterol lies with the replacement of the benzene ring with a pyridine ring (see Fig. 10.9). Carbuterol (marketed abroad) also has pharmacologic effects that are very similar to albuterol. However, carbuterol is less potent and has a shorter duration of effectiveness (approximately 4 hours). For these selective β_2-adrenoceptor agonists, the most common side effects are skeletal muscle tremor and palpitations.

The most recently saligenin bronchodilator approved by the Food and Drug Administration (FDA) (as of February 1994) that seems to have a promising future in the application of β_2-adrenoceptor therapy is salmeterol. Numerous clinical trials have compared the pharmacological properties of salmeterol with those of albuterol. The overwhelming consensus is that salmeterol is a superior β_2-adrenoceptor agonist in its efficacy and duration of activity. Salmeterol produces a greater and sustained increase in respiratory function, with a duration of activity two to three times that of albuterol—12 or more hours in most cases. Interestingly, some investigators referred to albuterol as the "short-acting" β_2-adrenoceptor agonist, a term that has never been associated with albuterol until the advent of salmeterol. The salmeterol-treated group of asthmatic patients experienced fewer symptoms of asthma and related events than the albuterol treated group. Smyth and colleagues (1993) indicate that salmeterol may be up to 10 times more potent than albuterol; 0.05 mg of salmeterol administered twice daily may be as effective as albuterol 0.5 mg administered every 4 to 6 hours. The one negative drawback of salmeterol is that it has a slower onset of action than albuterol. In the study by Simons and associates (1992), the increase in FEV_1 was significantly lower for salmeterol than for albuterol for the first one-half hour after administration. However, from 3 to 12 hours after administration, salmeterol's response greatly exceeded

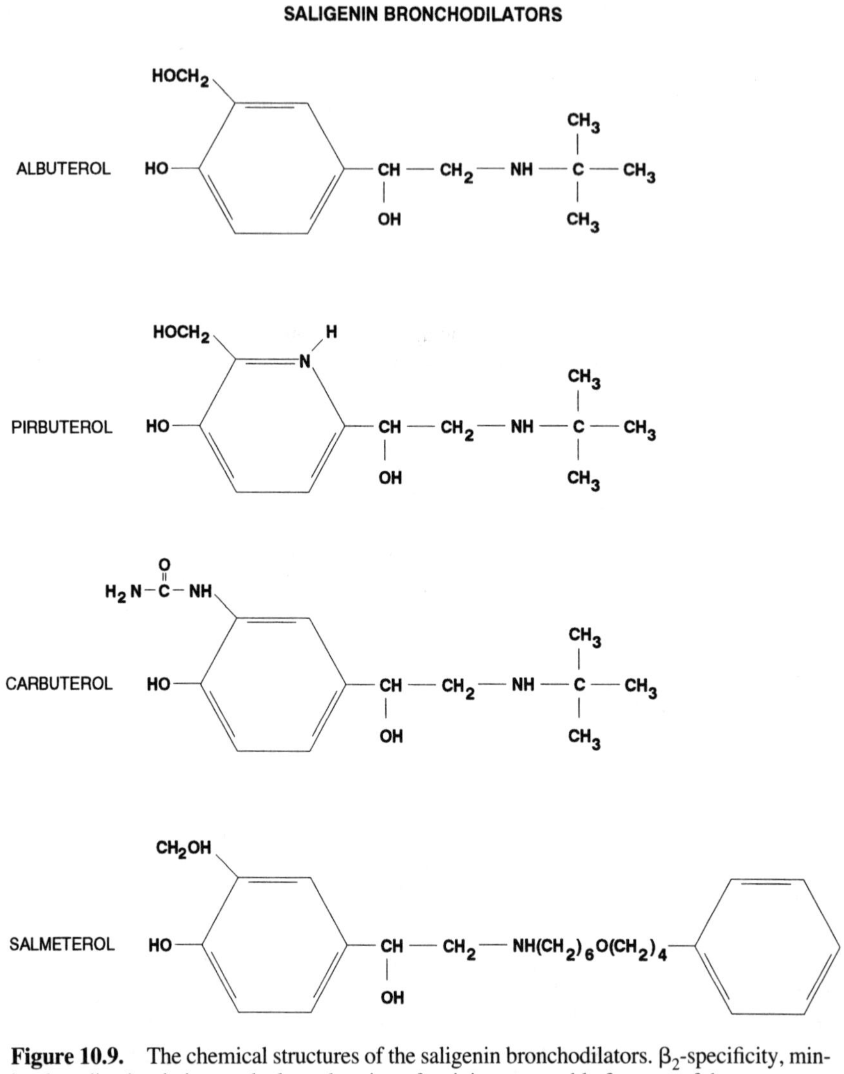

Figure 10.9. The chemical structures of the saligenin bronchodilators. β_2-specificity, minimal cardiostimulation, and a long duration of activity are notable features of these agents.

that of albuterol. Because of salmeterol's slower onset of action, which is an unusual characteristic for a β_2-adrenoceptor agonist, salmeterol would not be indicated for the rapid relief of acute bronchospasm. Regardless of the slower onset of action, a significantly lower incidence in nocturnal and daytime symptoms in salmeterol-treated asthmatics has been noted; therefore, salmeterol would be suitable for stable asthmatics or for those who experience nocturnal asthma. Adverse reactions to salmeterol were infrequent and mild; tremor and palpitations were reported in some of the patients who were administered higher than normal doses. Like other β_2-adrenoceptor agonists, salmeterol reduces vascular permeability, inhibits the release of mediators, and enhances mucociliary function. However, unlike the other β_2-adrenoceptor agonists, salmeterol exhibits this stimulatory effect with a higher efficacy and for up to 12 hours.

Miscellaneous Sympathomimetic (β_2-Adrenoceptor) Bronchodilators

Procaterol is a β_2-specific adrenoceptor agent that was synthesized by Yoshizaki and coworkers in 1976. It is unlike the agents previously mentioned in that it is a bicyclic compound (Fig. 10.10). Procaterol exhibits properties similar to the synthetic analogs of the catecholamine class of bronchodilators in that it is not metabolized by COMT and can be taken orally. Currently available in Canada, procaterol exhibits a higher potency and longer duration of activity (up to 8 hours) than albuterol.

Formoterol is an investigational agent that has pharmacological properties very similar to salmeterol. By nature of its bulky side chain (see Fig. 10.10), formoterol exhibits a very high affinity and selectivity for the β_2-adrenoceptor. For-

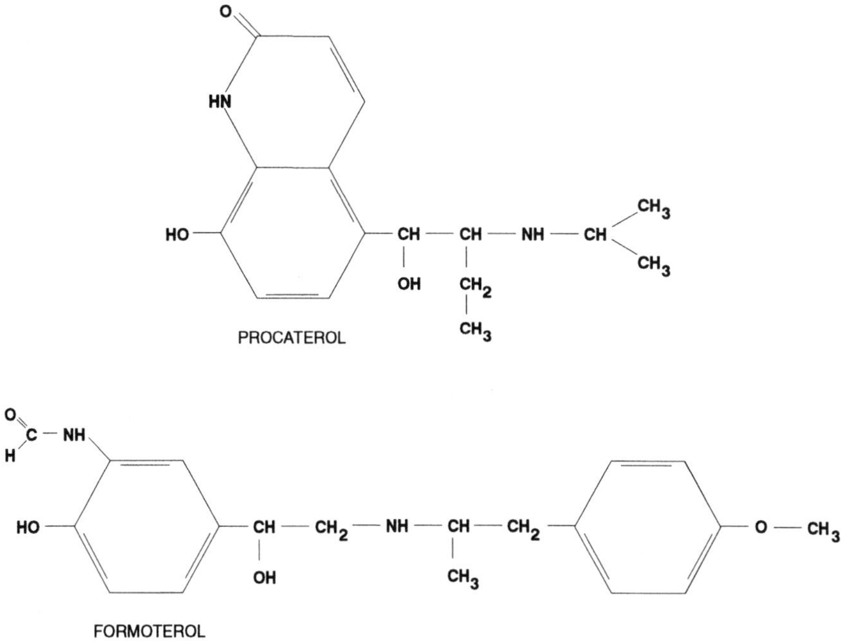

Figure 10.10. The chemical structures of procaterol and formoterol.

moterol has the added benefit of a duration of activity in excess of 12 hours. Comparatively, 12 μg of formoterol is equipotent to 50 μg of salmeterol. However, unlike salmeterol, formoterol has the clinical advantage of a rapid onset of action: within 1 minute after inhalation, formoterol produces a significant improvement in respiratory function. The most commonly reported side effect was tremor, which was especially noted in doses higher than 12 μg. Studies comparing the pharmacologic effects of formoterol with those of albuterol produced similar results as those studies comparing salmeterol with albuterol. These studies reported that the formoterol-treated patients not only had a sustained improvement in respiratory function but also had less daytime and nocturnal asthma symptoms than the albuterol-treated patients.

The recent development of new β_2-adrenoceptor agonists with a duration of action in excess of 12 hours may change the strategies in the treatment of bronchial asthma. These bronchodilating agents have not only brought forth a new concept to bronchodilator pharmacology but have also given clinicians viable alternatives for safe, effective, and long-lasting pharmacological manipulation of airway caliber.

Modes of Administration

As can be seen in Table 10.1, the β_2-adrenoceptor bronchodilators may be administered via the oral, inhalation, or parenteral (intravenous [IV], intramuscular [IM], subcutaneous [SC]) routes; the exception is that catecholamines cannot be administered orally. The inhaled route of β_2-adrenoceptor agonist administration is commonly preferred because: onset of action is very rapid (generally noted within 5 to 15 minutes); inhalation delivers the drug directly to the desired site of action—the airways; systemic side effects are minimal when these agents are administered in prescribed therapeutic doses; and administration by inhalation requires much smaller doses to achieve a desired therapeutic response. There is increasing evidence that β_2-adrenoceptor-mediated bronchodilation requires penetration of the aerosol into the smaller, peripheral airways (Newhouse and Ruffin 1978, Ingram et al. 1977, Hensley et al. 1978).

A deviation from standard therapy in which the bronchodilator is given as a single aerosolized dose 4 to 6 times per day is that of continuous nebulization. This mode of therapy is reserved for those seriously ill patients who exhibit severe asthma (e.g., status asthmaticus). Administration methods that have been used to deliver continuous nebulization include the following:

- Continuous refilling of a small volume nebulizer (SVN)
- Volumetric infusion pump with an in-line SVN
- Large reservoir, Vortran, high aerosol output nebulizer
- Small-particle aerosol generator (SPAG-2)

Table 10.1
β_2-Adrenoceptor Bronchodilators

Bronchodilator	Activity[a] α β1 β2	Preparations[b]	Dosages[c]	Onset (min)	Peak (min)	Duration (hours)
Noncatecholamine:						
Ephedrine (generic)	+2 +3 +3	PO: 25, 50 mg capsules IM, SC: 25 mg/ml, 50 mg/ml	25–50 mg b.i.d., t.i.d. 25–50 mg Children >2 yr: PO or SC: 3 mg/kg/day in 4–6 divided doses	PO: 15–60 IM: 10–20 SC: >20	120 ≤30 ≤30	3–5 ≤1 ≤1
Catecholamines:						
Epinephrine (Asthmahaler, Bronitin Mist, Bronkaid Mist, Primatine Mist, Medihaler-Epi, Sus-Phrine, Adrenalin)	+3 +4 +3	MDI: 0.16, 0.2, 0.27 mg/spray Nebulizer: 1:100 (10 mg/mL) IM, SC: 1:1000 (1 mg/mL); suspension—1:200 (5 mg/mL)	1–2 puffs q.i.d. 0.25–0.5 mL q.i.d. 1:1000—0.3 to 0.5 mL (repeat q 20 min to 4 h p.r.n.); 1:200—SC use only, 0.1 to 0.3 mL p.r.n. not more often than q 6 h Infants and children: IM, SC: 1:1000—0.01 mL/kg (repeat q 20 min to 4 h p.r.n.; 1:200—0.005 mL/kg SC p.r.n. not more often than q 6 h	Inhal: 3–5 IM: variable SC: 6–15	5–20 20–30	1–3 1–4 1–4
Ethylnorepinephrine (Bronkephrine)	+2 +2 +2	SC, IM: 2mg/mL	0.5–1 mL Children (dosage varies by age and weight): 0.1–0.5 mL	SC: 5–10 IM: 5–10	≤30 ≤30	1–2 1–2
Isoproterenol (Isuprel, Isuprel Glossets, Medihaler-Iso)	— +4 +4	MDI: 0.08, 0.13 mg/spray Nebulizer: 1:100 (10 mg/ml); 1:200 (5 mg/ml); 1:400 (2.5 mg/ml) IV: 1:5000 (0.2 mg/mL) SL: 10, 15 mg tablets	1–2 puffs q.i.d. 0.25–0.5 mL q.i.d. 0.01–0.02 mg, p.r.n. 10–20 mg, p.r.n. (not to exceed 60 mg/day) Children: Nebulizer: 0.25 mL of 1:200 solution SL: 5–10 mg, p.r.n. (not to exceed 30 mg/day)	Inhal: 2–5 IV: immediate SL: ≤30	5–30 <60	0.5–2 <1 1–2

Table 10.1—*continued*

Bronchodilator	Activity[a] α β_1 β_2	Preparations[b]	Dosages[c]	Onset (min)	Peak (min)	Duration (hours)
Isoetharine (Bronkometer, Bronkosol)	— +1 +3	MDI: 0.34 mg/spray	1–2 puffs q.i.d.	Inhal: 1–6	15–60	1–3
		Nebulizer: 1% (10 mg/ml); 0.5% (5 mg/ml)	0.25–0.5 mL q.i.d.			
		UD: varies from 0.62% to 0.25% in 2- to 4-mL single-dose vials	One vial per treatment q.i.d.			
Bitolterol (colterol) (Tornalate)	— +2 +4	MDI: 0.37 mg/spray	2–3 puffs q 4–6 hr, or 2 puffs q 8 hr (not to exceed 12 puffs/day)	Inhal: 3–4	30–60	5–8
		Nebulizer: 0.2%	1.25 mL t.i.d.			
Racemic epinephrine[f] (AsthmaNefrin, MicroNefrin, Vaponefrin)	+2 +3 +2	Nebulizer: 2.25%, 2% (equivalent to 1.125% and 1% epinephrine base, respectively)	0.25–0.5 mL q.i.d., p.r.n.	Inhal: 1–5	5–15	1–3
Resorcinols:						
Metaproterenol (Alupent, Metaprel)	— +2 +2	MDI: 0.65 mg/spray	2–3 puffs q 3–4 hr (not to exceed 12 puffs/day)	Inhal: 1–5	30–60	3–4
		Nebulizer: 5% (50 mg/mL)	0.3 mL (15 mg) t.i.d., q.i.d.	PO: 15–30	60	4
		UD: 0.4%, 0.6% in 2.5-mL single-dose vials	One vial per treatment t.i.d., q.i.d.			
		PO: 10, 20 mg tablets, 10 mg/5 mL syrup	20 mg t.i.d., q.i.d. Children 6–9 yr: PO: 10 mg t.i.d., q.i.d. Children <6 yr: PO: 1.3–2.6 mg/kg/day in divided doses of syrup			
Terbutaline (Brethaire, Brethine, Bricanyl)	— ± +4	MDI: 0.2, 0.25 mg/spray	2 puffs q 4–6 hr	Inhal: 5–30	30–60	3–6
		Nebulizer: 1% (10 mg/ml)[d]	5–10 mg q 4–6 hr[d]	PO: 30	120–240	4–8
		Turbuhaler: 0.5 mg/capsule	One capsule, p.r.n. (not to exceed 4 capsules/day)	SC: 5–15	30–60	1.5–4
		PO: 2.5, 5 mg tablets	2.5–5 mg q 6 hr (not to exceed 15 mg/day)			
		SC: 1 mg/mL[e]	0.25 mg (not to exceed 0.5 mg total dose in 4 hr)			
Saligenins:						
Albuterol, Salbutamol (Proventil, Ventolin, Proventil Repetabs, Volmax, Airet, Ventolin Nebules,	— ± +4	MDI: 0.09, 0.1 mg/spray	2 puffs q 4–6 hr			
		Nebulizer: 0.5% (5 mg/ml)	2.5 mg (0.5 mL) q 4–6 hr			
		UD: 0.083% (0.83 mg/ml) in 3-mL single-dose vials	One vial per treatment q 4–6 hr			
		Rotahaler: 0.2 mg/capsule	One capsule q 4–6 hr	Inhal: <15	30–60	3–6
		PO: 4 mg tablets; 4, 8 mg	2–4 mg t.i.d., q.i.d. (not to exceed 32 mg/day)	PO: ≤30	60–120	4–8

Ventolin Rotocaps)				ER tablets; 2 mg/5 mL syrup	4–8 mg q 12 hr 2–4 mg q t.i.d., q.i.d. Children 6–12 yr: PO: 2 mg t.i.d., q.i.d. (not to exceed 24 mg/day) Children 2–6 yr: PO: 0.1–0.2 mg/kg syrup t.i.d. (not to exceed 12 mg/day)			
Pirbuterol (Maxair)	—	±	+4	MDI: 0.2 mg/spray	1–2 puffs q 4–6 hr (not to exceed 12 puffs/day)	Inhal: 5	30–60	3–5
Salmeterol (Serevent)	—	±	+4	MDI: 0.025 mg/spray	2 puffs b.i.d. doses should be 12 hr apart	Inhal: 13–18	180–240	12–18
Some agents available abroad:								
Carbuterol (Bronsecur)				MDI: 0.1 mg/spray	1–2 puffs q 3 hr			
Fenoterol (Berotec)				MDI: 0.1, 0.2 mg/spray Nebulizer: 0.5% (5 mg/ml)	1–2 puffs b.i.d., t.i.d. 0.5–1.25 mg q.i.d.			
Formoterol				MDI: 0.006 mg/spray	2 puffs b.i.d.; doses should be 12 hr apart			
Hexoprenaline (Ipradol)				PO: 0.5 mg tablets	1–2 tablets t.i.d.			
Procaterol (Pro-Air)				MDI: 0.01 mg/spray PO: 0.025, 0.05 mg tablets; 0.025 mg/5 mL syrup	2 puffs t.i.d. 0.05 mg hs, or b.i.d.			
Reproterol (Bronchodil)				MDI: 0.5 mg/spray	1–2 puffs q 3–6 hr			
Rimiterol (Pulmadil)				MDI: 0.2 mg/spray	1–3 puffs, p.r.n. (not to exceed 8 doses daily)			
Tulobuterol (Brelomax, Respacal)				PO: 2 mg tablets; 1 mg/5 mL syrup	2 mg b.i.d., t.i.d.			

[a] — no activity; ± to +1, minimal or mild activity; +2, mild to moderate activity; +3 moderate activity; +4, strong activity.
[b] PO, by mouth; Inhal, by aerosol inhalation; IV, intravenous; IM, intramuscular; SC, subcutaneous; SL, sublingual; MDI, metered-dose inhaler; UD, unit dose; ER, extended release.
[c] Dosages are for adults and children >12 years old, unless otherwise stated.
[d] This form of terbutaline administration is not yet approved by the FDA but is being used abroad.
[e] This parenteral form of terbutaline is currently under investigation by the FDA for inhalational use.
[f] Racemic epinephrine is not normally used as a bronchodilator but as a decongestant for upper airway edema.

Both terbutaline and albuterol have been given by the methods outlined above. The reported dosages of terbutaline administered by continuous nebulization range between 1 and 12 mg/hr (average 6.9 mg/hr), whereas albuterol's range is 10 to 20 mg/hr (average 12.1 mg/hr); the duration of therapy is 1 to 24 hours for terbutaline and 1 to 10 hours for albuterol.

Reported side effects from continuous administration of a β_2 agonist include tremor, cardiac arrhythmias, hypokalemia, or hyperglycemia. Careful, continuous respiratory and cardiovascular monitoring is mandated when administering β_2 agonists via continuous nebulization.

Contraindications

Contraindications to the use of sympathomimetic bronchodilators include hypersensitivity to any component in the drug and cardiac arrhythmias associated with tachycardia.

Precautions

1. Excessive or unnecessary use of inhalants may lead to the development of paradoxical bronchospasm and increased airway resistance. Tolerance and tachyphylaxis may also occur. Some investigators have found that repeated and frequent dosing of a β_2-adrenoceptor agonist leads to a decreased responsiveness or duration of effectiveness with subsequent doses; the end result may be that the drug must be discontinued or that a higher dose of the drug may be needed to illicit the same effect that was noted with the initial dose. Tolerance and tachyphylaxis are key issues of concern for many clinicians worldwide who prescribe any β_2-adrenoceptor agonist for their patients with acute or chronic airflow obstruction. Subsensitivity resulting from continuous and prolonged administration of β_2-adrenoceptor stimulants is a highly debated issue and has been linked as a possible cause for the rise in deaths from asthma, as well as other adverse effects noted with β_2-adrenergic therapy, such as rebound bronchoconstriction, cardiotoxicity, and hypokalemic induced arrhythmias.

   Because of the controversy surrounding the long-term, continuous use of β_2-adrenoceptor agonist therapy, the current advice of many clinicians is that β_2-adrenoceptor agonist therapy should only be utilized on an as-needed basis for symptom relief. The reader is encouraged to review the literature on this highly controversial topic, especially the debate between Doctors Ziment (1993) and Skorodin (1993) concerning β2-adrenoceptor agonist tolerance, rebound bronchoconstriction, and tachyphylaxis.
2. Concomitant use with adrenergic β-blockers antagonizes the effects of bronchodilators and may also cause vasoconstriction and reflex bradycardia.
3. Use cautiously for patients with cardiovascular disease, including coronary

insufficiency, cardiac arrhythmias, and history of stroke and hypertension (owing to possible toxic symptoms). Also, use with caution for patients who are unusually hyperreactive to sympathomimetic agents.

4. If bronchial irritation, nervousness, or restlessness occurs, consider reducing the dosage.
5. Use cautiously for pregnant patients; several of these agents may cross the placental barrier.
6. Use in children—the safety and efficacy of several of these agents in children younger than 12 years of age have not been established.
7. Coadministered use of one sympathomimetic agent with another may produce unwanted additive effects.
8. As mentioned previously, catecholamines must be stored in light-resistant containers. Heat, light, or air will metabolize catecholamines into inert adrenochromes.
9. Use of catecholamines with:
   a. Digitalis may produce additive effects and ectopic pacemaker activity.
   b. Monoamine oxidase (MAO) inhibitors may create a hypertensive crisis.
   c. Diuretics and antihypertensive drugs may antagonize the effects of catecholamines.
10. If a sympathomimetic crisis occurs, the effects may be counteracted by injection of an α- or β_1-adrenoceptor blocker.
11. As mentioned previously, catecholamines are not effective when given orally, owing to inactivation in the GI tract and liver by the sulfatase enzymes.
12. Large doses of IV albuterol may worsen preexisting diabetes mellitus and ketoacidosis.
13. Large doses of salmeterol (up to 12 to 20 times the recommended dose) have been associated with prolongation of the QT interval, which may precipitate ventricular arrhythmias.
14. Do not use salmeterol to relieve acute bronchospastic attacks.
15. As mentioned, decreases in serum potassium (hypokalemia) have been noted with the use of these agents. Adverse cardiovascular effects may be noted.
16. Patients should be advised not to discontinue the use of corticosteroid therapy without the advice of a physician, even if they feel better with the use of a β_2-adrenoceptor bronchodilator (see Chapter 12).
17. Some of these agents contain sulfites (e.g., some solutions of isoetharine, isoproterenol, racemic epinephrine, and albuterol), which may precipitate allergic-type reactions in susceptible individuals. Sulfite-free agents should be used for these patients.
18. Metered-dose inhalers (MDIs) contain propellants that may induce adverse effects, especially for individuals with hyperreactive airways. The clinician should consider nebulized or dry-powder formulations in such cases. Ad-

verse effects (cardiotoxicity, bronchospasm) are most notable in cases of extreme overuse.

Adverse Reactions

Adverse reactions are significantly reduced with aerosol administration of these agents. The most common reactions include tremor and palpitations.

CNS: Anxiety, fear, apprehension, tremors, irritability, lightheadedness, headache, flushing, pallor, sweating, insomnia.

Cardiovascular: Hypertension, hypotension, arrhythmias, palpitations. Reflex tachycardia from peripheral vasodilation and cardiac stimulation are dose-related occurrences.

Pulmonary: Coughing, bronchospasm, pulmonary edema (IV use), respiratory difficulties.

GI: Nausea, vomiting, heartburn.

Overdosage

Inhalation: Intensification of the unwanted effects listed under *Adverse Reactions* may occur. May produce anginal pain and hypertension. Increased blood pressure may be noted initially and then pressure may drop, possibly causing shock. Treatment consists of supportive care and discontinuance of the drug. May use β-receptor blockers cautiously, bearing in mind the possibility of airway aggravation.

Systemic: Palpitations, tachycardia, bradycardia, heart block, chest pain, hypertension, nausea, vomiting, delirium, collapse, and coma. Treatment consists of rapid intervention to reduce the incidence of morbidity and mortality. Airway, ventilation, and cardiovascular circulation (cardiopulmonary resuscitation) may be indicated in cases of severe acute toxic reaction.

Dosage and Administration

Table 10.1 lists the preparations, dosages, and basic pharmacokinetics of the β_2-adrenoceptor bronchodilators.

ANTICHOLINERGIC (ANTIMUSCARINIC) BRONCHODILATORS

The predominant neural control of bronchomotor tone and submucosal gland secretion is through the vagally mediated pathways of the parasympathetic nervous system which, when stimulated, induce bronchial smooth muscle contraction and an increase in the production of secretions. The rationale for administering parasympatholytic (antimuscarinic) agents to patients with airflow obstruction is based on two primary postulates: 1) parasympathetic mediated bronchospasm is considered a primary component for some patients with airflow obstruction, and 2) airflow obstruction can be inhibited and/or reversed pharmacologically with antimuscarinic agents.

The prototypic parasympatholytic agent, atropine (a naturally occurring alkaloid found in plants of *Atropa belladonna* and *Datura* species) has been used for thousands of years for its CNS effects. Of interest is that as early as the 17th century in India, the fumes from burning *Datura* plants were inhaled to alleviate respiratory distress. In the early 18th century, this mode of therapy became a popular method in Britain to treat asthma. By the mid-19th century, Americans packed the *Datura* leaves into cigars, cigarettes, and pipes so the *Datura* leaves could be inhaled by smoking.

The introduction of the sympathomimetic bronchodilators in the late 1920s led to a reduction in the use of atropine to treat asthma. The use of antimuscarinic agents to treat bronchospasm has recently regained popularity. Not only has it been realized that many precipitators of bronchospasm can be best treated with the use of antimuscarinics, but safer, more effective agents, such as the quaternary ammonium compounds of atropine, have been developed that have significantly fewer CNS effects than atropine.

Mechanism of Action and Indications for Use

Upon stimulation, the vagal efferent nerves release the neurotransmitter acetylcholine from the presynaptic nerve terminal. Acetylcholine diffuses across the synaptic cleft and binds to the muscarinic receptors located within the tracheobronchial tree. Acetylcholine receptor sites are located in or adjacent to the respiratory epithelium, submucosal glands, mast cells, and airway smooth muscle. Autoradiographic mapping of muscarinic receptors has demonstrated a high density of these receptors in the smooth muscle of large central airways. The density of these receptors decreases as the airways become smaller; thus, proximal and distal bronchioles are nearly devoid of receptors.

After attachment of acetylcholine to the muscarinic receptor, a series of enzymatic reactions is initiated. As discussed in Chapter 2, muscarinic receptor activation leads to:

- Release of intracellular calcium (results in contraction of airway smooth muscle)
- Inhibition in the production of cAMP (favors contraction of airway smooth muscle)
- Increased intracellular levels of cGMP. An increase in the level of intracellular cGMP elicits an excitatory reaction in the lung: bronchial smooth muscle contraction and increased bronchial gland secretion (Fig. 10.11).

Also, in response to acetylcholine, various chemical mediators that abide within mast cells and inflammatory cells are released (e.g., histamine, chemotactic fac-

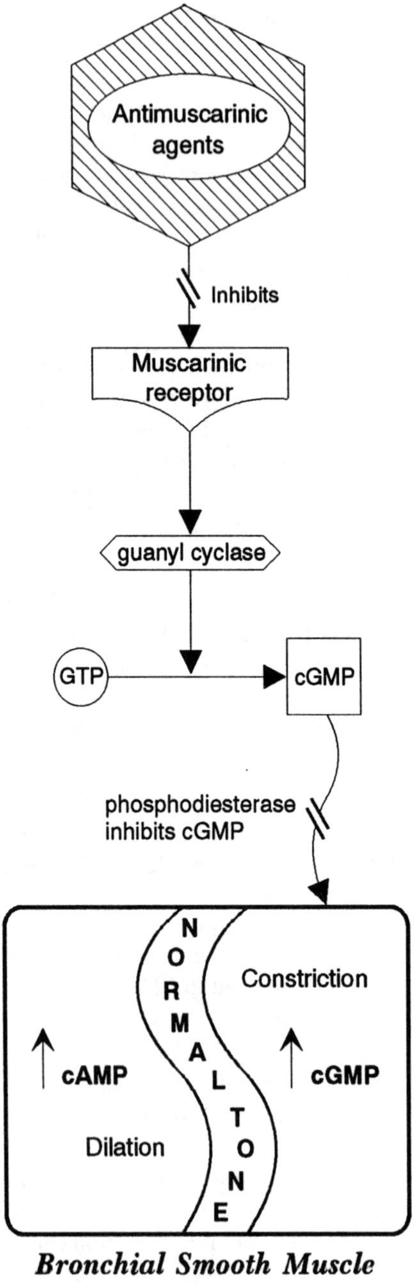

Figure 10.11. Pharmacologic control of bronchomotor tone with antimuscarinic agents.

tors, and the arachidonic acid metabolites: the leukotrienes, prostaglandins D_2 and $F_{2\alpha}$, and platelet-activating factor). These mediators initiate the inflammatory response in the lung: smooth muscle spasm, mucus secretion, and mucosal edema.

Antimuscarinic agents competitively inhibit acetylcholine from binding to the muscarinic receptor (see Chapter 2, Fig. 2.14) which, in turn, produces a parasympathetic (vagal) blockade. This action results in bronchodilation and a decrease in the production of tracheobronchial secretions as well as an increase in the heart rate (most notable with atropine). Results of several clinical trials indicate that the major sites of bronchodilator action for inhaled antimuscarinic agents are the large central airways (De Troyer et al. 1979, Hensley et al. 1978, McFadden et al. 1977, Marini et al. 1981).

Atropine, the prototypic antimuscarinic agent, is a drug that is indicated for use in a variety of conditions:

1. In cholinergic-mediated bronchospasm.
2. As a supplement in peptic ulcer therapy.
3. As a preoperative drying agent to control bronchial, nasal, pharyngeal, and salivary secretions.
4. As an antidote for mushroom poisoning (*Amanita muscaria* species) and chemical warfare nerve gases.
5. As a resuscitative measure during cardiac arrest (see Chapter 19). Also, because of atropine's vagolytic actions, it is especially suited for use for patients with hypotension associated with sinus bradycardia, junctional bradycardia, third-degree atrioventricular (AV) block, and second-degree AV block (Mobitz Types I and II).
6. To prevent reflex bradycardia such as that induced by oropharyngeal stimulation during intubation.

The various quaternary ammonium derivatives of atropine (atropine methonitrate, ipratropium bromide, glycopyrrolate, oxitropium bromide) are safe, effective agents that are indicated for reversal of cholinergic-mediated bronchospasm.

Specific Antimuscarinic Agents

Atropine is a tertiary ammonium alkaloid commonly used as the sulfate salt (Fig. 10.12). The plasma half-life is 2 to 3 hours, and the drug is eliminated by hepatic metabolism. Following an aerosol dose, onset of action and peak effects usually occur within 15 minutes and 60 to 120 minutes, respectively. The duration of action of atropine sulfate is 3 to 5 hours (dose dependent). The optimal effective aerosol dose of atropine sulfate with the least side effects is 0.025 mg/kg in adults and 0.05 mg/kg in children with airway obstruction. At this dose, dryness of the mouth is the most common reported side effect. Following administration, at-

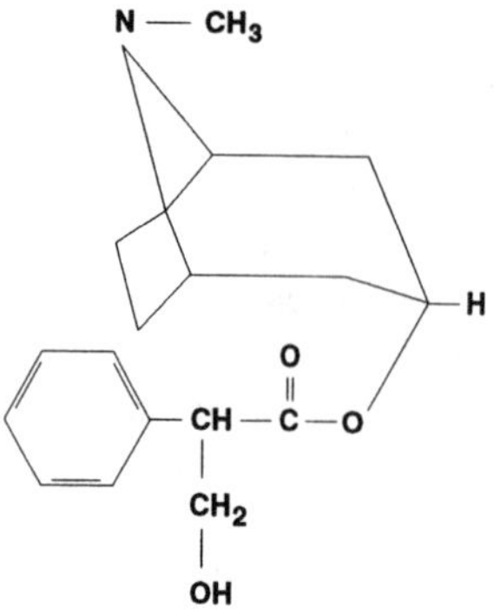

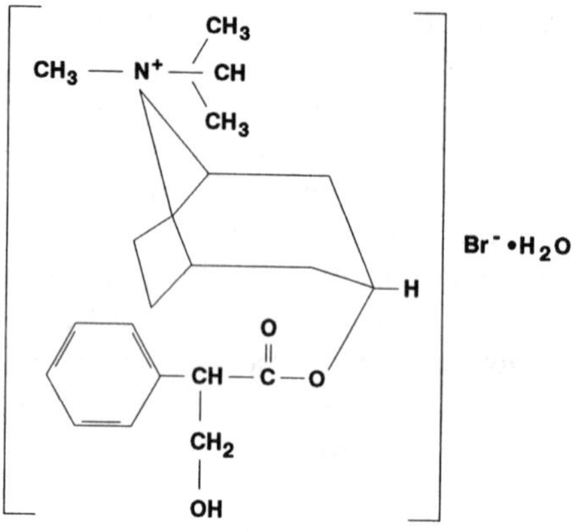

Figure 10.12. The chemical structures of atropine and ipratropium bromide. Atropine, a tertiary ammonium compound, readily crosses the blood-brain barrier and exerts central nervous system (CNS) side effects, whereas the quaternary ammonium compound, ipratromium bromide, does not penetrate the blood-brain barrier and does not exert CNS side effects.

ropine is widely distributed in the body and may elicit systemic side effects. As the dosage of atropine is increased, significant adverse effects may result: tachycardia, urinary retention, transient headache, visual blurring, mental confusion, depressed ciliary transport, and depressed mucociliary clearance. Many of these effects are the result of inhibiting the actions of the vagus nerve.

Atropine methonitrate (methylnitrate quaternary salt of atropine) has properties very similar to that of atropine sulfate with two notable exceptions: it is twice as potent as atropine and has a longer duration of activity. A 2-mg dose of atropine methonitrate in combination with fenoterol (0.4 mg) produces a similar increase in FEV_1 in asthmatic patients as 4 mg of atropine sulfate in combination with 0.4 mg fenoterol (Allen and Campbell 1980). The response with the atropine methonitrate combination also produced a significant increase in the FEV_1 for 6 hours, whereas the increase in the FEV_1 with the atropine sulfate combination was 4 hours. The recommended therapeutic dose of atropine methonitrate is 1.5 mg. At this dose, an onset of action occurs between 15 and 30 minutes, peak effects between 1 and 2 hours, with a duration of activity of 4 to 6 hours. Atropine methonitrate does not cross the blood-brain barrier; therefore, systemic side effects are minimal, even with an inadvertent overdose (Gross and Skorodin 1985). Atropine methonitrate is more popular in Europe, where it is also known as methylatropine nitrate.

Glycopyrrolate is a semisynthetic quaternary ammonium compound that has an onset of action of approximately 15 to 30 minutes. A therapeutic dose of 1.0 mg produces a peak response within 30 to 60 minutes. Glycopyrrolate has a relatively long duration of activity of 6 to 8 hours. Like all quaternary ammonium salts, glycopyrrolate does not cross the blood-brain barrier; therefore, it has minimal cardiovascular and CNS side effects as compared to atropine. Glycopyrrolate methylbromide (Robinul) is currently in the experimental phase as an aerosol antimuscarinic bronchodilator with the injectable solution (0.2 mg/mL) used for aerosol administration.

Ipratropium bromide is a quaternary isopropyl derivative of atropine (Fig. 10.12) that is currently the only FDA-approved antimuscarinic bronchodilator. When administered by way of inhalation, significant bronchodilation usually occurs within minutes. Ipratropium bromide usually produces 50% of the maximal bronchodilator response within 3 minutes, 80% within 30 minutes, and 100% at 1 to 2 hours (Engelhardt and Klupp 1975, Deckers 1975). Ipratropium bromide does not cross the blood-brain barrier as does atropine; therefore, it is a relatively safe bronchodilator when used in prescribed therapeutic doses. Optimal bronchodilation is achieved by doses of 0.04 to 0.08 mg with a resultant duration of activity of 4 to 6 hours. Side effects of ipratropium are minimal owing to poor systemic absorption from the respiratory tract. Dryness of the mouth is the most commonly reported side effect. Vision disturbances (after reportedly spraying a part of the dose into the eyes) has also been reported. Ipratropium bromide does not depress ciliary activity, change sputum viscosity, or retard mucociliary clearance as does atropine. By inhalation, ipratropium bromide (0.04 or 0.08 mg) is as effective a bronchodilator as atropine (2 mg) with a 30 to 50% longer duration of effectiveness (Spector and Ball 1975). Ipratropium bromide (trade name, Atrovent) is currently available for inhalation administration in MDI form as well as in solution for nebulization. Atrovent is a very popular antimuscarinic bronchodilator throughout the USA. Ipratropium bromide in combination with fenoterol (Duovent, Berodual) is currently available in Europe. This combination provides the simultaneous administration of an antimuscarinic and a β_2-adrenoceptor agonist.

Oxitropium bromide, quaternary ammonium derivative of scopolamine (hyoscine), is a relatively new antimuscarinic agent marketed abroad under the trade names of Oxivent, Tersigat, Ventilat, and Ventox. Comparatively, oxitropium is less potent than ipratropium; 0.2 mg of oxitropium is equivalent in effectiveness to 0.08 mg of ipratropium (Peel et al. 1984). However, oxitropium has a longer duration of activity than ipratropium, causing bronchodilation for up to 8 to 10 hours. Several clinical trials have shown that a dose of 0.2 mg is optimal in eliciting a maximal response and prolonged duration of activity (up to 10 hours). Onset of action of oxitropium varies from within 5 to 15 minutes with peak effects occurring between 1 and 2 hours. Oxitropium does not adversely affect mucociliary clearance, sputum production, or sputum viscosity. As with ipratropium bromide, the most commonly reported side effect is dryness of the mouth.

Contraindications

Hypersensitivity to atropine or its derivatives. Use with caution for patients with narrow-angle glaucoma, prostatic hypertrophy, and tachycardia as well as unstable cardiovascular status in acute hemorrhage and myocardial ischemia.

Precautions

Atropine

1. Not indicated for the initial treatment of acute bronchospastic attacks in which a rapid response is desired.
2. CNS stimulation may be noted with increased dosages.
3. Following inhalation, systemic absorption may occur. Nondetectable to highly significant symptoms of unwanted side effects may result.
4. Safety and efficacy of use for pregnant women and children have not been established.
5. Use in patients with chronic lung disease may precipitate drying of secretions and mucus plugging.
6. Use with extreme caution for patients with myasthenia gravis. However, atropine may be given to reverse the effects of cholinergic muscle stimulants in cases of overdose (see Chapter 14).

Ipratropium Bromide and Other Quaternary Ammonium Compounds

1. Not indicated for the initial treatment of acute bronchospastic attacks in which a rapid response is desired.
2. Safety and efficacy in children younger than 12 years of age have not been established.
3. Use cautiously for pregnant women and nursing mothers.

Adverse Reactions

Atropine

The most common side effects for nebulized atropine include dryness of mouth, possible thickening of secretions leading to mucus plugging, and an increase in the heart rate.

CNS: Headache, nervousness, drowsiness, dizziness, insomnia, fever, confusion, agitation.
Cardiovascular: Bradycardia (below normal doses), tachycardia (higher doses), palpitations, angina.
GI: Dry nose and mouth, thirst, nausea, vomiting, dysphagia, heartburn.
Side effects of atropine are dose related:

Dose	Effects
0.5 mg:	Slight decrease in cardiac function, slight dryness of mouth, reduced sweating.
1.0 mg:	Increased dryness of mouth, thirst, and cardiac rate. Slight dilation of pupil.
2.0 mg:	Rapid cardiac rate, palpitations, increased dryness of mouth, dilated pupils, slight blurring of vision.
5.0 mg:	Marked unwanted side effects as mentioned above, in addition to difficulty in swallowing, restlessness, fatigue, headache, difficulty in micturition, and decreased intestinal peristalsis.
10 mg or more:	Above symptoms markedly pronounced, in addition to: rapid and weak pulse; very blurred vision; hot, flushed, dry skin; ataxia; hallucinations; delirium; coma.

Ipratropium Bromide and Other Quaternary Ammonium Compounds

Most common: dry mouth. Other adverse reactions include insomnia, nervousness, dizziness, headache, nausea, blurred vision (when sprayed in the eyes), cough, palpitations, rash, exacerbation of symptoms. Cases of the onset of or worsening of narrow-angle glaucoma, acute eye pain, and hypotension have also been reported.

Overdosage

Atropine

As dosage is increased, adverse reactions are intensified, possibly leading to delirium, hallucinations, or coma. Individual tolerance varies; however, toxic effects are primarily dose related and are more commonly seen in children.

Treatment with IV physostigmine (reverses muscarinic blockade; see Chapter 14) is reserved for patients with severe drug-induced supraventricular tachycardia.

Ipratropium Bromide and Other Quaternary Ammonium Compounds

Overdosage by inhalation is unlikely because these agents are not well absorbed systemically.

Dosage and Administration

Table 10.2 summarizes the preparations, dosages, and basic pharmacokinetics of the antimuscarinic agents discussed in this section.

Table 10.2.
Antimuscarinic Bronchodilators

Bronchodilator[a]	Preparations[b]	Dosages[c]	Onset (min)	Peak (min)	Duration (hours)
Atropine sulfate	Nebulizer: 0.5% (5 mg/ml); 0.2% (2 mg/ml)	0.025 mg/kg t.i.d., q.i.d. (adult); 0.05 mg/kg t.i.d., q.i.d. (child)	15	60–120	3–5
Atropine methonitrate	Nebulizer: 0.5% (5 mg/ml)	1.5 mg t.i.d., q.i.d.	15–30	60–120	4–6
Glycopyrrolate (Robinul)	Nebulizer: 0.02% (0.2 mg/ml) (injectable solution)	1 mg t.i.d., q.i.d.	15–30	30–60	6–8
Ipratropium bromide (Atrovent)	MDI: 0.018, 0.02 mg/spray	2 puffs t.i.d., q.i.d.; up to 4 puffs t.i.d.	3–15	60–120	4–6
	Nebulizer: 0.025% (0.25 mg/ml)	0.25–0.5 mg q 4–6 hr			
Oxitropium bromide (Oxivent, Tersigat, Ventilat, Ventox)	MDI: 0.1 mg/spray	2 puffs b.i.d., t.i.d.	5–15	60–120	8–10

[a]The only antimuscarinic bronchodilator currently approved for use in the USA is ipratropium bromide (Atrovent).
[b]MDI, metered-dose inhaler.
[c]Dosages are for adults and children >12 years old, unless otherwise stated.

Clinical Application of β_2-Adrenoceptor and Antimuscarinic Agents

Comparative Bronchodilator Studies and Precipitators of Bronchospasm

Numerous clinical trials published to date have compared the efficacy of various antimuscarinic agents to various β_2-adrenoceptor agonists. β_2-adrenoceptor agonists and antimuscarinic agents are both highly effective bronchodilators for the treatment of reversible airway obstruction. On the basis of the available evidence, β_2-adrenoceptor agonists have a higher efficacy in the treatment of asthma, whereas patients with chronic obstructive pulmonary disease (COPD) generally benefit more from antimuscarinic agents. For the management of acute airway obstruction, the β_2-adrenoceptor agonist is preferred owing to its rapid onset of action.

In developing a pharmacotherapeutic approach to the treatment of airflow obstruction, the practitioner should have a sound understanding of the precipitators of airways obstruction. Characteristic aspects of patients with COPD include structural narrowing of the airways, loss of elastic recoil, and fibrotic distortion of the airways, combined with a degree of vagal bronchomotor tone. Some components of airway obstruction in COPD are irreversible—loss of elastic recoil and fibrotic distortion of airways—whereas other components of airway obstruction in patients with COPD are potentially reversible—mucous obstruction, airway inflammation, and bronchial smooth muscle contraction.

Although patients with COPD generally do not have a significant reversible component to their airway obstruction, many patients in this group exhibit at least a 10 to 20% improvement in their airflow rates after the administration of a bronchodilator. The interesting feature that is especially noted for patients with emphysema, even if airflow is not significantly improved, is that they tend to breathe at a lower lung volume after the administration of an antimuscarinic bronchodilator (i.e., these agents have a tendency to lower functional residual capacity [FRC]) (Hughes et al. 1982).

Many studies exist that correlate with the assumption that antimuscarinic agents produce a greater response in patients with COPD than a β_2-adrenoceptor agent. For example, Tashkin and colleagues (1986) conducted a multicenter clinical trial of 261 patients with clearly defined COPD and found that ipratropium not only achieved a greater response and duration of effectiveness over a β_2-adrenoceptor agonist but that ipratropium maintained the heightened response over the entire 90-day trial period as compared to the β_2-adrenoceptor agonist. Many investigators believe that vagal tone is the major reversible element of this disorder and conclude that an antimuscarinic agent should be first-line therapy.

Asthmatic patients' airways are hyperresponsive to a multitude of precipitators of bronchospasm. Mast cell degranulation with the resultant release of histamine and the formation of other various endogenous mediators of inflammation (serotonin, bradykinin, prostaglandins, and leukotrienes) play a vital role in regulating airway caliber in these patients. β_2-adrenoceptor agents are considered first-line therapy for these types of inflammatory mediators. Antimuscarinic agents are relatively ineffective or, at most, provide limited protection against bronchospasm induced by histamine, bradykinin, serotonin, or prostaglandin F_2.

β_2-adrenoceptor agents are also considered first-line therapy for exercise-induced and cold-air-induced bronchospasm, as well as allergens and exogenous irritants. However, for some patients with asthma, ipratropium and atropine effectively reduce the severity of exercise- and cold-air-induced bronchospasm if given prior to exercise or exposure to cold air. McFadden and associates (1977) found that two predominant airway sites cause the bronchoconstriction brought on by exercise. Five of the 12 asthmatic patients tested had predominantly large airway obstruction after exercise, whereas seven patients had predominantly small airway obstruction after exercise. In the large airway obstruction group, antimuscarinic therapy totally abolished the bronchospastic response to exercise, whereas antimuscarinic therapy in the small airway obstruction group was relatively ineffective in altering the response to exercise.

The experimental findings of several investigators indicate that antimuscarinics reliably protect against cholinergic (acetylcholine, methacholine) mediated bronchospasm and bronchospasm induced by certain irritants such as house dust, grass pollen, molds, animal hair, cigarette smoke, ozone, and citric acid. Some studies also indicate that patients whose asthma is brought on by psychogenic factors respond more favorably to antimuscarinic therapy than to β_2-adrenoceptor agonist therapy.

Nonselective β-blocking agents can precipitate severe bronchospasm in patients with asthma owing to the β_2-blockade and resultant loss of β-adrenergic opposition to parasympathetic tone. Antimuscarinic agents provide a moderate degree of protection in preventing and reversing such bronchospasm, whereas the β_2-adrenoceptor agonists are less effective.

Table 10.3 lists a summary of the precipitators of bronchospasm with the corresponding bronchodilator most effective to reverse the obstruction as discussed in this section.

Combination Therapy: β_2-Adrenoceptor and Antimuscarinic Agents

An overview of the published studies suggests that, when given by inhalation, there may be an additive bronchodilator effect when an antimuscarinic agent is coadministered with a β_2-adrenoceptor agonist. Some investigators have noted there may be an even higher efficacy of combination therapy with an antimuscarinic agent and a β_2-adrenoceptor agonist in the acutely ill patient, whereas others maintain that the severity of airflow obstruction does not affect the bronchodilator response.

Many of the studies presented reemphasize the heterogeneity of airway responses to all stimuli and indicate that effective prophylaxis should be directed at peripheral as well as large central airways. For many patients with airflow obstruction, the combined use of an antimuscarinic with a β_2-adrenoceptor agonist presents an opportunity to increase the efficacy and duration of response and/or

Table 10.3.
Summary of Precipitators of Bronchospasm and Efficacy of Inhaled Bronchodilators

Bronchoconstricting Stimulus	Antimuscarinic Agents	β_2-Adrenoceptor Agents
Asthma:		
Cholinergic agents (acetylcholine, methacholine)	Fully effective	Less effective
Beta blockers	Effective reversal	Less effective
Allergens-irritants	Moderately effective (studies vary from none to excellent)	Very effective
Exercise-induced, cold air	Moderately effective (more so in large doses or if given prior to exercise)	Very effective
Various mediators (histamine, serotonin, bradykinin, prostaglandin $F_{2\alpha}$)	Limited effectiveness (partially protective at most)	Moderate to very effective
Emotional (psychogenic) factors	Very effective	Less effective
Chronic Obstructive Disease:		
Bronchitis	Moderately effective	Moderately effective
Emphysema	Moderately effective	Less effective

to lower the incidence of side effects. The additional bronchodilation achieved by combination therapy may be related to differences in the pharmacological properties of each drug type or to differences in receptor sites within the airways. Owing to these differences in action, the effects of the two drugs may be additive.

If combination therapy is used, the sequence of administration may affect the response. In some cases, a higher efficacy and more prolonged effect were achieved when the antimuscarinic agent was administered prior to the β_2-adrenoceptor agonist. This is exemplified by the studies conducted by Leahy and associates (1983) and Bruderman and associates (1983). The results of these two studies are depicted in Figure 10.13. In these clinical trials, a significant and more prolonged effect resulted when ipratropium was given prior to the β_2-adrenoceptor agonist.

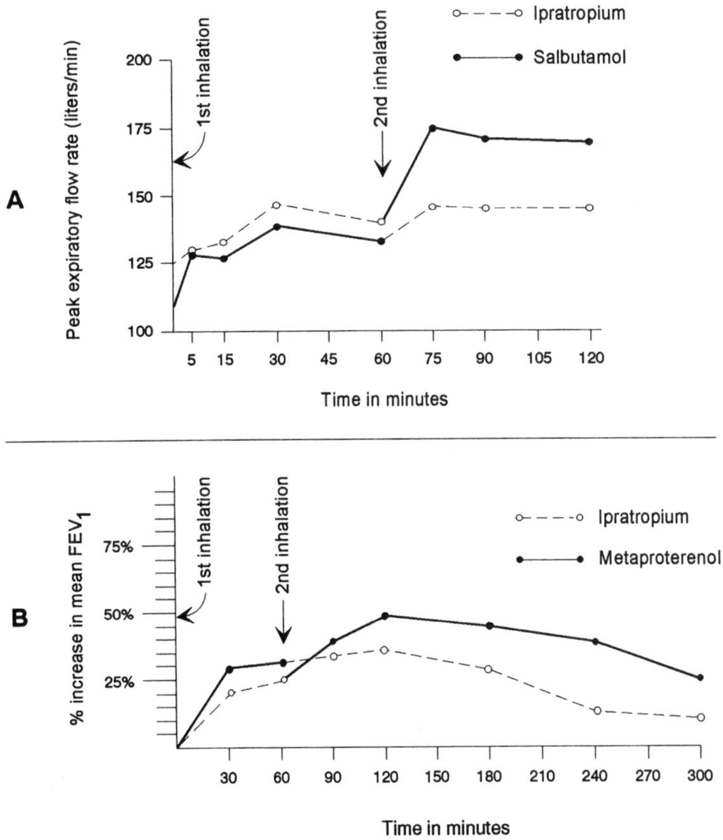

Figure 10.13. Comparative effects of sequencing ipratropium bromide with a β_2-adrenoceptor agonist. A higher efficacy is achieved when ipratropium bromide is administered prior to the β_2 agonist. Based on studies conducted by Leahy and associates, 1983 (*A*) and Bruderman and associates, 1983 (*B*).

The rationale for the higher efficacy and sustained response that is generated when ipratropium is administered prior to the β_2-adrenoceptor agonist is based on two primary postulates: 1) inhaled ipratropium dilates larger airways predominantly, whereas inhaled β_2-adrenoceptor agonists dilate the smaller, peripheral airways; hence, a more favorable deposition into the peripheral airways would result if the β_2-adrenoceptor agonist is given as a second inhalation, and 2) the additive effect of a β_2-adrenoceptor agonist may presumably only be obtained in the presence of decreased vagal tone. Antimuscarinics inhibit vagal efferent pathways and, therefore, can significantly counteract increased vagal influences. Once this vagal influence is negated by antimuscarinic administration, the β_2-adrenoceptor agonist may be able to elicit more effective results. On the basis of these studies, it seems that correct sequential administration of the two drug types plays a vital role in enhancing the effectiveness and duration of activity.

Whatever bronchodilator regimen is chosen for the patient, optimal therapy should lean toward maximum efficacy while minimizing adverse effects. In all situations, it must be remembered that patients are individuals and must have a regimen tailored to their needs.

XANTHINE BRONCHODILATORS

Caffeine, theophylline, and theobromine compose the group known as the xanthines. Their natural major source is, of course, beverages (coffee, cola, tea, and cocoa). Caffeine (1,3,7-trimethylxanthine), theophylline (1,3-dimethylxanthine), and theobromine (3,7-dimethylxanthine) are commonly referred to as *methylxanthines* owing to their methyl attachments and their chemical relation with the natural metabolite xanthine (Fig. 10.14). Although the methylxanthines are a naturally occurring class of plant alkaloids, most are produced synthetically and are related to the prototype theophylline. The pharmacologic properties of the methylxanthines (caffeine, theophylline) are quite diverse and include the following:

- Bronchial smooth muscle relaxation
- Uterine smooth muscle relaxation
- Vascular smooth muscle relaxation
- Coronary vasodilation
- Cerebral vasoconstriction
- Cardiac stimulation
- Central nervous system stimulation as well as stimulation of the medullary respiratory centers
- Enhancement of skeletal muscle contractility, including the diaphragm
- Augments the release of various secretory products from endocrine and exocrine tissues
- Inhibits secretion by mast cells
- Promotes diuresis

THE XANTHINES

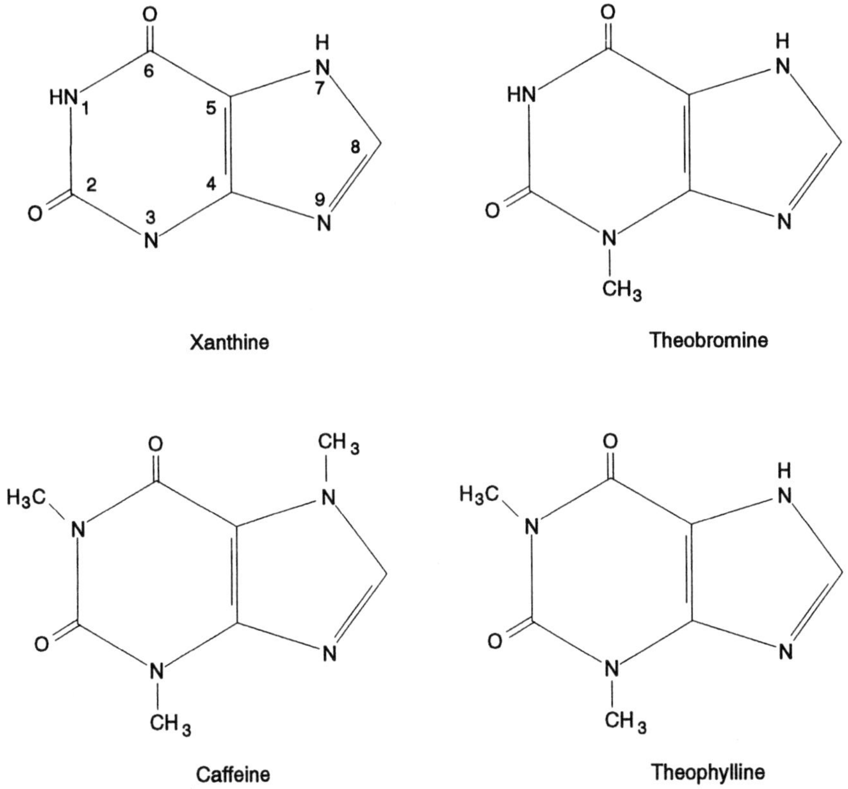

Figure 10.14. The chemical structure of xanthine and its derivatives.

Theophylline is most selective in its smooth muscle activity, whereas caffeine has the most marked CNS effects (see Chapter 15, Central Nervous System/Ventilatory Stimulants and Depressants). Theobromine is the least potent of these agents and is not used clinically; it is the major methylxanthine in chocolate. Of the methylxanthine group, only theophylline, its salts aminophylline and oxtriphylline, and dyphylline (1,3-dimethyl-7-[2,3-dihydroxypropyl]-xanthine, a covalently modified derivative) are currently approved for use for their bronchodilating property in the USA. An investigational agent of this class includes enprofylline (3-propylxanthine). Enprofylline is an agent that has been extensively researched in Europe for use in the treatment of bronchospasm in patients with asthma. Comparatively, enprofylline exhibits a fivefold increase in bronchodilator potency than theophylline with less CNS, renal, and cerebrovascular effects. However, tachycardia is more prominent with this agent than it is with theophylline. The following section focuses on the bronchodilating properties of theophylline and its derivatives.

Mechanism of Action and Indications for Use

For many years, theophylline's mechanism of bronchodilation was believed to be through phosphodiesterase inhibition, which would lead to the accumulation of cAMP. However, several clinical studies indicate that some forms of theophylline that have potent bronchodilator actions have little efficacy as phosphodiesterase inhibitors. Therefore, various other mechanisms have been proposed, but as yet, none have been established as being responsible for theophylline's bronchodilating effect. Other proposed mechanisms of bronchodilator action for theophylline include:

1. Inhibition of prostaglandin synthesis.
2. Interference with the uptake and storage of calcium.
3. Reduction in the uptake and/or metabolism of catecholamines.
4. Competitive antagonism at adenosine receptors.

Of the mechanisms listed above, the anti-adenosine action of theophylline seems to be the leading contender (Rall 1982). Receptors for adenosine are located in the plasma membranes of virtually every cell and consist of two subtypes: A_1 and A_2. There also appears to be two subtypes of A_2 receptors that reside in brain tissue: A_{2a} and A_{2b}. Activation of adenosine receptors by adenosine or various analogs of adenosine either activate (A_2 receptors) or inhibit (A_1 receptors) adenyl cyclase. Thus, stimulation of A_2 receptors, which leads to an increase in cAMP, mediates smooth muscle relaxation, whereas stimulation of A_1 receptors, which leads to a decrease in cAMP, brings about smooth muscle contraction.

The attachment of substituents at the nitrogen-1 position (Fig. 10.14) accounts for the xanthines' high affinity for adenosine receptors and subsequent adenosine antagonism. Theophylline is nonselective in its ability to antagonize the effects of adenosine at these adenosine specific receptors, in that it equally inhibits the binding of adenosine at both A_1 and A_2 receptors. By this mechanism, theophylline blocks bronchial smooth muscle contraction that is mediated by stimulation of A_1 receptors.

Although the proposed anti-adenosine mechanism may explain the actions of theophylline and its derivatives, other newer derivatives of xanthine (such as enprofylline) have demonstrated as good or better bronchodilating properties than theophylline while being relatively poor antagonists of adenosine (enprofylline lacks substituents at the nitrogen-1 position).

Theophylline is indicated to relieve moderate to severe airflow obstruction in acute asthma and to reduce the severity of symptoms associated with chronic asthma. Although theophylline's primary use has been for patients with asthma (especially those who experience nocturnal symptoms), its use for patients with moderate to severe COPD may be indicated, because theophylline not only reverses acute bronchospastic episodes in these patients but it can also significantly improve respiratory function and decrease dyspnea owing to its ability to improve pulmonary gas exchange, reduce respiratory muscle fatigue, stimulate the ventilatory drive, and stimulate and strengthen diaphragmatic contractility (Murciano et al. 1989). In addition, theophylline's positive inotropic effects are beneficial for patients with obstructive lung disease who also exhibit increased pulmonary arterial pressure as theophylline enhances both right and left heart systolic function while lowering pulmonary arterial pressure (Bukowskyj 1988).

Other actions of theophylline may be beneficial for patients with asthma and COPD. For some patients, the use of oral theophylline in conjunction with an inhaled β_2-adrenoceptor agonist or the antimuscarinic agent, ipratropium bromide, appears to enhance the efficacy of these inhaled agents (Boyers 1988, Kreisman et al. 1981). In addition, in sufficient concentration, theophylline inhibits antigen-induced release of histamine from lung tissue and improves mucociliary transport (Bukowskyj 1988).

Other nonbronchodilating indications for theophylline administration include:

- Cheyne-Stokes respiration to increase the regularity of respirations and as an adjunct in the treatment of neonatal apnea and bradycardia owing to theophylline's ability to elicit respiratory stimulation at the medullary level.
- To relieve paroxysmal dyspnea, stimulate the myocardium, and promote diuresis for patients with acute pulmonary edema.
- To strengthen diaphragmatic contractility and prevent respiratory muscle fatigue, particularly during weaning from mechanical ventilation and for patients after upper abdominal surgery.

Theophylline's primary effects on the various body systems are summarized in Table 10.4.

Contraindications

Hypersensitivity to the drug or any of its ingredients. May also be contraindicated for patients with active peptic ulcer, active gastritis, uncontrolled hypertension, coronary artery disease, angina pectoris, uncontrolled seizures, and uncontrolled arrhythmias.

Precautions

1. Dosages for theophylline and its derivatives are highly individualized. Ideal body weight must be used for dosage calculations. Dosage calculations must be adjusted according to the serum theophylline level.

Table 10.4
Main Effects of Theophylline on Body Systems

Organ System	Effects
Cardiovascular system	Cardiac muscle: increases heart rate, force of contraction, and cardiac output Blood vessels: Vasodilates coronary vessels (improves coronary blood flow) Vasodilates peripheral vessels (decreases peripheral vascular resistance) Vasoconstricts cerebral vessels (causes a marked increase in cerebrovascular resistance leading to a decrease in cerebral blood flow)
Gastrointestinal system	Stimulates gastric acid secretion: stimulates secretion of both acid and pepsin
Genitourinary system	Causes uterine smooth muscle relaxation
Muscoskeletal system	Stimulates skeletal muscle contraction: augments and strengthens the contractility of striated muscle
Central nervous system	Stimulates the central nervous system (CNS): as the dose is increased, signs of progressive CNS stimulation ensue: nervousness, anxiety, restlessness, insomnia, tremors, hyperesthesia Stimulates the medullary respiratory centers: enhances the ventilatory drive
Renal system	Promotes diuresis
Respiratory system	Relaxes bronchial smooth muscle Inhibits mediator release of histamine Stimulates respirations Enhances mucociliary transport Strengthens diaphragmatic contracility Reduces respiratory muscle fatigue

2. Slow infusion of aminophylline (10 to 20 minutes) must be maintained. Rapid IV infusion may result in hyperventilation, hypotension, syncope, cardiac collapse, and death.
3. Use with caution for patients with severe cardiac disease, severe hypoxemia, hepatic or renal disease, severe hypertension, acute myocardial injury, cor pulmonale, and congestive heart failure (CHF) and in elderly and neonatal patients. The volume of distribution, clearance, half-life, and excretion of these drugs may be altered in such a way as to produce toxic conditions, even with low doses.
4. The therapeutic blood level is close to the toxic level; careful monitoring of the patient is essential, including taking frequent vital signs and serum theophylline levels.
5. Concurrent use of xanthines with other xanthines or with β_2-adrenoceptor agonists may produce synergistic toxicity in patients with compromised cardiac function, resulting in life-threatening cardiac arrhythmias.
6. Certain types of drug interactions have been noted with the use of theophylline and its derivatives:

- The sedative effects of benzodiazepines may be antagonized by theophylline; however, coadministration may be beneficial to reverse excessive sedation produced by benzodiazepines.

- Catecholamine-induced arrhythmias have been noted with halothane and theophylline coadministration.
- Theophylline adverse reactions may be enhanced by concomitant administration of theophylline and tetracycline.
- Theophylline can reverse the effects of nondepolarizing neuromuscular blocking agents such as pancuronium and atacurium. This is a feature that should be realized when coadministering these agents.

Adverse Reactions

Side effects are dose-related occurrences and occur more commonly at serum theophylline levels >20 μg/mL.

CNS: Headache, insomnia, dizziness, seizures, depression, irritability, restlessness, convulsions, abnormal speech, abnormal behavior.
Cardiovascular: Hypotension, arrhythmias, palpitations, tachycardia, circulatory failure.
Pulmonary: Tachypnea, respiratory arrest.
GI: Nausea, vomiting, diarrhea, anorexia, epigastric pain, hematemesis.
Miscellaneous: Fever, flushing, hyperglycemia, rash.
Ethylenediamine in aminophylline can induce sensitivity reactions, including urticaria and exfoliative dermatitis.

Overdosage

Rapid IV infusion has caused severe cardiac arrhythmias and cardiac arrest. The first signs of toxicity may be convulsions or ventricular arrhythmias. In children, seizures and death may be the first signs of toxicity. Other toxic symptoms include a marked reaction from one or more of the effects listed under *Adverse Reactions*. Treatment consists of:

- Discontinuing the administration of the xanthine;
- Providing supportive care;
- Inducing vomiting (only if seizures have not occurred); and
- Guarding against the possibility of aspiration for patients with impaired consciousness, for infants, and for children.

If seizures have occurred:

- Maintain an airway (intubate if necessary);
- Provide oxygen;
- Administer activated charcoal;
- Give IV diazepam 0.1 to 0.3 mg/kg up to 10 mg; and
- Carefully monitor vital signs.

Theophylline Serum Levels

<5 μg/mL: no effect. Dose adjustment: administer a loading dose and reschedule maintenance doses.

5 to 10 μg/mL: mild bronchodilation, suboptimal therapeutic effects. Dose adjustment: increase theophylline to therapeutic range. IV—increase dose by approximately 25% (±50 mg). Oral—increase doses by 50 to 100 mg at 3-day intervals. Consider adding a β_2-adrenoceptor agent for an additive effect.

10 to 20 μg/mL: therapeutic target range (8 to 20 μg/mL recommended by the American Thoracic Society [1987]). Clinical effect: maximal bronchodilation. Dose adjustment: continue present dose, as tolerated.

20 to 30 μg/mL: mild to moderate toxicity: nausea, vomiting, diarrhea, headache, insomnia, irritability. Dose adjustment: decrease doses by 50 to 100 mg or skip one to two doses; decrease subsequent doses by 25% (±50 mg).

>30 μg/mL: severe toxicity: hyperglycemia, hypotension, cardiac arrhythmias, tachycardia, seizures, death. Dose adjustment: theophylline serum levels >30 μg/mL are considered a medical emergency—withhold theophylline, skip next two or three doses, and recheck serum levels for appropriate guidance in further dosing schedules. Consider the administration of activated charcoal.

Specific therapeutic levels and toxic levels are highly variable between patients. An increase in the dose of theophylline may be contraindicated when a patient elicits unwanted side effects, even though a serum theophylline level is less than 10 μg/mL. In this case, a β-adrenoceptor agonist may be given with low-dose theophylline to produce an additive effect of the two drugs. On the other hand, a patient may tolerate and need a higher serum theophylline level for clinical improvement. However, a serum theophylline level greater than 30 μg/mL constitutes a medical emergency in which theophylline administration is withheld and the patient is monitored for signs of toxicity.

Factors Affecting Theophylline Serum Levels

Various drugs or patient conditions may interact with theophylline to either increase or decrease serum levels. Some of the more common interactions include:

Agents and Conditions that Increase Theophylline Levels (Decreased Dosage Required): Influenza virus vaccine, oral contraceptives, cimetidine, loop diuretics (e.g., furosemide—may increase or decrease serum levels), calcium channel blockers (e.g., verapamil), nonselective β-blockers (e.g., propranolol), corticosteroids, ephedrine, interferon, thyroid hormones, isoniazid (may increase or decrease theophylline effects), quinolones, thiabendazole, disulfiram, allopurinol, macrolides, mexiletine.

Conditions that may increase theophylline levels resulting in an accumulation and possible toxic effects include hepatitis, CHF, renal failure, liver dysfunction, respiratory infections (e.g., pneumonia), alcoholism, fever, shock, hypoxia, severe COPD, cor pulmonale, and diets high in chocolate, cola, tea, and coffee.

Agents that Decrease Theophylline Levels (Increased Dosage Required): Cigarette and marijuana smoking (may require 50 to 100% increase in dosage), barbiturates, charcoal, ketoconazole, rifampin, isoniazid (may increase or decrease levels), loop diuretics (may increase or decrease levels), β-adrenoceptor agonists, thioamines, sulfinpyrazone, aminoglutethimide, hydantoins.

Conditions that may decrease theophylline levels necessitating an increased dosage include infants, children, women, adolescents with cystic fibrosis, high-protein low-carbohydrate diet, hyperthyroidism, diets high in charcoal-broiled beef.

Dosage Schedules

The loading doses of theophylline and its derivatives are based on lean body weight and on the assumption that for each 0.5 mg/kg of theophylline administered, a 1.0 μg/mL increase in serum theophylline will result (for a patient not previously receiving theophylline). Serum theophylline levels should be monitored before and after drug administration. Ideally, serum theophylline levels are measured 15 to 30 minutes after an IV loading dose, 1 to 2 hours after the administration of immediate-release preparations, and 5 to 9 hours after administration of the morning dose of sustained-release formulations. Any dose that is not tolerated is contraindicated.

Because of differing theophylline content, the salts of theophylline are not equivalent on a weight basis. Anhydrous theophylline is the only compound that has 100% theophylline content; therefore, all dosage regimens are based on anhydrous theophylline. Derivatives with low theophylline content are likely to produce less bronchodilation than those with high theophylline content. For example, aminophylline dihydrate has 79% theophylline content. Comparatively, one would need to administer 127 mg of aminophylline to achieve the same response that 100 mg of anhydrous theophylline gives. The following list indicates the approximate equivalent dose of each agent based on anhydrous theophylline dosage equivalents:

Theophylline Salts	Theophylline Content (%)	Equivalent Dose (mg)
Theophylline anhydrous	100	100
Theophylline monohydrate	91	110
Aminophylline anhydrous	86	116
Aminophylline dihydrate	79	127
Oxtriphylline	64	156

Aminophylline is a composite of theophylline with ethylenediamine that exerts its bronchodilating effect at the cellular level after it is converted to theo-

Table 10.5.
Xanthine Bronchodilators

Xanthine	Preparations	Dosing Schedule
Theophylline Preparations:		
Bronkodyl, Elixophyllin, Slo-Phyllin, Theolair, Quibron-T-Dividose	**Immediate-release capsules and tablets:** Varies from 100 to 300 mg	**For an acute attack:** 5 mg/kg initial loading dose, followed by maintenance dosages of 3 to 4 mg/kg q 6 hr to 8 hr.
Asmalix, Elixomin, Elixophyllin, Lanophyllin, Theolair, Aquaphyllin, Slo-Phyllin, Theoclear-80, Theostat-80, Accurbron, Aerolate	**Liquids:** Varies from 80 mg/15 mL to 150 mg/15 mL	
Aerolate, Elixophyllin SR, Slo-bid Gyrocaps, Slo-Phyllin Gyrocaps, Theo-24 (24 hours), Theobid Duracaps, Theoclear L.A., Theo-Dur Sprinkle, Theospan-SR, Theovent	**Timed-release capsules:** Varies from 50 mg to 300 mg; 12 to 24 hour timed release	*Older adults and patients with cor pulmonale:* Loading dose of 5 mg/kg then 2 mg/kg q 8 hr. *Patients with cardiac or liver disease:* Loading dose of 5 mg/kg then 1 to 2 mg/kg q 12 hr. *Preterm infants to <1 years old:* 1 to 1.5 mg/kg q 12 hr.
Theophylline SR, Constant-T, Quibron-T/SR, Respbid, Sustaire, Theochron, Theo-Dur (12 to 24 hours), Theolair-SR, Theo-Sav (8 to 24 hours), Theo-X (12 to 24 hours, Uniphyl (12 to 24 hours)	**Timed-release tablets:** Varies from 100 mg to 500 mg; 12 to 24 hour timed release.	**Chronic therapy:** *Initial dose:* 16 mg/kg/day or 400 mg/24 hours (whichever is less) of anyhydrous theophylline in divided doses administered at 6 to 8 hr intervals. May increase dose in 25% increments at 3 day intervals until desired clinical response is achieved (as long as tolerated), or until maximum dose is reached (see below).
Theophylline and 5% Dextrose	**Injection (IV theophylline):** 200, 400, or 800 mg/container	
		Maximum daily (24 hr) oral dose where serum levels are not measured: 1 to 9 years: 24 mg/kg/day 9 to 12 years: 20 mg/kg/day 12 to 16 years: 18 mg/kg/day >16 years: 13 mg/kg/day *Note: do not exceed listed dose or 900 mg, whichever is less.
Aminophylline (Theophylline Ethylenediamine) Preparations:		
Aminophylline	**Immediate-release tablets:** 100-mg tablets (equivalent to 79 mg theophylline), 200-mg tablets (equivalent to 158 mg theophylline)	**For bronchial asthma:** *Adults:* 600 to 1600 mg PO daily divided t.i.d., q.i.d. *Children:* 12 mg/kg PO daily

Phyllocontin	**Controlled-release (12 hr) tablets:** 225-mg tablets (equivalent to 178 mg theophylline)	divided t.i.d., q.i.d.
Aminophylline	**Oral liquid:** 105 mg/5 mL (equivalent to 90 mg theophylline)	**IV injection:** For an acute attack in patients not currently receiving any theophylline products administer a loading dose of 6 mg/kg given slowly (10 to 20 minutes), infused at a rate of no more than 25 mg/min. Monitor serum theophylline levels in order to accurately maintain therapeutic concentrations and to guide dosage requirements. Substitute oral therapy as soon as feasible.
Aminophylline, Truphylline	**Suppositories:** 250 mg (equivalent to 197.5 mg theophylline), 500 mg (equivalent to 395 mg theophylline)	
Aminophylline	**For IV use:** **Injection:** 250 mg/10 mL (equivalent to 197 mg theophylline)	**Maintenance Infusion Rates (mg/kg/hr):** *Patient Type* — *First 12 hr* — *After 12 hr* 6 mo to 9 yr — 1.2 — 1 9 to 16 yr — 1 — 0.8 Adults — 0.7 — 0.5 Elderly and patients with corpulmonale — 0.6 — 0.3 Patients with cardiac and liver disease — 0.5 — 0.1–0.2
Oxtriphylline (Choline Theophylline) Preparations:		
Choledyl	**Immediate-release tablets:** 100 mg (equivalent to 64 mg theophylline), 200 mg (equivalent to 127 mg theophylline)	*Adults and children 9 to 16 years old:* **PO:** 4.7 mg/kg (usual dose 200 mg) q 6 to 8 hr **Sustained-action (SA) tablets:** If total daily dose is established at 800 or 1200 mg, may take 1 SA tablet q 12 hr
Choledyl SA	**Sustained-action tablets:** 400 mg (equivalent to 254 mg theophylline), 600 mg (equivalent to 382 mg theophylline)	*Children 1 to 9 years old:* **PO:** 6.2 mg/kg q 6 hr
Choledyl	**Elixir:** 100 mg/5 mL (equivalent to 64 mg theophylline)	
Choledyl	**Pediatric syrup:** 50 mg/5 mL (equivalent to 32 mg theophylline)	
Dyphylline (Dihydroxypropyl Theophylline) Preparations:		
Dilor, Dyflex, Lufyllin, Neothylline	**Immediate-release tablets:** 200 mg, 400 mg	*Adults:* **PO:** Up to 15 mg/kg q 6 hr. **IM:** 250 to 500 mg q 6 hr; not to exceed 15 mg/kg q 6 hr. Solution must be injected slowly.
Lufyllin, Dilor	**Elixir:** *100 mg/15 mL:* Lufyllin. *160 mg/15 mL:* Dilor.	
Lufyllin, Dilor	**Injection (IM only):** 250 mg/mL	

phylline. Ethylenediamine enhances the solubility of the theophylline molecule, which makes aminophylline suitable for parenteral administration. The onset of action is within 15 minutes (IV loading dose), with a duration of action that varies with route and formulation.

Oxtriphylline is a choline salt of theophylline with actions and uses similar to theophylline. Oxtriphylline exerts its bronchodilating effects after it is converted to theophylline (oxtriphylline contains 64% theophylline). Comparatively, oxtriphylline is more stable, more soluble, and more predictably absorbed and produces less gastric irritation than aminophylline. Oxtriphylline is especially useful in long-term therapy for patients with asthma and COPD. The onset of action is dose related, usually within 45 minutes. The duration of activity is also dose related, approximately 4 to 8 hours.

Dyphylline (dihydroxypropyl theophylline) is a derivative of theophylline that is approximately one-tenth as potent as theophylline; however, adverse reactions are less prominent. Dyphylline is an alternative drug for patients who are sensitive to ethylenediamine. Measurements of serum theophylline levels will not measure dyphylline levels; specific serum dyphylline levels must be used to monitor therapy. The minimal effective therapeutic concentration is 12 μg/mL. The onset of action is dose related, usually within 45 minutes, with a duration of activity of approximately 4 to 6 hours.

The preparations and dosing schedules of the xanthine bronchodilators are summarized in Table 10.5.

REFERENCES/RECOMMENDED READING

Allen CJ, Campbell AH. Comparison of inhaled atropine sulphate and atropine methonitrate. Thorax 35:932, 1980.

American Academy on Allergy and Immunology—Committee on Drugs. Position statement: adverse effects and complications of treatment with beta-adrenergic agonist drugs. J Allergy Clin Immunol 75:443, 1985.

Barnes PJ, Basbaum CB, Nadel JA. Autoradiographic localization of autonomic receptors in airway smooth muscle: marked differences between large and small airways. Am Rev Respir Dis 127:758, 1983.

Bertino JS Jr, Walker JW. Reassessment of theophylline toxicity. Serum concentrations, clinical course, and treatment. Arch Intern Med 147:757, 1987.

Boyers MC. COPD in the ambulatory elderly; management update. Geriatrics 43:29, 1988.

Britton MG, Earnshaw JS, Palmer JB. A twelve month comparison of salmeterol with salbutamol in asthmatic patients. Eur Respir J 5:1062, 1992.

Brogden RN, Faulds D. Salmeterol xinafoate: a review of its pharmacological properties and therapeutic potential in reversible obstructive airways disease. Allergol Immunopathol (Madr) 20:72, 1992.

Bruderman I, Cohen-Aronovski R, Smorzik J. A comparative study of various combinations of ipratropium bromide and metaproterenol in allergic asthmatic patients. Chest 83:208, 1983.

Bukowskyj M. Theophylline, an overview. Ration Drug Ther 22:(1), 1988.

Carstairs JR, Nimmo AJ, Barnes PJ. Autoradiographic visualization of beta-adrenoceptor subtypes in human lung. Am Rev Respir Dis 132:541, 1985.

Choi OH, et al. Caffeine and theophylline analogues: correlation of behavioral effects with activity as adenosine receptor antagonists and as phosphodiesterase inhibitors. Life Sci 43:387, 1988.

Chung KF, Barnes PJ. Role of inflammatory mediators in asthma. Br Med Bull 48:135, 1992.

Deckers W. The chemistry of new derivatives of tropane alkaloids and the pharmacokinetics of a new quaternary compound. Postgrad Med J 51(Suppl 7):76, 1975.

Derom EY, Pauwels RA. Time course of bronchodilating effect of inhaled formoterol, a potent and long acting sympathomimetic. Thorax 47:30, 1992.

De Troyer A, Yernault JC, Rodenstein D. Effects of vagal blockade on lung mechanics in normal man. J Appl Physiol 46:217, 1979.

Drug Facts and Comparisons. 49th ed. St. Louis: Facts and Comparisons, 1995.

Dureuil B, et al. Effects of aminophylline on diaphragmatic dysfunction after upper abdominal surgery. Anesthesiology 62:242, 1985.

Engelhardt A, Klupp H. The pharmacology and toxicology of a new tropane alkaloid derivative. Postgrad Med J 51(Suppl 7):82, 1975.

Firstater E, Mizrochi E, Topilsky M. The effect of vagolytic drugs on airway obstruction in patients with bronchial asthma. Ann Allergy 46:332, 1981.

Foster WM, et al. Effect of adrenergic agents and their mode of action on mucociliary clearance in man. J Appl Physiol 41:146, 1976.

Gross NJ, Skorodin MS. Anticholinergic, antimuscarinic bronchodilators. Am Rev Respir Dis 129:856, 1984.

Gross NJ, Skorodin MS. Role of the parasympathetic system in airway obstruction due to emphysema. N Engl J Med 311:421, 1984.

Gross NJ, Skorodin MS. Massive overdose of atropine methonitrate with only slight untoward effects (letter). Lancet 2:386, 1985.

Hensley MJ, et al. Distribution of bronchodilation in normal subjects: beta agonist versus atropine. J Appl Physiol 45:778, 1978.

Higgins RM, Stradling JR, Lane DJ. Should ipratropium bromide be added to beta-agonists in treatment of acute severe asthma? Chest 94:718, 1988.

Hughes JA, et al. Effects of ipratropium bromide and fenoterol aerosols in pulmonary emphysema. Thorax 37:667, 1982.

Ingram RH, Wellman JJ, McFadden ER, Med J. Relative contributions of large and small airways to flow limitation in normal subjects before and after atropine and isoproterenol. J Clin Invest 59:696, 1977.

Ingram RH Jr, McFadden ER Jr. Localization and mechanisms of airway responses. New Engl J Med 297:596, 1977.

Jenne JW. Theophylline as a bronchodilator in COPD and its combination with inhaled β-adrenergic drugs. Chest 92(Suppl):7S, 1987.

Kreisman H, et al. Synergism between ipratropium and theophylline in asthma. Thorax 36:387, 1981.

Leahy BC, Gomm SA, Allen SC. Comparison of nebulized salbutamol with nebulized ipratropium bromide in acute asthma. Br J Dis Chest 77:159, 1983.

Mahler DA, et al. Sustained-release theophylline reduces dyspnea in nonreversible obstructive airway disease. Am Rev Respir Dis 131:22, 1985.

Marini JJ, Lakshminarayan S, Kradjan WA. Atropine and terbutaline aerosols in chronic bronchitis: efficacy and sites of action. Chest 80:285, 1981.

Marlin GE, Berend N, Harrison AC. Combined cholinergic antagonist and beta2-adrenoceptor agonist bronchodilator therapy by inhalation. Aust N Z J Med 9:511, 1979.

Mathewson H. Anticholinergic aerosols. Respiratory Care 28(4):467, 1983.

McFadden ER Jr, et al. Predominant site of flow limitation and mechanisms of postexertional asthma. J Appl Physiol 42:746, 1977.

McFadden ER Jr. Beta2 receptor agonist: metabolism and pharmacology. J Allergy Clin Immunol 68:91, 1981.

McNeill RS. Effect of a beta-adrenergic blocking agent, propranolol, on asthmatics. Lancet 2:1101, 1964.

Miech RP, Stein M. Methylxanthines. Clin Chest Med 7:331, 1986.

Murciano D, et al. Effects of theophylline on diaphragmatic strength and fatigue in patients with chronic obstructive pulmonary disease. N Engl J Med 311:349, 1984.

Murciano D, et al. A randomized, controlled trial of theophylline in patients with severe chronic obstructive pulmonary disease. N Engl J Med 320:1521, 1989.

Nair N, et al. Protection by ipratropium bromide and metaproterenol against methacholine and histamine bronchoconstriction. Clin Allergy 24:11, 1984.

Newhouse MT, Ruffin RE. Deposition and fate of aerosolized drugs. Chest 73:936, 1978.

Pearlman DS, et al. A comparison of salmeterol with albuterol in the treatment of mild-to-moderate asthma. N Engl J Med 327:1420, 1992.

Peel ET, et al. A comparison of oxitropium bromide and ipratropium bromide in asthma. Eur J Respir Dis 65:106, 1984.

Peel ET, Anderson G. A dose response study of oxitropium bromide in chronic bronchitis. Thorax 39:453, 1984.

Physicians' Desk Reference. 49th ed. Montvale, NJ: Medical Economics, 1995.

Pistelli R, et al. Selectivity of anticholinergic drugs on central and peripheral airways in normal subjects. Eur J Respir Dis 64(Suppl 128):499, 1983.

Popa V. Beta-adrenergic drugs. Clin Chest Med 7:313, 1986.

Rabe KF, et al. Comparison of the effects of salmeterol and formoterol on airway tone and responsiveness over 24 hours in bronchial asthma. Am Rev Respir Dis 147:1436, 1993.

Rall TW. Evolution of the mechanism of action of methylxanthines: from calcium mobilizers to antagonists of adenosine receptors. Pharmacology 24:277, 1982.

Reed CE. Adrenergic bronchodilators: pharmacology and toxicology. J Allergy Clin Immunol 76:335, 1985.

Ruffin RE, Montgomery JM, Newhouse MT. Site of beta adrenergic receptors in the respiratory tract. Chest 74:256, 1978.

Ruffin RE, et al. Combination bronchodilator therapy in asthma. J Allergy Clin Immunol 69:60, 1982.

Sears MR, et al. Regular inhaled beta-agonist treatment in bronchial asthma. Lancet 336:1391, 1990.

Simons FE, et al. Bronchodilator and bronchoprotective effects of salmeterol in young patients with asthma. J Allergy Clin Immunol 90:840, 1992.

Skorodin MS, et al. Oxitropium bromide, a new anticholinergic bronchodilator. Ann Allergy 56:229, 1986.

Skorodin MS. Beta-adrenergic agonists: a problem. Chest 103:1587, 1993.

Smith G. How to use theophylline for maximal benefit in pulmonary disease. Respiratory Therapy 13(4):31, 1983.

Smyth ET, et al. Interaction and dose equivalence of salbutamol and salmeterol in patients with asthma. BMJ 306:543, 1993.

Solis-Cohen S. The use of adrenal substance in the treatment of asthma. JAMA 34:1164, 1900.
Spector S, Ball RE Jr. Bronchodilating effects of aerosolized SCH 1000 and atropine sulfate in asthmatics. Chest 68:426, 1975.
Spitzer WO, et al. The use of beta-agonists and the risk of death and near death from asthma. N Engl J Med 326:501, 1992.
Stam J, Souren M, Zweers P. The onset of action of formoterol, a new beta 2 adrenoceptor agonist. Int J Clin Pharmacol Ther Toxicol 31:23, 1993.
Stiel I, Rivington R. Adrenergic agents in acute asthma: valuable new alternatives. Ann Emerg Med 12(8):493, 1983.
Svedmyr N. Theophylline. Am Rev Respir Dis 136(Suppl):568, 1987.
Tashkin DP, et al. Comparison of the anticholinergic bronchodilator ipratropium bromide with metaproterenol in chronic obstructive pulmonary disease. Am J Med 81(Suppl 5A):81, 1986.
Ullman A, et al. Onset of action and duration of effect of formoterol and salmeterol compared to salbutamol in isolated guinea pig trachea with or without epithelium. Allergy 47:384, 1992.
Viires N, et al. Effects of aminophylline on diaphragmatic fatigue during acute respiratory failure. Am Rev Respir Dis 129(3):396, 1984.
Vozeh S, et al. Theophylline serum concentration and therapeutic effect in severe acute bronchial obstruction: the optimal use of intravenously administered aminophylline. Am Rev Respir Dis 125(2):181, 1982.
Wanner A. Effect of ipratropium bromide on airway mucociliary functions. Am J Med 81(Suppl 5A):23, 1986.
Yoshizaki S, et al. Sympathomimetic amines having a carbostyril nucleus. J Med Chem 19:1138, 1976.
Ziment I. Respiratory Pharmacology and Therapeutics. Philadelphia: WB Saunders Co., 1978.
Ziment I. Beta-adrenergic agonist toxicity: less of a problem, more of a perception. Chest 103:1591, 1993.

PROPHYLACTIC ANTIASTHMATIC AGENTS 11

PATHOPHYSIOLOGY OF ASTHMA—AN OVERVIEW

Bronchial asthma is a condition characterized by increased irritability of the airways by various stimuli. As one of the most common pulmonary disorders, asthma is estimated to exist in 10% of all people. No one age group, population, or sex is exempt.

An acute asthma attack (regardless of cause) is characterized by bronchospasm, mucosal edema, and excessive mucus secretion with mucus plugging of the airway. There is also a noticeable increase in the production of eosinophils and neutrophils. In combination, the previously mentioned factors cause airway obstruction, hypoxemia, and hyperinflation. During an acute attack, respiratory distress is obvious. Dyspnea, cough with tenacious sputum production, chest tightness, and wheezing are present. Status asthmaticus is a life-threatening asthma attack that is refractory to conventional therapy (β_2-adrenoceptor drugs, theophylline). At this point, intravenous corticosteroids are required (see Chapter 12).

Also known as "reactive airway disease," bronchial asthma has two primary forms:

Atopic or extrinsic asthma: Allergic (immunologic) asthma. Approximately 50% of all individuals with asthma have this form of the disease. The causative agent precipitating an asthma attack is some external antigenic material. Common antigens (or allergens) include pollens, dust, smoke, perfumes, pets, or ragweed. Occasionally, foods (milk, eggs, chocolate) or drugs (aspirin) may precipitate an attack.

This form of asthma involves the immune system in antigen-antibody formation. An allergic individual exposed to an antigen or allergen induces antibody formation specific to the antigen. The antibody is then *sensitized* to that particular antigen. The antibody of interest in allergic asthma is immunoglobulin E (IgE), a circulating immunoglobulin that is synthesized by plasma cells in response to an initial exposure of antigen in a susceptible individual. Once IgE molecules become *sensitized* to a specific antigen, they fix themselves to the surface of mast cells in airway mucosa and basophils and other mast cells throughout the body. By this action, the mast cell becomes receptive.

The fixed IgE molecules are antigen-specific: upon reexposure to the antigen, a "bridging" occurs with the antigen-specific IgE complex bound to the receptive mast cell. This antigen-antibody reaction provokes a rapid influx of calcium ions into the mast cell and the activation of phospholipase enzymes within the cell. Phospholipase metabolizes membrane phospholipids to arachidonic acid, which is subsequently metabolized to prostaglandins (via the cyclooxygenase pathway) and to leukotrienes (via the lipoxygenase pathway) (see Chapter 2, *Local Control Substances*). Some of these products (e.g., $PGF_{2\alpha}$, thromboxanes, and the leukotrienes LTC_4, LTD_4, and LTE_4) are potent mediators that are responsible for the inflammatory reaction in allergic individuals. Along with the synthesis of the prostaglandins, thromboxanes, and leukotrienes, phospholipid metabolism by phospholipase triggers the production of platelet activating factor (PAF), another potent bronchospastic agent. As these newly synthesized mediators are released from the cell, other stored mediators such as histamine are also released. In allergic individuals, release of mediators produces airway smooth muscle contraction, mucosal edema, cellular infiltration, and mucus secretion with mucus plugging (i.e., an acute asthma attack).

Nonatopic or intrinsic asthma: Nonallergic (nonimmunologic) asthma. The asthma attack is precipitated either by some endogenous cause (nonallergic stimuli of unknown etiology) or in response to nonimmunologic stimuli such as infection, cold air, exercise, emotional upset, or stress. This form of asthma does not involve the immune response; however, nonimmunologic, nonallergic stimuli still evoke mast cell degranulation, which then causes an acute asthma attack. Figure 11.1 presents a schematic representation of the sequence of events that lead to an asthmatic response.

Of the inflammatory reactions (whether precipitated in extrinsic or intrinsic asthmatics), contraction of airway smooth muscle is most easily reversed by β_2-adrenoceptor, antimuscarinic, and/or theophylline therapy, whereas reversal of the edema and cellular infiltration requires sustained treatment with anti-inflammatory agents (see Chapter 12, Steroidal Anti-inflammatory Drugs). Prevention of the inflammatory occurrence or as a means to reduce the frequency and severity of the attack can be brought about by the prophylactic antiasthmatic agents cromolyn sodium (disodium cromoglycate) and nedocromil sodium.

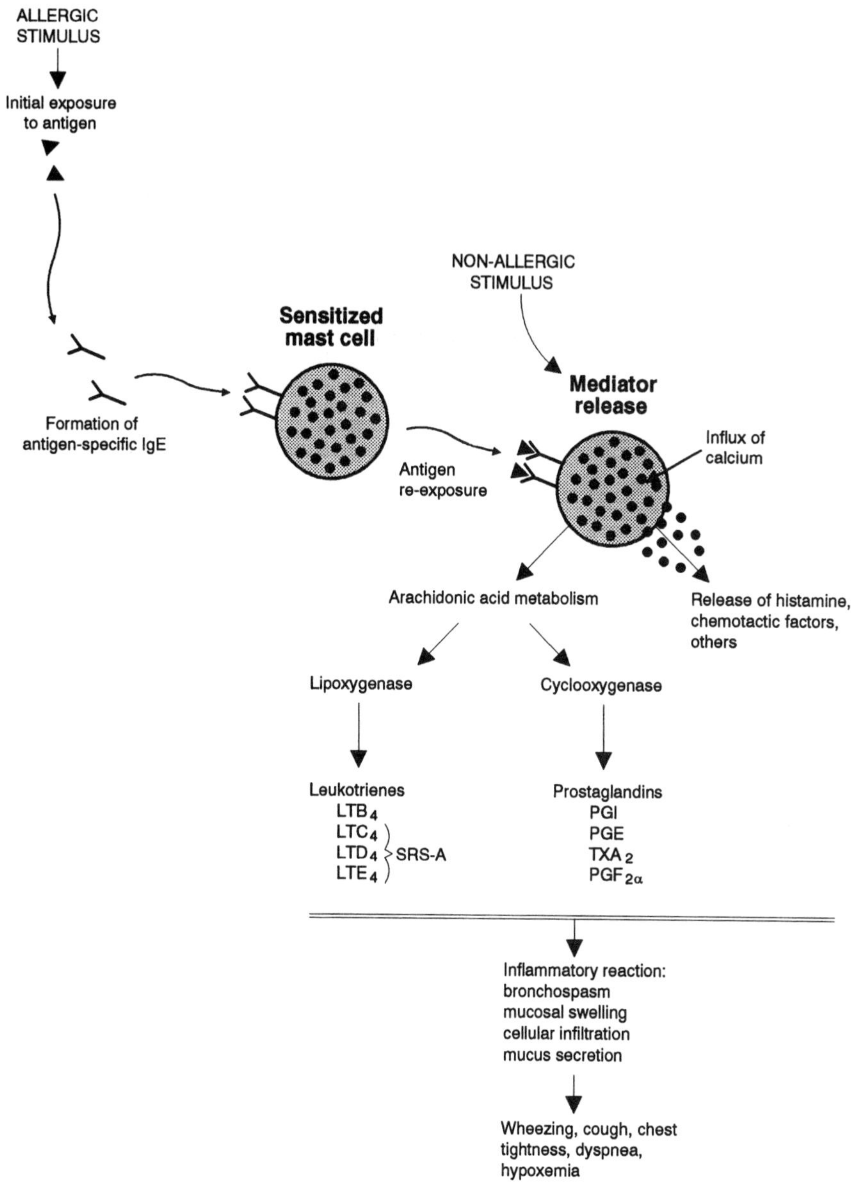

Figure 11.1. Schematic representation of the factors that lead to an asthmatic response.

SPECIFIC ANTIASTHMATIC AGENTS

CROMOLYN SODIUM: INTAL, AARANE, NASALCROM, GASTROCROM, OPTICROM

Mechanism of Action and Indications for Use

Cromolyn sodium (or disodium cromoglycate, as it is sometimes termed) is an antiasthmatic agent that produces its therapeutic effect in a unique and different manner from the other classes of agents used in airway disease. Several postulates have been formulated that may account for cromolyn's mechanism of action. Some of these postulates include:

- Inhibition of the influx of calcium into the mast cell, thereby preventing the degranulation of the mast cell and subsequent release of inflammatory mediators
- Inhibition of IgE-mediated mast cell degranulation
- Phosphodiesterase inhibition
- Inhibition of neural irritant receptors

Although cromolyn's mechanism of action has not been clearly defined, it does inhibit the degranulation of mast cells; mediator release is then prevented (Fig. 11.2). For this reason, cromolyn is known as a "mast cell stabilizer" or, currently, as a mediator release inhibitor (MRI). By inhibiting release of inflammatory mediators from mast cells within the airway mucosa and along bronchial blood vessels, cromolyn blunts both the immediate and late asthmatic reactions to inhaled or absorbed antigens.

The antiallergic activity of cromolyn is mainly prophylactic in that *pretreatment* is necessary for inhibition of mast cell degranulation. Cromolyn is poorly absorbed from the gastrointestinal tract and therefore is only effective when de-

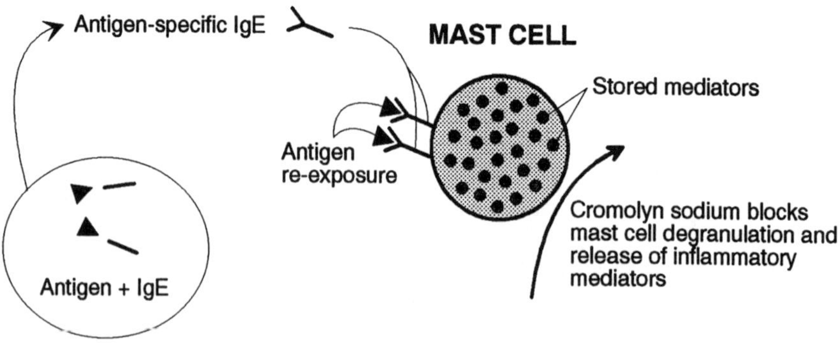

Figure 11.2. The inhibition of mast cell degranulation by cromolyn sodium.

posited directly into the airways. For use in asthma, cromolyn is applied topically to the airways either by inhalation of a microfine powder via the Spinhaler device (see Chapter 3, Fig. 3.7) or via aerosolized solution as described in Table 11.1. The nebulizer solution must be stored below 30°C (86°F) and protected from direct light. When administered by inhalation, approximately 10% of cromolyn is absorbed and most is excreted unchanged. The plasma level of cromolyn reaches its peak within 30 minutes with a duration of activity of 4 to 6 hours.

Inhaled cromolyn sodium is indicated for use to decrease the frequency and intensity of asthma attacks in both allergic and nonallergic asthma. Cromolyn sodium is also used for the treatment and prevention of allergic rhinitis (nasal solution, Nasalcrom) and for the prevention of exercise-induced bronchospasm. Because it is a prophylactic drug, cromolyn has no role in the treatment of acute asthma, especially status asthmaticus.

The complete prophylactic activity of cromolyn may take from 4 to 6 weeks before any symptomatic improvement occurs. At present, a therapeutic trial of 4 to 6 weeks is the only way of determining whether a patient will respond. In patients who do respond, regular and consistent use of cromolyn (20 mg four times daily) is at least as effective in controlling the symptoms of asthma as oral maintenance theophylline therapy.

Other uses of cromolyn include the treatment of allergic conjunctivitis (ophthalmic solution, Opticrom) and the treatment of mastocytosis (oral solution,

Table 11.1.
Dosages and Preparations of the Antiasthmatic Agents

Antiasthmatic Agent	Preparations	Dosage[a]
Cromolyn sodium Inhalation: Intal, Aarane Ophthalmic solution: Opticrom Nasal solution: Nasalcrom Oral solution: Gastrocrom	Inhal solution: 20 mg/2 mL liquid ampule Inhal capsules: 20 mg/dry powder capsule (to be used with Spinhaler) Metered-dose inhaler: 0.8 mg/inhalation Ophthalmic solution: 40 mg/mL (4%) Nasal Solution: 40 mg/mL (5.2 mg/spray) Oral Solution: 100 mg/capsule	1 ampule via small volume nebulizer q.i.d. (inhale <1 hr prior to exercise) 1 capsule via Spinhaler q.i.d. (inhale <1 hr prior to exercise) 2 puffs q.i.d. (inhale <1 hr prior to exercise) 1–2 drops in each eye 4–6 times daily 1 spray per nostril 3–6 times daily Dissolve 2 capsules in hot water, take orally q.i.d. 1/2 hour before meals and hs *Children 2–12 yr:* 1 capsule dissolved in hot water q.i.d., do not exceed 40 mg/kg/day
Nedocromil sodium (Tilade)	Metered-dose inhaler: 1.75 mg/inhalation	2 puffs q.i.d. (14 mg/day)

[a]Adult dose, unless otherwise specified.

Gastrocrom). Mastocytosis is a condition associated with mast cell infiltration of viscera as well as skin. Oral cromolyn has also been used for prevention of an allergic response to certain foods.

Contraindications

Contraindications to the use of cromolyn include hypersensitivity to the drug, acute asthmatic attacks, status asthmaticus.

Precautions

1. Cromolyn is not a bronchodilator and should not be used for the reversal of acute bronchospasm. Its primary advantage lies in its prophylactic activity. If bronchospasm occurs, the treatment should be stopped and the physician should be notified. Prior administration of a β_2-adrenoceptor agent is recommended if a patient develops bronchospasm and wheezing with the administration of nedocromil.
2. Cromolyn must be used regularly to achieve maximum effectiveness, even during symptom-free periods.
3. Cromolyn's therapeutic effect relies on topical application to the lungs. Proper inhalational technique is essential; therefore, patients should be properly instructed regarding correct method of use.
4. Cromolyn should be protected from light and stored between 2° and 30°C (36° to 86°F). Do not freeze.

Adverse Reactions

Cromolyn is generally well tolerated by patients. Adverse effects of cromolyn are minor and primarily localized to the site of application. Symptoms such as throat irritation, cough, mouth dryness, chest tightness, or wheezing may occur. Some of these symptoms (chest tightness, wheezing) may be prevented by inhaling a β_2-adrenoceptor agonist prior to cromolyn treatment. Other adverse reactions such as laryngeal edema, joint swelling and pain, angioedema, headache, rash, and nausea have also been reported with the use of cromolyn.

Dosage and Administration

The preparations and dosages of cromolyn are listed in Table 11.1.

NEDOCROMIL SODIUM: TILADE

Mechanism of Action and Indications for Use

Nedocromil sodium is the newest, second-generation antiasthmatic agent; it was approved for use in the USA in late December 1992. Although cromolyn has been more extensively studied than nedocromil, the two agents seem to share a similar mechanism of action and indications for use. Prior to exposure, treatment with nedocromil has been shown to reduce the bronchoconstrictor response caused by sulfur dioxide, inhaled neurokinin A, various antigens, exercise, fog, and cold air. Nedocromil, like cromolyn, inhibits the immediate and late reactions to inhaled or absorbed antigens.

Various clinical studies have shown that with the use of nedocromil, there is symptomatic improvement in controlling asthma and pulmonary function when it is added to an as-needed regimen of β_2-adrenoceptor therapy and beneficial effect could be detected in as little as 2 weeks of consistent use.

Contraindications

Contraindications to the use of nedocromil include hypersensitivity to the drug or other ingredients in the preparation.

Precautions

1. As with cromolyn, nedocromil is not a bronchodilator and should not be used for the reversal of acute bronchospasm. Its primary advantage lies in its prophylactic activity. If bronchospasm occurs, the treatment should be stopped and the physician should be notified. Prior administration of a β_2-adrenoceptor agent is recommended if a patient develops bronchospasm and wheezing with the administration of nedocromil.
2. Nedocromil must be used regularly to achieve maximum effectiveness, even during symptom-free periods.
3. As with cromolyn, nedocromil's therapeutic effect relies on topical application to the lungs. Proper inhalational technique is essential; therefore, patients should be properly instructed regarding the correct method of use.
4. Nedocromil should be stored between 2° and 30°C (36° to 86°F). Do not freeze.

Adverse Reactions

Nedocromil is a relatively safe drug and is generally well tolerated. Reported adverse effects are similar to those of cromolyn.

Dosage and Administration

Nedocromil's dosage and preparations are summarized in Table 11.1.

KETOTIFEN: ZADITEN

Ketotifen is a drug currently under investigation as an antiasthmatic agent. Ketotifen exhibits the same pharmacologic activities as cromolyn. However, ketotifen has the added advantage of oral administration. Clinical studies have shown that 1 mg of ketotifen given orally twice daily has the same effect as 20 mg of cromolyn given four times daily (via Spinhaler).

As with cromolyn, the complete prophylactic activity of ketotifen requires approximately 4 to 6 weeks. However, there are a few documented case studies in which ketotifen failed to provide prophylaxis in adults with intrinsic (nonallergic) asthma and in exercise-induced bronchospasm in children with asthma, in addition to causing marked sedation and drowsiness. Overdosage symptoms include mild abdominal pain, confusion, bradycardia, hyperexcitability, tachycardia, dyspnea, tachypnea, cyanosis, convulsions, and unconsciousness.

Although ketotifen may not replace established antiasthmatic drugs, it is a potential alternative in the prophylaxis of asthma. Ketotifen is already available in Britain and Europe. Pending further approval in the USA, Sandoz (new drug application filed in 1982) plans to market the drug under the name of Zaditen.

REFERENCES/RECOMMENDED READING

Aalbers R, et al. The effect of nedocromil sodium on the early and late reaction and allergen-induced bronchial hyperresponsiveness. J Allergy Clin Immunol 87:993, 1991.

Barnes PJ, Chung KF, Page CP. Inflammatory mediators and asthma. Pharmacol Rev 40:49, 1988.

Bernstein IL. Cromolyn sodium. Chest 87(Suppl):68S, 1985.

Brogden RN, Sorkin EM. Nedocromil sodium: an updated review of its pharmacological properties and therapeutic efficacy in asthma. Drugs 45:693, 1993.

Drug Facts and Comparisons. 49th ed. St. Louis: Facts and Comparisons, 1995.

Djukanovic R, et al. Mucosal inflammation in asthma. Am Rev Respir Dis 142:434, 1990.

Friedman MM, Kaliner MA. Human mast cells and asthma. Am Rev Respir Dis 135:1156, 1987.

Gonzales JP, Brogden RN. Nedocromil sodium: a preliminary review of its pharmacodynamic properties, and therapeutic efficacy in the treatment of reversible obstructive airways disease. Drugs 34:560, 1987.

Neal MG, et al. The pharmacokinetics of sodium cromoglycate in man after intravenous and inhalation administration. Br J Clin Pharmacol 22:373, 1986.

Physicians' Desk Reference. 49th ed. Montvale, NJ: Medical Economics, 1995.

ANTI-INFLAMMATORY AGENTS 12

This chapter focuses on the reactions that occur when the inflammatory response is activated as well as the primary drug groups that act to inhibit or suppress this process: steroidal anti-inflammatory drugs and nonsteroidal anti-inflammatory drugs (NSAIDS).

THE INFLAMMATORY RESPONSE

The body's defense against invasion by foreign materials (antigens) includes immune and inflammatory processes. The immune response is the body's natural defense mechanism in which specific foreign materials are neutralized, destroyed, or eliminated by white blood cells (see Appendix B, IV, G) and the production and activation of antibodies. The immune response is specific for a particular antigen, requires an initial exposure before it can be initiated, and can trigger the inflammatory reaction at a rapid rate.

The immune system has two distinct functional units: humoral immunity (HI) and cell-mediated immunity (CMI). In response to an antigen, either or both units of the immune system can activate lymphocytes and macrophages. The humoral immune response involves the activation of B lymphocytes (see Appendix B), which produce antigen-specific antibodies that act to remove or destroy the antigen. Currently, there are five major classes of antibodies (all antibodies are immunoglobulins, but as yet it is not known whether all immunoglobulins have antibody functions) that exist naturally in the body or are produced in response to a foreign invasion. Table 12.1 indicates their location and roles.

Cell-mediated immune response involves the production of T lymphocytes (see Appendix B) that are antigen specific in that each one responds to only one antigen. T lymphocytes remove or destroy antigens directly in this manner or they

Table 12.1.
Major Antibodies (Immunoglobulins) of the Immune System

Type	Location	Function
IgA	Serum (10 to 15%) Exocrine secretions (tears, saliva, sweat, milk, respiratory and intestinal mucosa)	Principal immunoglobulin in body secretions. Protects body lumens and mucosal surfaces from invasion of pathogenic bacteria and viruses. First-line defense in the prevention of respiratory infections. Individuals deficient in IgA are prone to recurrent respiratory infections. Presence of IgA in colostrum helps protect the nursing infant from infection.
IgD	Serum (trace amounts—prepared from the plasma of individuals with a high concentration of Rh antibodies)	Administered to an Rh-negative mother within 72 hours after delivery of an Rh-positive infant to prevent isoimmunization and hemolytic disease of the newborn in subsequent pregnancies.
IgE	Serum (trace amounts) Tissue bound (mast cells)	Primary immunoglobulin in immediate hypersensitivity (allergic) reactions. Attaches to mast cells in the respiratory and intestinal tracts after exposure to an antigen. Approximately 50% of individuals with allergic diseases (e.g., asthma) have increased IgE levels. Also known as "reaginic immunoglobulin" (participates in the formation of reagin) and "cytophilic immunoglobulin" (has a high affinity for cell surfaces; i.e., mast cell). See also Chapter 11, *Pathophysiology of Asthma.*
IgG	Serum (80%)	Principal immunoglobulin in human serum. Major immunoglobulin for antitoxins, bacteria, and viruses. Recruits phagocytic cells. Moves across the placental barrier to provide protection in the fetus and newborn. As gamma globulin, IgG may be given for temporary protection against hepatitis and other diseases.
IgM	Serum (5 to 10%)	Formed from almost every immune response during the early phase of the reaction. Most active immunoglobulin that participates in the agglutination of foreign particles. Controls the A, B, O, blood group antibody responses.

Ig, immunoglobulin.

may interact indirectly by invoking the assistance of phagocytic macrophages and neutrophils.

The inflammatory response is a vascular reaction in which fluid, chemical mediators, and cells are delivered to the site of injury. The chemical mediators of inflammation (e.g., histamine, leukotrienes, prostaglandins, thromboxanes, bradykinin, serotonin, platelet–activating factor) and their corresponding physiological effects have previously been presented in Chapter 2, *Local Control Substances.* The inflammatory process is generally the same regardless of cause and can involve two distinct phases:

Early (immediate hypersensitivity) phase: an acute transient phase characterized by local vasodilatation and increased capillary permeability. This phase has the classic triple response features that result when the skin is injured:

- Redness (caused by local vasodilatation of blood vessels)
- Flare or erythema (a flushed, red area surrounding the site of injury)
- Welt or wheal (an elevated area resulting from localized edema)

The immediate inflammatory response that occurs in the airways of asthmatic individuals results in bronchial smooth muscle contraction. Wheezing, cough, dyspnea, and hypoxemia are evident.

Late (delayed hypersensitivity) phase: a subacute phase that can occur several hours after antigen exposure. This phase is characterized by infiltration of leukocyte and phagocytic cells. In the airways of asthmatics, there is an increase in eosinophils and neutrophils, a sloughing off (desquamation) of airway cells, and an excessive proliferation (hyperplasia) of goblet cells. The result is mucus hypersecretion. Mucosal swelling (edema) also occurs due to increased vascular permeability. Subsequently, mucus plugging of the airway (secondary to retained secretions and the accumulation of cellular debris) and severe respiratory distress ensue and may lead to intubation and mechanical ventilation.

As mentioned previously, the above inflammatory sequence can be blocked or made less severe with the use of anti-inflammatory agents.

STEROIDAL ANTI-INFLAMMATORY AGENTS

Adrenocorticosteroids are naturally occurring hormones secreted by the adrenal cortex. These corticosteroids are classified into three groups according to their chemical structure and major physiological effects: 1) glucocorticosteroids (e.g., hydrocortisone, anti-inflammatory and immunosuppressive actions), 2) mineralocorticosteroids (e.g., aldosterone, maintains water and electrolyte balance), and 3) sex hormones (e.g., androgens and estrogens). Of main concern to the practitioner are the glucocorticoids used in cardiopulmonary care, all of which are analogs of hydrocortisone (cortisol).

Physiology of Glucocorticosteroid Production

The Hypothalamic-Pituitary-Adrenal (HPA) Transport System

The hypothalamus contains corticotropin-releasing hormone (CRH) which, when released, travels through a portal system of blood vessels to the pituitary gland. After reaching the pituitary gland, CRH stimulates the pituitary corticotrophs to secrete adrenocorticotrophic hormone (ACTH) into the bloodstream. ACTH then mediates the synthesis and release of glucocorticoids (primarily cortisol) at the adrenal cortex. The degree of ACTH stimulation at the adrenal cortex is a direct factor of plasma cortisol levels. Elevated plasma levels decrease ACTH secretion, and likewise, reduced plasma levels increase the secretion of ACTH. This feedback system is important in maintaining the normal plasma level of cortisol and functioning of the adrenal cortex (Fig. 12.1).

The rate at which cortisol is secreted by the adrenal cortex ranges between 10 and 30 mg/day. However, this secretory rate is not steady or constant. Cortisol is primarily secreted in response to stressful events (surgery, exercise, infection, in-

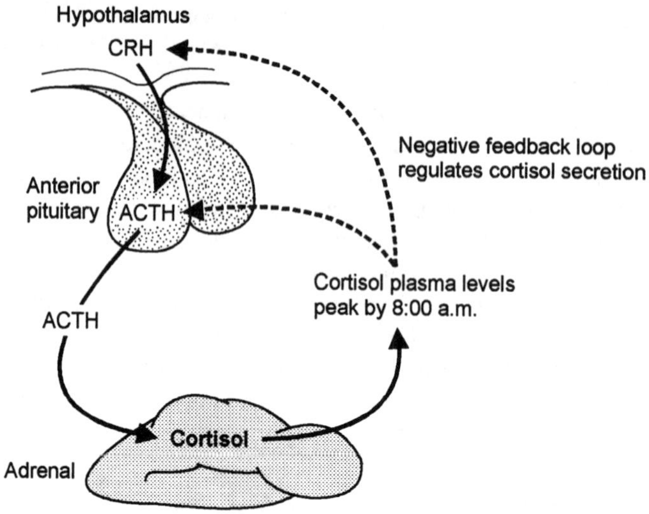

Figure 12.1. Schematic representation of the hypothalamic-pituitary-adrenal (HPA) transport mechanism. Negative feedback functions to control plasma cortisol levels.

jury, strong emotions, pain, fear, etc.) and on a regular circadian (24-hour cycle) or diurnal (daily) rhythm. Serum concentrations of cortisol gradually rise beginning at 3:00 or 4:00 AM, peak at approximately 8:00 AM (which blocks further production because of the feedback system just described), and then gradually decline to a minimum around midnight. Individuals who work at night have reversal to a nocturnal pattern (this may take several weeks to synchronize).

Mechanism of Action and Indications for Use

In the plasma, steroidal anti-inflammatory agents (glucocorticoids) are reversibly bound to two plasma proteins: corticosteroid-binding globulin (CBG) and albumin. Plasma-free glucocorticoids enter sensitive target cells by passive diffusion and react with receptor proteins in the cytoplasm, forming a steroid-receptor complex. The complex undergoes a modificational change and migrates to the nucleus of the cell, where it binds with steroid receptors on chromatin, which contains the genetic material of the nucleus, deoxyribonucleic acid (DNA). This interaction by glucocorticoids in the cell's nucleus results in transcription of new messenger ribonucleic acid (RNA) and new protein synthesis. The newly synthesized proteins mediate the cellular response associated with the glucocorticoid (Fig. 12.2).

The pharmacologic actions of glucocorticoids depend on the type of target cell involved. In addition, because of the time involved in the above described nuclear pathway, glucocorticoid effects may not be evident for several hours. The major influences that these agents have on bodily systems and tissues include the following:

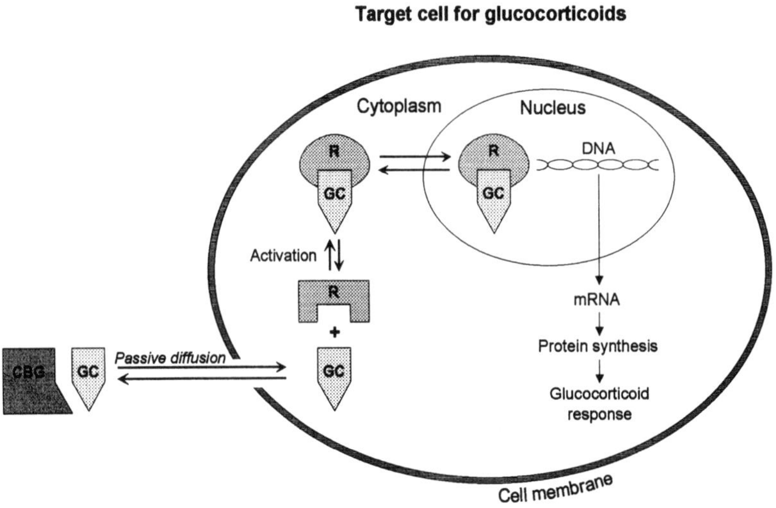

Figure 12.2. Nuclear pathway of glucocorticoid (GC) action. Plasma-free glucocorticoids move into the cytoplasm of target cells and bind to cytoplasmic receptor (R) proteins. The steroid-receptor complex undergoes a transitional change and migrates into the nucleus of the cell, where it modifies the formation of messenger RNA and, hence, protein synthesis. The newly synthesized proteins bring about the cellular responses associated with the glucocorticoid. CBG, corticosteroid-binding globulin.

- Anti-Inflammatory and Immunosuppressive Effects: Glucocorticoids have a profound capacity to prevent or suppress the manifestations of inflammation. This is due to the glucocorticoids' significant effects on the concentration, distribution, and function of peripheral leukocytes and to their inhibition of phospholipase activity. Glucocorticoids reduce the number of circulating lymphocytes, monocytes, eosinophils, and basophils by moving these cells from the vascular bed to lymphoid tissue, bone marrow, and spleen. This then reduces the number of these cells that reach the site of inflammation, which in turn causes a reduction in cell-mediated immunity and inflammation. Glucocorticoids also inhibit macrophage and leukocyte processing of antigens; thus, the ability of these cells to respond to antigens and mitogens is reduced. Glucocorticoid activity also leads to the increase in the concentration of lipocortins, enzymes that inhibit the activity of phospholipase. By this action, the conversion of phospholipid to arachidonic acid (see Chapter 11) is prevented, which in turn blocks the production of the highly inflammatory arachidonic acid metabolites, the prostaglandins and leukotrienes, as well as the potent bronchoconstrictor, platelet-activating factor. Glucocorticoids also reduce capillary permeability by reducing the amount of histamine released by basophils.

- Carbohydrate, Protein, and Fat Metabolism Effects: Glucocorticoids increase the synthesis of glucose from protein (gluconeogenesis), increase liver glycogen, increase plasma glucose concentration, and decrease peripheral glucose utilization. The increase in plasma glucose levels stimulates insulin release. In general, the body is being prepared for fasting during stress as it increases the production of glucose, decreases glucose use in muscle, and promotes glycogen storage. Glucocorticoids cause the redistribution of fat from the periphery to the face (produces a moon face appearance), to the back of the neck (produces a buffalo hump appearance), and to the supraclavicular region (results in truncal obesity).
- Electrolyte and Water Metabolism Effects: Glucocorticoids enhance sodium retention and potassium excretion (however, not to the extent that aldosterone does). If prolonged, the patient may exhibit hypokalemic alkalosis as well as weakness because of potassium loss. Glucocorticoids also promote renal excretion of calcium; osteoporosis may develop. In addition, inhibition of bone growth is a problem for children who are on long-term glucocorticoid therapy, resulting in a reduced adult height.
- Miscellaneous Effects: Glucocorticoids also influence the central nervous system (CNS). Individuals may experience euphoria, behavioral disturbances, and psychoses. In addition, large doses of these steroids may lead to peptic ulcers. Glucocorticoids have some effects on the development of the near-term fetus. There are structural and functional changes in the lungs as well as the production of surfactant (see Chapter 13) that is stimulated by glucocorticoids.

In addition to the above-mentioned effects, glucocorticoids exhibit activity that restores and enhances the response of the β_2-adrenoceptor to inhaled β_2-adrenoceptor agonists. Mechanisms that may be responsible for these effects include an up-regulation of β_2-adrenoceptors with an increase in their numbers and availability. Clinical studies have also shown that glucocorticoids can prolong endogenous circulating catecholamine activity by inhibiting the extraneuronal uptake (uptake-2) detailed in Chapter 2. As a result, there is a noticeable increase in sympathomimetic responsiveness. Glucocorticoids also help to control mucus volume, alter mucus composition, and increase mucociliary transport, which ultimately helps to alleviate mucus retention problems.

Glucocorticoids do not cure any disease. They are used predominantly for their anti-inflammatory properties and provide only symptomatic relief. However, they are nevertheless widely used to treat the acute, critical stages of chest disease and to control the symptoms of disabling chronic disorders. Glucocorticosteroids are indicated for use in such conditions as acute and chronic asthmatic attacks (only if conventional therapy has failed: β_2-adrenoceptor agents, theophylline, avoidance of provoking stimuli), status asthmaticus, severe chronic obstructive pulmonary disease (variable effect, may improve general sense of well-being without other objective signs of clinical improvement), hypersensitivity pneumonitis, active interstitial lung disease (sarcoidosis, collagen-vascular disorders, pneumoconioses, idiopathic interstitial pulmonary fibrosis), allergic bronchopulmonary aspergillosis, neonatal respiratory distress syndrome, adult respiratory distress syndrome (a controversial indication), aspiration pneumonitis, airway injury from inhalation of toxic gases, severe pneumocystis carinii pneumonia, miliary tuberculosis, laryngitis, tracheitis, and allergic rhinitis (available as nasal sprays). Systemic administration of steroids is indicated for an acute asthma attack and status asthmaticus, whereas aerosolized steroids are primarily used for control of severe asthma and in patients with chronic asthma. Table 12.2 lists the advantages and disadvantages of systemic and aerosol administration of glucocorticoids.

Other, nonrespiratory uses for the administration of glucocorticoid therapy include:

- Diagnosis and treatment of disturbed adrenal function such as that which occurs in acute or chronic (Addison's disease) adrenocorticol insufficiency and adrenocorticol hyperfunction (congenital adrenal hyperplasia).
- Stimulation of lung maturation in the fetus. Treatment of the mother with large doses of glucocorticoid reduces the incidence of infant respiratory distress syndrome in infants delivered prematurely.
- Other various nonadrenal disorders in which the glucocorticoid is used for its ability to suppress inflammatory and immune responses. This diverse group of

Table 12.2.
Comparison of Oral and Aerosol Glucocorticoids for Asthma[a]

	Oral	Aerosol
ADVANTAGES OF AEROSOL FORMULATIONS		
Development of Cushing's syndrome with optimal dose	Yes	No
Suppression of hypothalamic-pituitary-adrenal mechanism	Yes	No (doses of <1000 μg/day)
Development of a steroid-dependent state	High risk	Low risk
Local therapeutic effects	No	Yes
ADVANTAGES OF ORAL FORMULATIONS		
Ease of administration	Simple	Complex
Dosage schedules	Well dictated	Not well established
Cost	Inexpensive	Expensive
Hazards of therapy	Well documented	All hazards not fully known
Potential improper use (e.g., as a "bronchodilator")	Medium risk	High risk
Used for status asthmaticus	Yes	No
Risk of superinfection	Moderate	Greater risk
Local airway reaction	No	Hoarseness Coughing Throat irritation

[a]Adapted from Ziment I. Respiratory pharmacology and therapeutics. Philadelphia: WB Saunders, 1978.

diseases include certain eye diseases (e.g., acute uveitis, allergic conjunctivitis, optic neuritis, and choroiditis), gastrointestinal (GI) diseases (e.g., inflammatory bowel disease), hematologic disorders (e.g., acquired hemolytic anemia, leukemia, multiple myeloma), infections such as gram-negative septicemia, inflammatory conditions of bones and joints (arthritis, bursitis), neurologic disorders (cerebral edema, multiple sclerosis), renal disorders (nephrotic syndrome), skin diseases (atopic dermatitis, dermatoses, xerosis, mycosis fungoides), thyroid diseases (malignant exophthalmos, subacute thyroiditis), hypercalcemia and mountain sickness, and in the prevention and treatment of organ transplant rejection (in which immunosuppression is required).

Contraindications

Contraindications to the use of steroidal anti-inflammatory agents include hypersensitivity to any of the drug's ingredients, systemic fungal infections (because of their immunosuppressant actions, corticosteroids mask the symptoms of infection), psychoses, peptic ulcer, acute glomerulonephritis, herpes simplex of the eye, and severe diabetes mellitus.

Precautions

1. These agents are not direct bronchodilators; therefore, they are not indicated for the rapid relief of bronchospasm.
2. Prolonged therapy may lead to the suppression of the HPA transport system. This is why the dosage of the glucocorticoid, when administered for more than a few weeks, must be gradually tapered, allowing the HPA transport mechanism to return to its normal functioning level; otherwise, an adrenal crisis may occur and may potentiate the disease state. When tapering dosages, the patient should be monitored for steroid withdrawal syndrome: anorexia, nausea, vomiting, lethargy, headache, hypotension. Aerosol corticosteroids have less HPA suppression effects than systemic corticosteroids; however, if recommended dosages are exceeded (>1000 μg/day), the HPA transport mechanism may be influenced. As remission is maintained, a recommended dosing schedule for oral administration is alternate day therapy whereby double the daily dose is given as a single dose every other morning. This method not only mimics the natural diurnal rhythm of the HPA system by administering the drug early in the morning, it allows the transport system to function on the nonsteroid day, while also keeping the disease in a stable subacute state. The overall beneficial effects of alternate day therapy include minimal suppression of the HPA transport system, reduced risk for developing Cushing's syndrome (see below), lower incidence of withdrawal symptoms, and a reduced risk for growth suppression in children. The benefits of alternate day therapy are only gained with the administration of intermediate-acting glucocorticoids.

3. Use with caution in pregnancy. Use only if the benefits outweigh the potential risk to the fetus.
4. Prolonged therapy with moderate to high doses results in Cushing's syndrome, a condition that stimulates adrenal cortex hypersecretion, with the following Cushingoid effects: moon-like appearance of the face, edema, buffalo hump over back and neck, truncal obesity, weight gain, thin fragile skin susceptible to bruising, ecchymosis, and poor wound healing.
5. Administer PO forms with food to minimize ulcer activity.
6. To minimize side effects, local administration is preferred over systemic therapy when indicated.
7. Long-term steroid therapy requires the smallest dose that will produce the desired effects. Once symptoms are under control, glucocorticoid doses are gradually tapered by small decrements until the lowest dose that produces the desired clinical response is reached.
8. Intravenous corticosteroids are indicated only when the patient with asthma has failed to respond to conventional therapy (e.g., sympathomimetic bronchodilators, theophylline, and other nonsteroid medications).
9. Use with caution for patients with renal disease or impairment; edema may occur.
10. Certain disorders and drugs require adjustment of the administered dose. Conditions or drugs that may necessitate an increased dosage include liver disease (metabolic degradation of glucocorticoids occurs mostly in the liver), barbiturates, ephedrine, dilantin, rifampin, tranquilizers (e.g., diazepam, nitrazepam, hydroxyzine). Conditions or drugs that may require a decrease in the glucocorticoid dose include low serum albumin, cromolyn (slight decrease), certain antibiotics such as erythromycin, high-dose salicylates, and preparations with the preservative parabens.
11. Owing to the immunosuppression that results from glucocorticoid use, the patient's susceptibility to infection (especially nosocomial, viral, fungal) increases. Because immunosuppression tends to mask early signs and symptoms of infection, the infection may become systemic with little to no warning. The immunosuppression effect may also inhibit reactions to skin tests.
12. Moderate to large doses may elevate the blood pressure, induce salt and water retention, and increase excretion of potassium and calcium. Salt restriction and supplemental potassium may be necessary.

Adverse Reactions: Systemic Corticosteroids

Suppression of the HPA system and the adrenal cortex.

Fluid and Electrolyte Imbalance: Sodium and fluid retention, edema, hypokalemia, hypocalcemia, metabolic alkalosis.

Cardiovascular: Fat embolism, thromboembolism, cardiac arrhythmias, syncope, hypertension.

GI: Pancreatitis, abdominal distention, nausea, vomiting, increased appetite, weight gain, peptic ulcer, perforation of the small and large bowel.

CNS: Headache, vertigo, insomnia, restlessness, seizures, mood swings, depression, euphoria.

Musculoskeletal: Muscle wasting, muscle pain, osteoporosis, delayed wound healing.

Miscellaneous: Growth suppression, obesity, Cushingoid appearance, hyperglycemia, diabetes, and immunosuppression.

Adverse Reactions: Aerosol Corticosteroids

Local: Throat irritation, hoarseness, dry mouth, coughing, oropharyngeal fungal infection (Candida albicans or Aspergillus niger); rinsing and gargling with a mouthwash high in alcohol content (e.g., Listerine, Cepacol) after metered-dose inhaler (MDI) administration and using a spacer device may reduce the incidence of this infection.

Systemic: Suppression of the HPA mechanism (with excessive doses, >1000 μg/day).

Other: Bronchospasm (rare), rash (rare).

Overdosage

There are primarily two toxic effects from the use of these agents: acute adrenal insufficiency (caused by too rapid a withdrawal of the drug after long-term, prolonged therapy) and Cushingoid changes. For acute overdoses, treatment consists of gastric lavage or emesis and usual supportive measures.

Dosing Schedule

Hydrocortisone is the prototypic glucocorticoid, which is the synthetic derivative of the principal endogenous glucocorticoid, cortisol. Because of this, hydrocortisone is assigned a glucocorticoid potency of 1.0 and is the standard with which the various synthetic derivatives are compared. Several synthetic derivatives have been introduced into therapeutics because they have greater anti-inflammatory properties than hydrocortisone, with a longer duration of activity and without a significant mineralocorticoid effect (i.e., the newer agents have little to no sodium-retaining effects). The distinct advantages of each agent rely on the desired clinical effect, the glucocorticoid/mineralocorticoid potency, the duration of action, and the mode of administration. These facets are detailed in Table 12.3. Preparations most commonly used in cardiopulmonary disease are listed in Table 12.4. All dosages are highly individualized.

Table 12.3.
Pharmacologic Activity of Various Glucocorticoids

Glucocorticoid	Anti-Inflammatory Potency[a]	Topical Potency[a]	Sodium–Retaining Potency[a]	Plasma Half-life (minutes)	Biologic Half-life (hours)	Equivalent Oral Anti-inflammatory Dose (mg)	Routes of Administration
Short-acting:							
Cortisone	0.8	0	0.8	30	8–12	25	Oral, injectable, topical
Hydrocortisone	1.0	1	1	80–118	8–12	20	Oral, injectable, topical
Intermediate-acting:							
Methylprednisolone	5	5	0–0.8	78–188	18–36	4	Oral, injectable, topical
Prednisolone	4	4	0.8	115–212	18–36	5	Oral, injectable, topical
Prednisone	4	0	0.8	60	18–36	5	Oral
Triamcinolone	5	5[b]	0	200+	18–36	4	Oral, injectable, topical
Long-acting:							
Betamethasone	30	10	0	300+	36–54	0.6–0.75	Oral, injectable, topical
Dexamethasone	30	10	0	110–210	36–54	0.75	Oral, injectable, topical

[a]Potency relative to hydrocortisone.
[b]Acetonide: up to 100.

Table 12.4. Preparations and Dosages of the Glucocorticoids

Glucocorticoid	Preparations	Dosing Schedule[a]
Intravenous and Oral:		
Cortisone	Tablets: 5, 10, 25 mg Injection: 50 mg/mL	Initial dosage: 25 to 300 mg/day
Hydrocortisone (Cortisol) (Cortef, Hydrocortone)	Tablets: 5, 10, 20 mg	Initial dosage: 20 to 240 mg/day
Hydrocortisone cypionate (Cortef)	Oral suspension: 10 mg/5 mL	Initial dosage: 20 to 240 mg/day
Hydrocortisone sodium phosphate (Hydrocortone Phosphate)	Injection: 50 mg/mL	Initial dosage: 15 to 240 mg/day Acute diseases: may require higher than 240 mg/day
Hydrocortisone sodium succinate (A-Hydrocort, Solu-Cortef)	Injection: 100, 250, 500, 1000 mg per vial	Initial dosage: 100 to 500 mg, repeated at 2-, 4-, or 6-hour intervals (depends on patient response and clinical condition)
Prednisone (Orasone, Panasol-S, Deltasone, Prednicen-M, Sterapred, Prednisone Intensol Concentrate, Liquid Prep)	Tablets: 1, 2.5, 5, 10, 20, 50 mg Oral solution: 5 mg/mL, 5 mg/5 mL Syrup: 5 mg/5 mL	Initial dosage: 5 to 60 mg/day Alternate Day Therapy (ADT): twice the usual dose administered at 8:00 AM every other day (this conversion may be impaired in patients with liver disease. Prednisone is converted to prednisolone by the liver)
Prednisolone (Delta-Cortef, Prelone)	Tablets: 5 mg Syrup: 15 mg/5 mL	Initial dosage: 5 to 60 mg/day Multiple sclerosis: Treatment of acute exacerbations, 200 mg daily for 1 week, then 80 mg q.o.d. for 1 month
Prednisolone acetate (Key-Pred 25, Predcor-25, Articulose-50, Predaject-50, Predalone 50, Predcor-50, Predicort-50, Key-Pred 50)	Injection: 25, 50 mg/mL (not for IV use)	Initial systemic dosage: 4 to 60 mg/day, IM
Prednisolone sodium phosphate (Hydeltrasol, Key-Pred-SP, Pediapred)	Injection: 20 mg/mL Oral liquid: 5 mg/5 mL	Initial dosage: 4 to 60 mg/day
Triamcinolone (Aristocort, Atolone, Kenacort)	Tablets: 1, 2, 4, 8 mg Syrup: 4 mg/5 mL	Initial dosage: 4 to 48 mg (up to 100 mg/day in leukemia) Acute leukemia (children): 1 to 2 mg/kg
Triamcinolone diacetate (Aristocort Intralesional, Trilone, Amcort, Aristocort, Forte, Articulose LA, Cenocort Forte, Triam Forte, Triamolone 40, Tristoject)	Injection: 25, 40 mg/mL (not for IV use)	Initial systemic dosage: 40 mg IM per week
Triamcinolone acetonide (Tac-3, Kenalog-10, Cenocort A-40, Kenaject-40, Tac-40, Triam-A, Triamonide 40, Tri-Kort, Trilog)	Injection: 3, 10, 40 mg/mL (not for IV use)	Initial systemic dosage: 2.5 to 60 mg/day, IM
Methylprednisolone (Medrol)	Tablets: 2, 4, 8, 16, 24, 32 mg	Initial dosage: 4 to 48 mg/day Alternate Day Therapy (ADT): twice the usual dose administered at 8:00 AM every other day

Table 12.4.—*continued*

Glucocorticoid	Preparations	Dosing Schedule[a]
Methylprednisolone sodium succinate (A-Methapred, Solu-Medrol)	Powder for injection: 40, 125, 500, 1000, 2000 mg per vial	Initial dosage: 10 to 40 mg, IV Infants and children: not less than 0.5 mg/kg/24 hours For high dose therapy: 30 mg/kg IV, infused over 10 to 20 minutes, may repeat every 4 to 6 hours, not beyond 48 to 72 hours
Methylprednisolone acetate (Depo-Medrol, Adlone, depMedalone 40, Depoject, Depopred-40, Duralone-40, Medralone 40, M-Prednisol-40, Depopred-80, D-Med 80, Duralone-80, Medralone 80, M-Prednisol-80, Rep-Pred 80)	Injection: 20, 40, 80 mg/mL (not for IV use)	Asthma and allergic rhinitis: 80 to 120 mg, IM
Dexamethasone (Decadron, Dexameth, Dexone, Hexadrol)	Tablets: 0.25, 0.5, 0.75, 1, 1.5, 2, 4, 6 mg Elixir: 0.5 mg/5 mL Oral solution: 0.5 mg/0.5 mL, 0.5 mg/5 mL	Initial dosage: 0.75 to 9 mg/day
Dexamethasone acetate (Dalalone LA, Decadron-LA, Decaject-LA, Dexacen LA-8, Dexasone LA, Dexone LA, Solurex LA, Dalalone DP)	Injection: 8, 16 mg/mL (not for IV use)	Initial systemic dosage: 8 to 16 mg, IM (may repeat in 1 to 3 weeks)
Dexamethasone sodium phosphate (Dalalone, Decadron Phosphate, Decaject, Dexacen-4, Dexasone, Dexone, Hexadrol Phosphate, Solurex)	Injection: 4, 10, 20, 24 mg/mL	Initial systemic dosage: 0.5 to 9 mg daily Cerebral edema: initially, 10 mg IV; followed by 4 mg IM every 6 hours
Betamethasone (Celestone)	Tablets: 0.6 mg Syrup: 0.6 mg/5 mL	Initial dosage: 0.6 to 7.2 mg/day
Betamethasone sodium phosphate (Celestone Phosphate, Cel-U-Jec, Selestoject)	Injection: 4 mg/mL	Initial systemic and local dosage: up to 9 mg/day
Betamethasone sodium phosphate (BSP) and betamethasone acetate (BA) (Celestone Soluspan)	Injection: 3 mg of each compound/mL (not for IV use)	Initial systemic dosage: 0.5 to 9 mg/day [b]BSP provides prompt activity, whereas BA provides sustained activity
Respiratory Inhalants:		
Beclomethasone dipropionate (Beclovent, Vanceril)	MDI: 42 μg/inhalation	Adults: 2 inhalations t.i.d., q.i.d. or 4 inhalations b.i.d. (12 to 16 inhalations/day may be needed for severe asthma, the dosage is then adjusted downward according to patient response) (not to exceed 20 inhalations daily)[b] Children 6 to 12 years: 1 to 2 inhalations t.i.d., q.i.d. or 2 to 4 inhalations b.i.d. (not to exceed 10 inhalations daily)
Dexamethasone sodium phosphate (Decadron Phosphate Respihaler)	MDI: 84 μg/inhalation	Adults: 3 inhalations t.i.d., q.i.d. (not to exceed 12 inhalations daily) Children 6 to 12 years: 2 inhalations t.i.d., q.i.d. (not to exceed 8 inhalations daily)

Table 12.4.—*continued*

Glucocorticoid	Preparations	Dosing Schedule[a]
Triamcinolone acetonide (Azmacort)	MDI: 100 μg/inhalation	Adults: 2 inhalations t.i.d., q.i.d. (12 to 16 inhalations/day may be needed for severe asthma; the dosage is then adjusted downward according to patient response) (not to exceed 16 inhalations daily) Children 6 to 12 years: 1 to 2 inhalations t.i.d., q.i.d. (not to exceed 12 inhalations daily)
Fluinisolide (AeroBid, AeroBid-M)	MDI: 250 μg/inhalation	Adults: 2 to 4 inhalations b.i.d. (not to exceed 8 inhalations daily) Children 6 to 15 years: 2 inhalations b.i.d. (not to exceed 4 inhalations daily)
Intranasal Sprays:		
Dexamethasone sodium phosphate (Decadron Phosphate Turbinaire)	Nasal spray: 84 μg/spray	Adults: 2 sprays in each nostril b.i.d., t.i.d. Children: 1 or 2 sprays in each nostril b.i.d.
Flunisolide (Nasalide)	Nasal spray: 25 μg/spray	Adults: 2 sprays in each nostril b.i.d., t.i.d. Children: 1 spray in each nostril t.i.d. or 2 sprays in each nostril b.i.d.
Beclomethasone dipropionate (Beconase Inhalation, Vancenase Nasal Inhaler, Beconase AQ Nasal, Vancenase AQ Nasal)	Nasal spray: 42 μg/spray	Adults: 1 spray in each nostril b.i.d., t.i.d., or q.i.d. Children 6 to 12 years: 1 spray in each nostril t.i.d.
Triamcinolone acetonide (Nasacort)	Nasal spray: 55 μg/spray	Adults and children >12 years: 2 sprays in each nostril once a day
Budesonide (Rhinocort)	Nasal spray: 32 μg/spray	Adults and children ≥6 years: 2 sprays in each nostril b.i.d. or 4 sprays in each nostril once a day

[a]Adult dosage, unless otherwise stated.
[b]The patient should be advised not to exceed the maximum daily dose. Otherwise, HPA suppression and Cushingoid effects may be pronounced.
IM, intramuscular; IV, intravenous; MDI, metered-dose inhaler.

Intravenous Glucocorticoids

Although hydrocortisone is available in tablets for oral administration and in lotions, creams, and ointments for topical application, its intravenous preparation (Solu-Cortef) is preferred in the treatment of status asthmaticus and other various acute chest diseases owing to its relative rapid onset of action (symptomatic relief occurs in approximately 1 hour). However, peak effects do not occur until approximately 5 hours; therefore hydrocortisone's effectiveness mainly depends on prompt intervention in the emergency room. Intravenous methylprednisolone (Solu-Medrol), an intermediate-acting glucocorticoid, is occasionally administered rather than hydrocortisone in hypersensitivity reactions, status asthmaticus, aspiration pneumonitis, and acute respiratory distress syndrome (ARDS) because it has five times the glucocorticoid activity of hydrocortisone and little to no mineralocorticoid activity, resulting in less sodium retention and potassium loss. Dexamethasone (Decadron) is yet another intravenously administered agent that is a long-acting glucocorticoid that lacks sodium-retaining activity. It has approximately 20 to 30 times the potency of hydrocortisone, with a duration of activity of approximately 72 hours. This agent is primarily reserved for situations in which a strong anti-inflammatory agent is required and in which fluid or sodium retention is undesirable (e.g., cerebral edema secondary to tumor, unresponsive shock). The main disadvantage of dexamethasone is its relatively long duration of activity, which extends the HPA transport system suppression, making it unsuitable when a quick recovery of the HPA transport system is wanted.

Oral Glucocorticoids

Prednisone is usually the oral drug of choice because it is relatively inexpensive and intermediate-acting. The acutely ill patient is switched to oral prednisone as soon as feasible. Acute disease exacerbations are kept in control with daily administrations of about 40 to 60 mg. High-dose therapy is usually required for 1 to 3 days, and then is tapered to about 5 to 10 mg every 1 to 2 days and then by as little as 1 to 5 mg/month for the steroid-dependent individual. Daily doses are gradually reduced to once per day or once every other day (administered at 8:00 AM to mimic the normal HPA transport system). Some individuals with severe chronic disease may require long-term glucocorticoid therapy indefinitely to control acute exacerbations. For patients with liver disease, oral prednisolone is highly preferred owing to the liver's inability to convert prednisone to prednisolone, the biologically active form.

Aerosol Glucocorticoids

Several inhaled glucocorticoids are available, as shown in Table 12.4. All inhaled glucocorticoids are available only by MDI administration. Dexamethasone is the oldest of the inhaled glucocorticoids. It is a long-acting agent that has a 30-fold increase in anti-inflammatory action over hydrocortisone. Beclomethasone was the second agent marketed in the USA. It exhibits a significantly higher potency than dexamethasone with a lower systemic effect. Two or four puffs q.i.d. or b.i.d. permits most patients to either discontinue or reduce their oral glucocorticoid dose. In terms of HPA suppression, 500 to 600 μg/day of inhaled beclomethasone is equivalent to 20 mg of oral prednisone administered on alternate days. Triamcinolone and flunisolide are the two newest agents available in the USA for the treatment of chronic asthma. Triamcinolone comes packaged with its own built-in spacer. Budesonide is an investigational agent not yet approved for use in the USA.

An inhaled glucocorticoid is generally initiated during the slow tapering of oral prednisone. An overlap is necessary (at least 2 to 4 weeks) to prevent adrenal failure. Some symptoms that may accompany oral withdrawal include nasal stuffiness and postnasal drip. This is primarily the result of the loss of the systemic glucocorticoid effect on the nasal mucosa. The patient may need coadministration of an antihistamine or nasal decongestant or an intranasal glucocorticoid preparation to clear nasal passages and reduce postnasal drip. With the success of these inhaled glucocorticoid preparations in treating severe asthma, there has been an increase in the use of these agents in the treatment and management of mild asthma (with concomitant use of a β_2 adrenoceptor agonist).

Other uses for aerosol glucocorticoids include intranasal application to control perennial and seasonal rhinitis and to decrease the size of nasal polyps. These preparations are available as nasal sprays as listed in Table 12.4.

NONSTEROIDAL ANTI-INFLAMMATORY DRUGS (NSAIDS)

Nonsteroidal anti-inflammatory drugs (NSAIDS) have been so named to distinguish them from glucocorticoids. The primary anti-inflammatory effects of NSAIDS stem from their ability to inhibit cyclooxygenase and thereby prevent the conversion of arachidonic acid to prostaglandins, thromboxane, or prostacyclin. Because these agents of arachidonic acid metabolism, as discussed in Chapter 2, induce symptoms of inflammation and possibly enhance the effects of bradykinin and histamine, a reduction in their formation should be beneficial in relieving some of the inflammatory process. NSAIDS do not appear to inhibit or suppress the total inflammatory response owing to their inability to block the arachidonic/lipoxygenase pathway, which brings about the formation of the highly reactive leukotrienes.

NSAIDS have long been used for their analgesic (reduces pain), antipyretic (reduces elevated temperature), and anti-inflammatory effects (primarily in the treatment of arthritic diseases and other inflammatory joint conditions to reduce the inflammation and swelling associated with these conditions). NSAIDS have also been used to treat patent ductus arteriosus (usually indomethacin). The patency of the ductus arteriosus is favored by low oxygen tension and prostaglandin E_2. By inhibiting the formation of this prostaglandin, indomethacin promotes closure and alleviates the associated symptoms of cardiac failure in the premature infant or newborn. In addition, the results of several clinical studies provide evidence that aspirin reduces the incidence of coronary artery thrombosis in patients at risk for or recovering from myocardial infarction and coronary artery bypass grafts. The reason for this is explained by the inhibition of platelet aggregation secondary to inhibition of thromboxane formation (see Chapter 2, Table 2.6).

Major side effects of these agents include gastric upset (these agents should be taken with meals), renal insufficiency (acute renal failure, interstitial nephritis, nephrotic syndrome), rash, dizziness, headache, and anxiety. Serious hematologic effects include agranulocytosis and aplastic anemia.

Although aspirin (the prototypic NSAID) and other nonsteroidal anti-inflammatory drugs share common pharmacologic effects in the prevention of inflammation, in that these agents block prostaglandin formation, they are generally not well tolerated by individuals with asthma. NSAID intolerance is a frequent provoking factor in severe acute asthma that may ultimately lead to mechanical ventilation or death (Picado et al. 1989). The resulting intolerance from aspirin ingestion in allergic individuals has been defined as acute urticaria-angioedema, bronchospasm, severe rhinitis, or shock occurring within 3 hours of aspirin ingestion. The mechanisms for aspirin intolerance are not clearly understood. For asthma, one possibility seems to be that these agents potentiate the arachidonic/lipoxygenase pathway formation of the highly reactive bronchoconstrictor leukotrienes because the arachidonic/cyclooxygenase pathway formation of prostaglandins is blocked. On the other hand, Fairfax and colleagues (1982) found that pretreatment with NSAIDS, such as aspirin or indomethacin, inhibited the late asthmatic response in certain individuals with asthma who appeared to benefit symptomatically from continuous treatment with aspirin. Thus, it is not possible to know which patient will respond in a specific way, because it seems that some asthmatic patients derive benefit from the use of NSAIDS and others do not.

Table 12.5 lists some of the more commonly used NSAIDS along with their recommended anti-inflammatory dosage.

Table 12.5.
Anti-Inflammatory Dosages of Aspirin and Some Newer Nonsteroidal Anti-Inflammatory Drugs (NSAIDS)

Drug	Half-life (hours)	Recommended Anti-Inflammatory Dose[a]
Salicylates:		
Aspirin (acetylsalicylic acid, ASA)	0.25	1500 mg t.i.d.
Propionic acids:		
Fenoprofen (Nalfon)	2.5	600 mg q.i.d.
Flurbiprofen (Ansaid)	3.8	300 mg t.i.d.
Ibuprofen (Advil, Motrin)	2	600 mg q.i.d.
Ketoprofen (Orudis, Oruvail)	1.8	70 mg t.i.d.
Naproxen (Aleve, Anaprox, Naprosyn)	14	375 mg b.i.d.
Oxaprozin (Daypro)	58	1800 mg q.d.
Acetic acids:		
Etodolac (Lodine)	6.5	300 mg q.i.d.
Indomethacin (Indocin)	4–5	70 mg t.i.d.
Ketorolac (Toradol)	4–10	10 mg q.i.d.
Nabumetone (Relafen)	26	2000 mg q.d.
Sulindac (Clinoril)	8	200 mg b.i.d.
Tolmetin (Tolectin)	1	400 mg q.i.d.
Diclofenac (Cataflam, Voltaren)	1.1	75 mg q.i.d.
Oxicams:		
Piroxicam (Feldene)	57	20 mg q.d.
Pyrazoles:		
Phenylbutazone (Azolid)	68	100 mg q.i.d. (not recommended for chronic use)
Fenamates:		
Meclofenamate (Meclomen)	3	100 mg q.i.d.

[a]Adult dose.

REFERENCES/RECOMMENDED READING

Barnes PJ, Adcock I. Anti-inflammatory actions of steroids: molecular mechanisms. Trends Pharmacol Sci 14:436, 1993.

Baxter JD. Minimizing the effects of glucocorticoid therapy. Adv Intern Med 35:173, 1990.

Baxter JD, Forsham PH. Tissue effects of glucocorticoids. Am J Med 53:573, 1972.

Cott GR, Cherniack RM. Steroids and steroid-sparing agents in asthma. N Engl J Med 318:634, 1988.

DiRosa M, et al. Multiple control of inflammation by glucocorticoids. Agents Actions 17:284, 1985.

Drug Facts and Comparisons. 49th ed. St. Louis: Facts and Comparisons, 1995.

Fairfax AJ. Inhibition of the late asthmatic response to house dust mite by non-steroidal anti-inflammatory drugs. Prostaglandins Leukot Med 8:239, 1982.

Flower RJ, Blackwell GJ. Anti-inflammatory steroids induce biosynthesis of a phospholipase A_2 inhibitor which prevents prostaglandin generation. Nature 278:456, 1979.

Funder JW. Adrenal steroids: new answers, new questions. Science 237:236, 1987.

Helfer EL, Rose LI. Corticosteroids and adrenal suppression: characterising and avoiding the problem. Drugs 38:838, 1989.

Hench PS. Introduction: cortisone and ACTH in clinical medicine. Proc Staff Meet Mayo Clin 25:474, 1950.

Henry D. Assessing the benefits and risks of drugs. The example of NSAIDS. Aust Fam Physician 19(3):378, 1990.

Iamandescu IB. NSAIDS-induced asthma: peculiarities related to background and association with other drugs or non-drugs etiological agents. Allergol Immunopathol 17(6):285, 1989.

Keller-Wood ME, Dallman MF. Corticosteroid inhibition of ACTH secretion. Endocr Rev 5:1, 1984.

Knox AJ, Mascie-Taylor BH, Muers MF. Acute hydrocortisone myopathy in severe asthma. Thorax 41:411, 1986.

Physicians' Desk Reference. 49th ed. Montvale, NJ: Medical Economics, 1995.

Picado C, et al. Aspirin-intolerance as a precipitating factor of life-threatening attacks of asthma requiring mechanical ventilation. Eur Respir J 2(2):127, 1989.

Toogood JH. Steroid and cromolyn for treatment of chronic asthma. Chest 82S:42S, 1982.

Truhan AP, Ahmed AR. Corticosteroids: a review with emphasis on complications of prolonged systemic therapy. Ann Allergy 62:375, 1989.

Mucokinetic Agents and Surface-Active Agents 13

This chapter details agents that alter the composition and/or volume of airway secretions (mucokinetic agents) to promote expectoration and airway patency and agents that are used to lower the surface tension of bubbly, frothy secretions and alveoli (surface-active agents). In addition, an introductory explanation of the physiology associated with these agents precedes the discussion of the agents.

Key Terms

(The following key terms are highlighted in **bold** when they first occur in the text of this chapter.)

adhesivity—refers to the ability of two unlike substances to become attached. Mucus has been described as being "gummy," "sticky," or "tacky" because it has the ability to adhere to other substances. The more viscous (thick, tenacious) the mucus, the greater its adhesive property. Adhesivity corresponds to the strength that must be applied to achieve the separation between the adhesive fluid (the mucus) and the adherent surface (the mucosa).

cohesive—refers to the ability of two like substances to become attached. Mucoprotein strands cross-link (bind) with each other to become a complex viscoelastic material. Cohesive forces also reflect the ability of other like substances, such as water molecules, to adhere to each other.

Curschmann's spirals—coiled spirals of mucus seen in sputum of patients with asthma.

elastic—reflects the ability of a substance to deform (change its shape, stretch) when a force is applied and then to return to its original shape when the force is removed (like a rubber band). Mucus generally possesses high elasticity, one of its rheologic (see below) properties.

endogenous—originating from within the body.

exogenous—originating from outside the body.

exudates—matter (such as pus or serum) that penetrates through vessel walls and collects in adjoining tissue.

glycoprotein—a compound consisting of a carbohydrate and protein (synonym in this chapter: mucoprotein).

hyperviscosity—extremely thick, tenacious, dehydrated.

inspissated—thickened by evaporation or dehydration.

macromolecule—a large molecule, such as a protein, polymer, or polysaccharide.

mucoid—a secretion containing mucopolysaccharides, mucoproteins.

mucopurulent—containing mucus and pus.

mucostasis—stopping the secretion of mucus.

mucoviscidosis—cystic fibrosis, a condition of thickened mucus.

osmotic—the passage of solvent (water, saline) through a semipermeable membrane that separates solutions of different concentrations.

purulent—containing pus (product of inflammation that consists of leukocytes and the debris of dead cells), gives sputum a yellow color. If sputum is blue or green, it indicates the presence of *Pseudomonas aeruginosa*.

recombinant—by chemical or biological means, a strain that receives chromosomal parts from different parental strains (the result of combining genetic material from different sources).

reconstitution—returning a substance previously altered for preservation and storage to its original form.

rheological—pertains to rheology, the study of the deformation and flow of materials. Mucus has rheological properties in that it has elasticity (the ability to deform) and viscosity (the ability to flow).

surface tension—the tension or force that is present at the surface of a liquid in contact with a gas. Surface tension holds the liquid surface intact at the liquid-gas interface.

tonicity—the osmotic pressure or tension of a solution, usually relative to that of blood or body fluids.

viscoelastic—having the property of being both viscous and elastic.

viscosity—resistance to flow or alteration of shape by a substance. A highly viscous substance, such as mucus in disease states, resists flow and has a tendency to be “sticky” or “gummy.”

wettability—a surface property of mucus that characterizes its ability to spread when deposited onto a solid surface.

ALVEOLAR EPITHELIUM AND THE MUCOCILIARY SYSTEM

The respiratory epithelium is the layer of cells lining the luminal surface of the respiratory tract. The epithelium may be simple (consisting of a single layer) or stratified (consisting of several layers of cells). The cells of the epithelium may be flat and scale-like (squamous), cube-shaped (cuboidal), or tall and cylindrical (columnar).

The source of support for the epithelium comes from the underlying connective tissues (lamina propria), to which the epithelial tissues are firmly attached by a permeable but adhesive basement membrane. No blood vessels are located in epithelial tissues; therefore, the epithelial tissues rely on the capillaries located in the underlying connective tissues for nourishment of food and oxygen and for removal of waste products. The ability of well nourished epithelial cells to regenerate is exceptional; the cells may replace themselves as often as every 24 hours. General functions of the respiratory epithelium include protection, filtration, absorption, and secretion.

There are four primary types of respiratory epithelium (Fig. 13.1):

1. Simple squamous epithelium:

- Consists of a single layer of thin, flat cells.
- Highly adapted to allow diffusion and filtration.
- Lines the alveolar ducts, alveolar sacs, and alveolar portions of the respiratory bronchioles, through which oxygen and carbon dioxide diffuse without difficulty.

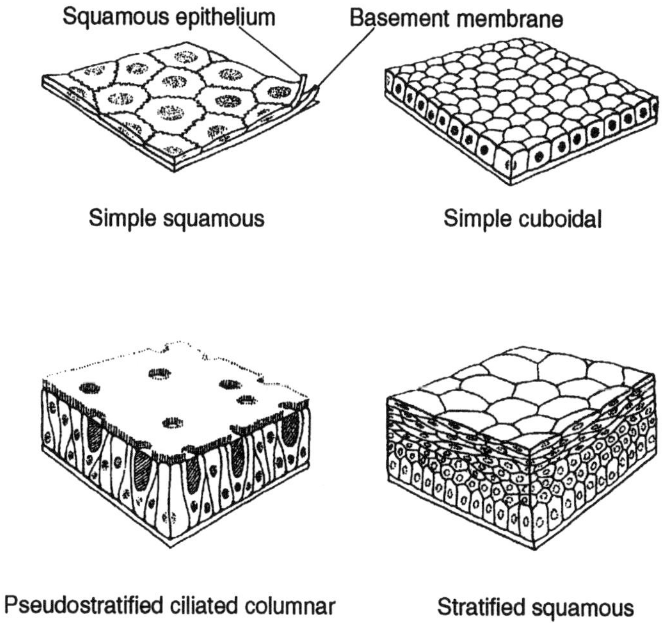

Figure 13.1. Three-dimensional representation of the respiratory epithelial tissues.

2. Simple cuboidal epithelium:

- Consists of a single layer of cells that resemble cubes.
- Performs the functions of secretion and absorption.
- Primarily lines the bronchioles, the terminal bronchioles, and the respiratory bronchioles (nonalveolar portions).

3. Stratified squamous epithelium:

- Consists of several layers of cells; cuboidal to columnar shape in the deeper layers; squamous cells in the superficial layers.
- Functions as a protective epithelium for the underlying tissues.
- Lines the vestibular section of the nose, oropharynx, laryngopharynx, and the larynx above the true vocal cords.

4. Pseudostratified ciliated columnar epithelium:

- Cylindrical cells one layer thick; all cells are attached to the basement membrane; however, some cells do not reach the free surface of the tissue. The stratification appearance is a result of different levels of nuclei within the pseudostratified cells.
- Functions to secrete and move mucus.
- Located along the basement membrane of the epithelium are basal cells that are involved in mucosal repair and serve to replenish the ciliated and goblet cells when needed.
- Lines most of the respiratory passages (respiratory section of the nose, paranasal sinuses, nasopharynx, larynx below the true vocal cords, trachea, all bronchial segments, some of the bronchiolar generations).

The respiratory epithelium (in particular, the pseudostratified ciliated columnar epithelium) contains numerous submucosal (or bronchial) glands and surface goblet cells that synthesize, store, and release mucus (Fig. 13.2). Submucosal glands, located below the epithelium in the submucosal layer (lamina propria) of the tracheobronchial tree, are the major source of mucus secretion; the total volume is approximately 40 times more than the volume produced by the goblet cells. The parasympathetic (vagal) nerve fibers innervate submucosal glands; cholinergic activation results in an increase in mucus production. The mucous and serous cells of the submucosal gland secrete their contents within the gland; this secretion is mixed within the gland and then transported onto the airway lumen.

Goblet cells, located in the epithelium, accumulate granules of mucus that eventually form a large mass within the cell, causing the cell to become swollen

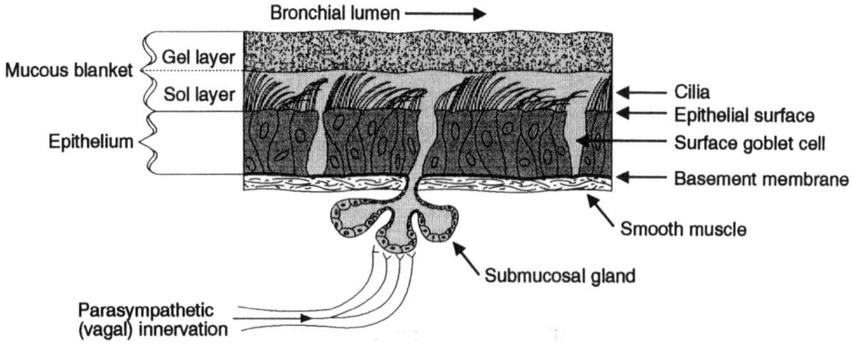

Figure 13.2. Cross-sectional view of the bronchial wall displaying the mucociliary system in the lung.

and distorted. Upon rupture of the cell, mucus is liberated onto the airway surface. Goblet cells are stimulated into action through irritants; the result is an increase in mucus production. There are approximately 6800 goblet cells per square millimeter of mucosa.

Mucus is composed of 95% water, 2% glycoprotein, 1% carbohydrate, and trace amounts of lipid, deoxyribonucleic acid (DNA), and cellular debris. In normal conditions, the glands and secretory cells in the mucous lining produce approximately 100 ml of mucus per day. The major portion of the 100 ml of mucus produced in healthy individuals is reabsorbed in the bronchial mucosa, whereas the rest is usually swallowed unnoticed. One of the main missions linked to mucus is to form a continuous filter and barrier at the cell-air interface, thus lubricating and protecting the epithelial cells from invasion and injury by inhaled contaminants in the environment. Another mission of mucus is to trap, transport, and remove (during coughing) foreign materials (e.g., inhaled particles, microorganisms, cellular debris, dead cells, toxic agents) from the airway.

Clara cells, located in the terminal bronchioles, are secretory cells that have functions that are not clearly known. The secretions may aid in coating the inner lumen of the bronchioles and alveoli. They may also have enzymes that help detoxify inhaled toxic substances.

The mucociliary system (mucociliary escalator) functions as the normal defense mechanism to remove mucus, debris, and other particles from the tracheobronchial tree. In the upper airways, mucus is moved downward toward the pharynx; in the lower airways, mucus is moved upward toward the pharynx, where it is expectorated or swallowed. Factors such as dehydration, smoking, alcohol ingestion, hypoxia, positive pressure ventilation, general anesthetics, high inspired oxygen fraction, atmospheric pollutants, and parasympatholytics (atropine) may impair clearance, rendering the lungs susceptible to infection.

Pseudostratified ciliated columnar epithelium contains numerous ciliated cells; each ciliated cell has 200 to 250 hairlike processes (cilia) projecting from the surface of the epithelium. The cilia function as a clearance mechanism for mucus, foreign particles, and debris. The cilia move material in a metachronal wave fashion; this process is referred to as the "ciliary escalator." It is estimated that there are approximately 1 to 2 billion cilia per square centimeter of mucosa. Cilia are about 6 to 7 micrometers in length, beat at approximately 20 strokes per second, and move the mucous layer at a rate of 2 cm/minute.

The component parts of the mucus blanket are subdivided into two distinct layers (see Fig. 13.2). The *sol* layer is the fluid bottom layer adjacent to the epithelial surface and is where ciliary activity occurs. The *gel* layer is the more viscous layer lining the top of the sol layer, which the cilia extend into to propel the gel layer's contents (Fig. 13.3).

Sputum refers to expectorated secretions and is the material raised from the lower respiratory tract (lungs and bronchi) during deep coughing. Sputum contains mucus, oropharyngeal, nasopharyngeal, and lingual secretions; therefore, sputum and mucus are not synonyms. In a healthy individual, normal flora of the respiratory tract (e.g., alpha-hemolytic streptococci, Neisseria species, and diphtheroids) appear in sputum samples.

Defense of the Airways

As mentioned, the mucociliary escalator provides the major defense of the respiratory tract against accumulation of particulates and infection; however, other components of the airway defense mechanism help prevent infection: alveolar clearance, prevention of deposition of particulates in the airways, and the reflexes of the airways that illicit a cough or bronchoconstriction.

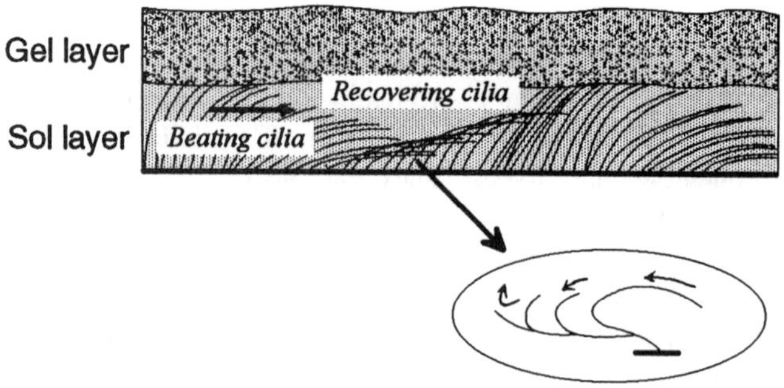

Figure 13.3. The action of the ciliary escalator. The forward power stroke of the cilia propels the viscous gel layer with its mucus, foreign particles, and other debris in one direction only, whereas the backward recovering motion (inset) takes place entirely within the more fluid sol layer, thereby preventing a retrogressive motion of the gel layer.

Alveolar Clearance: The principal alveolar defense mechanism against particulates is macrophage activity. Macrophages are scavengers of foreign particles, dead cells, and other debris that function to digest these substances. Another alveolar defense component that plays a role in removal of particulates from the lung includes the lymphatic system, which transports the particulates engulfed in macrophages.

Prevention of the Deposition of Particulates in the Airways: A normal individual inspires approximately 10,000 to 12,000 liters of air daily. Each liter of inspired air contains millions of particles suspended in it. The first site of deposition of the larger particles is the nose, which removes particles 100 to 5 microns in size. These particles are filtered out by the nares or are trapped by the nasal mucosa. Also, the larger median mass and high linear velocity of these particles induce rainout in the nose. Through impaction, particles 5 to 2 microns in size are deposited proximal to the alveoli and are removed by the mucociliary transport system. Particles 2 to 1 micron in size and those less than 0.25 micron in size can enter the alveoli and settle there; these particles are removed primarily by the phagocytic action of the alveolar macrophages. Particles 1 to 0.25 micron in size are considered stable in that they have minimal settling abilities.

Reflexes of the Airways: Stimulation of the sensory receptors of the trigeminal nerves (fifth cranial nerve) innervating the upper respiratory tract results in the sneeze. Stimulation of the vagal nerve sensory endings innervating the larynx, trachea, or larger bronchi or stimulation of the glossopharyngeal nerve in the pharynx would activate the cough reflex. Stimulating the vagally mediated irritant receptors in the airways can trigger bronchospasm, which also serves as a defense mechanism. Bronchospasm causes contraction of the airways, thereby limiting the deposition of particles into the distal airways.

PROPERTIES OF MUCUS

Respiratory mucus is a complex biological material that possesses distinct physiochemical properties. Mucus is primarily a high molecular weight **glycoprotein** (**macromolecule**) that consists of a polypeptide core (long chains of amino acids [proteins]) to which carbohydrate (saccharide) side chains are attached (Fig. 13.4). The formation of a long, thread-like mucus strand is brought about by various chemical bonds. Intramolecular bonding, known as dipeptide bonds, connect adjacent amino acid groups, whereas intermolecular bonding (such as disulfide bonds and hydrogen bonds) cross-link adjacent strands to each other.

Mucus possesses specific **rheological** characteristics in that it has flow and deformation properties. The ability of mucus to flow through a tube (i.e., the airways) relates to its viscous nature. Normal mucus has a relatively low **viscosity** and easily moves up and out of the airways during coughing or during the forward beat of the cilia. Mucus is also highly **elastic** in that it will deform (change its

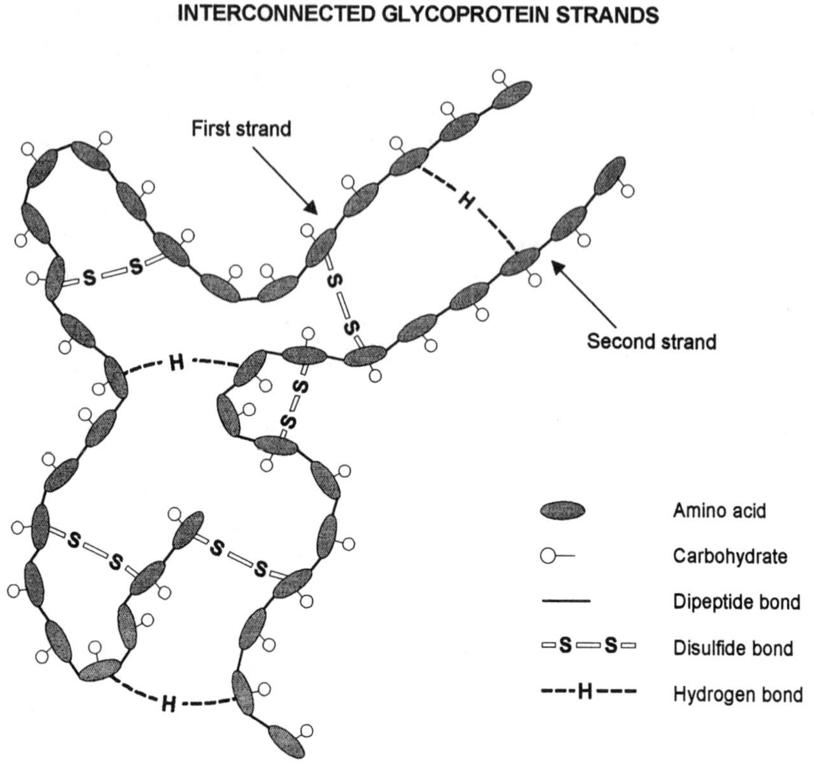

Figure 13.4. Schematic representation of interlinking and cross-linking of glycoprotein strands. (Adapted from Cottrell GP, Surkin HB. Pharmacology for respiratory care practitioners. Philadelphia: F.A. Davis Company, 1995.)

shape, stretch) when a force is applied to it but will return to its normal shape after the force is removed (as during the recovery period of breathing, after cessation of coughing, or after forward propulsion by the cilia). Because of these **viscoelastic** properties, mucus behaves as both a liquid and a solid. As a liquid (because of its viscous nature), mucus flows forward under the force applied by the cilia. As a solid (because of its elastic nature), mucus stretches from the forward power stroke of the cilia. It then snaps forward and returns to its normal shape as the cilia's force is removed.

In addition to the rheological characteristics, the respiratory mucus has surface properties, such as **adhesivity** (stickiness or tackiness) and **wettability**. These properties are important in that they help determine the capacity of mucus to protect, hydrate, and lubricate the underlying airway epithelium. These characteristics also help in mucus transport, either by the ciliary or cough mechanism.

MUCUS PRODUCTION IN DISEASE STATES

During pulmonary infection, in chronic bronchitis, asthma, and especially in cystic fibrosis, there is a decrease in the water component of mucus and an increase in macromolecule secretion, resulting in the dry weight of mucus being from 5 to 10 times higher than normal (Boucher et al. 1988). Consequently, a marked **hyperviscosity** and an increase in adhesivity are observed. The overall effect is a negative action on the mucociliary transport rate, which brings about retained secretions with mucus plugging, airway obstruction, atelectasis, and bacterial invasion.

Mucus Production in Pulmonary Infections

Bacterial pneumonia is an acute inflammation of the lung parenchyma characterized by an outpouring of exudates and white blood cells in response to the bacterial invasion. The sputum of patients with pneumonia varies from being scant or totally absent at the beginning of the infection, to being thick, tenacious, and **purulent** as the disease progresses. It may also be green (indicating old, retained secretions), bloody, or rusty in color. Dullness to percussion and impaired breath sounds may be detected over the diseased area.

Mucus Production in Chronic Bronchitis

Chronic bronchitis is defined as chronic excessive mucus production manifested by an increase in sputum production for at least 3 consecutive months each year for 2 or more successive years. Sputum obtained from patients with chronic bronchitis is usually thick, gray, and **mucoid,** unless an infection is present, and then it is **mucopurulent**. The mucus hypersecretion is a reflection of the increase in the number of mucus-secreting glands as well as submucosal gland hypertrophy.

Mucus Production in Asthma

Eosinophilic infiltrates are common in the sputum of patients with asthma. There is an increase in the production of thick, viscid secretions owing to an increased number of goblet cells and hypertrophy of mucous glands. Cough is at first nonproductive, at the early onset of an asthmatic attack, but becomes more and more productive of stringy casts (**Curschmann's spirals**) and mucoid sputum near the end of the attack. Lack of airflow from the accompanying bronchospasm leads to mucus plugging. Purulent-appearing sputum may be misleading, because large numbers of eosinophils will give the sputum this appearance. A bacterial infection is present if there are a significant number of neutrophilic white blood cells in the sputum.

Mucus Production in Cystic Fibrosis

Cystic fibrosis (CF; also known as **mucoviscidosis**) is an inherited recessive disorder characterized by abnormally thick secretions from the exocrine glands.

There is both hypertrophy and hypersecretion of airway glands in which thick, tenacious mucus is produced. The thick, dehydrated mucus and subsequent impairment of mucosal cilia is mediated from abnormal transepithelial electrolyte transport due to a faulty chloride channel (i.e., sodium and water are drawn into airway epithelial cells from the airway surface owing to the impaired chloride ion movement across airway epithelium to the airway lumen—by this mechanism, mucus becomes dehydrated and viscous).

Because patients with cystic fibrosis are prone to repeated, chronic pulmonary infections, the secretions of patients with cystic fibrosis are chronically infected and attract neutrophils. The abnormal viscoelastic, purulent nature of cystic fibrosis secretions are primarily the result of two macromolecules: dehydrated mucus glycoproteins and DNA. The extracellular DNA comes from the nuclei of degenerating polymorphonuclear neutrophils, which accumulate in response to chronic bacterial infections. An enzyme preparation (rhDNase) that selectively cleaves or digests this extracellular DNA has recently been approved by the Food and Drug Administration (FDA) (December 30, 1993). As a result of the action of rhDNase, mucus viscosity is reduced.

METHODS OF MUCOKINETICS

Because the increase in mucus production and changes in physiochemical properties are defensive responses to biological, chemical, or physical stimuli, the primary therapeutic maneuvers are to eliminate the offending cause and optimize tracheobronchial clearance of secretions. Although this may seem obvious, it is not very easily achieved in clinical practice; thus, **mucostasis** is corrected by the use of drugs that fluidize the mucus and improve mucociliary transport.

During the last several years, the discovery of new mucokinetic agents has resulted in a plethora of terms to explain their activity on mucus. As can be seen in Table 13.1, some terms are used to describe the same properties with only a slight alteration in the definition. This has led to some confusion in mucus pharmacology, because various classifications have been proposed based on these terms.

An alternative approach in setting up a classification scheme for mucokinetic agents is to classify the biological site of action. There are several known methods of altering the biochemical nature of mucus. Each method exemplifies a specific mode of action that tends either to lessen the viscosity of mucus, to control the production of mucus, or to liquefy secretions to facilitate bronchial hygiene. The first method presented in this chapter lowers the viscosity and elasticity of mucus by replacing the disulfide bond ($\overline{SS}$) of the mucoprotein with its own free sulfhydryl (SH) group (acetylcysteine). The second method presented enhances an increased topical pH in the lung mucosa, which weakens the saccharide side chains of the mucoprotein, thereby decreasing mucus viscosity (sodium bicarbonate). The third method humidifies and liquefies pulmonary secretions by directly adding liquid to the tracheobronchial tree (hydrating agents). Finally, the

Table 13.1.
Terminology Use In Mucus Pharmacology

Term	Definition
Bronchomucotropic	Any agent that stimulates bronchial glands to enhance their output of mucoid secretion
Bronchorrheic	Any agent that increases the transepithelial secretion of water; may result in excessive liquefication of secretions
Ciliary excitant	Any agent that stimulates the cilia to move at a faster rate and/or more effective beat
Detergent	Any agent that diminishes the adhesiveness of secretions to mucosal surfaces via a surface-active effect
Diluent	Any agent that liquefies and dilutes secretions by adding water
Expectorant	Any agent that acts on bronchial glands via the vagal reflex pathway: increases their output of mucoid secretions
Fluidifier	A generic term used to describe an agent that increases mucous mobility and transport
Hydrating agent	Any agent that adds water to respiratory secretions
Liquefier	Same as Mucolytic
Mucoactive	Indicates all drugs that have a beneficial effect on respiratory secretions
Mucolytic	Any agent that dissolves, digests, or liquefies mucus by altering the mucoprotein structure and/or DNA
Mucokinetic	Pertains to all drugs that promote the transport and clearance of respiratory secretions
Mucomodifying	Same as Mucoactive
Mucoregulator	Any agent that initiates the synthesis of more normal biochemical components of mucus
Mucosecretolytic	Same as Fluidifier
Mucospissic	Any agent that thickens or diminishes the fluidity of abnormally hypoviscous (thin) mucus (the term "inspissated" means "thickened")
Secretolytic	Same as Fluidifier
Surfactant agent	Any agent that stimulates type II alveolar cell secretion
Tensioactive	Same as Detergent
Wetting agent	Same as Detergent

Adapted from Braga PC, Allegra L. Drugs in Bronchial Mucology. New York: Raven Press, 1989.

fourth method presented selectively cleaves and digests extracellular DNA that accumulates in purulent sputum; by this action, the viscoelasticity of mucus is reduced (recombinant human DNase). Also included in this chapter is propylene glycol, which disrupts the mucoprotein by breaking the hydrogen bonds.

SPECIFIC THERAPEUTIC MUCOKINETIC AGENTS

ACETYLCYSTEINE: MUCOMYST, MUCOSAL

Mechanism of Action and Indications for Use

Acetylcysteine, a compound $C_5H_9NO_3S$, is a derivative of the naturally occurring amino acid L-cysteine as well as a thiol derivative because of its sulfur-containing properties. Acetylcysteine replaces the disulfide ($\overline{SS}$) bonds of mucoproteins with its own free sulfhydryl (SH) groups, thus lowering both the viscosity and elasticity of mucus (Fig. 13.5). The mucolytic action of acetylcysteine significantly increases with increasing pH (7.0 to 9.0). Acetylcysteine is indicated as adjuvant therapy for tenacious, viscid, or **inspissated** mucus in disease states such as chronic emphysema, acute and chronic bronchitis, asthma, tuberculosis, bronchiectasis, pneumonia, tracheobronchitis, and atelectasis caused by mucus obstruction. It is also indi-

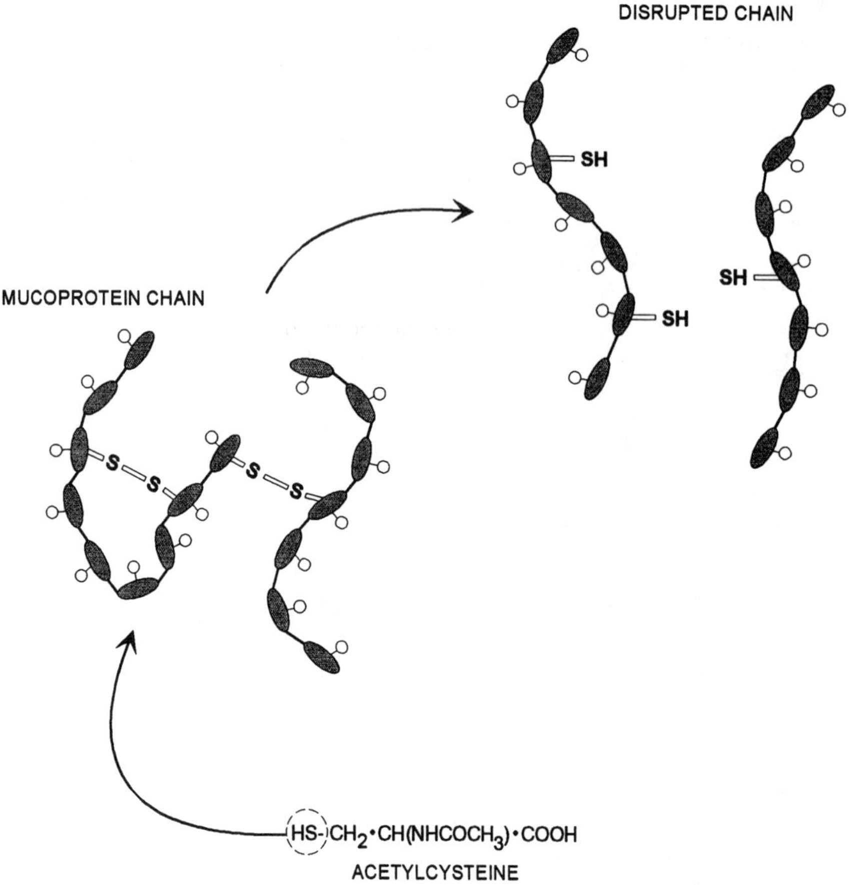

Figure 13.5. Acetylcysteine effects on the mucoprotein structure.

cated for pulmonary complications of cystic fibrosis, tracheostomy care, and complications associated with surgery. Acetylcysteine is also used for diagnostic bronchial studies such as bronchograms, bronchospirometry, and bronchial wedge catheterization.

In acetaminophen poisoning, acetylcysteine (administered orally, not by aerosol) is indicated as an antidote to lessen hepatic injury that may occur.

Contraindications

Contraindications to the use of acetylcysteine include hypersensitivity to the drug and patients at risk of gastric hemorrhage.

Precautions

1. After the administration of acetylcysteine, there may be an increased volume of liquefied bronchial secretions. For patients who demonstrate a weak or ineffective cough, tracheal suctioning may be necessary.
2. If bronchospasm occurs, acetylcysteine should be discontinued, given concurrently, or given before a fast-acting β_2-bronchodilator (preferred choice).
3. Admixture incompatibility: acetylcysteine may inactivate a number of antibiotics (e.g., tetracycline, chlortetracycline, oxytetracycline, erythromycin, lactobionate, amphotericin B, and sodium ampicillin) when mixed in the same solution. However, the topical application of acetylcysteine in the lung and the simultaneous administration of these antibiotics by other routes of administration do not adversely affect each other. Iodized oil, chymotrypsin, trypsin, and hydrogen peroxide are also incompatible with acetylcysteine.
4. Acetylcysteine produces a characteristic foul-smelling odor (i.e., "rotten egg" odor) that is caused by the liberation of hydrogen sulfide (H_2S).
5. Because it releases hydrogen sulfide, acetylcysteine adversely reacts with rubber, copper, iron, and cork. Most conventional types of nebulizers made of plastic or glass are safe to use for purposes of administering the drug. The following materials do not adversely affect acetylcysteine and therefore are also safe to use: aluminum, chromed metal, tantalum, sterling silver, or stainless steel. Silver may tarnish after exposure to acetylcysteine, but this is not harmful to the drug action or to the patient.
6. Opened vials should be stored in a refrigerator and discarded in 96 hours.
7. Using a face mask may result in stickiness on the face after nebulization; this may be removed with water.

Adverse Reactions

The most important adverse reaction that may occur with the aerosolized form of acetylcysteine is the precipitation of bronchospasm (this is especially noted in patients with hyperreactive airways). As previously stated, prior or concurrent administration of a fast-acting β_2-adrenoceptor is recommended. Other adverse reactions include stomatitis, nausea, vomiting, rhinorrhea, fever, and drowsiness.

Dosage and Administration

Onset of action: <1 minute.
Peak effects: 5 to 10 minutes.
Dosage form:
Inhal solution: 10%, 20%.
Combination form: 10% acetylcysteine in combination with 0.05% isoproterenol.

Dosage:

Recommended dosage: 3 to 5 ml of 20% solution equally diluted with sterile water for injection, U.S.P., or with normal saline given three to four times daily via nebulization; or 6 to 10 ml of 10% solution (undiluted) three to four times daily via nebulization.

Combination form: 3 to 5 ml four times daily by nebulization.

Direct installation into the lungs of an intubated patient: 1 to 2 ml of 10% or 20% solution (may be given as often as every 1 to 4 hours).

For diagnostic bronchograms: 1 to 2 ml of 20% solution or 2 to 4 ml of 10% solution, given before or during the procedure.

For acetaminophen overdosage: Loading dose, 140 mg/kg. Maintenance dose, 70 mg/kg for a total of 17 doses.

SODIUM BICARBONATE

Mechanism of Action and Indications for Use

Sodium bicarbonate ($NaHCO_3$) is a weak base (pH 7.4 to 8.5) that, when inhaled, directly increases bronchial pH. The net effect of elevating bronchial pH is a weakening and rupturing of the saccharide side chain of the mucoprotein structure. This then produces a decrease in mucus viscosity. Sodium bicarbonate may be combined with other drugs for immediate use and may be used as a diluent for acetylcysteine to potentiate the effects of acetylcysteine, which are enhanced in the alkaline environment.

Contraindications

Use with caution if delivering large amounts and higher concentrations. May cause hypernatremia or metabolic alkalosis.

Adverse Reactions

Adverse reactions are noted only when solutions of more than 2% are used. May cause bronchomucosal and oropharyngeal irritation. Concurrent administration of bronchodilators may be used to prevent bronchospasm.

Dosage and Administration

Sodium bicarbonate is available for inhalation in concentrations of 1.4%, 5%, and 7.5%. Recommended strength for less irritating effects is equal dilution of the 5% solution, producing a 2.5% solution. For nebulization, 2 to 5 ml every 4 to 8 hours. For intratracheal installation, 5 to 10 ml as needed. Alkalosis may occur if the drug is overused.

Note: When administering sodium bicarbonate concomitantly with a bronchodilator, the solution must be mixed immediately before administration and any remaining solution must be discarded. In an alkaline environment, such as that with sodium bicarbonate, bronchodilators are inactivated. Color changes of the drug occur owing to a breakdown of products (sputum may then have a red tinge when expectorated).

HYDRATING AGENTS

STERILE DISTILLED WATER: Aerosolized inhaled water is partially absorbed into the cell, owing to the cell's diffusion gradient. The remainder of solution that is not absorbed into the cell hydrates secretions, thereby liquefying secretions and promoting expectoration. Sterile distilled water is indicated to humidify dry inspired gases and especially to provide humidification when the upper airway is bypassed.

NORMAL PHYSIOLOGIC SALINE: Isotonic solution (0.9% of NaCl) that denotes the same **tonicity** as body fluids. There is no diffusion of water into or out of the cell membrane, owing to the equal tension generated on both sides of the semipermeable cell membrane. Because there is no net flow of water across the cell membrane, the inhaled aerosol particles tend to remain stable in size throughout the tracheobronchial tree and impact the more distal airways. Normal saline minimizes tracheobronchial irritation and is less irritating than water. Normal saline is indicated for use as a diluent with bronchodilators and for use by itself to liquefy secretions through direct instillation of the lungs in the intubated patient.

HYPERTONIC SALINE: A solution of NaCl that is greater than 0.9%. Hypertonic saline has a greater **osmotic** pressure than body fluids and therefore causes diffusion of water out of the cell. This may generate cellular dehydration and overhydration of the intracellular space. Due to the influx of cellular water, the inhaled aerosol particles tend to increase in size throughout the tracheobronchial tree and impact in the upper and middle portions of the airway. Hypertonic saline is primarily indicated to stimulate a productive cough and for sputum induction. This solution is very irritating to the airway and may cause bronchospasm.

HYPOTONIC SALINE: A solution of NaCl that is less than 0.9% (usually 0.45% of NaCl). Due to the cell's diffusion gradient, hypotonic saline solution is absorbed into and through the cellular membrane; therefore, the inhaled aerosol particles become smaller throughout the tracheobronchial tree and tend to impact the more distal airways. Hypotonic saline solution is generally indicated when other more irritating solutions are contraindicated or for patients on restricted sodium intake. This concentration of NaCl seems to be less irritating to the airway and least affects airway resistance.

Contraindications

Large amounts of saline and water solutions are contraindicated for patients with congestive heart failure and in neonates. Large amounts of these solutions may lead to fluid overload and peripheral edema. For patients with sodium restriction, care should be taken not to exceed the daily limitation through the administration of saline solutions. When total electrolyte administration is contraindicated, saline solutions should not be given.

Adverse Reactions

Miscellaneous: Fluid overload, edema (primarily noted with hypertonic saline solutions and in neonates).

Pulmonary: Bronchospasm, coughing, swelling of secretions that may result in airway occlusion, atelectasis (primarily noted with hypertonic saline solutions).

Some patients may not be able to tolerate the "salty" taste of hypertonic saline solutions. Gagging, choking, nausea, or vomiting may occur.

DORNASE ALFA (RECOMBINANT HUMAN DEOXYRIBONUCLEASE I, RHDNASE): PULMOZYME

Mechanism of Action and Indications for Use

Proteolytic enzymes (such as pancreatic dornase) have been noted to decrease the viscoelastic properties of purulent secretions by attacking either the polypeptide core of the mucoprotein structure or DNA (a component of purulent sputum that is released from the nuclei of degenerating polymorphonuclear neutrophils—the substance responsible for the increased viscoelastic properties of mucus). **Recombinant** human deoxyribonuclease I (rhDNase) is an enzyme that has a mechanism of action similar to pancreatic dornase in that it selectively cleaves and digests extracellular DNA, which accumulates in response to chronic bacterial infections. rhDNase is a highly purified solution that is produced by genetically engineered Chinese Hamster Ovary (CHO) cells containing DNA encoding for the human enzyme, deoxyribonuclease I (DNase).

For patients with cystic fibrosis, retention of viscid purulent sputum contributes to both exacerbations of infections and reduced pulmonary function. In several clinical trials, rhDNase hydrolyzed extracellular DNA in purulent sputum from patients with cystic fibrosis and significantly reduced the viscoelasticity of these secretions. Consequently, there is an associated improvement in mucociliary clearance and in pulmonary function parameters, as well as a decrease in the frequency and severity of respiratory infections (secondarily, the need for intensive antibiotic therapy, either at home or in the hospital, is reduced). Other symptomatic improvements have also been observed. Such improvements include diminished dyspnea, cough, sputum production, and fatigue in addition to an increase in appetite, improved sleeping habits, and exercise tolerance. Recent studies indicate that rhDNase seems to be more effective than acetylcysteine for patients with cystic fibrosis with infected sputum (Shak et al. 1990).

Contraindications

Contraindications to the use of rhDNase include hypersensitivity to dornase, Chinese Hamster Ovary cell products, or any component of the product.

Precautions

1. rhDNase must be stored in the refrigerator at 2° to 8°C and protected from strong light (do not expose to room temperature for a total of 24 hours). Discard the solution if it is cloudy or discolored.
2. rhDNase contains no preservatives. The entire ampule must be used or discarded once opened.
3. DO NOT mix or dilute rhDNase with other drugs in the nebulizer. Adverse physiochemical or functional changes (such as drug degradation) may occur. Concomitant medications such as inhaled bronchodilators may be given either before or after rhDNase administration. There are currently no recommendations available regarding the order in which rhDNase and other nebulized medications should be delivered.
4. The rhDNase must be administered on a continuous (i.e., daily) basis in order to maintain a full therapeutic effect. A decline in pulmonary function parameters (FEV_1) has been observed within 24 to 48 hours after cessation of treatment.
5. Safety and efficacy in children <5 years old have not been established.
6. Clinical trials have been performed with the following nebulizers and compressors:

   Hudson T Updraft II Nebulizer/DeVilbiss Pulmo-aide Compressor
   Marquest Acorn II Nebulizer/DeVilbiss Pulmo-aide Compressor
   Pari LC Jet Nebulizer/Pari Proneb Compressor

   Both the Hudson and Marquest nebulizers are disposable (i.e., intended for single patient use), whereas the Pari nebulizer is a durable and reusable nebulizer that can be used multiple times with proper care and cleaning. For optimal safety and efficacy, it is currently recommended that one of the above aerosol delivery systems be used for the administration of rhDNase. Researchers have found that these three systems have about a 25% (range, 23% to 28%) respirable delivery. Ultrasonic nebulizers and battery-powered compressors (cannot generate sufficient power) are not recommended for use with rhDNase. The safety and efficacy of rhDNase administration with other aerosol delivery systems have not been determined.

7. The patient should be instructed in the proper use and maintenance of the nebulizer and compressor. rhDNase should be administered as any other nebulizer treatment:

- Hands should be washed thoroughly before assembling equipment.
- The surface where the equipment will be assembled should be clean.
- The patient should be sitting upright and should be breathing at a normal rate and depth through the mouth (a nose clip should be used if the patient is having difficulty breathing only through the mouth).
- To reduce the risk of infection, manufacturer's guidelines for disinfection and disposal of the equipment should be followed.

Adverse Reactions

Significant adverse reactions are primarily dose related (e.g., 10 mg twice daily). The most common occurrences include hoarseness, pharyngitis, laryngitis, rash, chest pain, and conjunctivitis. There were no episodes of anaphylaxis. Some patients developed serum antibodies (IgG) to rhDNase (approximately 5% of studied patients). Other adverse reactions (some of which may reflect the underlying lung disease) include:

Body as a Whole: Abdominal pain, asthenia, fever, flu symptoms, malaise, sepsis.
Respiratory: Apnea, bronchiectasis, bronchitis, change or increase in sputum, increase in cough, dyspnea, hemoptysis, pulmonary function decrease, nasal polyps, pneumonia, pneumothorax, rhinitis, sinusitis, wheeze.
GI: Intestinal obstruction, gallbladder disease, pancreatic disease.
Metabolic/Nutritional: diabetes mellitus, hypoxia, weight loss.

Dosage and Administration

Dosage form:
Inhal solution: 2.5 mg in 2.5 ml ampule (1 mg/ml of rhDNase with 0.15 mg/ml calcium chloride dihydrate and 8.77 mg/ml sodium chloride)
Dosage: Recommended dose for most patients with cystic fibrosis is 2.5 mg single-use ampule inhaled once daily using a recommended nebulizer. Some patients (e.g., adults older than 23 years of age) may have a greater reduction in frequency of respiratory infections when receiving 2.5 mg twice daily.

PROPYLENE GLYCOL

Mechanism of Action and Indications for Use

Propylene glycol is a hygroscopic agent that absorbs moisture and resists dehydration. Propylene glycol disrupts the mucoprotein structure by breaking hydrogen bonds. It also stabilizes aerosol particles by preventing evaporation, thereby improving distal deposition in the airway.

Propylene glycol (2 to 25%) may be indicated when other inhalational therapy produces less than desired effects.

Contraindications

Propylene glycol inhibits the growth of the *Mycobacterium tuberculosis* species in sputum; therefore, its use is contraindicated when obtaining a sputum sample to check for tuberculosis organisms.

Adverse Reactions

Excessive doses may cause coughing and irritation of the proximal airways.

Dosage and Administration

Nebulize 1 to 2 ml of 2% solution concurrently with a bronchodilator or another mucokinetic agent. For very viscous secretions: nebulize 10 to 20% of propylene glycol solution for 20 minutes.

OTHER MUCOKINETIC AGENTS

S-carboxymethylcysteine (Viscorex, Mucodyne) and sodium 2-mercaptoethane sulfonate (Mistabron) are two mucolytic agents currently marketed abroad that have actions and effects similar to that of acetylcysteine. Other cysteine derivatives currently being investigated for their mucolytic properties include nesosteine and erdosteine. Seaprose (Flaminase, Puropharma) is a new proteolytic enzyme derived from *Aspergillus melleus* that is currently undergoing investigation in Europe. It works as other proteolytic enzymes, in that it acts directly on the mucoprotein structure and DNA to reduce the viscosity of mucus (see Chapter 9, Cough and Cold Preparations).

SURFACE-ACTIVE AGENTS

Surface-active agents currently have three potential uses:

- To reduce the adhesiveness (tackiness) of mucus.
- To reduce the surface tension of frothy, bubbly secretions that typically accompany pulmonary edema.
- As replacement therapy (**exogenous** surfactants) for missing or deficient pulmonary surfactant levels in infant respiratory distress syndrome (IRDS).

PHYSIOLOGIC NATURE OF SURFACE-ACTIVE AGENTS

Surface tension is the tension or force that is present at the surface of a liquid in contact with a gas. Surface tension holds the liquid surface intact at the liquid-gas interface. Surface tension reflects the mutual attraction of like molecules to each other, thus producing a **cohesive** attraction that causes a liquid bubble to assume the most compact, smallest surface area to the surrounding medium. This phenomenon explains the tendency for fluids, such as drops of oil, water, or even soap bubbles, to form their characteristic spherical shapes.

The force required to keep a liquid film, with gas inside and out (such as an alveolus or bubbly, frothy secretions), intact is a reflection of not only the amount of surface tension but also the internal distending pressure and the radius of the substance. The above relationships can be illustrated in the following formula, known as LaPlace's Law:

$$\text{Pressure} = (4 \times \text{Surface Tension}) / \text{Radius}$$

From the above formula, it can be seen that surface tension and distending pressure are directly proportional (i.e., when one rises in value, the other also rises), whereas the radius of the sphere is indirectly proportional (i.e., when one falls in value, the other one rises) to the distending pressure. Thus, as the radius of the sphere decreases, the pressure required to keep the sphere open increases, and vice versa.

Surface-active agents have the ability to lower the surface tension and thus the internal distending pressure that exists inside a liquid bubble. Subsequently, the liquid bubble expands as the radius is increased. By this mechanism, bubbly, frothy secretions dissipate, or collapse, resulting in the liquefication of the secretions. Likewise, because alveoli have a liquid lining, lower surface tensions result in stable, expanded alveoli.

SPECIFIC SURFACE-ACTIVE AGENTS

ALCOHOL: ETHANOL, ETHYL ALCOHOL

Mechanism of Action and Indications for Use

Alcohol is a surface-active agent that has a surface tension of approximately half that of bubbly, frothy respiratory tract secretions. Thus, alcohol applied topically to these secretions correspondingly lowers their surface tension. By lowering the surface tension, the frothy bubbles collapse and liquefy, thus improving ventilation and gas exchange. Ethyl alcohol may be indicated for use in acute pulmonary edema; however, the use is rare owing to the advent of more sophisticated and useful drugs (cardiotonics, diuretics).

Contraindications

Contraindications to the use of alcohol include patients on Antabuse therapy.

Adverse Reactions

Pulmonary: Lung mucosa irritation, bronchospasm.

CNS: Depression, sedation, decrease in ventilatory drive (corresponding effects to a slightly intoxicated state).

Other: Local dehydration.

Dosage and Administration

Ethyl alcohol: By way of nebulization or direct tracheal instillation in an intubated patient: 5 to 15 ml of 30% to 50% solution (short treatments are recommended).

Note: Do not use isopropyl or denatured alcohol.

Tyloxapol (Alevaire) and sodium ethasulfate (Tergemist) are no longer recommended for use in the control of pulmonary secretions due to the lack of proof of efficacy as stated by the FDA (they have been removed from the market). These agents were previously used in respiratory care as mucus-wetting (detergent) agents.

EXOGENOUS SURFACTANTS

THE GAS EXCHANGE SITES AND PULMONARY SURFACTANT

Alveoli are the primary sites for gas exchange; a total estimate of 300,000,000 alveoli exist in the adult. This arrangement greatly increases the surface area of the lung; the total cross-sectional area available for gas exchange averages 70 square meters (40 to 100 m^2). Each alveolus is surrounded by a network of capillaries and supported by elastic and reticular fibers. Gas is exchanged between the lung and the blood by diffusion through the thin walls of the alveoli and capillaries.

In order for oxygen to get from the alveolus to the hemoglobin molecule, it must pass through the surfactant layer lining the internal surface of the alveolus, the alveolar epithelium, the interstitial space, the capillary basement membrane and capillary endothelium, the plasma, the red blood cell membrane, and into the red blood cell cytoplasm, where it will bind to the hemoglobin molecule. Carbon dioxide diffusion takes the same path, except in reverse order (from the hemoglobin molecule to the alveolus) (see Fig. 8.1).

As mentioned above, oxygen must pass through the surfactant layer, the alveolar epithelium, the interstitial space, and the capillary endothelium before entering the capillary bloodstream; these are the primary constituents of the alveolar-capillary membrane. The alveolar-capillary membrane is about 0.5 to 1.0 micrometer thick in healthy adults and does not produce any significant barrier to gas diffusion. Respiratory disease may increase the membrane's thickness, which would hinder gas exchange.

Surfactant coats the internal alveolar surface. Surfactant serves as an air-water interface that considerably lowers the surface tension of the fluid that lines the alveoli. High surface tension forces the alveoli into small, compact shapes with a tendency for collapse at end-expiration when they are at their smallest size. By lowering the surface tension, surfactant promotes stability and expansion of the alveoli (prevents alveolar collapse—atelectasis). Surfactant also increases the compliance of the lung, which then makes it easier to inflate the lung with each breath.

Surfactant consists of a mixture of proteins (12%, approximately half is specific for surfactant whereas the rest is contaminating protein from the plasma or lung tissue), neutral lipids (8%), and phospholipids (80%). The most important substance of surfactant, which is the primary surface-active compound, is a phospholipid called dipalmitoylphosphatidylcholine (DPPC; also known as lecithin). Three unique surfactant proteins have been identified: SP-A, SP-B, and SP-C. All three proteins are synthesized by type II alveolar cells (see below). SP-A, a high-molecular-weight glycoprotein, functions with other surfactant proteins and lipids to improve surface properties. SP-A also regulates secretion of surfactant and its exocytosis from the type II alveolar cells. Additionally, SP-A plays a vital role in surfactant reuptake by type II alveolar cells for recycling and repeated use. SP-B and SP-C, low-molecular-weight, hydrophobic proteins, facilitate the dispersion and adhesion of lipid throughout the air-liquid interface within alveoli to form the surfactant monolayer.

The alveolar epithelium consists of two primary cell types lying on a basement membrane (Fig. 13.6). Type I cells (squamous pneumocytes) are very flat, thin cells composing the majority (more than 90%) of the alveolar surface. Type I cells are responsible for structural support of the alveoli and for gas exchange. Spaces between these cells, the pores of Kohn, allow collateral communication (i.e., movement of gases) between adjacent alveoli; there is a noted increase in the size and number of pores with increasing age.

Type II cells (granular pneumocytes) have microvilli, are cuboidal in shape, are primary secretory cells, and form the remaining (5% to 10%) of the alveolar sur-

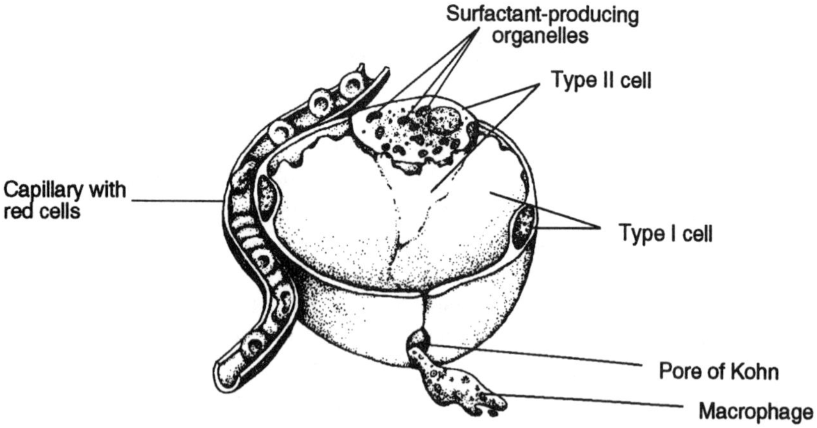

Figure 13.6. Schematic representation of the alveolus and its epithelium. Note that most of the surface is the cytoplasmic extension of type I cells. (From Shapiro BA, et al. Clinical Application of Respiratory Care. 4th ed. St. Louis: Mosby-Year Book, Inc., 1991. Reproduced with permission.)

face. These cells are the primary source for the production and recycling of surfactant. Type II cells rapidly reproduce in cases of injury to aid in alveolar repair.

Type III cells (alveolar macrophages) are free-roaming cells located in the luminal space of the alveolus responsible for phagocytosis (ingests bacteria, dead cells, and other foreign material).

PULMONARY SURFACTANT THERAPY

Historically, Kurt von Neergaard was the first to propose that lung expansion was dependent on alveolar surface tension. His work was published in 1929 in a paper entitled "New notions on a fundamental principle of respiratory mechanics: the retractile force of the lung, dependent on the surface tension in the alveoli" (translated from German). However, it wasn't until the mid-1950s when further work was performed on this topic. In 1958, Clements, who demonstrated that lungs contain a substance that lowers surface tension, identified the major component of pulmonary surfactant, DPPC. In 1959, Avery and Mead reported that saline extracts from the lungs of preterm infants with infant respiratory distress syndrome (IRDS) lacked the low surface tension characteristics of pulmonary surfactant. Soon thereafter, several attempts were made to treat IRDS with aerosolized surfactant, all of which were unsuccessful. In 1972, Enhorning and Robertson administered surfactant, via the intratracheal route, into the lungs of preterm animals. The surfactant they used had been recovered from the air spaces of mature animal lungs. The result of this investigation was the discovery that exogenously administered surfactant significantly improved lung expansion and ventilation in preterm animals. In 1980, Fujiwara and colleagues successfully progressed to using a surfactant prepared from an organic solvent extract of bovine lung (Surfactant TA) to treat 10 infants with severe IRDS. By 1985, there were significant decreases in pneumothorax and neonatal death rates from using surfactants prepared from bovine alveolar lavage or human amniotic fluid. Although still investigational, widespread use of exogenously administered surfactant began in 1989. The first synthetic lung surfactant (Exosurf) was approved in 1990 by the FDA for the treatment of IRDS. In 1991, the first natural animal lung surfactant (Survanta) was approved for general use in the USA. Thus, the surfactants in clinical use today are of two general classes: surfactants prepared from mammalian lungs and synthetic lung surfactants.

The animal surfactants have phospholipid components similar to that of natural human pulmonary surfactant. They also contain some SP-B and SP-C, but no SP-A. The surfactant developed in Japan by Fujiwara as Surfacten (Surfactant TA) and subsequently approved for use in the USA as Survanta (Beractant, Ross Laboratories) is obtained by mincing bovine lungs in saline and then extracting the lipids, SP-B, and SP-C with organic solvents. DPPC, palmitic acid, and triglyceride are then added to improve the surface-active property of the extract. An even bigger improvement in the surface properties of these organic-solvent extracts of lung tissue can be brought about by removing the neutral lipids by chromatography. Curosurf (Chiesi Farmaceutici, Parma, Italy), a surfactant undergoing investigation in Europe, is such an extract. Although not currently approved for use in the USA, surfactants obtained from organic-solvent extracts of alveolar-lavage fluid are being extensively tested. Such surfactants (e.g., CLSE and Infrasurf, Forest Laboratories) need no supplementation or removal of components.

Two synthetic surfactants have been investigated in several clinical trials, one of which (Exosurf, Burroughs Wellcome Co.) has been approved for use in the USA. Exosurf is a protein-free mixture of DPPC (85%), hexadecanol (9%), and tyloxapol (6%). A 7:3 mixture of DPPC and phosphatidylglycerol (ALEC, United Kingdom) is currently being tested in England. As previously stated, DPPC is the primary surface-active phospholipid of surfactant; the other ingredients of these synthetic surfactants are added to enhance and facilitate dispersion and surface adsorption (attachment and adhesion to the inner alveolar surface). The primary advantages of synthetic surfactants over natural animal surfactants are the elimination of possible organic contaminants (e.g., foreign material, infectious microbes) and, owing to their protein-free mixtures, in risks of immunologic reactions and infections. However, because the synthetic surfactants lack the natural surfactant proteins, they do not seem to be equivalent in their performance as compared to the performance illicited from the natural animal surfactants (Jobe 1993).

At this time, there is not a clear understanding of how to stimulate the production of **endogenous** surfactant or what kind of surfactant preparations can be used that may positively affect endogenous surfactant production. In addition, it is not clearly known if exogenously administered surfactant affects the metabolism of the endogenously produced surfactant. However, it is known that the reuptake and recycling mechanism of surfactant by type II alveolar cells, as previously described, leads to a storage pool for exogenously administered surfactant for repeated recycling and reuse, which seems to be the basis for the success of exogenously administered surfactant preparations.

Surfactant depletion, or loss of production, may occur with various lung diseases (e.g., emphysema, neonatal and adult respiratory distress syndrome), certain drugs, repeated bronchial lavage, irritants (cigarette smoke, toxic chemicals), aspiration of fluids, near drowning, or after exposure to high concentrations of oxygen. Inadequate production of surfactant may precipitate stiff lungs (low compliance) and areas of atelectasis whereby very high airway pressures would be required to inflate and maintain the lungs.

Approximately 70% of deaths among preterm newborns are caused by immature lungs failing to produce sufficient quantities of surfactant. Synonymous names associated with this condition not only include IRDS but also surfactant deficiency disease (SDD) and hyaline membrane disease (HMD). Without a doubt, the use of surfactant therapy in preterm infants is the most intensively, thoroughly studied new therapy in neonatal care. Since the induction of surfactant replacement therapy, there has been a significant decrease in the general infant mortality rate from IRDS in the USA. There has also been a striking decrease in IRDS-associated complications, such as air leaks (pneumothorax, pulmonary interstitial emphysema [PIE]). The tendency for reduced air leaks is noticeably greater with animal surfactants (Jobe 1993).

Surfactant replacement therapy is effective as evidenced by its immediate effects such as improved gas exchange and oxygenation with concomitant decreases in peak inspiratory pressure settings, ventilatory rate, and FIO_2; its medium-term effects such as improvement of lung mechanics (compliance) and reduced air leak; and its long-term effects such as an increase in the survival rate.

Currently, there are three primary approved indications for surfactant replacement therapy via intratracheal administration:

- Prevention of IRDS in very low birth weight infants (1350 grams).
- Prevention of other, larger infants (>1350 grams) with corresponding evidence of immature lungs and who are at risk for developing IRDS.
- Rescue treatment of infants who have already developed IRDS.

NEW APPLICATIONS OF PULMONARY SURFACTANT THERAPY

Surfactant therapy has been shown or is speculated to be beneficial in a variety of respiratory disorders other than IRDS. At present, there is no FDA approval for the following potential applications of surfactant therapy:

- Meconium, blood, amniotic fluid, or gastric aspiration (Auten et al. 1991, Moses et al. 1991, Blanke and Jorch 1993, Thomas et al. 1994)
- Pneumonia and congenital infectious pneumonia (Holm et al. 1991)
- Adult respiratory distress syndrome (ARDS) (Buheital, Scharf, and Harms 1992, Stubbig et al. 1992, Holm and Matalon 1989)
- Congenital diaphragmatic hernia (Glick et al. 1992)
- Pulmonary hypoplasia (Glick et al. 1992)
- Surfactant therapy in conjunction with high-frequency ventilation (Davis et al. 1992)
- Surfactant therapy before or in conjunction with extracorporeal membrane oxygenation (ECMO) (Bui et al. 1992)

AVAILABLE SURFACTANT PREPARATIONS

COLFOSCERIL PALMITATE (SYNTHETIC LUNG SURFACTANT): EXOSURF NEONATAL

Mechanisms of Action and Indications for Use

The mechanisms of action and indications for use are the same as those for all exogenous surfactants, as previously described (see *Pulmonary Surfactant Therapy*).

Contraindications

There are currently no known contraindications for surfactant replacement therapy for infants.

Precautions

1. Administer only by instillation into the trachea. Aerosol delivery is currently undergoing investigation (Lewis et al. 1991). Constant bedside attention for at least 30 minutes after drug administration and frequent blood gas sampling are essential.
2. After administration, colfosceril can rapidly improve oxygenation and lung compliance; therefore, the ventilator settings (e.g., peak inspiratory pressure setting, ventilator rate, FIO_2) must be immediately adjusted downward; otherwise, lung overdistention and fatal pulmonary air leak may occur, as well as hyperoxia and a reduced brain blood flow (from marked hypocarbia). Close monitoring by trained personnel and vigilant clinical attention is required for all patients before, during, and after the administration of colfosceril.
3. Reflux of colfosceril into the endotracheal tube has been observed during dosing and may be the result of too rapid administration. If reflux occurs, stop drug administration and (if necessary) increase the inspiratory pressure setting by 4 to 5 cm H_2O until colfosceril is no longer present in the endotracheal tube.
4. A transient drop in oxygen saturation (>20%) has been noted during dosing. If this occurs, stop drug administration and increase the inspiratory pressure setting by 4 to 5 cm H_2O and/or increase the FIO_2 for 1 to 2 minutes.
5. Markedly impaired ventilation and airway obstruction may occur during or shortly after colfosceril administration. This may be caused by mucous plugging of the endotracheal tube, especially if secretions are prominent before drug administration. Suctioning of all infants before drug administration should reduce this occurrence. If the patient cannot be successfully ventilated or suctioned because of an occluded endotracheal tube, the tube must be removed and replaced immediately. It is important to note that the infant should not be suctioned for 2 hours after colfosceril is administered, except when clinically necessary.
6. Complete prescribing information from the manufacturer should be reviewed before drug administration.
7. Exogenous surfactant treatment is not a substitute for attempts to increase fetal lung maturation and thus prevent IRDS by delaying preterm delivery or by using maternal glucocorticoid therapy. Additionally, maternal glucocorticoid therapy seems to improve the response to surfactant treatment in preterm infants with IRDS (Robertson 1993).

Adverse Reactions

The following adverse reactions have been reported. These adverse effects may be caused by the drug itself, by the dosing procedure (see below), or by the resultant therapeutic effect of the drug:

- Intraventricular hemorrhage
- Pulmonary air leak (pneumothorax, pneumopericardium, pneumomediastinum, pulmonary interstitial emphysema) (see Precaution no. 2)
- Death
- Patent ductus arteriosus
- Necrotizing enterocolitis
- Pulmonary hemorrhage (primarily noted in infants with a birth weight less than 700 grams and those with a patent ductus arteriosus)
- Congenital pneumonia
- Nosocomial pneumonia
- Nonpulmonary infections (sepsis, death from sepsis, meningitis, other)
- Major anomalies
- Hypotension
- Hyperbilirubinemia
- Exchange transfusion
- Thrombocytopenia (that required platelet transfusion)
- Persistent fetal circulation
- Seizures
- Apnea
- Airway obstruction (see Precaution no. 5)
- Oxygen desaturation (see Precaution no. 4)

Dosage and Administration

Accurate determination of birth weight is important to accurate dosing. Colfosceril is packaged as a lyophilized powder for injection. The following components are contained in a 10-ml vial:

108 mg colfosceril palmitate
12 mg cetyl alcohol
8 mg tyloxapol

Solutions containing buffers or preservatives should not be used for **reconstitution**. Reconstitute each vial, immediately before use, with 8 ml of the accompanying diluent (preservative-free sterile water for injection). Reconstituted colfosceril is a milky white suspension with a total volume of 8 ml per vial. Various sizes of endotracheal adapters (2.5, 3, 3.5, 4, and 4.5 mm), each with a special right-angle Luer-lock sideport, are supplied with each vial of colfosceril. An adapter that corresponds to the internal diameter of the endotracheal tube should be selected and fitted on the endotracheal tube.

The recommended single dose of colfosceril is 5 ml/kg of birth weight of the reconstituted suspension. This dose is administered in two equally divided doses of 2.5 ml/kg and instilled intratracheally through the endotracheal adapter that fits on the endotracheal tube. Each half-dose is administered slowly over 1 to 2 minutes (without interruption of mechanical ventilation). The dose is given in small bursts that are synchronized with inspiration. This dose is administered with the infant in the midline position. After this half-dose has been administered, the infant's head and torso are turned 45° to the right for 30 seconds while continuing mechanical ventilation. After the infant is turned back to the midline position, the second half-dose (2.5 ml/kg) is given in an identical fashion as the first half-dose. The turning maneuvers allow gravity to assist in distributing the drug throughout the lungs. It is essential to continuously monitor ECG and oxygen saturation during dosing.

For Prophylactic Treatment: The first dose is administered as a single 5 ml/kg dose as soon as possible after birth. Second and third doses are administered 12 and 24 hours later to all infants who remain on mechanical ventilation at those times. If the infant weighs more than 1600 grams, at least two vials will be needed for each dose (5 ml/kg × 1.6 kg = 8 ml).

For Rescue Treatment: Administer in two 5 ml/kg doses. The initial dose is given as soon as possible after the diagnosis of IRDS is confirmed. The second dose is administered 12 hours later, if the infant is receiving mechanical ventilation at the time of dosing. Some institutions have given more than two doses as rescue treatment.

BERACTANT (NATURAL LUNG SURFACTANT): SURVANTA

Mechanisms of Action and Indications for Use

The mechanisms of action and indications for use are the same as those for all exogenous surfactants, as previously described (see *Pulmonary Surfactant Therapy*).

Contraindications

There are currently no known contraindications for surfactant replacement therapy in infants.

Precautions

The precautions for natural lung surfactant are as previously stated for colfosceril.

Adverse Reactions

The adverse reactions for natural lung surfactant are as previously stated for colfosceril.

Dosage and Administration

Accurate determination of birth weight is important to accurate dosing. Beractant is packaged in single-use vials containing 25 mg phospholipids per ml suspended in 0.9% sodium chloride solution. Additionally, there are 0.5 to 1.75 mg triglycerides, 1.4 to 3.5 mg free fatty acids, and <1 mg protein per ml. Each single-use vial contains 8 ml suspension (200 mg of phospholipids/vial). Beractant does not require reconstitution as does colfosceril, because it already is in suspension. The color of beractant is off-white to light brown. Beractant must be kept refrigerated (2° to 8°C) and protected from light. The suspension should be taken out of the refrigerator at least 20 minutes before administration or warmed in the hand for at least 8 minutes. Do not shake the vial; if settling occurs, gently swirl the vial. Discard any unused portion.

The recommended dose of beractant is 100 mg of phospholipids per kg of birth weight. Because there are 25 mg of phospholipids per ml in the beractant suspension, this equates to a dose of 4 ml/kg of birth weight (100 mg/kg ÷ 25 mg/ml = 4 ml/kg). Four doses may be administered in the first 48 hours of life (preferably, the first dose is given within the first 15 minutes of birth). Each dose should not be given more frequently than every 6 hours.

Dosing Regimen: Beractant is administered intratracheally via a 5-Fr. end-hole catheter that is inserted just beyond the tip of the endotracheal tube (do not advance the catheter any farther; otherwise, endobronchial administration may result). To ensure homogenous distribution of the drug, each single dose is divided into fourths and administered with the infant in a different position each time the quarter dose is given. In many clinical trials, the sequence of positioning the infant was as follows:

head and body slightly down, head turned to the right
head and body slightly down, head turned to the left
head and body slightly up, head turned to the right
head and body slightly up, head turned to the left

The first quarter-dose is gently administered through the catheter over 2 to 3 seconds. The catheter is removed from the endotracheal tube and the infant is manually ventilated or returned to the ventilator for at least 30 seconds or until stable. Each subsequent dose is given in a similar fashion after the infant has been repositioned. However, the manufacturer's literature does not recommend handbag manual ventilation for the repeat doses. During the dosing procedure, ventilator settings may need to be adjusted to maintain adequate oxygenation and ventilation.

REFERENCES/RECOMMENDED READING

Aitken MI, et al. Effect of inhaled recombinant human DNase on pulmonary function in normal and cystic fibrosis patients: phase I study. JAMA 267:1947, 1992.

Auten Rl, et al. Surfactant treatment of full-term newborns with respiratory failure. Pediatrics 87:101, 1991.

Avery ME, Mead J. Surface properties in relation to atelectasis and hyaline membrane disease. Am J Dis Child 97:517, 1959.

Basbaum C, et al. Cellular mechanisms of airway secretions. Am Rev Respir Dis 137:479, 1988.

Blanke JG, Jorch G. Surfactant therapy in severe neonatal respiratory failure—multicenter study—II. Surfactant therapy in 10 newborn infants with meconium aspiration syndrome. Klin Padiatr 205(2):75, 1993.

Boucher RC, et al. Evidence for reduced Cl^- and increased Na^+ permeability in cystic fibrosis human primary cell cultures. J Physiol (Lond) 405:77, 1988.

Braga PC, Ziment I, Allegra L. Drugs in Bronchial Mucology. New York: Raven Press, 1989.

Buheital G, Scharf J, Harms D. Experiences with surfactant therapy of adult respiratory distress syndrome. Monatsschrift Kinderheilkunde 140(9):629, 1992.

Bui KC, et al. Phospholipid and surfactant protein A concentrations in tracheal aspirates from infants requiring extracorporeal membrane oxygenation. J Pediatr 121:271, 1992.

Clarke SW. Management of mucus hypersecretion. Eur J Respir Dis 153(Suppl):136, 1987.

Clements JA. Surface tension of lung extracts. Proc Soc Exp Biol Med 95:170, 1957.

Cottrell GP, Surkin HB. Pharmacology for Respiratory Care Practitioners. Philadelphia: F.A. Davis Company, 1995.

Davis JM, et al. High-frequency jet ventilation and surfactant treatment of newborns with severe respiratory failure. Pediatr Pulmonol 13:108, 1992.

Drug Facts and Comparisons. 49th ed. St. Louis: Facts and Comparisons, 1995.

Dulfano JJ, Adler KB. Physical properties of sputum. VII. Rheologic properties and mucociliary transport. Am Rev Respir Dis 112:341, 1975.

Enhorning G, Robertson B. Lung expansion in the premature rabbit fetus after tracheal deposition of surfactant. Pediatrics 50:58, 1972.

Enhorning G, et al. Improved ventilation of prematurely delivered primates following tracheal deposition of surfactant. Am J Obstet Gynecol 132:529, 1978.

Fujiwara T, et al. Artificial surfactant therapy in hyaline membrane disease. Lancet 1:55, 1980.

Giordano AM, Holsclaw D, Litt M. Mucus rheology and mucociliary clearance: normal physiologic state. Am Rev Respir Dis 118:245, 1978.

Girod S, et al. Role of the physiochemical properties of mucus in the protection of the respiratory epithelium. Eur Respir J 5(4):477, 1992.

Glick PL, et al. Pathophysiology of congenital diaphragmatic hernia, III. Exogenous surfactant therapy for the high risk neonate with CDH. J Pediatr Surg 27:866, 1992.
Glick PL, et al. Pathophysiology of congenital diaphragmatic hernia, II. The fetal lamb CDH model is surfactant deficient. J Pediatr Surg 27:382, 1992.
Hills BA. The role of lung surfactant. Br J Anaesth 65:13, 1990.
Holm BA, Enhorning G, Notter RH. A biophysical mechanism by which plasma proteins inhibit lung surfactant activity. Chem Phys Lipids 49:49, 1988.
Holm BA, Matalon S. Role of pulmonary surfactant in the development and treatment of adult respiratory distress syndrome. Anesth Analg 69:805, 1989.
Holm BA, et al. Inhibition of pulmonary surfactant function by phospholipases. J Appl Physiol 71:317, 1991.
Holm BA. Surfactant replacement therapy. New levels of understanding. Am Rev Respir Dis 148:834, 1993.
Hubbard RC, et al. A preliminary study of aerosolized recombinant human deoxyribose I in the sputum of cystic fibrosis patients. N Engl J Med 326:812, 1992.
Jeanneret-Grosjean A, et al. Sampling technique and rheology of human tracheobronchial mucus. Am Rev Respir Dis 137:707, 1988.
Jobe AH. Pulmonary surfactant therapy. N Engl J Med 328(12):861, 1993.
Kaliner M, et al. Human respiratory mucus. J Allergy Clin Immunol 73:318, 1984.
King M, Macklem PT. Rheological properties of microliter quantities of normal mucus. J Appl Physiol 42:797, 1977.
Lewis JF, et al. Aerosolized surfactant treatment of preterm lambs. J Appl Physiol 70:869, 1991.
Lewis JF, et al. Nebulized vs. instilled exogenous surfactant in an adult lung injury model. J Appl Physiol 71:270, 1991.
Liechty EA, et al. Reduction of neonatal mortality after multiple doses of bovine surfactant in low birth weight neonates with respiratory distress syndrome. Pediatrics 88:19, 1991.
Lopez-Vidriero MT. Biochemical basis of physical properties of respiratory tract secretions. Eur J Respir Dis 71(Suppl 153):130, 1987.
Lundgren JD, Shelhamer JH. Pathogenesis of airway mucus hypersecretion. J Allergy Clin Immunol 85(2):399, 1990.
Marin MG. Pharmacology of airway secretion. Pharmacol Rev 38:273, 1986.
Merritt TA, Hallman M. Surfactant replacement: a new era with many challenges for neonatal medicine. AJDC 142:1333, 1988.
Moses D, et al. Inhibition of pulmonary surfactant function by meconium. Am J Obstet Gynecol 164:477, 1991.
Pavia DP. Effects of pharmacologic agents on the clearance of airway secretions. Sem Resp Med 5(4):345, 1984.
Physicians' Desk Reference. 49th ed. Montvale, NJ: Medical Economics, 1995.
Ramsey BW. A summary of the results of the Phase III multicenter clinical trial: aerosol administration of recombinant human DNase reduces the risk of respiratory tract infections and improves pulmonary function in patients with cystic fibrosis. Pediatr Pulmonol 9(Suppl):152, 1993.
Ramsey BW, Dorkin HL. Consensus conference: practical applications of Pulmozyme. Pediatr Pulmonol 17(6):404, 1994.
Robertson B. Corticosteroids and surfactant for prevention of neonatal RDS. Ann Med 25(3):285, 1993.
Sackner MA. Effect of respiratory drugs on mucociliary clearance. Chest 73(Suppl):958, 1978.

Shah PL, Scott SF, Hodson ME. Report on a multicenter study using aerosolized recombinant human DNase I in the treatment of cystic fibrosis patients with severe pulmonary disease. Pediatr Pulmonol 9(Suppl):157, 1993.

Shak S, et al. Recombinant human DNase I reduces the viscosity of cystic fibrosis sputum. Proc Natl Acad Sci U S A 87:9188, 1990.

Stubbig K, et al. Surfactant administration in acute respiratory failure. Anaesthesist 41(9):555, 1992.

The OSIRIS Collaborative Group. Early versus delayed neonatal administration of synthetic surfactant—the judgment of OSIRIS. Lancet 340:1363, 1992.

Thomas NL, et al. The use of exogenous surfactant in three pediatric patients following gastric aspiration. Respiratory Care 39(9):912, 1994.

Turner-Warwick M, Openshaw P. Sputum in asthma. Postgrad Med J 63(Suppl 1):79, 1987.

Wanner A. The role of mucus in chronic obstructive pulmonary disease. Chest 97(Suppl 2):11, 1990.

Wanner A, Rao A. Clinical indications for and effects of bland, mucolytic, and antimicrobial aerosols. Am Rev Respir Dis 122:79, 1980.

Wellcome Medical Division. Exosurf NEONATAL (Colfosceril Palmitate for Suspension) Product Monograph. Kirkland, Quebec: Burroughs Wellcome, Inc., 1991.

Zahm JM, et al. Adhesive properties of airway secretions in cystic fibrosis. Am Rev Respir Dis 137:303, 1988.

Agents that Affect Skeletal Muscle Contraction 14

The agents presented in this chapter affect the somatic motoneurons of the peripheral nervous system. This system innervates striated muscle fibers such as the biceps, triceps, deltoids, and diaphragm (i.e., body movements, posture, lifting, and breathing functions). The action of these skeletal muscles are both movements under conscious voluntary control and reflex movements, as opposed to the involuntary movements of the smooth muscle cells innervated by the autonomic nervous system.

Two classes of drugs will be detailed in this chapter.

- Cholinergic muscle stimulants (indirectly facilitate muscle contraction)
- Neuromuscular blocking agents (directly inhibits muscle contraction)

To fully comprehend how these drugs work, it is helpful to have an understanding of the impulse transmission occurring at the myoneural junction. Therefore, an introductory explanation of skeletal muscle contraction precedes the presentation of the drugs.

Physiology of Skeletal Muscle Contraction

A motor neuron originates from the spinal cord and extends to the muscle it innervates, where it then branches into several muscle fibers (Fig. 14.1). Upon stimulation, the nerve fibers shorten as a unit and the muscle contracts. Flaccidity is the relaxed state of the muscle when no impulse transmission is occurring. The neuromuscular junction (detailed in Fig. 14.2) is the area between the motor nerve fiber and the skeletal muscle fiber. The motor endplate is the chemical receptor area for the neurotransmitter acetylcholine (ACh). These receptors are designated as cholinergic nicotinic (N_M) receptors (see Chapter 2, Fig. 2.6).

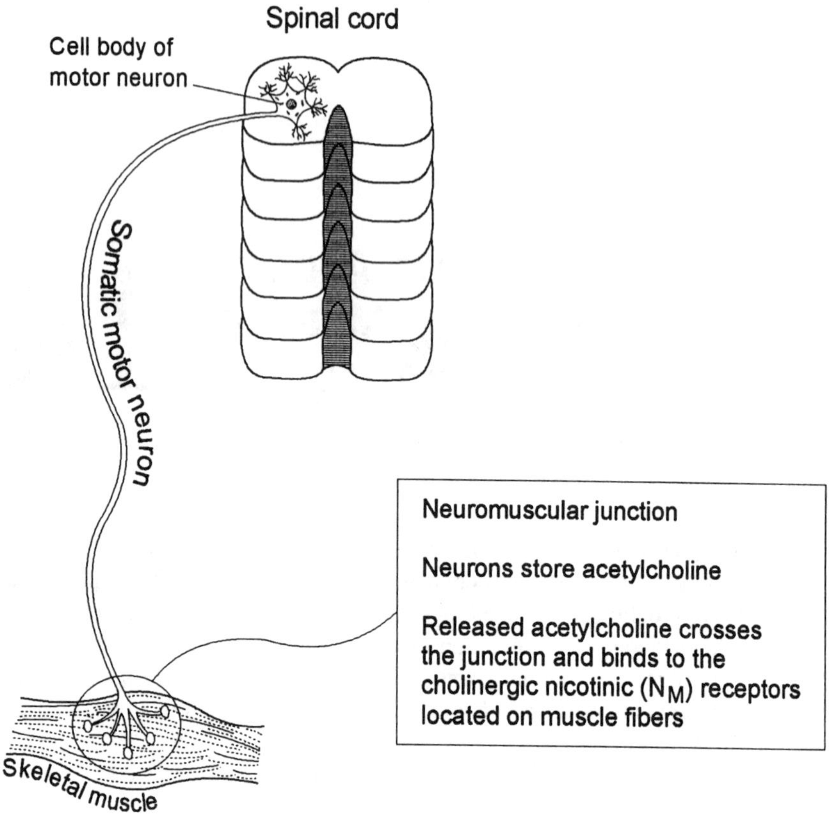

Figure 14.1. Somatic motor neuron innervating skeletal muscle.

Impulse transmission into the axon terminal of the motor neuron results in the liberation of ACh from its storage vesicles. Released ACh enters and crosses the neuromuscular junction to specifically bind with the N_M receptors on the motor endplate. When the motor endplate is chemically stimulated by acetylcholine, a transient change in the membrane permeability is brought about that allows the influx of sodium ions. The influx of sodium ions across the nerve fiber membrane reverses the polarity of the muscle fiber, causing depolarization to occur. Once in the depolarized mode, the muscle fiber releases calcium. The release of calcium then initiates muscle contraction. As long as calcium is allowed to remain free, the muscle contraction continues. As depolarization ceases, calcium is taken back into its storage sacs in the muscle fiber; contraction of the muscle ceases, repolarization occurs, and the membrane returns to its resting level. The entire event of muscle stimulation, depolarization, and repolarization occurs in approximately 20 milliseconds (Fig. 14.3).

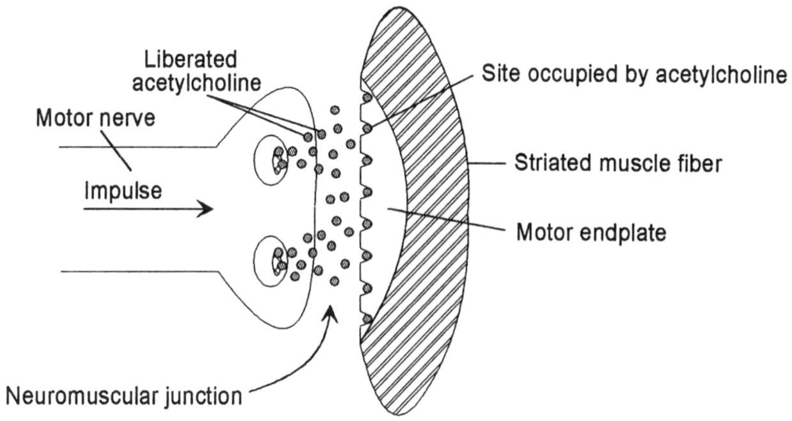

Figure 14.2. Impulse transmission across the neuromuscular junction.

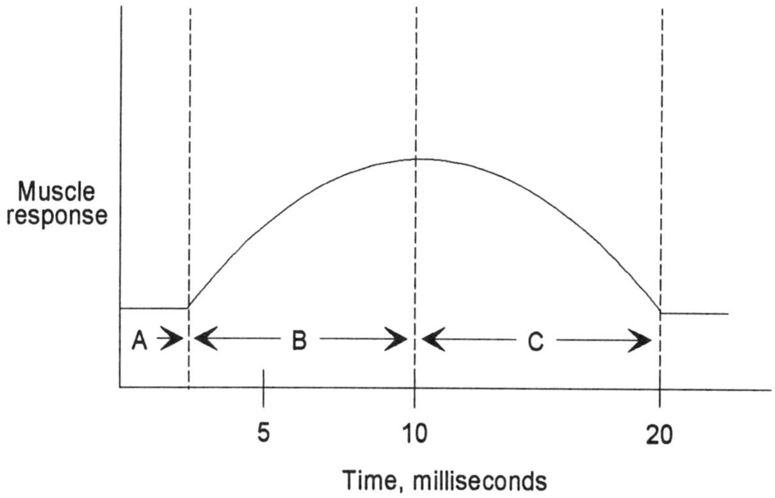

Figure 14.3. Skeletal muscle contraction. A, latent period; B, contraction; C, relaxation.

Acetylcholinesterase (AChE; also known as specific or true ChE) is an enzyme found in high concentrations in cholinergic neurons (dendrites, axons), in the immediate vicinity of cholinergic synapses, and in other tissues. AChE has the ability to rapidly hydrolyze, and thus inactivate, ACh after it has been released from cholinergic neurons. By this action, the stimulus is aborted and the muscle returns to its relaxed state.

CHOLINERGIC MUSCLE STIMULANTS

Mechanism of Action and Indications for Use

Cholinergic muscle stimulants indirectly potentiate acetylcholine's duration of action at various cholinergic receptor sites by inhibiting the hydrolysis of this mediator by the enzyme AChE (Fig. 14.4). By this action, the transmission of impulses are facilitated at the myoneural junction, enhancing muscular strength and response to repetitive nerve stimulation. Owing to their mechanism of action, these agents are also known as anticholinesterases (anti-ChE) or AChE inhibitors.

Cholinergic muscle stimulants are especially useful in the diagnosis and treatment of myasthenia gravis. Myasthenia gravis (also known as Goldflam disease) is a neuromuscular disease characterized by marked muscular weakness and progressive fatigability. An autoimmune process causes production of antibodies that decrease the number of functional nicotinic receptors at the motor endplate of skeletal muscle. The net effect is that nerve impulses fail to induce normal muscle contraction. The muscles of the face and neck are initially involved at the onset of the disease. The patient may complain of difficulty in chewing, swallowing, or talking. Drooping eyelids and intermittent double vision are also usually present. As the disease progresses, the muscles of the trunk and extremities fail to produce sufficient contraction. Some cases of myasthenia are mild, whereas others may be rapidly fatal, leading to respiratory failure and death. Exacerbations of

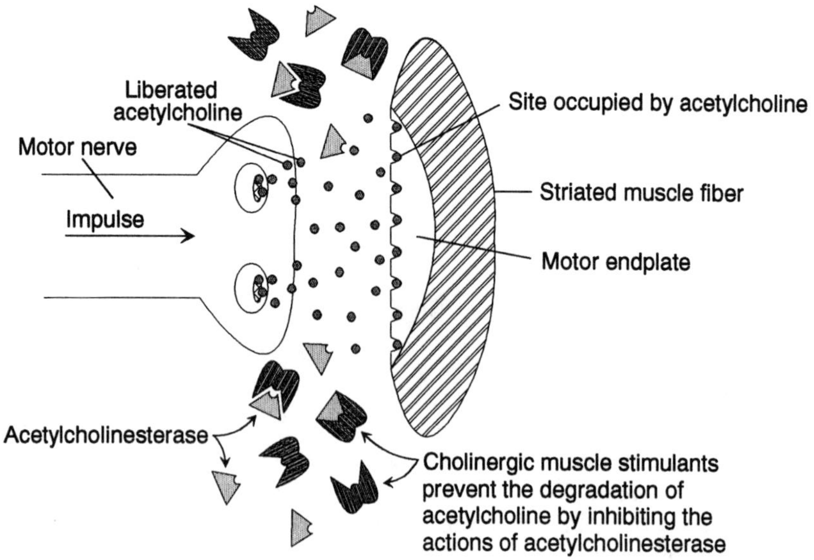

Figure 14.4. Conceptual representation of the actions of cholinergic muscle stimulants at the myoneural junction.

the disease may occur without warning, or the patient may exist in a state of remission for several years.

Patients with myasthenia gravis usually exhibit a dramatic improvement in muscle strength after administration of a cholinergic muscle stimulant. Neostigmine, pyridostigmine, and ambenonium are the standard drugs of choice in the symptomatic treatment of myasthenia gravis. They all have the ability to increase the response of myasthenic muscle to repetitive nerve transmission. This is due to their direct inhibition of AChE at neuromuscular junctions, thus preserving and augmenting endogenous ACh's activity at the cholinergic receptor. Additionally, because ACh is not inactivated in the neuromuscular junction by AChE, a greater cross-sectional area of the motor endplate is exposed to ACh stimulation, which also results in an enhanced performance from muscles.

The dosages of these drugs must be carefully titrated. An excessive dose may result in a cholinergic crisis characterized by general weakness, a condition that may be confused with the symptoms of myasthenia gravis. The generalized weakness is a result of the now nonresponsive, overstimulated motor endplates of skeletal muscle fibers from repetitive ACh stimulation. Edrophonium is the drug of choice to differentiate whether the patient is exhibiting a myasthenic crisis or a cholinergic crisis (see below). Additionally, cholinergic muscle stimulants are *not* selective to just enhancing the activity of ACh at the N_M receptors. These agents have the ability to affect any cholinergic synapse in which AChE abides. This means that impulse transmission at the cholinergic receptors of the autonomic ganglia (N_N receptors), as well as those of the muscarinic type, may be potentiated. Intravenous atropine should be given immediately if a severe muscarinic reaction occurs. Muscarinic stimulation can be especially hazardous in the patient with asthma owing to the potential for severe bronchospasm.

Because these agents are not cholinergic receptor selective, they have uses other than as muscle stimulants. Other pharmacologic properties of these agents can be predicted by knowing where ACh is released by nerve impulses and what the concomitant physiologic reaction is when these receptors are activated (see Chapter 2, Tables 2.3 and 2.4). As previously stated, acetylcholine is the transmitter for all nicotinic receptors (N_N, autonomic ganglia; N_M, neuromuscular junctions) as well as all muscarinic receptors of the parasympathetic system and those select few muscarinic receptors of the sympathetic system (e.g., sweat glands, blood vessels in skeletal muscles). The therapeutic usefulness of cholinergic muscle stimulants has found favor with treating glaucoma, atony (lacking normal tone or strength; failure to contract normally) of the smooth muscle of the intestinal tract and urinary bladder, and termination of the action of nondepolarizing neuromuscular blocking agents (see following section on *Neuromuscular Blocking Agents*). Physostigmine is a useful agent used to reverse the severe antimuscarinic effects resulting from atropine overdose (see below). It is also useful in phenothiazine and tricyclic antidepressant poisoning (see Chapter 15). Unlabeled uses include the treatment of delirium tremens (DTs) and Alzheimer's disease, a condition characterized by dysfunctional cholinergic neurons. Edrophonium has been used for alleviating sudden onset of supraventricular tachycardia (SVT).

Contraindications

Contraindications to the use of cholinergic muscle stimulants include hypersensitivity to these drugs and intestinal and urinary obstructions.

Precautions

1. Use with extreme caution for patients with asthma, epilepsy, bradycardia, recent coronary occlusion, hyperthyroidism, cardiac arrhythmias, or peptic ulcer owing to the possible aggravation of symptoms or increase in the severity of these diseases with cholinergic agonist use.
2. Anticholinesterase insensitivity may occur with repeated use of these drugs. Reduce or withhold dosage until the patient again becomes sensitive. Monitor patient for myasthenic crisis.
3. Have atropine sulfate readily available for possible overdose of these agents (see below, *Overdosage*) or when large doses are given, prior injection of atropine sulfate is recommended. Additionally, atropine or other belladonna derivatives may be used concomitantly with cholinergic muscle stimulants to overcome the muscarinic symptoms associated with these drugs.
4. Overdosage may result in cholinergic crisis, which may be confused with exacerbation of myasthenic symptoms: use edrophonium to differentiate between the two (see below). Withhold the drug if symptoms are caused by cholinergic crisis.
5. When using these agents to reverse the effects of nondepolarizing neuromuscular blocking agents, ensure adequate recovery of spontaneous ventilation and neuromuscular transmission before discontinuing ventilatory assistance.
6. Concomitant use of corticosteroids may decrease the AChE effects of these agents. Consequently, AChE effects may be potentiated after stopping corticosteroid use.
7. Drugs that suppress or interfere with neuromuscular transmission (such as local or general anesthetics, antiarrhythmics) should be used with caution, if at all, for patients with myasthenia.

Adverse Reactions

CNS: Convulsions, dysphonia, dizziness, drowsiness, loss of consciousness, headache.

Cardiovascular: Bradycardia, tachycardia, other arrhythmias, decreased cardiac output, hypotension, cardiac arrest, syncope.

Pulmonary: Increased tracheobronchial secretions, laryngospasm, bronchoconstriction, dyspnea, respiratory depression, respiratory arrest.

GI: Increased salivary, gastric, and intestinal secretions, nausea, vomiting, dysphagia, increased peristalsis, diarrhea, abdominal cramps.

Miscellaneous: Urinary frequency and urgency, diaphoresis, rash, flushing, allergic reactions, anaphylaxis.

Overdosage

Marked pronouncement of parasympathomimetic actions; cardiac arrhythmias, increased GI stimulation, abdominal cramps, diarrhea, vomiting, excessive salivation, blurring of vision, paralysis of voluntary muscles. Also, conversion of a myasthenia crisis to a cholinergic crisis has been noted with excessive use of anticholinesterase drugs.

Treatment consists of discontinuing all cholinergic medications and administering from 0.5 to 1.0 mg of atropine IV. A total dose of 5 to 10 mg of atropine may be required. Monitor patient for supportive treatment such as assisted respirations, intubation, oxygen, etc.

SPECIFIC CHOLINERGIC MUSCLE STIMULANTS
Indications, Dosage, and Administration

AMBENONIUM CHLORIDE: MYTELASE

Indications: Administered orally to treat myasthenia gravis. Ambenonium has a longer duration of action than other anticholinesterase agents and, therefore, requires less frequency of use. It produces less side effects and is the preferred drug for patients who are allergic to the bromide ion found in other cholinergic muscle stimulants.

Onset of action: 20 to 30 minutes.

Duration: 3 to 8 hours.

Dosage form: PO: 10-mg tablets.

Dosage:

Adults: 5 to 25 mg three to four times daily. Start with 5 mg and increase gradually to determine optimal dose. Dosage must be adjusted at 1- to 2-day intervals to avoid accumulation and overdosage.

EDROPHONIUM CHLORIDE: TENSILON, ENLON, REVERSOL

Indication: Used in the diagnosis of myasthenia gravis; however, because of its short duration, edrophonium is not useful in the maintenance or continued treatment of patients with myasthenia. This drug is also used as a nondepolarizing muscle relaxant antagonist.

Onset of action: <1 minute IV; 2 to 10 minutes IM.
Duration: 0.08 to 0.33 hours IV; 0.17 to 0.67 hours IM.
Dosage form: IV, IM solution: 10 mg/ml.
Dosage:
Adults: For diagnosis: Inject 2 mg IV in 15 to 30 seconds; if no reaction occurs after 45 seconds, inject 8 mg more. Test may be repeated after 30 minutes. Patients with myasthenia will show an increase in muscle strength in 1 to 3 minutes, which lasts for 5 to 10 minutes. If a cholinergic reaction occurs (increased muscarinic side effects, muscle weakness), discontinue test and administer atropine 0.4 to 0.5 mg IV. For IM administration of edrophonium, inject 10 mg.
Children: For diagnosis: Up to 34 kg, inject 1 mg IV; more than 34 kg, inject 2 mg. If no response occurs after 45 seconds, administer an additional dose of up to 5 mg IV for children weighing less than 34 kg and for children weighing more than 34 kg, administer up to 10 mg IV in 1-mg increments every 30 to 45 seconds. For IM administration, inject 2 mg for patients weighing up to 34 kg and 5 mg for patients weighing more than 34 kg. There is a 2- to 10-minute delay in reaction.
Infants: Give 0.5 mg IV. Alternately, give 0.04 mg/kg initially, then in 1-mg increments if no response occurs within 1 minute. 10 mg is the maximum dose (0.2 mg/kg).
For differential diagnosis of myasthenic crisis vs. cholinergic crisis: Adults: inject 1 to 2 mg; if the crisis is myasthenic, the test will clearly improve respirations in the patient. If the crisis is cholinergic (indicating an overdose of medication), edrophonium will increase secretions and further weaken respiratory muscles. Only initiate this test if assisted ventilation and intubation are immediately available.
As a nondepolarizing neuromuscular blocking agent (curare) antagonist: administer 10 mg IV over 30 to 45 seconds. Repeat when necessary. Maximal dose is 40 mg.

NEOSTIGMINE: PROSTIGMIN

Indication: For symptomatic control of myasthenia gravis. May be used to diagnose myasthenia gravis; however, edrophonium is preferred owing to its rapid onset and brief duration. Neostigmine is also used as an antidote for nondepolarizing neuromuscular blocking agents.
Onset of action: 4 to 8 minutes IV; 20 to 30 minutes IM; 45 to 75 minutes PO.
Duration: 2 to 4 hours IV, IM, PO.
Dosage form: IV, IM, SC solution: 0.25 mg/ml (1:4000) in 1-ml vials; 0.5 mg/ml (1:2000) in 1 and 10-ml vials; 1 mg/ml (1:1000) in 10-ml vials. **PO:** 15-mg tablets.
Dosage:
Adults: **IM, SC:** Inject 1 ml of the 1:2000 solution (0.5 mg), adjust subsequent

dosages according to patient response. **PO:** Varies from 15 to 375 mg/day according to the response of the patient. Average dose is 150 mg in a 24-hour period.

Children: **IV, IM, SC:** 0.01 to 0.04 mg/kg dose every 2 to 3 hour as needed. **PO:** 2 mg/kg daily in three to four divided doses.

For diagnosis of myasthenia gravis: Adults: 0.022 mg/kg IM; Children: 0.04 mg/kg IM.

As a nondepolarizing neuromuscular blocking agent (curare) antagonist: administer 0.5 to 2 mg IV over 30 to 45 seconds. Repeat when necessary. Maximal dose is 5 mg. Administer atropine (0.6 to 1.2 mg) several minutes before neostigmine to minimize muscarinic side effects.

PYRIDOSTIGMINE BROMIDE: MESTINON, REGONOL

Indication: Given orally, pyridostigmine is the most widely used cholinergic muscle stimulant for the treatment of myasthenia gravis. Individualized doses are necessary because of the wide variance in the drug's absorption, biotransformation, and elimination among patients. Pyridostigmine is also used to reverse nondepolarizing muscle relaxant effects.

Onset of action: 2 to 5 minutes IV; <15 minutes IM; 20 to 30 minutes PO.

Duration: 2 to 4 hours IV, IM; 3 to 6 hours PO.

Dosage form: IV, IM solution: 5 mg/ml; **PO:** 60-mg tablets; 180-mg sustained release tablets; 60 mg/5 ml syrup.

Dosage:

Adults: **IV, IM:** Given when oral therapy is not practicable or for exacerbation; 1/30th of the oral dose, either IM or very slowly IV. **PO:** Must be individualized; 600 mg/day (range: 60 to 1500 mg).

Children: **IM:** For newborn infants of myasthenic mothers; 0.05 to 0.15 mg/kg. **PO:** 7 mg/kg daily in divided doses (five to six doses).

As a nondepolarizing neuromuscular blocking agent (curare) antagonist: administer 0.1 to 0.25 mg/kg. Repeat when necessary. Maximal dose is 10 to 20 mg IV. Give atropine (0.6 to 1.2 mg IV) immediately before pyridostigmine to minimize muscarinic side effects.

PHYSOSTIGMINE SALICYLATE: ANTILIRIUM

Indication: As an antidote to reverse toxic central nervous system (CNS) effects produced by anticholinergic drugs (including tricyclic antidepressants). Physostigmine may also counteract the CNS depressant effects of diazepam. Unlabeled use includes treatment of delirium tremens (DTs) and Alzheimer's disease.

Onset of action: Peak effects are noted within 5 minutes.

Duration: Approximately 1 hour.
Dosage form: IM, IV: 1 mg/ml.
Dosage:
Adults: **For overdosage of anticholinergics:** 2 mg IV or IM. Give IV administration no more than 1 mg/minute. Repeat dosage if life-threatening signs occur (arrhythmias, convulsions, coma).
Children: **For life-threatening occurrences only:** 0.02 mg/kg by IM or slow IV injection. Maximum dose is 2 mg.
Post anesthesia: 0.5 to 1 mg IM or slow IV administration. May repeat at 10- to 30-minute intervals if the desired response is not achieved.

NEUROMUSCULAR BLOCKING AGENTS

Mechanism of Action and Indications for Use

Neuromuscular blocking agents have the ability to combine with, and thus occupy, the cholinergic N_M receptors but do not trigger muscle contraction (i.e., they have affinity for these receptors but lack efficacy). By this action, muscle immobility (paralysis) ensues. Because these agents occupy the receptors of the motor endplate, ACh binding to these receptors is blocked (Fig. 14.5)

Appropriate doses of these agents produce a rapid onset of motor weakness

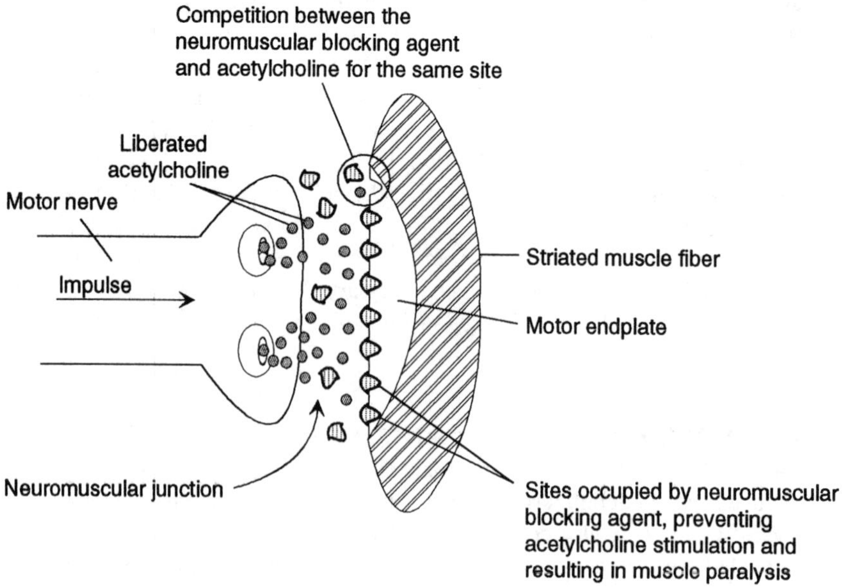

Figure 14.5. Competitive inhibition by nondepolarizing neuromuscular blocking agents.

progressing to total flaccid paralysis. Muscles capable of rapid movement, such as the muscles of the jaws, fingers, and eyes, are affected before those of the limbs, neck, and trunk. Ultimately, paralysis moves to the intercostal muscles and, finally, to the diaphragm, and respiration ceases. Recovery of these muscles from paralysis occurs in the reverse order, such that the diaphragm is ordinarily the first to regain function.

Neuromuscular blocking agents consist of two classes: nondepolarizing agents and depolarizing agents. Nondepolarizing agents are antagonists that actually compete with the agonist, ACh, for the receptors of the motor endplate; thus, they are known as competitive inhibitors (depicted in Fig. 14.5). These agents are called *nondepolarizing* because when they occupy the receptors of the motor endplate, they prevent it from depolarizing. Many of these agents are also called curariform, or curare-like, because their mode of action resembles the poison curare. Older nondepolarizing agents (those that are curare-like) are nonselective in their ability to antagonize cholinergic nicotinic receptors; thus, the autonomic ganglionic (N_N) receptors are also blocked from stimulation.

Owing to their competitive nature, the nondepolarizing agents form reversible bonds with the nicotinic receptors; thus, their effect can be reversed by having more ACh available in the neuromuscular junction for receptor competition, bonding, and subsequent stimulation. The cholinergic muscle stimulants (e.g., edrophonium, neostigmine, physostigmine; see previous section) are especially useful in increasing the duration of action of ACh in the neuromuscular junction through their interaction with AChE. By this mechanism, more ACh is made available to compete with the nondepolarizing agents for occupation of the available receptors of the motor endplate. Effective reversal of the nondepolarizing agent's skeletal muscle blockade, resulting in the return of normal muscle contraction, occurs when there is a sufficient quantity of ACh present in the neuromuscular junction for receptor bonding and stimulation. Anesthesiologists sometimes employ this method of using cholinergic muscle stimulants upon completion of surgery to reverse and decrease the duration of action of nondepolarizing agents. Additionally, an antimuscarinic agent (such as atropine) is coadministered to negate the stimulation of muscarinic receptors that results from ACh accumulation at these specific receptors.

Depolarizing neuromuscular blocking agents are called such because these agents initially instigate motor endplate depolarization, thus causing total body muscle contraction when they combine with the cholinergic N_M receptors. In this respect, depolarizing agents mimic the actions of ACh and act as ACh would if it were present in excessive amounts. In fact, these agents bear a structural resemblance to ACh. Succinylcholine, the prototypic depolarizing agent, is actually two ACh molecules linked end-to-end (Fig. 14.6).

A noticeable feature of depolarizing agents is the transient muscular fascicu-

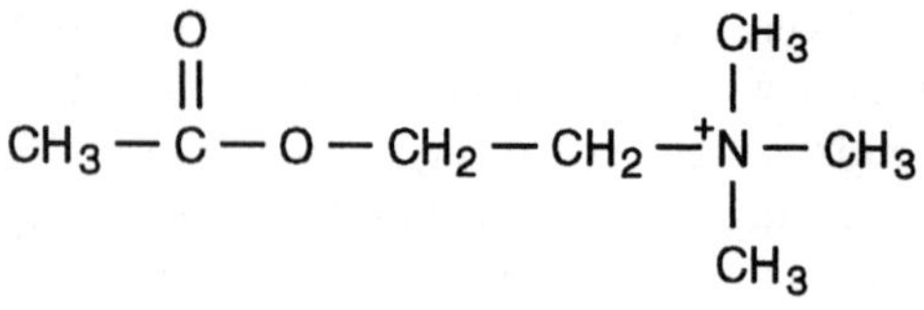

$$CH_3-\overset{\overset{O}{\|}}{C}-O-CH_2-CH_2-\overset{\overset{CH_3}{|}}{\underset{\underset{CH_3}{|}}{N^+}}-CH_3$$

Acetylcholine

$$CH_2-\overset{\overset{O}{\|}}{C}-O-CH_2-CH_2-\overset{\overset{CH_3}{|}}{\underset{\underset{CH_3}{|}}{N^+}}-CH_3$$
$$|$$
$$CH_2-\overset{\overset{O}{\|}}{C}-O-CH_2-CH_2-\overset{\overset{CH_3}{|}}{\underset{\underset{CH_3}{|}}{N^+}}-CH_3$$

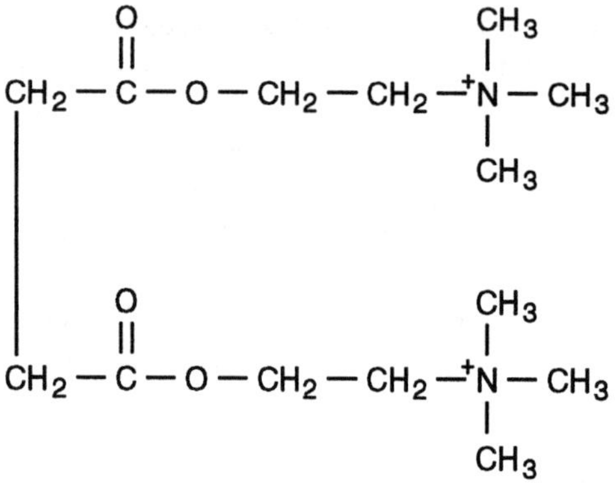

Succinylcholine

Figure 14.6. Structural relationship between acetylcholine and succinylcholine. Succinylcholine, originally called diacetylcholine, is simply two molecules of acetylcholine linked through the acetate methyl groups.

lations or skeletal muscle tremors ("twitching," especially noted over the chest and abdomen unless the patient is anesthetized) that result from initial stimulation of the motor endplate. The initial stimulation is soon followed by muscle paralysis. A blockade is produced in which any further stimulation to the muscle is prevented until the depolarizing agent's bonding to the receptor is terminated. Only when the effect wears off or is hydrolyzed by pseudocholinesterase (butyrylcholinesterase, a plasma and liver cholinesterase) is the muscle allowed to return to its normal state of activities. An interesting aspect of these drugs is that with increasing concentrations or prolonged administration, the neuromuscular block converts slowly from a depolarizing to a nondepolarizing type, termed *phase-I* and *phase-II* block.

Cholinergic muscle stimulants are not effective antidotes, or reversal agents, for the effects produced by depolarizing neuromuscular blocking agents. These agents have a synergistic activity when coadministered with depolarizing agents and may potentiate the blockade. This is because depolarizing agents not only act as ACh does, but they also illicit a type of neuromuscular blockade in which the motor endplate is nonresponsive to further stimulation. This condition is similar to ACh overdose, in which the motor endplate becomes desensitized to repetitive stimulation resulting in further muscle weakness. Therefore, allowing the accumulation of ACh in the neuromuscular junction, which is the ultimate action of cholinergic muscle stimulants, would not be beneficial. In addition, because depolarizing agents are rapidly hydrolyzed by pseudocholinesterase and thus have a relatively short duration of action (approximately 5 to 10 minutes), it is generally not practicable to employ means for reversal. However, neuromuscular blockade by succinylcholine may be prolonged for patients with an abnormal variant of plasma pseudocholinesterase (due to genetic disturbances, hepatic disease, or nutritional disturbances) or patients who have a deficiency of the enzyme. Clinically, this produces prolonged paralysis and apnea that may last for several hours, instead of minutes. In cases such as these, a nondepolarizing agent may be needed to counteract the depolarizing agent's effect.

Neuromuscular blocking agents are indicated for use as an adjunct to anesthesia to induce skeletal muscle relaxation during surgery, during endotracheal intubation, and as an aid in the prevention of laryngospasm. These agents are also used as an aid to electroshock therapy to prevent fractures and to reduce the severity of convulsions, as an aid to decrease muscle spasms during seizures and tetanus, and as an aid to diagnose myasthenia gravis (only tubocurarine, and when the results of tests with cholinergic muscle stimulants prove inconclusive). Nondepolarizing agents are also indicated for use to facilitate prolonged mechanical ventilation among patients who otherwise would be difficult to ventilate.

The total pharmacological properties of neuromuscular blocking agents vary with respect to each agent. However, one feature that is classic to these agents is their lack of CNS effects. This is primarily due to the inability of tubocurarine (curare) and other quaternary neuromuscular blocking agents to penetrate the blood-brain barrier. The debate on whether these agents possess significant CNS effects was put to rest by Smith (an anesthesiologist) who, in 1947, permitted himself to receive intravenously two and one-half times the normal dose of tubocurarine. Adequate artificial ventilation was maintained throughout the test time of the procedure. Smith reported that at no time was there any lapse of consciousness, clouding of sensorium, analgesia, or any kind of disturbance of the special senses. Smith also reported that, despite adequate ventilation, he felt shortness of breath and a sensation of choking, which was caused by the accumulation of unswallowed saliva in the back of the throat. Smith relayed that the sensation was decidedly unpleasant. By this account, paralytic agents are not central stimulants, depressants, or analgesics: patients still feel pain and are alert when under the influence of these agents, unless an analgesic or sedative has been coadministered.

Neuromuscular blocking agents vary in their potencies to produce ganglionic blockade at the cholinergic N_N receptors as well as inhibiting the cholinergic N_N receptors of the adrenal medulla. The clinical result of ganglionic blockade is a drop in blood pressure and a rise in the heart rate (tachycardia). As previously stated, nondepolarizing agents that are curare-like (tubocurarine, metocurine) have a tendency to illicit such effects owing to their nonselective stimulation of both types of cholinergic nicotinic (N_N and N_M) receptors. Newer agents, such as pancuronium, atracurium, and especially vecuronium, at normal doses do not produce ganglionic blockade. Gallamine and pancuronium have a tendency to selectively block the vagus nerve at cardiac postganglionic muscarinic sites, which may result in sinus tachycardia, cardiac arrhythmias, and hypertension. Of the depolarizing agents, succinylcholine at normal clinical doses rarely causes effects attributable to ganglionic blockade. This is primarily due to the fact that depolarizing agents initially stimulate, not inhibit, cholinergic nicotinic receptors. Thus, depolarizing agents have a tendency to manifest bradycardia (from stimulating the parasympathetic ganglionic receptors) or hypertension (from stimulating the sympathetic ganglionic receptors).

Some of these agents, especially tubocurarine, cause the release of histamine from storage sites. The clinical picture associated with histamine release is bronchospasm, hypotension, and excessive bronchial and salivary secretions. Additionally, rapid intravenous injection of some of these agents may produce a severe enough fall in blood pressure to be life-threatening. This effect results from a dual interaction between the peripheral vasodilation caused by histamine release and sympathetic ganglionic blockade.

The overall untoward responses of these agents include prolonged apnea, cardiovascular collapse, and those resulting from histamine release. Because the neuromuscular blocking agents are potentially hazardous drugs, they should only be administered by anesthesiologists and practitioners who have been trained in their use and in a setting in which respiratory and cardiovascular resuscitation are immediately available.

Contraindications

The neuromuscular agents that have iodide or bromide are contraindicated for patients sensitive to these compounds. Additionally, agents that release histamine should not be given to patients with asthma. Use with extreme caution, if at all, for patients with myasthenia gravis.

Relative contraindications to succinylcholine use include patients with severe burns, tetanus, spinal cord injuries, or multiple trauma, because severe ventricular arrhythmias or cardiac arrest may occur due to the increase in plasma potassium levels (hyperkalemia) following depolarization of the sensitized denervated muscle.

Precautions

1. Respiratory depression and apnea may follow the use of these drugs. Endotracheal intubation with assisted respirations should be immediately available.
2. These drugs have no effect on pain threshold or consciousness. Use only with adequate anesthesia.
3. Use with caution for patients with myasthenia gravis and patients with cardiovascular, renal, hepatic, pulmonary, or endocrine dysfunction owing to prolonged muscle weakness and hypotension.
4. Use with extreme caution for patients in which histamine release is a known hazard.
5. Have antidotes readily available (neostigmine, edrophonium, pyridostigmine for reversal of nondepolarizing agents). Atropine should be administered before the anticholinesterase to counteract the action on muscarinic receptors that results from anticholinesterase administration.
6. The effects of succinylcholine may be potentiated with the administration of anticholinesterase drugs such as neostigmine or pyridostigmine.

Adverse Reactions

Most Frequent: Sustained pharmacologic action of the drug.

Cardiovascular: Bradycardia, tachycardia, blood pressure changes, cardiac arrest, arrhythmias.

Pulmonary: Respiratory depression, apnea, bronchoconstriction (with histamine release).

GI: Excessive salivation.

Overdosage

Administering greater than normal doses of neuromuscular blocking agents may lead to sustained apnea, cardiovascular collapse, prolonged muscle weakness, and/or release of histamine. Treatment consists of ventilatory support and the administration of an anticholinesterase such as neostigmine, pyridostigmine, or edrophonium (only effective for antagonizing the effects of nondepolarizing blocking agents). Atropine should be administered before the anticholinesterase to counteract the action on muscarinic receptors that results from anticholinesterase administration.

Dosage and Administration

The pharmacologic profile of these agents are summarized in Table 14.1. Preparations and dosages are listed in Table 14.2.

Table 14.1.
Pharmacologic Activity of the Neuromuscular Blocking Agents

Drug	Onset of Action (minutes)	Duration of Action (minutes)[a]	Potency	Effect on Autonomic Ganglia	Effect on Cardiac Muscarinic Receptors	Tendency to Release Histamine[c]
Nondepolarizing Agents:						
Atracurium	3–5	20–40	2	None	None	Mild
Doxacurium	4–5	30–60	7	None	None	None
Gallamine	1–2	30–60	0.2	None	Strong block	None
Metocurine	1–2	25–90	2	Mild block	None	Mild
Mivacurium	2–4	10–20	4	None	None	Mild
Pancuronium	1–2	20–60	5	None	Moderate block	Rare
Pipecuronium	3–5	20–60	5	None	None	None
Rocuronium	1–2	20–35	0.8	None	None	Rare
Tubocurarine	1–2	25–90	1	Mild to moderate block	None	Moderate
Vecuronium	2–3	20–35	6	None	None	Rare
Depolarizing Agents:						
Succinylcholine	approx 1	5–10	N/A[d]	Stimulates	Stimulates	Mild

[a]Spontaneous recovery from the neuromuscular blockade is dose-dependent; the higher the dose, the longer the recovery time. Recovery may be considerably longer than the time noted above and is highly dose-dependent and variable in individuals.
[b]Potency relative to tubocurarine.
[c]Histamine release is related to the dose administered and the speed of injection (i.e., higher doses and rapid injections are more likely to cause the release of histamine).
[d]Not applicable to the potency of tubocurarine. Succinylcholine works by a different mechanism (it is a depolarizing agent).

Table 14.2.
Preparations and Dosages of the Neuromuscular Blocking Agents

Drug	Preparations	Dosage
Nondepolarizing Agents:		
Atracurium besylate (Tracrium)	***IV solution:*** 10 mg/ml in 5- and 10-ml vials	*Adults and children > 2 years:* 0.4 to 0.5 mg/kg initial dose by IV bolus. Maintenance dose, 0.08 to 0.1 mg/kg given within 20 to 45 minutes after initial dose, then every 12 to 25 minutes, as required. *Children <2 years old;* 0.3 to 0.4 mg/kg
Doxacurium chloride (Nuromax)	***IV solution:*** 1 mg/ml in 5-ml vials	*Adults:* Highly individualized dose, 0.05 mg/kg initial dose. Maintenance dose, 0.005 and 0.01 mg/kg given approximately 100 minutes after initial dose, then every 30 to 45 minutes, as required. *Children >2 years:* 0.03 to 0.05 mg/kg
Gallamine triethiodide (Flaxedil)	***IV solution:*** 20 mg/ml in 10-ml vials	*Adults and children >1 month:* initially, 1 mg/kg to maximum of 100 mg. Maintenance dose, 0.5 to 1 mg/kg given 30 to 40 minutes after initial dose, then every 30 to 40 minutes, as required *Children:* Infants up to 1 month: initially 1 mg/kg. Maintenance dose: 0.5 mg/kg. *Note:* A precipitate will form if gallamine is mixed with anesthetic gases. Do not administer solution with a visible precipitate. The presence of respiratory acidosis diminishes the blocking effects of gallamine, and alkalosis enhances the blocking action of gallamine.
Metocurine iodide (Metubine iodide, generic)	***IV solution:*** 2 mg/ml in 20-ml vials	*Adults:* Initially 0.2 to 0.4 mg/kg for endotracheal intubation. Supplemental doses average 0.5 to 1 mg. For electroshock therapy: 1.75 to 5.5 mg (average dose 2 to 3 mg). *Note:* When used with succinylcholine, an additive effect is noted. Do not mix metocurine with alkaline solutions (barbiturates), for a precipitate may occur.
Mivacurium chloride (Mivacron)	***IV solution:*** 2 mg/ml in 5-ml and 10-ml vials ***Infusion:*** 0.5 mg/ml in 50 ml dextrose 5% in water (D_5W)	*Adults:* Initially, 0.15 mg/kg IV push over 5 to 15 seconds. Maintenance dose, 0.1 mg/kg given 15 minutes after initial dose, then every 15 minutes, as required. *For continuous infusion:* 4 μg/kg/minute begun simultaneously with the initial dose, or 9 to 10 μg/kg/minute started after spontaneous recovery from initial dose.
Pancuronium bromide (Pavulon)	***IV solution:*** 1 mg/ml in 2-, 5- and 10-ml vials. 2 mg/ml in 2- and 5-ml vials, syringes	*Adults and children:* Initially, 0.04 to 0.1 mg/kg. Maintenance dose, 0.01 mg/kg q 30 to 60 minutes. *For endotracheal intubation:* 0.06 to 0.1 mg/kg IV bolus. (Maximum neuromuscular blocking action occurs in 2 to 3 minutes).
Pipecuronium bromide (Arduan)	***Powder for injection:*** 10 mg/ml in 10-ml vials	*Adults:* initially, 70 to 85 μg/kg. Maintenance dose, 10 to 15 μg/kg every 50 minutes

Table 14.2.—*continued*

Drug	Preparations	Dosage
Rocuronium bromide (Zemuron)	***Injection:*** 10 mg/ml in 5-ml vials	*Adults:* initially, 0.6 to 1.2 mg/kg. Maintenance dose, 0.1 to 0.2 mg/kg q 30 minutes *For continuous infusion:* initial rate is 0.01 to 0.012 mg/kg/minute only after evidence of spontaneous recovery occurs *Children:* initially, 0.6 mg/kg. Maintenance dose, 0.075 to 0.125 mg/kg every 10 minutes
Tubocurarine chloride (Generic)	***IV solution:*** 3 mg (20 units)/ml in 10- and 20-ml vials and 5-ml syringes	*Adults and children:* Initially, 0.2 to 0.5 mg/kg; then 0.04 to 0.1 mg/kg (average initial dose, 40 to 60 units). *For endotracheal intubation:* 0.5 to 0.6 mg/kg. *For electroshock therapy:* 1.1 units/kg given slowly over 60 to 90 seconds (initial dose is 20 units (3 mg) less than calculated dose). *For diagnosis of myasthenia gravis:* Very small doses produce an intense exaggeration of this syndrome (usually 1/15 to 1/5 of the electroshock therapy dose). The test is usually terminated within 2 to 3 minutes with the administration of neostigmine. Precaution: carefully monitor patient. *Note:* Respiratory acidosis and hypokalemia enhance the neuromuscular blocking effect and respiratory alkalosis diminishes the blocking action.
Vecuronium bromide (Norcuron)	***IV solution:*** 10-mg powder in 5-and 10-ml vials with diluent	*Adults:* Individualized dose: 0.08 to 0.1 mg/kg as IV bolus. Maintenance dose: 0.01 to 0.015 mg/kg 25 to 40 minutes after the initial dose. Thereafter, given in 12- to 15-minute intervals as required. *Children 10 to 17 years of age:* Same as adult dose *Children 1 to 10 years of age:* May require a slightly higher dose and more frequent supplementation than adults. Not recommended in neonates
Depolarizing Agents:		
Succinylcholine chloride (Anectine, Sucostrin, Quelicin)	***IV, IM solution:*** 20 mg/ml in 10-ml vials. 50 mg/ml in 10-ml amps. 100 mg/ml in 10-ml vials. ***Powder for injection:*** 100 mg powder in 5-ml vial with diluent. ***Powder for infusion:*** 500 mg or 1 g per vial	*Adults:* ***IV:*** initially 0.3 to 1.1 mg/kg (average dose is 25 to 75 mg), then 0.04 to 0.07 mg/kg at appropriate intervals to maintain required degree of relaxation. ***IM:*** up to 2.5 mg/kg; not to exceed 150 mg total dose *For continuous infusion:* 2.5 to 4.3 mg/minute *Children:* ***IV:*** 2 mg/kg for infants and younger children. 1 mg/kg for older children. ***IM:*** 3 to 4 mg/kg; not to exceed 150 mg per dose *Note:* Succinylcholine is not generally used to facilitate mechanical ventilation due to its very short duration of action (rapidly hydrolyzed by pseudocholinesterase).

REFERENCES/RECOMMENDED READING

Agoston S, et al. Clinical pharmacokinetics of neuromuscular blocking drugs. Clin Pharmacokinet 22:94, 1992.
Aquilonius S-M, Hartvig P. Clinical pharmacology of cholinesterase inhibitors. Clin Pharmacokinet 11:236, 1986.
Bevan DR, et al. Reversal of neuromuscular blockade. Anesthesiology 77:785, 1992.
Donati F, Smith CE, Bevan DR. Dose-response relationships for edrophonium and neostigmine as antagonists of moderate and profound atracurium blockade. Anesth Analg 68:13, 1989.
Drug Facts and Comparisons. 49th ed. St. Louis: Facts and Comparisons, 1995.
Engel WK. Myasthenia gravis: corticosteroids and anticholinesterases. Ann N Y Acad Sci 274:623, 1976.
Ertama PM. Histamine liberation in surgical patients following administration of neuromuscular blocking drugs. Ann Clin Res 14:27, 1982.
Fambrough DM, Drachman DB, Satyamurti S. Neuromuscular junction in myasthenia gravis: decreased acetylcholine receptors. Science 182:293, 1973.
Katz B, Thesleff S. A study of desensitization produced by acetylcholine at the motor endplate. J Physiol (Lond) 138:63, 1957.
Miller RD, Savarese JJ. Pharmacology of muscle relaxants and their antagonists. In: Miller RD, ed. Anesthesia, 4th ed. New York: Churchill Livingstone, 1994.
Nilsson E. Physostigmine treatment in various drug-induced intoxication. Ann Clin Res 14:165, 1982.
Physicians' Desk Reference. 49th ed. Montvale, NJ: Medical Economics, 1995.
Smith SM, et al. The lack of cerebral effects of d-tubocurarine. Anesthesiology 8:1, 1947.
Tortora GJ, Anagnostakus NP. Principles of anatomy and physiology. New York: Harper & Row, 1990.

Central Nervous System/Ventilatory Stimulants and Depressants 15

Drugs acting on the central nervous system (CNS) have been used since the days of primitive man to relieve a variety of disorders and are still the most widely used pharmacologic agents. Agents in this group include prescription as well as nonprescription drugs. Socially acceptable stimulants and mild depressants, such as caffeine, alcohol, nicotine, and sleep aids, are widely used in many countries. These agents have a tendency to illicit a sense of well-being, pleasure, relaxation, or comfort to the user. Because some of these drugs are addictive and may cause severe emotional disturbances, dysfunction, or disease when used in excess, many societies have found it necessary to control their use and availability.

The unique quality of drugs acting on the CNS make them therapeutically useful and practical in relieving pain, fever, and insomnia as well as in suppressing seizures, preventing disorders of movement, and reducing the desire to eat or the tendency to vomit. Without general anesthetics, modern surgery would be impossible, and without analgesics, some postsurgical patients would experience tremendous pain. CNS agents are also therapeutically useful in treating or controlling anxiety attacks, mania, depression, and schizophrenia.

In addition to their CNS effects, some of the above-mentioned agents stimulate or depress the ventilatory drive, especially when used in excess. Thus, drugs that exert CNS effects are a special consideration to cardiopulmonary practitioners who interact closely with patients and their ability to breathe.

This chapter focuses on agents that either stimulate or depress CNS and/or ventilatory function. Owing to the many groups of drugs presented in this chapter, the following topics will be presented in sections:

SECTION I: CNS/Ventilatory Stimulants
SECTION II: Opioid Agonists and Antagonists

SECTION III: Nonopioid Analgesics
SECTION IV: Sedative-Hypnotic Agents
SECTION V: Anesthetic Agents
SECTION VI: Psychotherapeutic Agents
SECTION VII: Anticonvulsant Agents

As a basis for understanding the actions of the drugs described in this chapter, an introduction to the functional organization of the CNS and its synaptic transmitters precedes the presentation of the drugs.

THE CENTRAL NERVOUS SYSTEM—AN OVERVIEW

Divisions and Functions of the Spinal Cord

The CNS is composed of two subsystems: the brain and the spinal cord. The spinal cord is an elongated mass of nervous tissue (Fig. 15.1) with primary functions to serve as a center for spinal reflexes and to relay information from all body areas to the brain and then conduct the messages from the brain to all body areas. In its function to serve as a conduction pathway, the spinal cord makes use of ascending tracts to conduct impulses to the brain and descending tracts that conduct impulses from the brain to various levels of the spinal cord.

The spinal cord is covered and protected by three layers or membranes known as meninges. The dura mater is the outermost membrane; the arachnoid membrane lies directly under the dura; and the innermost layer of the meninges, called the pia matter, closely lines the spinal cord. The subarachnoid space, existing between the arachnoid and the pia mater, is filled with spinal fluid or, more accurately, cerebrospinal fluid, because this liquid is also found in the cranial subarachnoid spaces. Inflammation of the meninges is termed meningitis. It may involve any one or more of the meninges and may be caused by the invasion of a variety of infectious organisms such as the tubercle bacillus, meningococcus, streptococcus, or staphylococcus (see Chapter 16).

The spinal cord consists of 31 pairs of spinal nerves. Each nerve is numbered according to its segmental location. As shown in Figure 15.1, there are eight pairs of cervical nerves, 12 pairs of thoracic nerves, five pairs of lumbar nerves, five pair of sacral nerves, and one pair of coccygeal nerves. Each spinal nerve innervates the spinal cord with a *sensory* root (dorsal root; contains afferent nerve fibers that conduct nerve impulses from the periphery *to* the spinal cord, and thus to the brain) and a *motor* root (ventral root; contains efferent nerve fibers that serve to conduct impulses *away* from the spinal cord and to the periphery). As sensory and motor roots reach their point of origin (intervertebral foramen; corresponds to their spinal cord segment of origin), they combine to form a spinal nerve. Thus, all spinal nerves are mixed nerves, containing both sensory (input) and motor (output) fibers.

The distribution of the spinal nerves is such that the first four cervical nerves

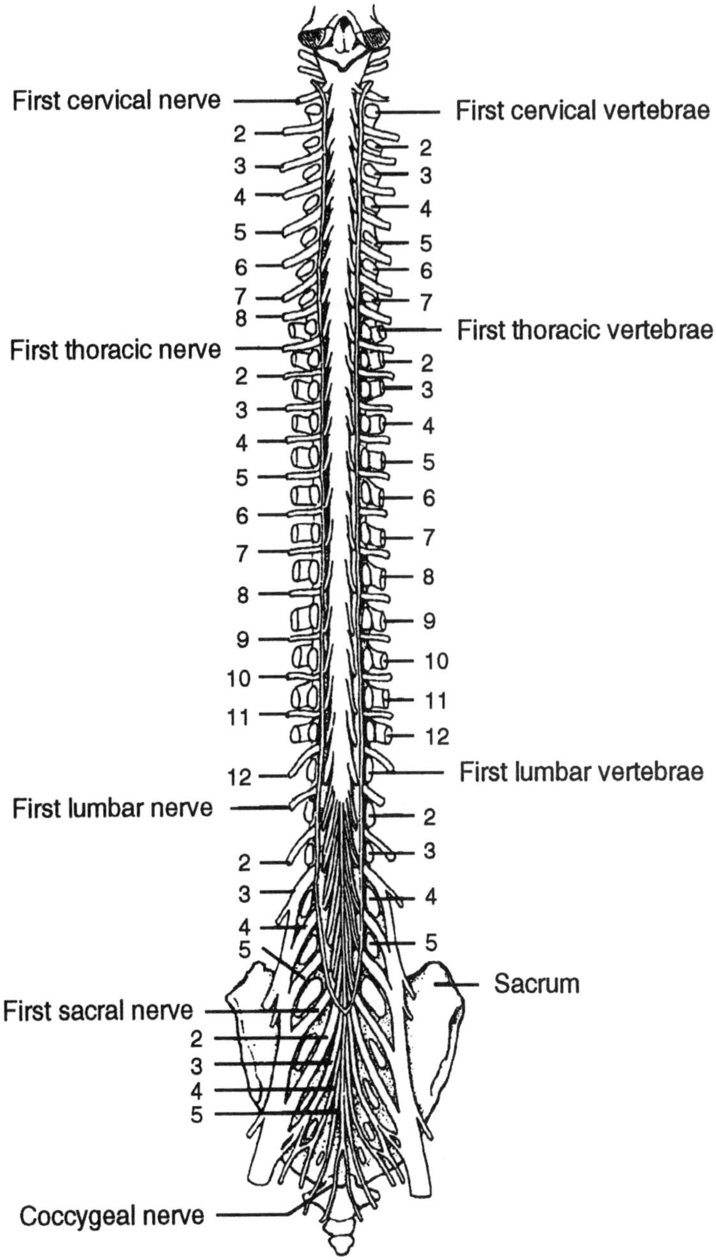

Figure 15.1. The spinal cord. Spinal nerves are numbered on the left; vertebrae on the right.

form the cervical plexus that lies deep in the neck on each side. Branches from this segment are distributed to the muscles and skin of the neck as well as the posterior part of the scalp. The phrenic nerve is considered the most important branch of this plexus because it innervates the diaphragm. Damage to this nerve, or crushing of the spinal cord above the level of the phrenic nerve, results in respiratory paralysis as the brain can no longer reach the phrenic nerves; the diaphragm ceases to function, resulting in respiratory failure.

The last four cervical and first thoracic spinal nerves form the brachial plexus, which supplies many of the neck and shoulder muscles as well as the muscles of the arms. Damage to these nerves will result in paralysis of the neck, shoulders, or arms. The 12 thoracic spinal nerves, with the exception of the first, are known as intercostal nerves because they run through the intercostal spaces in the thorax as well as to the muscles of the abdominal wall and overlying skin.

The first four lumbar spinal nerves form the lumbar plexus, which supplies motor and sensory fibers to the lower abdominal wall, the external genitalia, and part of the lower extremity. The largest branch of this plexus is the femoral nerve. The fourth and fifth lumbar nerves and the first three sacral spinal nerves form the sacral plexus. Branches of these nerves supply the muscles in the buttocks, perineum, and lower extremities. The main branch of this plexus is the sciatic nerve, which is the largest and longest nerve in the body. Sciatica is a type of neuritis (inflammation of a nerve) that is characterized by sharp, shooting pains along the course of the sciatic nerve. The second, third, and fourth sacral spinal nerves contribute to the pudendal plexus, which branches to supply the levator ani muscle, the skin, and other structures of the perineum. At times, this nerve may be blocked by drugs to facilitate childbirth.

The thoracic and upper lumbar spinal nerves also give rise to the visceral efferent branches or preganglionic autonomic nerve fibers of the sympathetic system, as discussed in Chapter 2 (see Fig. 2.5). The second through fourth sacral nerves of the spinal cord, as well as cranial nerves III, VII, IX, and X, form the parasympathetic branch.

The spinal nerves also serve as important reflex centers. Examples of spinal reflexes are the stretch reflexes (e.g., knee jerk) and the flexor reflexes (e.g., pulling your body away from a harmful object). Testing of various reflexes is an extremely important part of a physical examination because if they are normal, the reflex center in the CNS, the efferent fibers, and the muscles are all functioning normally.

Fractures, dislocations of vertebrae, or other trauma such as bullet wounds or crushing injuries may result in a complete transection or severing of the spinal cord. In such cases, the skeletal muscles distal to the level of injury will be paralyzed, and all feeling to the supplied muscles will be lost because the descending and ascending pathways have been interrupted. If the transection originates below the fifth cervical segment, the patient will continue to breathe because the phrenic nerves to the diaphragm have not been damaged. However, paralysis below this point is complete, even to the point of losing spinal reflexes.

Divisions and Functions of the Brain

The brain consists of three primary divisions: the forebrain, the midbrain, and the hindbrain (Fig. 15.2). The forebrain is composed of two major subdivisions: the cerebrum and the diencephalon. An external layer of gray matter, the cerebral cortex, covers the cerebrum. The cerebral cortex consists of 10 to 14 billion neurons and is responsible for regulating bodily functions and activities such as skeletal muscle movement, hearing, speech, vision, memory, learning, and discrimination of pain, temperature, and touch. The functions and activities listed above may be profoundly affected by drugs that exert their influence on cortical activity.

The diencephalon of the forebrain contains the thalamus and the hypothalamus (see Fig. 15.3). The hypothalamus regulates visceral activities innervated by both

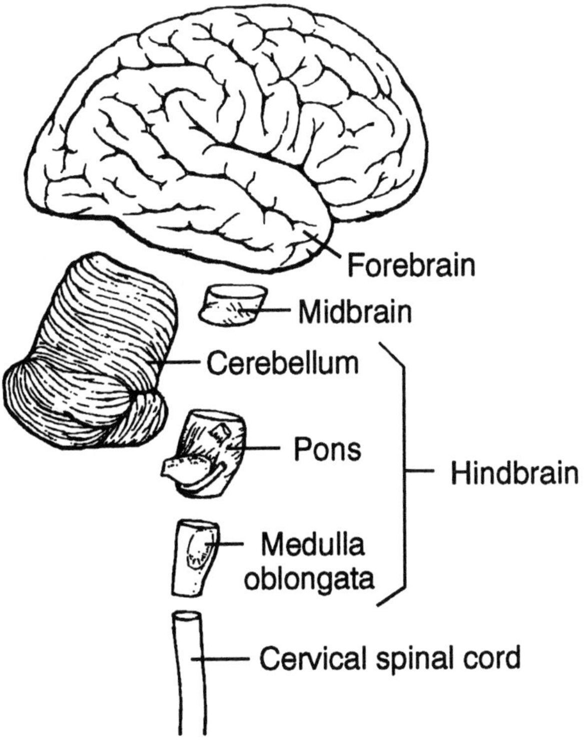

Figure 15.2. The primary divisions of the brain. Various parts of the brain have been separated to show detail.

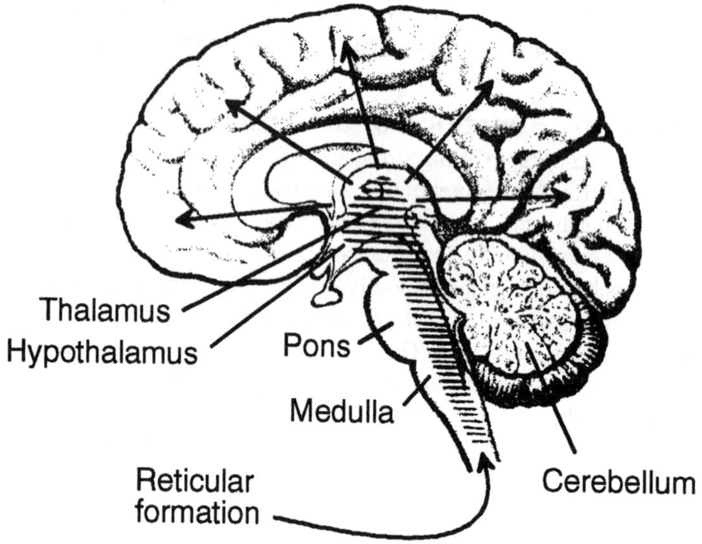

Figure 15.3. Diagram of the reticular formation, radiating from the brain stem to the cortical regions.

the sympathetic and parasympathetic divisions of the autonomic nervous system (see Chapter 2, *Autonomic Control by Higher Centers*). The hypothalamus is also the primary regulating center for endocrine gland secretion, body temperature, sleeping-waking mechanisms, behavior and emotional responses, and arterial blood pressure. It contains an extensive network of neurons that connect not only with the autonomic centers but with the thalamus and the cerebral cortex.

The hypothalamus is considered the most important component of the limbic system as far as behavior and emotions are concerned. The limbic system is a heterogeneous mixture of several brain structures at or near the edge (limbus) of the medial wall of the cerebral hemisphere. It also includes the interconnections of these structures as well as their connections with the hypothalamus. The limbic system influences the endocrine and autonomic motor systems and is a motivational and mood modulator. It is activated by motivated behavior and arousal such as divergent emotions and basic drives of extreme anxiety, fear, anger, aggression, rage, hunger, pleasure, and sex. The overall effect of these mood states is that the hypothalamic action systems are aroused and the body's defensive forces are called into action; this is especially noted in stressful situations in which the hypothalamic response is to release CRH to ultimately elevate cortisol levels (see Chapter 12, *The Hypothalamic-Pituitary-Adrenal Transport System*). Many antipsychotic and antianxiety drugs have the ability to suppress the limbic system and thus put the brain in a "tranquil" or subdued state.

The thalamus, which composes the bulk of the diencephalon, is an important relay center for impulse conduction from all body parts to the cerebral cortex. It functions to sort incoming sensory messages from the periphery and then relay these messages to the cerebral cortex. The activities of the thalamus are partly controlled by the state of consciousness and crude awareness. Drugs that stimulate or depress the activities of the thalamus alter the relay of impulse transmission to the cerebral cortex.

The midbrain, pons, and medulla oblongata (and the cerebellum because it is attached to the pons and medulla) collectively form the lower portion of the brain, commonly referred to as the brain stem. The midbrain serves as a conduction pathway to higher brain centers and also as a reflex center for visual, auditory, postural, and righting reflexes. These reflexes are concerned with constricting the pupil of the eye in response to bright light (visual reflex), turning the head to hear sounds that originate at one side of the body (auditory reflex), positioning the head in relation to the trunk and with adjustment of the extremities and eyes to the position of the head (postural reflex), and orientation of the head in relation to space (men and animals like to keep their heads up—righting reflex).

The hindbrain consists of the cerebellum, the pons, and the medulla oblongata. The pons (meaning "bridge") is located between the midbrain and the medulla and, like the midbrain, the pons serves as a conduction pathway to the higher brain centers. The pons contains the sensory and motor neurons of cranial nerves V (trigeminal), VI (abducens), VII (facial), and VIII (acoustic). The lower portion of the pons contains neurons that assist in the regulation of respiration and is known as the secondary respiratory coordinating center, with the medulla as the primary respiratory coordinating center.

There are two primary collections of neurons in the pons that assist the medullary respiratory center: the apneustic center and the pneumotaxic center (Fig. 15.4). The primary function of these two centers is to smoothly coordinate the changeover from inspiration to expiration and vice versa. Thus, these centers are responsible for the regularity of respiratory rhythm. As shown in Figure 15.4, the apneustic center stimulates the inspiratory neurons of the medullary respiratory center, causing inspiration. The pneumotaxic center, after stimulation from the medullary inspiratory center, acts on the expiratory center in the medulla and, at the same time, inhibits the apneustic center, thus allowing expiration to occur. Any trauma to these centers of the pons, or surgical removal of the pons, results in an apneustic type of breathing pattern in which there is a sustained inspiratory effort.

The medulla oblongata, in addition to being a conduction pathway, also contains the body's vital centers such as the cardiac center (regulates the rate of the heart beat), the vasomotor center (constricts or dilates blood vessels), and the respiratory center (regulates rate and depth of breathing). Drugs that affect the medulla may profoundly alter any one or more of these vital centers. The medulla

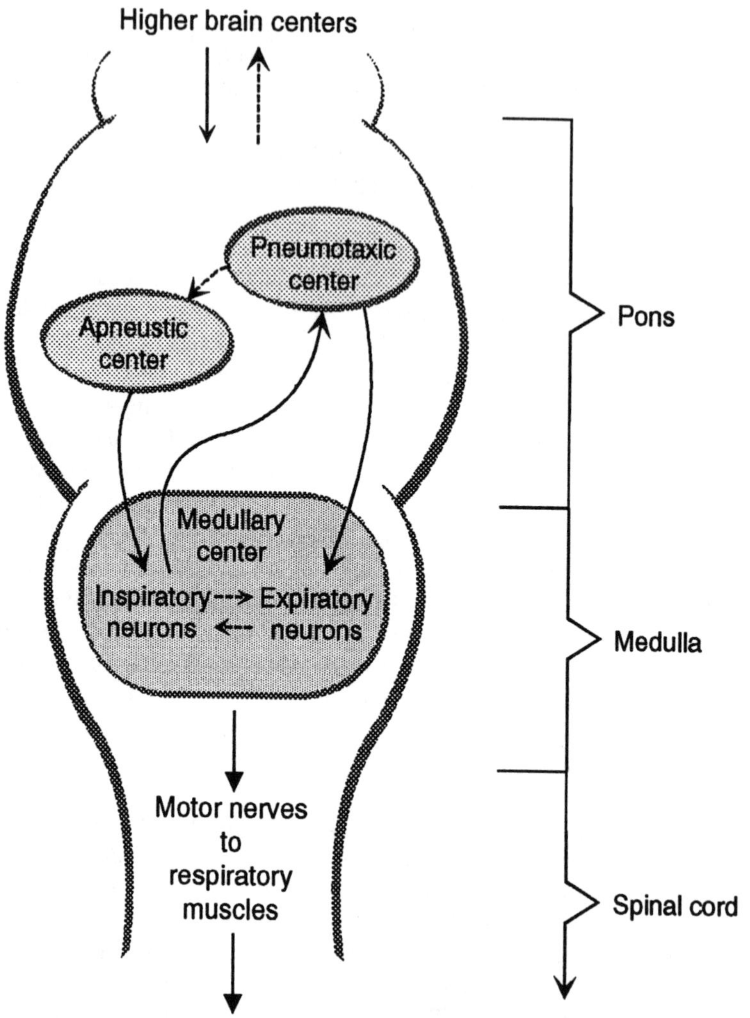

Figure 15.4. Conceptual representation of the interactions between the primary centers of the medulla and the secondary coordinating centers in the pons. Stimulation is represented by solid arrows (——→), and inhibition is represented by dashed arrows (– – →). See text for details.

contains the sensory and motor neurons of cranial nerves IX (glossopharyngeal), X (vagus), XI (accessory), and XII (hypoglossal).

Located on or near the ventral surface of the medulla are highly specialized receptors called central chemoreceptors. These receptors, when stimulated into action by chemical changes in their liquid environment, dispatch afferent nerve impulses to the respiratory center of the medulla. The overall result of this stimulation is that one begins to breathe rapidly and deeply. The central chemoreceptors activate in response to elevated hydrogen ion (low pH) and carbon dioxide content of the cerebrospinal fluid. As the excess carbon dioxide is blown off and the pH returns to a more normal level, the central chemoreceptors turn off their stimulus to the respiratory center and breathing returns to normal.

The central chemoreceptors do not activate in chronic hypercapnic states in which there is a normalized pH. Thus, the only stimulus to breathe comes from the peripheral chemoreceptors located in the arch of the aorta and in the carotid bodies. These chemoreceptors are more sensitive to a decrease in the amount of oxygen dissolved in the plasma (PaO_2) than they are to an excess of carbon dioxide and hydrogen ions. Thus, whenever the PaO_2 becomes too low (hypoxemia), these chemoreceptors excite the medullary respiratory center into action (see also Chapter 8, *Hazards of Oxygen Therapy*).

The cerebellum ("little brain") is attached to the brain stem (midbrain, pons, medulla oblongata) and the spinal cord by three paired bundles of nerve fibers, the cerebellar peduncles. The cerebellum serves primarily to coordinate involuntary muscular activity and muscle tone.

Located throughout the brain stem, extending from the medulla to the lower portion of the thalamus, are nuclei that run in various directions. These nuclei compose the reticular formation (Fig. 15.3). The upper portion of the formation and its pathway to the thalamus and the cerebral cortex are denoted as the reticular activating system (RAS). Stimulation of this system by afferent input from various pathways or the external environment results in the activation of the cerebral cortex, producing a state of alertness and attention. The RAS also acts to filter repetitive, extraneous sensory input, such as the droning of a fan or reading this chapter with the radio or television on. By this mechanism, the RAS prevents sensory overload and allows one to concentrate on the task at hand. However, when an unexpected noise occurs, such as the ringing of the telephone, the RAS will immediately alert one to the change in environment. The RAS also acts as a mediator in modulating the rate and depth of ventilation in response to various incoming stimuli. Lesions or damage in the area of the RAS result in a decreased level of consciousness (coma) due to the corresponding lack of input to the cerebral cortex. Additionally, drugs that depress (sedate, such as the sedatives and hypnotics) or those that stimulate (enhance consciousness, alertness) act in part, or totally, by altering the functional capability of the RAS.

The extrapyramidal system, which consists of descending fibers arising from cortical and subcortical motor centers, is responsible for coordinating balance and fine skeletal muscle movement. Some of the psychotherapeutic drugs (e.g., antipsychotic agents) frequently cause extrapyramidal reactions that may lead to immobility (akinesia), fixed positioning of the limbs (rigidity), sudden violent movement of the arms and head (dystonia), restlessness (akathisia), and rhythmic, clonic muscular activity (tremors).

Central Neurotransmission and Neurotransmitters

In most cases, impulse transmission between CNS neurons is chemically mediated at synapses. The events involved in the release of CNS neurotransmitters are similar to those described in Chapter 2 (see Fig. 2.2). Two types of neuronal pathways have been described for CNS neurons: excitatory and inhibitory (Fig. 15.5). All neuronal pathways in the CNS cause the release of neurotransmitters in response to incoming impulses. However, inhibitory neuronal pathways have a two-part mechanism of action: excitation and inhibition. This is because the axon of an inhibitory neuron synapses with the axon terminal of an excitatory neuron. When stimulated, the inhibitory neuron will release its neurotransmitter substance (excitatory action), which will then inhibit (inhibitory action) the release of the excitatory neuron's neurotransmitter substance. As shown in Figure 15.5, the inhibitory neuron, upon activation, will abort impulse transmission in the excitatory neuron.

Virtually all drugs that affect the CNS produce their action by modifying some aspect of chemical synaptic transmission (see Fig. 2.18). The selectivity of drug action is based almost entirely on the fact that different neurotransmitters are used by different groups of CNS neurons. A number of neurotransmitters have been localized to the brain and are listed in Table 15.1. Some of the agonists and antagonists listed in Table 15.1 are still in the experimental phase and are not in clinical use at this time.

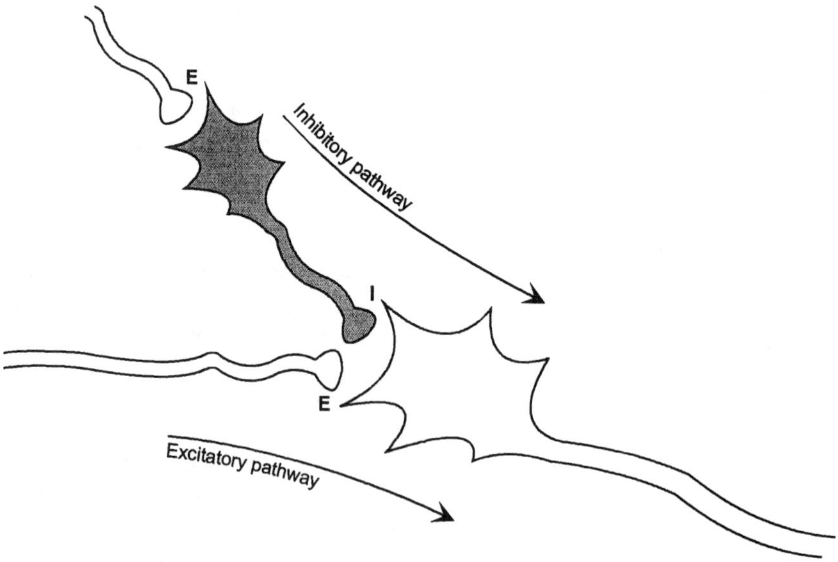

Figure 15.5. Inhibitory and excitatory pathways in the central nervous system. The inhibitory pathway is responsible for blocking impulse transmission of an excitatory neuron. I = inhibition; E = excitation.

Table 15.1.
Nonpeptide Neurotransmitters in the Central Nervous System

Transmitter	Location	Receptor Subtypes and Agonist	Antagonists	Receptor Mechanism
Acetylcholine	Cell bodies at all levels: probable long and short connections	Muscarinic (M_1): muscarine	Pirenzepine, atropine	Excitatory
		Muscarinic (M_2): muscarine, bethanechol	Atropine	Inhibitory
	Motoneuron-Renshaw cell*	Nicotinic: nicotine	Dihydro-β-erythroidine	Excitatory
Dopamine	Cell bodies at all levels: short, medium, and long connections	Dopaminergic (D_1): SKF 38393	Phenothiazines, SCH 23390	Inhibitory; increases cAMP
		Dopaminergic (D_2): apomorphine, quinpirole	Phenothiazines, butyrophenones	Inhibitory; decreases cAMP
Epinephrine	Midbrain and brain stem to diencephalon	Probably the same as for norepinephrine (see below)	Probably the same as for norepinephrine (see below)	Probably the same as for norepinephrine (see below)
GABA	Supraspinal interneurons; spinal interneurons involved in presynaptic inhibition	$GABA_A$: muscimol	Bicuculline, picrotoxin	Inhibitory
		$GABA_B$: baclofen	CGP 35348, 2-OH saclofen	Inhibitory
Glutamate; aspartate	Interneurons; relay neurons at all levels	Quisqualate, AMPA	CNQX	Excitatory
		N-Me-D-aspartate (NMDA)	CPP	Excitatory
		Kainate	Lactonized kainate	Excitatory
Glycine	Spinal interneurons and some brain stem interneurons	Taurine, β-alanine	Strychnine	Inhibitory
Histamine	Posterior hypothalamus	H_1: histamine	Mepyramine	?
		H_2: 2-Thiazolylethylamine	Cimetidine	Activates adenyl cyclase
		H_3: ?	Thioperamide	?
Norepinephrine	All levels; long axons from pons and brainstem	α_1: phenylephrine	Prazosin	Excitatory
		α_2: clonidine	Yohimbine	Inhibitory
		β_1: dobutamine, isoproterenol	Atenolol, practolol	Excitatory
		β_2: terbutaline, albuterol	Butoxamine	Inhibitory
Serotonin (5-Hydroxytryptamine)	Midbrain and pons to all levels	5 HT_{1A}: LSD, 8-OH-DPAT	Metergoline, spiperone	Inhibitory
		5-HT_{2A}: LSD, DOB	Ketanserin	Excitatory
		5-HT_3: 2-methyl-5-HT, phenylbiguanide	ICS 205930, ondansetron	Excitatory
		5-HT_4: BIMU8	GR 1138089	Excitatory

*Small cells with short axons that serve to connect motor nerve axons with each other.

AMPA, DL-α-3-hydroxy-5-methylisoxazole-4-propionate; BIMU8, (endo-*N*-8-methyl-8-azabicyclo[3,2,1]oct-3-yl)-2,3-dihydro-3-isopropl-2-oxo-1*H*-benzimidazol-1-carboxamide hydrochloride; CGP 35348, 3-aminopropyl (diethoxymethyl)phosphoric acid; CNQX, 6-cyano-7-nitroquinoxaline-2,3-dione; CPP, 3-(2-carboxypiperazin-4-yl)propyl-1-phosphoric acid; DOB, 5-brom-2,5-dimethoxyamphetamine; GABA, gamma-aminobutyric acid; GR 113808, [1-[2-](methylsulfonyl)amino]ethyl]-4-piperidinyl]methyl-1-methyl-1*H*-indole-3-carboxylate; 8-OH DPAT, 8-hydroxy-2(di-*n*-propylamino)tetralin.

Adapted from Gilman AG, Goodman LS, Rall TW, Murad F. Goodman and Gilman's The Pharmacological Basis of Therapeutics. 8th ed. New York: McGraw Hill, Inc., 1993; and Katzung BG. Basic and Clinical Pharmacology. 6th ed. Norwalk: Appleton & Lange, 1995.

I
CNS/Ventilatory Stimulants

The most commonly used centrally acting stimulants are a class of drugs known as analeptics. Broadly defined, analeptic agents are drugs that stimulate the CNS. Important sites of action of these agents include the reticular activating system, vital respiratory centers in the medulla, and carotid chemoreceptors. Analeptic agents have two primary beneficial effects: they promote generalized arousal, and they increase the rate and depth of ventilation.

A great many drugs can act as analeptics and stimulate the CNS; however, only a select handful are therapeutically useful or safe. This is because CNS stimulants have a tendency to enhance reflex excitability (especially in higher than normal doses), which can lead to convulsions. Some drugs that were previously used as analeptic agents (e.g., pentylenetetrazol, picrotoxin, nikethamide) are no longer widely used owing to their narrow margin of safety between the stimulating dose and the convulsant dose. These analeptics are primarily used as tools for basic research on convulsions and neurotransmission. Strychnine is an analeptic agent of toxicologic interest only. Amphetamines, anorexiants, and nonprescription diet aids also have CNS stimulant effects; however, these agents have no therapeutic usefulness as ventilatory stimulants. Currently, drugs that are in clinical use as CNS/ventilatory stimulants include doxapram, caffeine, theophylline, medroxyprogesterone, almitrine, and protriptyline.

General uses of these agents as CNS/ventilatory stimulants include:

- Reversal of drug-induced CNS/ventilatory depression from drug overdose.
- Stimulation of respiration in patients experiencing drug-induced postanesthesia respiratory depression or apnea.
- Chronic pulmonary disease associated with acute hypercapnia.
- Assistance with weaning patients from mechanical ventilation.
- Management of obstructive sleep apnea (OSA). This disorder is characterized by episodic periods of apnea occurring during sleep. Such occurrences are usually due to airway obstruction caused by the gradual loss of normal skeletal muscle tone, including upper airway structures and respiratory muscles of ventilation. During the apneic period, rapid hypercapnia and hypoxia ensue, which then wake the patient. The continual cycles of apnea followed by waking during the hours of sleep result in a somnolent or drowsy individual during normal waking hours. Over time, as a compensatory mechanism, the patient will develop polycythemia from the transient hypoxia that occurs during sleep (see Fig. 8.3). Eventually, the patient may exhibit cor pulmonale (right heart failure), pulmonary hypertension, and edema.

  Obstructive sleep apnea typically occurs in obese individuals, whose upper airways have a tendency to collapse during sleep. Collectively, the manifestations of obesity-somnolence-hypoventilation-polycythemia are known as

Pickwickian syndrome. This name originates from the fat boy who exhibited these same symptoms in Charles Dicken's *The Pickwick Papers*.

- Treatment of apnea of prematurity. Apneic episodes lasting more than 15 seconds and accompanied by bradycardia are sometimes frequent occurrences in preterm infants. In some cases, neonatal apnea is a result of a severe systemic illness, whereas in other cases, there is not a clearly defined cause. The repetitive episodes of apnea lead to hypoxia and possibly neurological damage.

The following section details the drugs currently in use for their CNS/ventilatory stimulant abilities.

DOXAPRAM HYDROCHLORIDE: DOPRAM, STIMULEXIN

Mechanism of Action and Indications for Use

Doxapram is a powerful respiratory stimulant that elicits widespread CNS activation. In particular, doxapram enhances the rate and depth of respiration by directly activating the medullary respiratory center as well as indirectly stimulating the aortic and carotid peripheral chemoreceptors. The degree of stimulation is directly dose related, and the duration of stimulation is seldom more than 5 or 10 minutes.

Doxapram is indicated for use to stimulate respiration for postanesthetic patients, for patients being weaned from mechanical ventilation, for drug-induced CNS depression, and for patients with chronic obstructive pulmonary disease (COPD) associated with acute hypercapnia. Doxapram has also been used in patients with OSA.

Low-dose doxapram has also been used in neonatal apnea refractory to xanthine therapy. Doxapram has been shown to be therapeutically effective in some cases of neonatal apnea in eliminating the apneic episodes or by significantly reducing the number of episodes to a shorter duration and/or making them less frequent. The use of doxapram in the treatment of neonatal apnea is currently investigational in the USA.

Contraindications

Contraindications to the use of doxapram hydrochloride include hypersensitivity to doxapram, epilepsy, convulsive states, severe hypertension, cerebrovascular accidents, head injury, respiratory insufficiency due to pneumothorax, flail chest, pulmonary embolism, airway obstruction, dyspnea, asthma, and pulmonary fibrosis. Preparations that contain benzyl alcohol are contraindicated for use in newborns.

Precautions

1. Administer cautiously with sympathomimetic amines or monoamine oxidase inhibitors; additive pressor effects may result.

2. Postanesthetic precaution: doxapram is neither an antagonist to neuromuscular relaxant drugs nor a narcotic antagonist. Ensure patent airway and oxygenation before use.
3. Safety and efficacy for use in children have not been established.
4. Use with extreme caution for patients with COPD because of possible arrhythmias secondary to hypoxia. Additionally, because doxapram increases the work of breathing, there is a concomitant increase in myocardial oxygen consumption, which may further worsen hypoxia.
5. Use seizure precautions after the administration of these drugs.

Adverse Reactions

CNS: Convulsions, headache, apprehension, dizziness, hyperactivity.

Pulmonary: Cough, dyspnea, tachypnea, laryngospasm, bronchospasm, rebound hypoventilation.

Cardiovascular: Arrhythmias, abnormal ECG, chest pain, flushing, tightness in chest.

GI: Nausea, vomiting, diarrhea.

GU: Urinary retention, spontaneous voiding, proteinuria.

Overdosage

Overdose symptoms include respiratory alkalosis and hypocapnia with tetany and apnea. Excessive CNS stimulation may result in convulsions. Treatment consists of supportive care. There is no specific antidote for overdosage of doxapram; however, intravenous (IV) barbiturates, oxygen, and resuscitative equipment should be readily available and used when indicated.

Dosage and Administration

Doxapram is available in 20 mg/ml IV injection form and has a duration of activity of 3 to 4 minutes.

For postanesthetic use: Doxapram is given as a single intravenous bolus of 0.5 to 1 mg/kg, as divided doses given at 5-minute intervals. Do not exceed 1.5 mg/kg as a single injection or 2 mg/kg total when given as multiple injections at 5-minute intervals.

For COPD associated with acute hypercapnia: Infusion is initiated at 1 to 2 mg/min (0.5 to 1 ml/min). May increase to a maximum of 3 mg/min, if necessary. Arterial blood gas analysis before administration and at least every 30 minutes during the 2-hour infusion is highly recommended to ensure the adequacy of ventilation.

For apnea of preterm infants: Treatment is initiated by the continuous infusion of 0.5 mg/kg per hour. The dose is increased at intervals of 24 to 48 hours until it reaches 2 mg/kg per hour or until the frequency of apneic periods is reduced to two per 6 hours or less.

CAFFEINE, THEOPHYLLINE

Mechanism of Action and Indications for Use

As previously stated in Chapter 10 (see Table 10.4), theophylline is not only a potent bronchodilator but is also a CNS stimulant. Both theophylline and caffeine are xanthines that can significantly enhance the central ventilatory drive resulting in an increased rate and depth of ventilation. This action seems to be related to the ability of these drugs to produce an increased responsiveness of the medullary respiratory centers to increasing carbon dioxide levels and hypoxia. The resultant increase in ventilatory rate and depth corresponds linearly at any given value of alveolar PCO_2. Additionally, an added benefit of these agents is that, at therapeutic concentrations, both theophylline and caffeine improve and strengthen diaphragmatic contractility, thus reducing respiratory muscle fatigue and the sensation of dyspnea. Proposed mechanisms for this action include the possible role of xanthines in the mobilization of intracellular Ca^{2+} or an improved neuromuscular transmission.

As ventilatory stimulants, theophylline and caffeine have therapeutic usefulness in the management of apnea of prematurity, in weaning of infants from mechanical ventilation, and in improving pulmonary function and dyspnea in patients with COPD.

Contraindications

Contraindications to theophylline and caffeine include hypersensitivity to any xanthine, peptic ulcer, and underlying seizure disorders. Do not use combinations of caffeine that contain sodium benzoate for neonates. (See Chapter 10, *Xanthine Bronchodilators*.)

Precautions

1. Aggressive treatment with parenteral caffeine may illicit a further depressed state in the already depressed patient. Do not exceed 1 gram as a single dose.
2. Higher blood glucose levels may occur as a result of caffeine use.
3. Although therapeutic and toxic blood levels vary among patients, caffeine has a relatively wider margin of safety and a longer half-life than theophylline. In premature infants, the average half-life of caffeine is more than 50 hours, whereas the mean values for theophylline range between 20 and 36 hours. These features should be considered when administering these agents, especially for neonates.
4. Large quantities of these agents may reactivate duodenal ulcers owing to their

ability to induce gastric acid secretion. (See Chapter 10, *Xanthine Bronchodilators*.)

Adverse Reactions

Most Common: Nausea, vomiting. As the dose of either theophylline or caffeine is increased, signs of progressive CNS stimulation occur. These include nervousness, anxiety, restlessness, insomnia, tremors, and hyperesthesia. Use of these agents, as with any analeptic, may lead to convulsions. (See also Chapter 10, *Xanthine Bronchodilators*.)

Overdosage

Early symptoms of overdose are manifest by the adverse reactions listed above. Severe toxicity may result in focal and generalized convulsions. Such seizures may be refractory to anticonvulsant therapy. The short-term lethal dose of caffeine appears to be 5 to 10 grams; however, toxic signs may be observed after the ingestion of 1 gram.

Dosage and Administration

Caffeine: **Formulations:** Tablets: 100, 150, 200 mg. Injection: 250 mg/ml in 2-ml ampules (equal parts caffeine and sodium benzoate).

Adults: **PO:** 100 to 200 mg every 3 to 4 h, as needed. **IV, IM:** 500 mg (250 mg caffeine) IM, or slow IV injection in emergency respiratory failure. A maximum single dose of 1 gram (500 mg caffeine) may be administered; however, the usual and maximum safe dose is 500 mg. Total dose administered in 24 hours should not exceed 2.5 g.

For neonatal apnea: Initial dose of 10 mg/kg caffeine followed by a maintenance dose of 2.5 mg/kg/dose. Adjust maintenance dose according to serum concentrations.

Theophylline: **Preparations:** see Chapter 10, *Xanthine Bronchodilators*.

For patients with COPD: 10 mg/kg/day.

For neonatal apnea and bradycardia of prematurity: Initial dose of 5 to 6 mg/kg followed by a maintenance dose of 1 mg/kg/dose. Adjust maintenance dose according to serum concentrations.

MEDROXYPROGESTERONE ACETATE (MPA): AMEN, CURRETAB, DEPO-PROVERA, PROVERA

Mechanism of Action and Indications for Use

MPA is an oral progesterone that has the ability to stimulate alveolar ventilation and enhance the ventilatory response to hypercapnia and hypoxia. MPA's mechanism of action is similar to that of the xanthines in that MPA increases the sensitivity of the medullary respiratory centers to respond to hypercapnia and hypoxia. MPA is essentially useful in stimulating respirations in patients with OSA (see above).

Adverse Reactions

Most Common: Nervousness, insomnia, dizziness, depression, nausea, headache, breast tenderness, menstrual irregularities. Prolonged therapy may cause impotency in males.

Dosage and Administration

MPA: 20 mg three times daily sublingual.

ALMITRINE DIMESYLATE: VECTARION

Almitrine is an analeptic agent currently available only in Europe that is used to improve ventilation and oxygenation in patients with COPD. Almitrine's mechanism of action is similar to that of doxapram in that it also stimulates carotid body chemoreceptors. Almitrine has distinct advantages over doxapram: it is effective orally and has a prolonged duration of activity. Adverse effects include headache, diarrhea, abdominal pain, fatigue, peripheral sensory neuropathy, and in some patients, a worsening of dyspnea. Almitrine's dosage in patients with COPD ranges between 50 and 100 mg b.i.d.

PROTRIPTYLINE HYDROCHLORIDE: VIVACTIL

Protriptyline is a tricyclic antidepressant (TCA) currently undergoing investigation as an agent for the management of obstructive sleep apnea. Technically, protriptyline is not an analeptic agent or ventilatory stimulant; however, it does exhibit properties that make it therapeutically useful in reducing apneic episodes in patients with severe, unmanageable OSA. Protriptyline, like other TCAs, decreases the total time spent in rapid-eye-movement (REM) sleep (see *Psychotherapeutic Drugs* presented later in this chapter). REM sleep is highly associated with the loss of upper airway muscle tone and the onset of apnea in patients with OSA. Thus, by suppressing REM sleep, protriptyline reduces the frequency of the obstructive apneic periods occurring during sleep. For complete prescribing information, see *Psychotherapeutic Drugs* presented later in this chapter.

II
Opioid Agonists and Antagonists

Opium is obtained from the seed pod of the opium poppy (*Papaver somniferum*) and contains more than 20 distinct alkaloids. In 1806, the principal alkaloid from opium was isolated and named morphine, after Morpheus, the Greek god of dreams. Other alkaloids derived from opium include codeine, thebaine, and papaverine.

The alkaloids found in opium and their related semisynthetic derivatives are collectively known as opiates, whereas the synthetics and naturally occurring (endogenous) morphine-like compounds are referred to as opioids. The word opioid has also been coined to refer to antagonists of morphine-like drugs (see next section) and to the receptors that are specific to morphine and its related class of drugs.

Three distinct classes of naturally occurring (endogenous) opioids have been identified: the enkephalins, the endorphins, and the dynorphins. There are five types of opioid receptors with which these endogenous opioid peptides have specificity to. These receptors are designated as mu (μ), kappa (κ), delta (δ), sigma (σ), and epsilon (ϵ) receptors. Some types of opioid receptors may even have subtypes, just as are found in several other systems (e.g., adrenergic and cholinergic systems).

Mu receptors are named after morphine owing to morphine's high affinity to this type of receptor. The endorphins ("endogenous morphine") interact primarily with this receptor type. Analgesia at the supraspinal level, euphoria, respiratory depression, and physical dependency are properties of the mu receptor. The kappa receptor, named after ketocyclazocine, is involved with spinal analgesia, diuresis, and thermoregulation; dynorphin seems to be the endogenous opioid for this receptor. The enkephalins have primary affinity to the delta receptor. Delta receptors produce effects very similar to the mu receptors. The sigma receptor seems to be related to the dysphoric, hallucinogenic, and cardiac stimulant effects of opioids. The epsilon receptor, not clearly defined as yet, seems to illicit an opioid type of euphoria when stimulated.

Of the five opioid receptor types described above, only three have been isolated and cloned: mu, kappa, and delta. These three primary receptors are the major action sites for the opioid analgesics. All three receptor types are widely distributed throughout the CNS and all three seem to function by exerting inhibitory modulation of synaptic transmission in the CNS, resulting in reduced transmitter release. The depressed transmitter release has been demonstrated for many types of neurotransmitters, including norepinephrine, dopamine, acetylcholine, and serotonin. Although not clearly defined or understood as yet, these receptors seem to be coupled to the regulatory G proteins introduced in Chapter 2. Thus, it can be anticipated that receptor stimulation leads to inhibition of adenyl cyclase and changes in Ca^{2+} and K^+ flux.

The opioids are classified into three major categories according to their activities at the opioid receptors: 1) agonists, 2) mixed agonist-antagonists, and 3) antagonists.

The opioid agonists include morphine and all of the drugs that exhibit morphine-like effects. These agents have both affinity and efficacy for the opioid receptors, thus mimicking the actions of the endogenous opioids. The mixed agonist-antagonists have affinity and efficacy at some opioid receptors but antagonistic activity at others. The antagonists have affinity for opioid receptors but do not activate them.

OPIOID AGONISTS AND MIXED AGONIST-ANTAGONISTS

Mechanism of Action and Indications for Use

Opioid agonists are sometimes referred to as "narcotics." Derived from the Greek word for "stupor," narcotics, in a pharmacological context, are drugs that depress the CNS and produce a state of stupor or sleep. In a legal context, narcotics are any drugs that can cause dependence. "Narcotics" is a term that can also refer to a group of individuals who are addicted to narcotic agents.

As previously stated, a number of alkaloids are present in opium. Alkaloids of opium that are important for their analgesic activity include morphine, codeine, and thebaine. Although thebaine is not clinically in use because it evokes strychnine-like convulsions, it is the precursor of many semisynthetic opiate agonists (e.g., etorphine) and antagonists (e.g., naloxone). Morphine, the oldest narcotic analgesic, is the standard by which all other opioid analgesics are compared. Codeine is synthesized commercially from morphine. Many semisynthetic derivatives are made by modifying the morphine molecule. Such derivatives include apomorphine (a potent emetic and dopaminergic agonist), heroin, hydromorphone, oxymorphone, hydrocodone, and oxycodone. Synthetic compounds include methadone, meperidine, fentanyl, alfentanil, sufentanil, levorphanol, and propoxyphene. The therapeutic usefulness of one agent over another reflects the degree of potency relative to morphine and its duration of activity.

Morphine and related μ-, δ-, and κ-receptor agonists produce their primary effects on the CNS and bowel. The effects of opioid receptor stimulation are quite diverse. Some of the more important CNS effects include:

- **Analgesia.** Opioid agonists effectively suppress the cortical processes that would interpret the afferent signal as pain. Thus, the threshold for pain is elevated, making the pain less intense and all-consuming. For this reason, the opioid agonists are more commonly referred to as opioid or narcotic analgesics.
- **Euphoria.** Typically, after administration of opioid agonists, a patient in pain or an addict experiences a pleasant, floating sensation. Also, relief of distress and anxiety often accompany opioid administration. However, normal subjects or patients not in pain often experience dysphoria, a disquieted state associated with restlessness and a feeling of malaise.
- **Sedation.** Drowsiness, mental confusion, and impairment of reasoning ability are frequent occurrences of opioid administration, especially when administered in larger than normal doses. The combination of opioid agonists with

other central depressant drugs, such as the sedative-hypnotic agents, may produce profound sedation or depression of the CNS. Marked sedation often occurs more frequently with the alkaloids of opium, such as morphine, than with the synthetic compounds.

- **Ventilatory depression.** All of the opioids can produce significant ventilatory depression by inhibiting the activity of the medullary respiratory center. The most important aspect of ventilatory depression is the suppressed response by the central chemoreceptors to increasing levels of carbon dioxide. Carbon dioxide retention is responsible for the cerebral vasodilation and increased intracranial pressure that accompanies the administration of these agents, in particular, after the administration of morphine. At toxic doses, sensitivity to oxygen may also decrease. The ventilatory depression accompanying the use of opioids is primarily dose-related.
- **Cough suppression.** A well recognized fact of opioid administration, especially codeine, is the ability to suppress the central cough reflex. (See Chapter 9, *Cough and Cold Preparations.*)
- **Miosis.** Morphine and most μ and κ opioid agonists cause constriction of the pupils. This effect is often valuable in diagnosing opioid overdose.
- **Nausea and vomiting.** Morphine-like drugs cause unpleasant side effects such as nausea and vomiting that are caused by the stimulation of the chemoreceptor trigger zone (CTZ) for emesis. The CTZ is located in the area of the medulla. Most often, this effect occurs in ambulatory patients.

Other bodily systems that are affected by the use of opioid agonists include the cardiovascular system, the gastrointestinal tract, and the genitourinary tract. In the supine patient, opioids usually have no effect on blood pressure or cardiac rate or rhythm. However, therapeutic doses of these agents do produce peripheral vasodilation and reduce peripheral resistance. In effect, when the supine patient sits or stands up, orthostatic hypotension and fainting may occur. Histamine release, which occurs with morphine and some other opioids, may also play a role in producing hypotension.

Morphine and morphine-like compounds usually suppress the secretion of hydrochloric acid in the stomach, although stimulation sometimes occurs. In addition, relatively low doses of these agents, especially morphine, decrease gastric motility. By this mechanism, gastric emptying is delayed, sometimes as much as 12 hours, prolonging the absorption of orally administered drugs. Constipation may also occur.

Renal function is suppressed by the use of opioid agonists. This effect is believed to be due to the decrease in renal plasma flow that accompanies the use of these agents. The net effect is a reduced urinary output by the kidneys. Miscellaneous effects of opioid agonists include flushing and warming of the skin accompanied by sweating and itching. Various central effects as well as histamine release may be responsible. Owing to histamine release by some of these agents, patients with asthma may experience bronchospasm.

Opioid agonists are clinically indicated:

- To relieve moderate to severe pain.
- As a preoperative medication because of their sedative, anxiolytic, and analgesic properties.
- As an adjunct during anesthesia.
- For management and sedation of intubated patients.
- In the treatment of patients with acute pulmonary edema due to left ventricular failure. Morphine is especially useful for patients with acute pulmonary edema due to left ventricular failure. Morphine relieves the dyspnea and anxiety that accompany acute pulmonary edema as well as causes a reduction in cardiac preload (reduces venous return to the right heart) and afterload (decreased peripheral resistance) that is associated with left ventricular failure.
- For detoxification and maintenance of the chronic relapsing heroin addict. Methadone, in particular, is the agent of choice for detoxification of a heroin addict. Its relatively long-acting, slower withdrawal signs and symptoms, and lower tolerance and physical dependency properties make it a useful drug in detoxifying heroin addicts.
- Some of these agents are also used for their antitussive effects (see Chapter 9) and their antidiarrheal effects.

The mixed agonist-antagonists include pentazocine, dezocine, nalbuphine, buprenorphine, and butorphanol. Pentazocine, the oldest of the mixed agonist-antagonists, is a primary kappa agonist with weak mu-receptor properties. Dezocine has a high affinity for mu receptors, with less affinity for kappa receptors. Nalbuphine is a strong kappa receptor agonist but a mu receptor antagonist. Buprenorphine is a potent and long-acting mu receptor agonist. Its long-acting ability is reflected by its slow dissociation from the mu receptor. However, this feature makes naloxone (see below) ineffective as a reversal agent for buprenorphine overdose. Butorphanol is a kappa agonist that produces analgesia similar to that produced by nalbuphine and buprenorphine. However, butorphanol exhibits a higher degree of sedation than either of the above-mentioned agents.

The mixed agonist-antagonists produce analgesia in addition to sedation when given in therapeutic doses. Severe ventilatory depression is less common with these agents than with pure agonists. If ventilatory depression does occur, it may be effectively reversed by the use of naloxone (see below) but not by other agonist-antagonists, such as nalorphine. Hallucinations, nightmares, and anxiety have been reported after use of these agents. When given higher than normal doses, patients may experience sweating, dizziness, and nausea.

Contraindications

Contraindications to the use of opioid agonists and mixed agonist-antagonists include hypersensitivity to opium or its derivatives, diarrhea caused by poisoning, acute bronchial asthma, upper airway obstruction, and acute hypercapnia. Contraindications to morphine (epidural or intrathecal) include infection at the injection site, patients on anticoagulant therapy. Contraindications to levorphanol include acute alcoholism and increased intracranial pressure. Contraindications to meperidine include use of monoamine oxidase inhibitors (MAO).

Precautions

1. With repeated use, tolerance, psychological dependence, and physical dependence may occur.
2. Use with extreme caution for patients with head injury and patients with increased intracranial pressure. Along with the respiratory depressant effects, these agents have the ability to increase intracranial pressure owing to the elevated carbon dioxide levels associated with opioid use.
3. Use with extreme caution for patients with asthma and patients with other pulmonary disease owing to the agent's ability to severely diminish respiratory drive, increase airway resistance, and suppress the cough mechanism.
4. Use with caution in elderly individuals, debilitated patients, and children.
5. Do not use concurrently with alcohol or other CNS depressants.

Adverse Reactions

Major Hazards: Respiratory depression, apnea, circulatory depression, respiratory arrest, shock, cardiac arrest.

Most Frequent: Lightheadedness, dizziness, sedation, nausea, vomiting, sweating.

CNS: Euphoria, dysphoria, delirium, insomnia, agitation, anxiety, fear, hallucinations, disorientation, lethargy, coma, mood changes, headache, tremor, convulsions.

Cardiovascular: Tachycardia, bradycardia, hypotension, hypertension, palpitations, arrhythmias, syncope, peripheral circulatory collapse, facial flushing.

Pulmonary: Respiratory depression, apnea, respiratory arrest, bronchospasm.

GI: Dry mouth, anorexia, constipation.

Overdosage

Symptoms of severe overdosage occurring by IV injection include apnea, circulatory collapse, convulsions, cardiopulmonary arrest, and death. Complications of overdose include hypotension, bradycardia, hypothermia, pulmonary edema, pneumonia, and shock. Treatment consists of maintaining an adequate airway with intubation and assisted respiration if necessary. Naloxone (Narcan, a narcotic antagonist; see below) is the preferred drug for reversal of opioid overdose symptoms.

Dosage and Administration

The pharmacologic activity, dosage, and administration of the opioid analgesics are listed in Table 15.2.

OPIOID ANTAGONISTS

Mechanism of Action and Indications for Use

Opioid antagonists reverse opioid-induced CNS and ventilatory depression by competitively binding to the opioid receptor sites. The pure opioid antagonists, naloxone and naltrexone, are morphine derivatives with a relatively high affinity for μ-receptors. These antagonists of opioid receptors can completely and dramatically reverse CNS and ventilatory depression caused by morphine and morphine-like compounds within 5 minutes after administration. Naloxone, in the absence of narcotics, does not produce any pharmacologic activity, except for a slight drowsiness. Therefore, naloxone is not effective in reversing CNS/ventilatory depression caused by nonnarcotic drugs, barbiturates, or anesthetics. Naloxone has been shown to be therapeutically useful for reversing alcoholic coma and dementia of the Alzheimer type, as well as in the treatment of schizophrenia.

Naltrexone, because of its long duration of activity, is primarily in clinical use as a maintenance drug for narcotic addicts in a rehabilitation program. A single dose will effectively block all of the effects of a dose of heroin. Recent studies indicate that naltrexone may also be clinically useful in decreasing the craving for alcohol in chronic alcoholics (Volpicelli 1992).

Contraindications

Contraindications to the use of opioid antagonists include hypersensitivity to these drugs. Contraindications to naltrexone include acute liver disease, hepatitis, or use of opioid analgesics.

Precautions

1. Maintain supportive therapy such as a patent airway and assisted respirations when indicated.
2. Administer with caution for patients who are known to be physically dependent on narcotic drugs, including newborns and mothers with narcotic dependence.
3. Safety and efficacy for children have not been established.

Table 15.2.
The Opioid Analgesics

Opioid	Dosage (mg)[a] IV	IM	PO	Onset (minutes)[b]	Peak (hours)[b]	Duration (hours)[b]	Pharmacologic Properties[c]
Opioid angonists:							
Morphine sulfate (Astramorph PF, Duramorph, Infumorph 200, MSIR, MS Contin, Roxanol SR, Oramorph SR, RMS)	4–15 (diluted in 4 to 5 ml water)	4–15	30–60	15–60 (epidural)	0.5–1 (epidural)	3–7 (epidural)	1++, 2+++, 3++, 4++, 5++
Codeine	NA	15–60	15–60	10–30	0.5–1	4–6	1+, 2+++, 3+, 4+, 5+
Hydromorphone hydrochloride (Dilaudid)	2–4	2–4	1–6	15–30	0.5–1	4–5	1++, 2+++, 3++, 4+, 5++
Levorphanol tartrate (Levo-Dromoran)	2–3	NA	2–3	30–90	0.5–1	6–8	1++, 2++, 3++, 4++, 5++
Oxycodone hydrochloride (Roxicodone)	NA	NA	5 (or 5 mL)	15–30 (PO)	1 (PO)	4–6 (PO)	1++, 2+++, 3++, 4++, 5++
Oxymorphone hydrochloride (Numorphan)	0.5	1–1.5	NA	5–10	0.5–1	3–6	1++, 2+, 3+++, 5+++
Alfentanil hydrochloride (Alfenta)	8–50 μg/kg	NA	NA	immediate	NDA	0.5–0.75	1++
Fentanyl (Sublimaze)	0.05–0.1	0.05–0.1	NA	7–8	NDA	1–2	1++, 3+
Meperidine hydrochloride (Demerol)	15–35 mg/hr	50–150	50–150	10–45	0.5–1	2–4	1++, 2+, 3++, 4+, 5++
Methadone hydrochloride (Dolophine)	NA	2.5–10	15–20; 40 mg max	30–60	0.5–1	4–6	1++, 2++, 3++, 4+, 5+

Propoxyphene hydrochloride (Darvon, Dolene)	NA	NA	65	30–60 (PO)	2–2.5 (PO)	4–6 (PO)	1+, 3+, 4+, 5+
Sufentanil citrate (Sufenta)	1–30 μg/kg	NA	NA	1.3–3 (IV)	NDA	NDA	1+++
Mixed agonist-antagonists:							***Relative antagonist activity:***
Buprenorphine hydrochloride (Buprenex)	0.3	0.3	NA	15	0.5	6	Equipotent with naloxone
Butorphanol tartrate (Stadol)	0.5–2	1–4	NA	<10	0.5–1	3–4	30x pentazocine or 1/40 naloxone
Dezocine (Dalgan)	2.5–10	5–20	NA	≤30 (≤15 IV)	0.5–2.5	2–4	Greater than pentazocine
Nalbuphine (Nubain)	10–20	10–20	NA	<15 (2–3 IV)	1 (0.5 IV)	3–6	10x pentazocine
Pentazocine hydrochloride (Fortral, Talwin)	30	30	50–100	15–20 (2–3 IV, 15–30 PO)	0.25–1 (1–3 PO)	3	Weak

NA = Not available.
NDA = No data available.
[a]Dosage intervals usually every 4 hours. Dosage range given for a 70-kg adult.
[b]IM administration values unless otherwise stated.
[c]1 = Analgesic activity: 1+ = mild activity; 1++ = moderate activity; 1+++ = strong activity.
2 = Antitussive activity: 2+ = mild activity; 2++ = moderate activity; 2+++ = strong activity.
3 = Ventilatory depression: 3+ = mild depression; 3++ = moderate depression; 3+++ = strong depression.
4 = Sedative activity: 4+ = mild sedation; 4++ = moderate sedation; 4+++ = strong sedation.
5 = Physical dependence: 5+ = mild dependence; 5++ = moderate dependence, 5+++ = strong dependence.

4. Naloxone is not effective against ventilatory depression caused by nonopioid drugs.

Adverse Reactions

An abrupt reversal of opioid-induced depression may cause nausea, vomiting, sweating, tachycardia, hypertension, and tremors. In postoperative patients, an excessive dose of naloxone may induce significant reversal of analgesia, hypotension, hypertension, pulmonary edema, and ventricular tachycardia or fibrillation.

Overdosage

Overdose should be treated symptomatically; resuscitation equipment should be available.

Dosage and Administration

The opioid antagonists are listed in Table 15.3.

III
Nonopioid Analgesics

ACETAMINOPHEN

ACEPHEN, TYLENOL, DATRIL, NEOPAP, PANADOL

Mechanism of Action and Indications for Use

The nonopioid analgesics include the nonsteroidal anti-inflammatory drugs (NSAIDS) previously presented in Chapter 12 (see Table 12.5) and acetaminophen. Acetaminophen is a para-aminophenol derivative that is a weak prostaglandin inhibitor in peripheral tissues; therefore, it does not exhibit anti-inflammatory effects. It is one of the more important nonopioid drugs for the

Table 15.3.
The Opioid Antagonists

Opioid Antagonist	Dosage Form	Dose[a]	Onset (min)	Duration (hr)
Naloxone hydrochloride (Narcan)	IV, IM, SC: 0.4, 1 mg/ml	0.4 to 2 mg initially, may repeat IV at 2- to 3-minute intervals[b]	<5	1–4
Naltrexone hydrochloride[c] (Trexan)	PO: 50-mg tablets	50 mg/day	60	24–72

[a]Total dose varies with patient and the degree of respiratory depression.
[b]Dosage range given is for reversal of narcotic overdosage.
[c]Indicated only for the prevention of narcotic use in former narcotic addicts.

treatment of mild to moderate pain when an anti-inflammatory action is not desired. Acetaminophen is essentially equivalent to aspirin in its analgesic properties; however, acetaminophen differs from aspirin in that it lacks aspirin's anti-inflammatory properties. Additionally, acetaminophen does not inhibit platelet aggregation, affect prothrombin response, or produce gastrointestinal ulceration. Acetaminophen also exhibits antipyretic activity owing to its direct action on the hypothalamic heat-regulating centers.

For mild analgesia, acetaminophen is the drug of choice for patients who are allergic to aspirin, patients who have a history of peptic ulcer, or patients with hemophilia. Acetaminophen is also therapeutically useful for patients in whom bronchospasm is precipitated by aspirin. Acetaminophen is also preferred over aspirin for children with viral infections. Additionally, acetaminophen is clinically useful for reducing fever caused by the common cold, "flu," and other bacterial and viral infections.

Contraindications

Contraindications to acetaminophen include hypersensitivity to the drug.

Precautions

1. Acetaminophen has the potential for producing hepatotoxicity and nephrotoxicity, especially when administered in larger than normal doses or over an extended period of time.
2. The therapeutic effects of acetaminophen may be reduced when administered concomitantly with the following agents: barbiturates, rifampin, carbamazepine, hydantoins, or sulfinpyrazone.

Adverse Reactions

Acetaminophen rarely causes severe toxicity or side effects, except as listed above. The following have been known to occur:

Hematologic: Hemolytic anemia, neutropenia, leukopenia, thrombocytopenia, pancytopenia.
Allergic: Skin eruptions, fever, urticarial and erythematous skin reactions.
Miscellaneous: Hypoglycemia, jaundice.

Overdosage

Acute toxic states are manifest by nausea, vomiting, drowsiness, confusion, hypotension, and cardiac arrhythmias as well as jaundice and acute hepatic and renal failure. The minimal toxic dose is 10 grams (140 mg/kg). The minimum lethal dose is 15 grams (200 mg/kg). Oral acetylcysteine (Mucomyst) is a specific antidote for acetaminophen poisoning (IV administration may induce anaphylaxis).

Dosage and Administration

Acetaminophen is available in a variety of formulations, including tablets (160, 500, 650 mg), chewable tablets (80 mg), suppositories (80, 120, 125, 300, 325, 650 mg), capsules (80, 160, 500 mg), granules (80 mg), liquids (160 mg/5 ml, 500 mg/15 ml, with and without alcohol), solutions (100 mg/ml, 120 mg/2.5 ml), suspensions (80 mg/0.8 ml, 160 mg/5 ml), and elixirs (80 mg/5 ml, 120 mg/5 ml, 130 mg/5 ml, 160 mg/5 ml, 325 mg/5 ml). The normal dosage for adults ranges between 325 and 650 mg every 4 to 6 hrs or 1 g three to four times per day. Patients are cautioned not to exceed 4 g/day.

IV
Sedative-Hypnotic Agents

A therapeutically useful *sedative* (*anxiolytic*) should relieve anxiety and produce a calming action with little to no effect on motor or mental functions, whereas a *hypnotic* should produce drowsiness and enhance the onset and maintenance of a natural-like sleep. Hypnotic agents depress the CNS to a higher degree than sedatives. However, sedatives may exhibit hypnotic effects when administered in higher doses. The two most important classes of sedative-hypnotic agents are the barbiturates and the benzodiazepines. The benzodiazepines have virtually replaced the barbiturates as sedative-hypnotic agents primarily because they have a much wider margin of safety and because their potential for chronic abuse is much lower. The barbiturates still have clinically important uses as anticonvulsant agents in controlling epilepsy and for induction of anesthesia. The overall clinical uses of the sedative-hypnotic agents include:

- Relief of anxiety
- Hypnosis
- For sedation and amnesia before and during surgery and other medical procedures such as endoscopy and bronchoscopy
- For treatment of epilepsy and seizure states
- To induce muscle relaxation in certain types of neuromuscular disorders
- For treatment in psychiatry

BARBITURATES

Mechanism of Action and Indications for Use

Barbiturates interfere with the relay of all sensory impulses to the cerebral cortex by inhibiting the ascending impulse conduction in the reticular formation. In addition, low doses of these agents appear to potentiate the effects of gamma aminobutyric acid (GABA), the major inhibitory neurotransmitter in the CNS. Barbiturates induce all levels of CNS divergence from mild sedation to deep coma or anesthesia. All barbiturates also depress the activity of the medullary respiratory center, resulting in a diminished ventilatory drive. When used in excessive amounts, barbiturates also suppress the hypoxic drive. Consequently, the degree of ventilatory depression and CNS depression is primarily dose related. Barbiturates are classified as long-acting, intermediate-acting, short-acting, or ultrashort-acting according to their onset of action and duration of effect.

As previously stated, barbiturates have been largely replaced by the safer benzodiazepines as sedative-hypnotic agents; however, barbiturates are sometimes used in the short-term (less than 2 weeks) treatment of insomnia and as preanesthetic sedatives. Other uses of barbiturates include the emergency treatment of convulsions such as occur with tetanus, eclampsia, cholera, meningitis, status epilepticus, cerebral hemorrhage, and toxic reactions by convulsant drugs (e.g., strychnine). Phenobarbital is the most frequently used barbiturate because of its anticonvulsant efficacy. These agents are also used in the treatment of tonic-clonic and cortical focal seizures (see *Section VII*).

The ultrashort-acting barbiturates are especially useful for the induction of anesthesia, as an adjunct with other anesthetic agents, and for IV anesthesia during short surgical procedures. IV thiopental is indicated to control convulsive states and for neurosurgical patients with increased intracranial pressure when adequate ventilation is provided.

Contraindications

Contraindications include barbiturate sensitivity, liver disease, impaired renal function, patients with severe respiratory distress, respiratory disease in which dyspnea, obstruction, or cor pulmonale is present, acute or chronic pain, and nephritis. Subcutaneous administration is contraindicated owing to tissue irritation that may lead to necrosis.

Precautions

1. Barbiturates are habit forming. With continued use, tolerance and psychological and physical dependence may occur.
2. Use with caution for patients who have suicidal or drug histories or who are mentally depressed.
3. Use with caution for elderly patients, debilitated patients, and children (increased adverse reactions may occur).
4. Rapid IV administration may cause respiratory depression, apnea, laryngospasm, and severe hypotension.

Adverse Reactions

CNS: Somnolence, agitation, confusion, ataxia, vertigo, CNS depression, lethargy, nervousness, anxiety, delirium.

Pulmonary: Hypoventilation, respiratory depression, apnea, laryngospasm, bronchospasm.

Cardiovascular: Bradycardia, hypotension, syncope.

GI: Nausea, vomiting, constipation, diarrhea, epigastric pain.

Other: Injection into or near peripheral nerves may produce permanent neurological deficit.

Hypersensitivity: Skin rash, angioneurotic edema, serum sickness.

Acute Intoxication: Unsteady walk, slurred speech, confusion, irritability, insomnia.

Overdosage

Serious poisoning is produced by a 1-g oral dose of barbiturates; 2 to 10 g may cause death. CNS and respiratory depression may progress to Cheyne-Stokes respirations, along with tachycardia, hypotension, decreased body temperature, and coma. Shock syndrome may occur, which is manifested by apnea, circulatory collapse, respiratory arrest, and possible death. With extreme overdosage, a "flat" EEG may result, which is reversible if hypoxic damage has not occurred. Pneumonia, pulmonary edema, cardiac arrhythmias, congestive heart failure, and renal failure are possible complications to barbiturate overdose. Treatment consists of providing supportive care, maintaining an airway, intubating with assisted ventilation if necessary, and monitoring of vital signs and fluid balance. Emesis may be induced if the patient has not lost consciousness, with care taken to prevent aspiration. If renal function is normal, forced diuresis may be induced. In severe barbiturate overdose, hemodialysis may be necessary.

Dosage and Administration

Table 15.4 lists the various barbiturates.

BENZODIAZEPINES

Mechanism of Action and Indications for Use

Benzodiazepines are more commonly the drugs of choice used for sedative or hypnotic effects due to their efficacy and safety as demonstrated by considerable clinical documentation and experience. Benzodiazepines exert their effect on subcortical levels of the CNS—primarily on the limbic system (emotional and behavioral responses) and on the reticular formation. However, benzodiazepines do not relatively affect the cerebral cortex as do the barbiturates. Benzodiazepines seem to directly facilitate the actions of the inhibitory neurotransmitter, gamma

Table 15.4.
The Barbiturates

Barbiturate	Sedation	Dose (mg)[a] Hypnotic[b]	Anticonvulsant	Onset (min)	Duration (hr)
Long-acting:					
Phenobarbital (Solfoton, Luminal Sodium)	PO: 30–120/day IV, IM: 30–120/day	PO: 100–320 IV, IM: 100–320	PO: 100–300/day IV: 10–15 mg/kg/day	30–60	10–16
Mephobarbital (Mebaral)	PO: 32–200/day	—	PO: 400–600/day		
Intermediate-acting:				45–60	6–8
Amobarbital (Amytal Sodium)	PO: 60–150/day	PO: 50–200 IM: 50–200	—		
Aprobarbital (Alurate)	PO: 120/day	PO: 40–80 (up to 160)	—		
Butabarbital (Butasol Sodium)	PO: 45–120/day	PO: 50–100	—		
Short-acting:				10–15	3–4
Secobarbital (Seconal Sodium)	PO: 200–300 (1–2 hr before surgery)	PO: 100–200 IM: 50–250	—		
Pentobarbital (Nembutal Sodium)	PO: 40–120/day	PO: 100–200 IM: 150–200 IV: 100 initially	—		
Ultrashort-acting:		***For anesthesia:***		<1	1/2
Thiopental sodium (Pentothal)	—	IV: 50–75 (2–3 ml of 2.5% solution), may be repeated	IV: 75–125		
Thiamylal sodium (Surital)	—	IV: 3–6 ml of 2.5% solution	—		
Methohexital sodium (Brevital Sodium)	—	IV: 1–1.5 mg/kg	—		

[a]Usual adult dose. Daily doses are usually given three to four times/day in equally divided doses.
[b]Usually given as a one-time dose for insomnia just before bedtime.

aminobutyric acid (GABA). At least two benzodiazepine receptor subtypes have been isolated in the brain: BZ_1 and BZ_2. BZ_1 is associated with sleep mechanisms, whereas BZ_2 interacts with memory, motor, sensory, and cognitive functions. The results produced include antianxiety effects, muscle relaxation, sedative or hypnotic effects, and anticonvulsant effects. The benzodiazepines exert minimal effects on the medullary respiratory center, which makes them safer to use than the barbiturates.

Benzodiazepines are indicated for the management of anxiety disorders, in the treatment of sleep disorders (insomnia), as hypnotics, for the induction of anesthesia, in the management of seizure states, as muscle relaxants (higher doses of benzodiazepines depress transmission at the skeletal neuromuscular junction, thereby relieving muscle spasms), for the management of acute alcohol withdrawal, as sedation for ventilator patients, and before and during medical procedures such as endoscopy and bronchoscopy.

Contraindications

Contraindications include hypersensitivity to benzodiazepines, psychoses, acute alcoholic intoxication, and shock or coma with depression of vital signs.

Precautions

1. Use with caution for patients with liver and/or renal disease (dosage may need to be reduced).
2. Continued use may lead to dependence.
3. Owing to the potentiation of adverse reactions use with caution in elderly individuals, patients with limited pulmonary reserve, very ill individuals, and children.
4. Avoid alcohol or other CNS depressants with use of these agents.

Adverse Reactions

CNS: Sedation, sleepiness, depression, lethargy, apathy, fatigue, disorientation, confusion, delirium, headache, slurred speech, stupor, coma, syncope, vertigo, nervousness, irritability.

Pulmonary: Respiratory disturbances (decreased tidal volume, respiratory rate, apnea).

Cardiovascular: Bradycardia, tachycardia, cardiovascular collapse, hypertension, hypotension (rare), palpitations, edema.

GI: Constipation, diarrhea, dry mouth, heartburn, nausea, anorexia, vomiting, increased salivation, gastritis.

Psychiatric: Behavior problems, hysteria, psychosis, suicidal attempt.

Other: Hiccups, fever, diaphoresis, paresthesis, muscular disturbances.

Overdosage

Fatalities resulting from oral ingestion are not well documented. The oral agents rarely produce serious respiratory or circulatory depression. Overdose symptoms include somnolence, confusion, ataxia, hypotonia, hypotension, seizures, respiratory depression, apnea, and coma. Treatment consists of inducing vomiting and monitoring respiration, pulse, and blood pressure. Maintain an adequate airway at all times. With normal kidney function, induce forced diuresis. In critical situations, hemodialysis may be necessary.

Flumazenil (Romazicon), approved for use in the USA in December 1991, is a competitive benzodiazepine receptor antagonist available for IV administration. Flumazenil effectively reverses the CNS depressant and sedative effects produced by benzodiazepines. The onset of reversal is usually evident within 1 to 2 minutes after the injection is completed. Flumazenil has a mean half-life of approximately 54 minutes; clearance is primarily through hepatic metabolism. Flumazenil does not block or antagonize the CNS effects of other sedative-hypnotic agents, opioids, or general anesthetics. Flumazenil is currently the only approved agent in use for benzodiazepine overdose.

The recommended initial dose of flumazenil (for known or suspected benzodiazepine overdose) is 0.2 mg (2 ml) administered IV over 30 seconds. If the patient does not regain consciousness after waiting 30 seconds, a second dose of 0.3 mg (3 ml) may be administered over another 30 seconds. Additional doses of 0.5 mg (5 ml) may be administered over 30 seconds at 1-minute intervals to a cumulative dose of 3 mg.

Dosage and Administration

Table 15.5 lists the benzodiazepines.

NONBARBITURATE NONBENZODIAZEPINE SEDATIVE-HYPNOTIC AGENTS

Several agents that are neither barbiturates or benzodiazepines exhibit CNS properties that induce sedation or produce hypnotic effects. However, the benzodiazepines remain the agents of choice in the treatment of anxiety and insomnia. Zolpidem (Ambien) is a newer sedative-hypnotic agent that is an imidazopyridine derivative with a mechanism of action similar to the benzodiazepines. Although structurally unrelated to the benzodiazepines, zolpidem binds with the BZ subtype receptors to facilitate GABA-induced inhibition. Zolpidem is primarily used to treat insomnia. As with all sedative-hypnotic agents, the patient is cautioned against coadministration with alcohol or other CNS depressants. Adverse reactions noted with the use of zolpidem include nausea, vomiting, diarrhea, dry mouth, headache, dizziness, abnormal dreams, lightheadedness, influenza-like symptoms, allergy, rash, and palpitations. Zolpidem overdose may be treated with flumazenil (see above, under *Benzodiazepine, Overdosage*); however, because the mean half-life of zolpidem (2½ hours) is longer than that of flumazenil, repeated doses may be necessary.

Older sedative-hypnotic agents, such as the alcohols (ethchlorvynol, chloral hydrate), piperidine derivatives (glutethimide, methyprylon), ureides (acetylcarbromal), carbamates (meprobamate), phenothiazine compounds (propiomazine), and paraldehyde essentially have been replaced by the safer, more effective benzodiazepines and thus currently are rarely used. Although sedative doses can be given, these agents are primarily intended to be hypnotic agents (agents that will produce drowsiness and facilitate sleep). Table 15.6 lists the adult sedative and hypnotic oral doses of the above-mentioned agents.

Table 15.5.
The Benzodiazepines

Benzodiazepine	Adult Dose
Alprazolam (Xanax)	***For anxiety or panic disorders:*** initial dose: 0.25–0.5 mg t.i.d. Titrate to a maximum dose of 4 mg/day, given in divided doses.
Chlordiazepoxide (Librium)	***For mild to moderate anxiety:*** PO: 5 or 10 mg t.i.d., q.i.d. ***For severe anxiety:*** PO: 20 or 25 mg t.i.d., q.i.d.. IV, IM: 50 to 100 mg initially, then 25 to 50 mg t.i.d., q.i.d. if necessary. ***For acute alcohol withdrawal:*** PO, IV, IM: 50 to 100 mg (up to 300 mg/day).
Clonazepam (Klonopin)	***As an adjunct in seizure control:*** initial dose: 0.5 mg t.i.d. Maximum daily dose is 20 mg/day.
Clorazepate (Tranxene)	***For relief of anxiety:*** 30 mg/day in divided doses (range: 15–60 mg/day). ***As an adjunct in the management of partial seizures:*** initial dose: 7.5 mg t.i.d. Dosage is gradually increased at weekly intervals. Maximum daily dose is 90 mg.
Diazepam (Valium, Zetran, Valrelease)	***For anxiety disorders:*** PO, IV, IM: 2–10 mg, repeat in 3 to 4 hours, if necessary. ***For acute alcohol withdrawal:*** PO, IV, IM: 10 mg initially, then 5–10 mg in 3 to 4 hours, if necessary. ***For skeletal muscle spasm:*** PO, IV, IM: 5–10 mg initially, then 5–10 mg in 3 to 4 hours, if necessary. ***For status epilepticus and severe seizures:*** IV preferred: 5–10 mg initially, may repeat at 10- to 15-minute intervals up to a maximum dose of 30 mg. ***For sedation or muscle relaxation:*** 2–10 mg/dose every 3 to 4 hours, as needed. ***As an adjunct in convulsive disorders:*** PO: 2–10 mg b.i.d., q.i.d. Sustained-release preparations: PO: 15–30 mg once daily.
Estazolam (ProSom)	***For insomnia:*** PO: 1–2 mg before bedtime.
Flurazepam (Dalmane)	***For insomnia:*** PO: 15–30 mg before bedtime.
Halazepam (Paxipam)	***For relief of anxiety:*** PO: 20–40 mg t.i.d., q.i.d. (range: 80–160 mg/day).
Lorazepam (Ativan)	***For relief of anxiety or sedation:*** PO: 2–3 mg/day given b.i.d., t.i.d. IV: 2 mg. IM: 0.05 mg/kg (up to a maximum dose of 4 mg). ***For insomnia:*** PO: 2 to 4 mg at bedtime.
Midazolam hydrochloride (Versed)	***For sedation and memory impairment before surgical or medical procedures:*** IV, IM: 0.07–0.08 mg/kg (1–5 mg is the usual adult dose), given 1 hour before procedure. ***For induction of general anesthesia:*** IV: 0.3–0.35 mg/kg (up to 0.6 mg/kg total dose), given over 20–30 seconds. For maintenance of anesthesia: use incremental doses of approximately 25% of the dose initially administered.
Oxazepam (Serax)	***For relief of anxiety:*** PO: 10–30 mg t.i.d., q.i.d.
Prazepam (Centrax)	***For relief of anxiety:*** PO: 20–60 mg/day, given in divided doses.
Temazepam (Restoril)	***For insomnia:*** PO: 15–30 mg before bedtime.
Triazolam (Halcion)	***For insomnia:*** PO: 0.125–0.5 mg before bedtime.
Quazepam (Doral)	***For insomnia:*** PO: 7–5–15 mg before bedtime.

There are several over-the-counter (OTC) compounds that can be administered to enhance the induction of sleep. These drugs are known as nonprescription sleep aids. The primary, active ingredient in these formulations is diphenhydramine or doxylamine. Both are antihistamines (H_1 blockers) that can induce a significant degree of sedation. For more information about these antihistamines, see Chapter 9.

Table 15.6.
Nonbarbiturate/Nonbenzodiazepine Sedative-Hypnotic Agents

Drug	Hypnotic Dose*	Sedative Dose*	Onset (min)	Duration (hrs)
Acetylcarbromal (Paxarel)	—	250–500 mg b.i.d., t.i.d.	NDA	NDA
Chloral hydrate (Noctec)	0.5–1 g	250 mg t.i.d. after meals	30	NDA
Ethchlorvynol (Placidyl)	500 mg	100–200 mg b.i.d., q.i.d.	15–60	5
Glutethimide (Various)	250–500 mg	—	30	4–8
Methyprylon (Noludar)	200–400 mg	50–100 mg, up to q.i.d.	45	5–8
Paraldehyde (Paral)	10–30 ml	5–10 ml	10–15	8–12
Propiomazine hydrochloride (Largon)	—	10–20 mg	NDA	NDA
Zolpidem tartrate (Ambien)	10 mg	—	NDA	NDA

NDA = No data available.
*Usual adult oral dose.

V
Anesthetic Agents

GENERAL ANESTHETIC AGENTS

The history of surgical anesthesia dates to 1846, when William Morton, a Boston dentist (and medical student) introduced under public demonstration the first general anesthetic agent, diethyl ether. The next year, Simpson, a Scottish obstetrician, introduced chloroform. Some 20 years later, the anesthetic properties of nitrous oxide ("laughing gas") were discovered (which had been first suggested by Davy in the 1790s). The advent of modern anesthesia dates to the 1930s, when the ultrashort-acting barbiturate thiopental was used intravenously to induce anesthesia. In the 1940s, curare was used in conjunction with anesthetic agents to achieve skeletal muscle relaxation. Halothane, the first modern halogenated hydrocarbon, was introduced as an inhaled anesthetic in 1956. Halothane remains the standard by which other, newer inhaled anesthetic drugs are compared.

Before 1846, surgery was generally considered a last resort, and for good reason. Strong men were needed, with various restraints and wooden bite blocks, to forcefully restrain patients from moving or leaving the surgical table. Often, patients were given drugs such as alcohol, hashish, and opium derivatives to soothe their anxiety before the surgical procedure and thus offer some consolidation. Some patients received a blow to the head, were strangled, or had their limb packed in ice or a tourniquet applied to dull the pain that would accompany the surgical procedure. Fortunately, modern anesthetic agents have eliminated the need for the above-mentioned practices.

The state of "general anesthesia" is characterized by certain primary attributes:

- Hypnosis and amnesia
- Analgesia
- Skeletal muscle relaxation
- Loss of consciousness and diminution of autonomic reflexes

The extent to which the above attributes are induced depends on the anesthetic agent itself, the dosage, and the clinical condition of the patient.

Two primary types of anesthetic protocols are used for surgical interventions in most institutions: *conscious sedation* and *balanced anesthesia*. Conscious sedation is a protocol employed for minor, short procedures and involves the use of benzodiazepines in conjunction with local anesthetics (see below). Balanced anesthesia is a protocol more appropriate for longer, extensive procedures and involves the use of a combination of agents, such as barbiturates with nitrous oxide and IV opioids. The goal is to induce a balance of deep anesthesia (total CNS depression) with the use of the above-mentioned agents. Additionally, before surgery, part of the anesthesia procedure is to administer medications to sedate and to relieve anxiety and to relieve preoperative pain if present. The barbiturates, benzodiazepines, and the opioid derivatives are especially useful for the above-mentioned effects (see *Sections II and IV* of this chapter). A secondary beneficial effect of these agents when used preoperatively is that the total dose requirement of a general anesthetic is reduced.

Antimuscarinic agents, such as atropine, scopolamine, or glycopyrrolate, are given preoperatively to control the production of secretions before and during surgery as well as to overcome or minimize the undesirable side effects of the general anesthetic agents, which include bradycardia, coughing, and postanesthetic vomiting (antiemetic agents, such as droperidol and hydroxyzine, are especially useful for preventing postanesthetic vomiting). Neuromuscular blocking agents, including pancuronium and succinylcholine (see Chapter 14), are not only given to facilitate endotracheal intubation, but to produce muscle flaccidity during the surgical procedure. Although some of the general anesthetic agents induce adequate relaxation of skeletal muscles, some surgeries require total, complete muscle paralysis to prevent any type of reflex muscle contraction or laryngospasm.

Signs and Stages of Anesthesia

In 1920, Arthur Guedel, a noted pioneer in anesthesia, described four stages of anesthesia that correlate with the increasing depth of anesthesia or CNS depression. Guedel's observations relate primarily to the effects produced by diethyl ether, an agent that has a relatively slow onset of central action owing to its high solubility in blood. Because the newer anesthetic agents have a significantly faster onset of action, all four stages may not be immediately recognized or may be obscured. Nevertheless, the progressive anesthetic effects of diethyl ether are still the basis for which all general anesthetics are compared and assessed. The four stages of increasing depth of CNS depression primarily involve the changes that occur in respiration, muscle tone, and reflex activity.

I. *Stage of Analgesia:* Initially, immediately after administration of a general anesthetic, the patient will experience relief from pain. During the latter part of stage I, the patient will also exhibit amnesia.
II. *Stage of Excitement:* During this stage, the patient exhibits delirium and excitation. The ventilatory pattern is erratic both in volume and rate, and retching and vomiting may ensue. As the anesthesia becomes sequentially deeper, the patient may struggle. For the above reasons, it is necessary to limit the duration of this stage. Combined, stage I and stage II are known as the induction period. Because these stages cannot be avoided, special inducing agents are administered for the patient to pass rapidly through these stages. Midazolam (Versed, see Table 15.5) has become popular as a preanesthetic medication owing to its relatively fast onset of action and short duration as well as its propensity to produce amnesia with few side effects.
III. *Stage of Surgical Anesthesia:* The surgical procedure is performed during this stage of anesthesia. If the eyelids blink in response to eyelash stroking, if the patient is swallowing, or if the ventilatory pattern is erratic, surgical anesthesia is not present. As anesthesia is deepened, these responses are abolished and surgery may be safely initiated. Four planes of stage III have been described that relate to pupil size, pupil reflexes to light, ocular movements, tearing, and responses of the respiratory rate and blood pressure to a surgical incision. As the patient moves from plane I to plane IV, these key responses or reflexes are reduced and finally abolished as the CNS is progressively depressed.
IV. *Stage of Medullary Depression:* Severe respiratory depression, apnea, marked hypotension, or asystole signals the presence of stage IV. Full cardiopulmonary support is mandated, because without it, death rapidly ensues.

Types of General Anesthetics

General anesthetics are administered by way of inhalation or by intravenous injection. Both types of general anesthetics depress all portions of the CNS. There is no single, selective site or focus of action. These agents facilitate the inhibitory effects of GABA, depress the reticular activating system, inhibit the action potential of general sensory and motor neurons of the cerebrum and cerebral cortex. At moderate to high doses, general anesthetics will block stimulation of the medullary vital centers.

Inhalational Agents

Inhalational general anesthetics include the gases nitrous oxide (N_2O), halothane, enflurane, isoflurane, desflurane, methoxyflurane, cyclopropane, and ethylene. Of these available agents, nitrous oxide, desflurane, and isoflurane are commonly used in the USA. Halothane is frequently used for pediatric anesthesia. Methoxyflurane is sometimes used in obstetric anesthesia but not for prolonged surgeries owing to its nephrotoxicity. Chloroform is generally not used currently because of its hepatotoxicity. Additionally, cyclopropane and diethyl ether are not given because of their highly flammable and explosive properties.

Pharmacokinetic Properties of Inhaled Anesthetics

The depth of anesthesia induced by an inhalational agent depends directly on the partial pressure or tension of the anesthetic in the brain, which reflects the tension of the agent in arterial blood. The rates of anesthetic induction and recovery also are dependent on the tension of the anesthetic agent in the brain and arterial blood. Five primary factors determine the tension of the anesthetic gas in the brain and arterial blood: 1) the solubility of the drug, 2) the concentration of the anesthetic agent in inspired gas, 3) the pulmonary ventilation rate, 4) the pulmonary blood flow, and 5) the concentration gradient between arterial and mixed-venous blood.

- Drug Solubility: An essential feature of an anesthetic gas is its solubility. Solubility reflects the uptake of the inhaled drug from the lungs to arterial blood to the brain. The blood:gas partition coefficient, or λ, is an index that is useful in determining the uptake properties of an anesthetic gas. The blood:gas partition coefficient represents the ratio of anesthetic concentration when it is in equilibrium with both the blood and gas phases. A low blood:gas partition coefficient signifies that the anesthetic agent is poorly soluble; thus, the arterial tension of the inhaled gas will rise at a relatively fast pace, the drug will reach the brain faster, and the induction of anesthesia will occur at a fast rate. For example, the blood:gas partition coefficients for nitrous oxide, halothane, and methoxyflurane are 0.47, 2.3, and 12, respectively. This indicates that nitrous oxide has a relatively fast onset of action, whereas methoxyflurane, even after 40 minutes, will reach only 20% of the equilibrium concentration. The high blood:gas partition coefficient of methoxyflurane suggests that this agent is very soluble in blood; therefore, more molecules dissolve before the tension changes significantly, and tension of the gas in arterial blood rises very slowly.
- Anesthetic Concentration in Inspired Gas: Higher concentrations of the inhaled anesthetic gas in a total mixture of inspired gases has direct effects on both the tension in the alveoli and rate of increase in its tension in arterial blood. The advantage of this feature lies with those anesthetic agents that have

relatively moderate to high solubility. By increasing the concentration of the agent, the onset of induction will be faster. Once adequate anesthesia is achieved, the concentration of the agent may then be reduced, sometimes by half its initial amount, to maintain anesthesia.

The *minimum alveolar concentration (MAC)* of an anesthetic agent is a measure of its potency and is defined as the concentration in the alveoli that results in immobility in 50% of patients when exposed to a noxious stimulus such as a surgical incision. A dose of 1 MAC will prevent movement in 50% of individuals in response to surgical incision; doses of 0.5 to 2.0 MAC are necessary to achieve anesthesia in most of the population. In effect, MAC reflects the ED50 of the drug (see Chapter 4). The higher the MAC (percent), the lower the potency of the drug. A MAC value greater than 100% for nitrous oxide indicates that this drug is the least potent of the inhaled anesthetic agents (Table 15.7).

- Pulmonary Ventilation Rate: Hyperventilating a patient by increasing both the rate and depth of ventilation (i.e., the minute ventilation) will result in a direct and significant rise in anesthetic gas tension in arterial blood. Thus, the rate of induction will occur at a faster rate. Because blood has a high capacity for highly soluble anesthetic gases, a more dramatic rise in anesthetic gas tension will occur. This is especially noted with those agents with a blood:gas partition coefficient > 1.
- Pulmonary Blood Flow: Any changes in the rates of blood flow to and from the lungs will influence the transfer of the inhaled anesthetic gas from the alveoli to the pulmonary vasculature system. High cardiac output states move blood at a faster rate and thus have a tendency to not allow enough time for the blood to receive the anesthetic agent as it passes the pulmonary circulation. As a result, the induction of anesthesia will occur at a slower rate. Normal, or even low, cardiac output conditions move blood at a slower rate than high output states; therefore, the transfer of the anesthetic agent from the alveoli to the bloodstream will result in a sequential rise in arterial tension.
- Arteriovenous Concentration Gradient: After the anesthetic gas is taken up by the pulmonary circulation, it circulates to the tissues, where it is then passed from the blood to the tissues. With each passage through the body, eventually an equilibrium will be reached in which the mixed-venous blood returning to the lungs contains more anesthetic. After a few minutes of inhaling an anesthetic gas, the gradient, or difference between arterial (or alveolar) and mixed-venous gas tension will decrease. Because the rate of diffusion across the alveolar capillary membrane is dependent on the arterial to mixed-venous gas tension, an already saturated system will result in a lower transfer rate of the gas between alveoli and blood. Thus, the volume of gas transferred to arterial blood decreases as time passes.

Table 15.7.
Pharmacokinetic Data of Inhalational Anesthetic Agents

Anesthetic	Blood:Gas Partition Coefficient (λ)	Brain:Blood Partition Coefficient	Minimum Alveolar Concentration (MAC) (percent)	Comments
Desflurane (Suprane)	0.42	1.3	7.30	Desflurane is a volatile liquid inhalational anesthetic that is not recommended for induction of anesthesia in infants and children owing to the high incidence of laryngospasm, coughing, breathholding, and secretions. However, after induction with other agents, desflurane may be used to maintain anesthesia in infants and children. For induction in adults: starting concentration is 3% with increments of 0.5% to 1% every two to three breaths. Anesthesia is usually produced within 2 to 4 minutes. Carrier gas may be O_2 or N_2O/O_2. Concentrations of desflurane >1 MAC may increase heart rate.
Enflurane (Ethrane)	1.90	1.4	1.68	Induction and recovery from anesthesia is rapid. Mild production of secretions is noted with the use of this agent. Progressive increases in the depth of anesthesia produce increasing hypotension. May cause renal damage owing to the release of fluoride ion. For induction of anesthesia: 2% to 4.5% will produce anesthesia in 7 to 10 minutes. Maintenance concentrations should not exceed 3%.
Halothane (Fluothane)	2.30	2.9	0.75	Induction and recovery are rapid. Halothane is not a respiratory irritant and does not ordinarily cause an increase in salivary or bronchial secretions. Halothane causes bronchodilation. Hypoxia, acidosis, or apnea may occur with deep anesthesia. Halothane produces moderate muscle relaxation. The induction dose varies and ranges between 0.5% to 1.5%. May be administered with O_2 or N_2O/O_2.
Isoflurane (Forane)	1.40	2.6	1.15	Induction and recovery are rapid. This agent is noted to be a profound respiratory depressant and hypotensive agent. Respiratory depression and hypotension may be partially reversed by surgical stimulation. Coadministration with N_2O may block or reduce the arterial hypotension seen with isoflurane alone. Induction dose ranges between an inspired concentration of 1.5% to 3%. Surgical anesthesia is produced in 7 to 10 minutes.
Methyoxyflurane (Penthrane)	12.00	2.0	0.16	Does not produce appreciable skeletal muscle relaxation. Usually used in combination with O_2 or N_2O/O_2. May cause renal failure or damage owing to the release of fluoride ion. For induction, concentrations of up to 2% are used.
Nitrous oxide	0.47	1.1	105	Most commonly used anesthetic gas. Because it is a weak anesthetic agent, it is usually used in combination with other anesthetics. It does not induce skeletal muscle relaxation. Hypoxia is a major feature of this agent; therefore, at least 20% oxygen must be used in conjunction with nitrous oxide. In high concentrations, nitrous oxide may cause vomiting, respiratory depression, and death. Nitrous oxide is supplied in blue cylinders.

As can be expected, elimination of inhalational anesthetics and the time to recover from anesthesia depend on the same factors that are important in the above-mentioned uptake phases: drug solubility in blood and tissue, pulmonary ventilation, and pulmonary blood flow. As ventilation with anesthetic-free gas washes out the lung, the arterial blood tension decreases, and so also that of the tissues. Because of the high blood flow to the brain, the anesthetic gas washes out of brain tissue at a relatively fast rate. This is especially noted with the comparably insoluble agents such as nitrous oxide. The major route of elimination of inhaled anesthetics is through exhalation of the respiratory cycle. Anesthetic gases are also eliminated via metabolism by enzymes of the liver and other tissues and through urinary excretion. Additionally, small amounts of the gas diffuse across the skin and mucous membranes.

Organ system effects of inhaled anesthetics are quite diverse. Effects on the cardiovascular system include a decrease in mean arterial pressure that is directly proportional to the anesthetic's concentration in the alveoli. Bradycardia may occur through direct depression of the atrial rate (halothane) or the patient may exhibit tachycardia (isoflurane). Enflurane and halothane manifest marked myocardial depressant effects, whereas isoflurane has a lesser effect on myocardial function.

All inhaled anesthetics are ventilatory depressants. The depressant effect varies with each agent; isoflurane and enflurane are the most potent depressors of ventilation. The inhaled anesthetics also depress mucociliary function, which may result in pooling of secretions leading to atelectasis and pulmonary infections. However, most inhaled anesthetics exhibit bronchodilator properties, which makes them potentially useful in the treatment of status asthmaticus.

Most inhaled anesthetics increase cerebral blood flow because they decrease cerebral vascular resistance. This is usually an undesirable side effect, especially for patients with head injuries or brain tumors. The increase in cerebral blood flow correspondingly increases cerebral blood volume, which in turn increases intracranial pressure. If the patient is hyperventilated before administration of the anesthetic gas (to reduce $PaCO_2$), the increase in intracranial pressure from the inhaled anesthetic can be minimized.

To varying degrees, inhaled anesthetics decrease blood flow to the kidneys and liver. Hepatotoxicity and nephrotoxicity are features associated with halothane and methoxyflurane, respectively. Isoflurane, halothane, and enflurane are potent uterine smooth muscle relaxants. This effect may be a desirable trait when profound uterine relaxation is required for intrauterine manipulation of the fetus during delivery.

Table 15.7 summarizes some pharmacokinetic properties of the inhaled anesthetics as well as the usual dose administered for induction and maintenance of anesthesia.

Intravenous Agents

The ultrashort-acting barbiturates are used not only as preanesthetic medications but for the induction and maintenance of anesthesia (see Table 15.4). Likewise, the benzodiazepine midazolam (Versed) is therapeutically useful as a preanesthetic agent for sedation and memory impairment of perioperative events as well as for conscious sedation before short diagnostic or endoscopic procedures. Lorazepam and diazepam have also been used in anesthetic procedures (see Table 15.5). The above-mentioned benzodiazepines are occasionally used in combination with other anesthetic agents as part of balanced anesthesia.

The opioid analgesics, given in higher than normal doses, have been used to achieve anesthesia. IV morphine and fentanyl have been used at doses of 1 to 3 mg/kg and 50 to 100 μg/kg, respectively. These opioid analgesics seem to be especially useful for patients with minimal circulatory reserve, such as patients undergoing cardiac surgery.

Nonbarbiturate nonbenzodiazepine intravenous general anesthetics include propofol, etomidate, ketamine, and droperidol. Propofol is a rapidly acting IV sedative-hypnotic agent used for induction and maintenance of anesthesia, as a component of balanced anesthesia, as well as for continuous sedation and control of stress for intubated adult patients in intensive care units (ICUs). Propofol's main advantage of use lies in its brevity of action, which allows rapid recovery from anesthesia. Additionally, postanesthetic nausea and vomiting are minimal. In a dose-dependent fashion, propofol may induce apnea, hypotension, and bradycardia. Injection site pain and vein irritation are sometimes observed.

IV injection of etomidate produces hypnosis rapidly, usually within 1 minute after administration, and recovery usually occurs within 3 minutes. The primary use of etomidate is as an inducing agent and as a supplement to subpotent anesthetic agents such as nitrous oxide in oxygen. Etomidate exhibits fewer cardiovascular and respiratory depressant effects than the barbiturates and does not increase intracranial pressure as the inhaled anesthetics. Etomidate does not possess any analgesic properties; therefore, premedication with opioids may be required. Etomidate has a high incidence of causing nausea and vomiting, pain on injection, and involuntary muscle contractions. Etomidate may also cause adrenocorticol suppression. Prolonged infusion may precipitate hypotension, electrolyte imbalance, as well as oliguria.

Ketamine is indicated for use as a sole anesthetic agent for short diagnostic or surgical procedures in which skeletal muscle relaxation is not required, for the induction of anesthesia before administration of other general anesthetic agents, and to supplement low-potency agents such as nitrous oxide. Although ketamine is a potent analgesic and desirable anesthetic under most circumstances, it illicits significant hypertensive effects, tachycardia, increased cerebral blood flow, and psychological manifestations that range between pleasant dream-like states to hallucinations and delirium after anesthesia. Premedication with IV diazepam (0.2 to 0.3 mg/kg) reduces the incidence of this "emergence phenomena." Owing to the above-mentioned effects, ketamine is contraindicated for patients in whom increases in blood pressure would be a serious hazard, patients with head injuries, and patients with psychiatric disorders.

Droperidol produces marked tranquilization, sedation, and antiemetic effects. It also causes mild α-adrenoceptor blockade and peripheral vascular dilatation. Because of this, it reduces the pressor effects of epinephrine, resulting in hypotension and decreased peripheral vascular resistance. Following IV or IM administration, droperidol's action occurs in 3 to 10 minutes; however, the full effects may not be realized for 30 minutes. Droperidol usually has a duration of activity of 2 to 4 hours and alterations of consciousness may last for as long as 12 hours. Droperidol is especially useful to produce tranquilization and reduce the incidence of nausea and vomiting in medical and surgical procedures. Droperidol is also used as a premedicating agent, inducing agent, and as an adjunct in the maintenance of general anesthesia. Droperidol in conjunction with an opioid analgesic (e.g., fentanyl), produces neuroleptanalgesia that will aid in enhancing a tranquil state as well as reducing anxiety and pain before the medical or surgical procedure.

Other intravenous general anesthetics include a combination of an antimuscarinic agent for antisecretory effects and an opioid analgesic, such as morphine or meperidine, for sedation administered before the medical or surgical procedure.

The nonbarbiturate nonbenzodiazepine general anesthetics, along with their dosages, are listed in Table 15.8. For the general anesthetic dosages of barbiturates and benzodiazepines, see Tables 15.4 and 15.5, respectively.

LOCAL ANESTHETIC AGENTS

In contrast to general anesthetics, local anesthetics render various regions of the body insensitive to pain without any associated loss of consciousness. The history of local anesthesia begins with cocaine, an alkaloid derived from the *Erythroxylon coca* plant. Cocaine was first introduced into clinical use in 1884 as a topical ophthalmic anesthetic for patients undergoing operations for glaucoma. For the next 30 years, cocaine was the agent of choice because it was the only local anesthetic available, even though it was found to have strongly addictive CNS properties. Because of these properties, cocaine's current clinical use is severely restricted. In 1905, procaine, the first safe local anesthetic suitable for injection, was synthesized. For 50 years, procaine was the most widely used local anesthetic until the advent of lidocaine, the first amide-type local anesthetic, which is currently considered the agent of choice for infiltration. Lidocaine also has important uses as an antiarrhythmic agent (see Chapters 18 and 19). In 1963, bupivacaine, a long-acting amide-type local anesthetic, was introduced into clinical practice. Current therapeutic local anesthetics are either esters (procaine, benzocaine, chloroprocaine, tetracaine) or amides (lidocaine, prilocaine, mepivacaine, bupivacaine, etidocaine).

Table 15.8.
Nonbarbiturate Nonbenzodiazepine General Anesthetic Agents

General Anesthetic	Adult Dose	Onset (min)	Duration (min)
Droperidol (Inapsine)	***For premedication:*** IM; 2.5–10 mg (1–4 ml) 30–60 minutes preoperatively. ***As an induction agent:*** IV; 0.22–0.275 mg/kg with analgesic or general anesthetic. ***Maintenance dosage in general anesthesia:*** IV; 1.25–2.5 mg.	3–10 (up to 30)	120–240
Etomidate (Amidate)	***For induction of general anesthesia:*** IV; 0.2–0.6 mg/kg given over a period of 30 to 60 seconds.	1	3–5
Ketamine hydrochloride (Ketalar)	***For induction of general anesthesia:*** IV; 1–4.5 mg/kg. IM; 6.5–13 mg/kg. ***Maintenance dosage in general anesthesia:*** repeat in increments of half to full initial dose.	IV: 0.5 IM: 3–4	IV: 5–10 IM: 12–25
Propofol (Diprivan)	***For induction of general anesthesia:*** IV; 1–2.5 mg/kg. ***Maintenance infusion:*** IV; 0.1–0.2 mg/kg/min (6–12 mg/kg/hr). ***For light anesthesia, with nitrous oxide:*** IV; 3–5 μg/ml. ***For deep anesthesia, with nitrous oxide:*** IV; 4–7 μg/ml. ***For light ICU sedation:*** IV; 0.5–1 μg/ml. ***For deep ICU sedation:*** IV; 1–1.5 μg/ml.	0.7	Dose dependent
Combined Products:			
Droperidol with fentanyl (Innovar)	***Premedication:*** IM; 0.5–2 ml 45–60 minutes before surgery. ***Adjunct to general anesthesia:*** 0.1 ml/kg by slow IV to produce neuroleptanalgesia. ***For diagnostic procedures:*** IM; 0.5–2 ml 45–60 minutes before procedure. For prolonged procedures, give 0.5–1 ml IV with caution and without a general anesthetic.		
Atropine with meperidine (Atropine and Demoral)	***For preoperative sedation and antisecretory effect:*** individualized dosage. Administer appropriate dose, IM 30–90 minutes before beginning anesthesia.		
Atropine with morphine	***For preoperative sedation and antisecretory effect:*** IV, IM, or SC; 0.25–2 ml		

Mechanism of Action and Indications for Use

All local anesthetics have a similar mechanism of action and effect. The only difference or advantage of use lies with their potency, onset, duration, selectivity, and metabolism in the body.

Impulse transmission through nerves are mediated by the opening and closing of certain *voltage-gated ion channels*. These ionic channels are normally closed but will open in response to a change in voltage at the membrane. Of particular importance are the voltage-sensitive channels through which sodium and potassium ions enter and leave cells. Nerve axons in the resting state maintain a transmembrane potential of about −60 to −90 mV. This resting potential is brought about by the relative concentrations and permeabilities of sodium ions (extracellular component) and potassium ions (intracellular component) across the membrane. While in the resting state, the membrane is not permeable to sodium, but it is permeable to potassium ions through selective potassium channels. When an impulse stimulates the nerve, the resting potential or transmembrane potential becomes less negative, which allows the influx of sodium ions through the now open sodium channels, and cell depolarization occurs. At the peak of depolarization (approximately +30 mV), potassium channels open fully, allowing potassium ions to leave, resulting in repolarization. At the same time, sodium channels are closing, thus preventing more sodium from entering. This sequence of depolarization and repolarization occurs in about 1 to 2 ms and is known as an *action potential.* After repolarization, the sodium-potassium pump again reestablishes the transmembrane ionic gradients by transporting sodium out of the cell and allowing potassium back into the cell.

Local anesthetics prevent sodium influx after binding with sodium channels. By this mechanism, local anesthetics slow or prevent depolarization, which will eventually block the conduction of the action potential in nerve fibers. When the ability to generate an action potential is abolished, nerve fibers are essentially deadened to stimulation, resulting in a total loss of sensation to touch, temperature, and pressure, as well as pain and/or motor function from those nerves to which the local anesthetic was applied.

Different types of nerve fibers differ in their susceptibility to local anesthetic blockade. Nerve fibers are classified and grouped according to their axon diameter, whether they are myelinated, and their relative conduction velocity (in meters/second). Nerve fibers are placed in one of three fiber type groups: A, B, or C (Table 15.9). Local anesthetics have a high affinity for blocking fiber types B and C first, the smaller type A delta fibers next. Type A alpha fibers are the last to lose their function. Table 15.9 summarizes the physiologic response to blockade of these specific fiber types. Generally, the order of loss of function after exposure to a local anesthetic is: pain, temperature, touch, proprioception, skeletal muscle tone. In summary, the small, unmyelinated fibers (Type C) are blocked first by local anesthetics and the larger, myelinated fibers last (Type A).

Absorption of the local anesthetic away from the administration site may produce undesired systemic effects. Therefore, phenylephrine or epinephrine, potent vasoconstrictor agents (i.e., α-adrenoceptor agonists), are sometimes added to the anesthetic solution to diminish blood flow at the injection site, which not only reduces systemic absorption but also allows the local anesthetic to persist at the injection site for a longer period of time.

The ester type of local anesthetics (e.g., procaine) have relatively short durations of activity owing to their rapid degradation by plasma pseudocholinesterase (the average half-lives of these agents are usually less than 1 minute). The amide types (e.g., lidocaine) are largely metabolized in the liver and then excreted in the urine. As a consequence, toxicity from the amide type of local anesthetics may occur in patients with liver dysfunction. The amides' half-lives are considerably longer than the ester types, approximately 1.8 hours (lidocaine).

Local anesthetics are usually administered at their desired anatomic sites of action or in proximity to the nerves to be blocked and include the following clinical applications:

Table 15.9.
Classification of Nerve Fibers and Susceptibility to Block

Fiber Group	Location/Function	Axon Diameter (μm)	Myelinated	Conduction Velocity (m/sec)	Sensitivity to Block	Local Anesthetic Effects
Type A	Somatic motor and sensory fibers	Large	Heavy myelination			Blockade of these fibers results in the loss of the sensation of sharp pain, proprioceptive loss, loss of thermal and tactile sensation, and skeletal muscle relaxation.
Alpha - α	Proprioception*, motor	12–20		70–120	Mild	
Beta - β	Touch, pressure	5–12		30–70	Medium	
Gamma - γ	Muscle, spindles	3–6		15–30	Medium	
Delta - δ	Temperature, pain	2–5		12–30	Medium to strong	
Type B	Preganglionic autonomic fibers	Medium <3	Light myelination	3–15	Strong	Blockade of these fibers results in autonomic paralysis.
Type C		Small	No myelination			Blockade of these fibers results in loss of the sensations of itch, tickle, dull pain, and thermal sensation, as well as autonomic paralysis.
Dorsal root	Pain	0.4–1.2		0.5–2.3	Strong	
Sympathetic	Sympathetic postganglionic fibers	0.3–1.3		0.7–2.3	Strong	

*Awareness of posture, movement, and changes in equilibrium.
Adapted from Katzung BG. Basic and Clinical Pharmacology. 6th ed. Norwalk: Appleton & Lange, 1995.

- Topical administration for surface anesthesia: The local anesthetic is applied to mucous membranes of the nose, mouth, throat, tracheobronchial tree, eyes, urinary tract, or gastrointestinal tract to provide surface anesthesia. Formulations of topical anesthetics include ointments, creams, gels, jellies, sprays, lotions, liquids, viscous solutions, and aerosols. Many of these agents are available as OTC drugs.

  Lidocaine (Xylocaine, 1% solution) administered into the tracheobronchial tree of an intubated patient either by direct instillation through the endotracheal tube or by nebulization of the solution has been effective in overcoming reflexive gagging, coughing, and bronchospasm that accompanies patients with hyperreactive airways or those patients who experience reflex irritation due to movement of the endotracheal tube. By the same mechanism, lidocaine is therapeutically useful during bronchoscopy or endoscopy. Lidocaine (2.5% or 5% ointment or viscous solution) is also applied to the mucous membranes of the nose for its numbing effect before nasal intubation or bronchoscopy for the nonintubated patient. In addition, lidocaine is used as an anesthetic lubricant on endotracheal tubes, nasal airways, nasogastric tubes, bronchoscopic tubes, and endoscopic tubes. Benzocaine (Solarcaine, Unguentine) is a popular local anesthetic for application to the skin for superficial abrasions, minor burns, chickenpox, prickly heat, insect bites, and eczema. Topical local anesthetics are also useful in relieving sore throats.
- Peripheral nerve block: Depositing a local anesthetic onto or in proximity to individual nerves or groups of nerves called plexuses will result in anesthesia of the peripheral motor, sensory, and autonomic neural pathways. This technique, as well as spinal and epidural anesthesia, is referred to as regional anesthesia. Several types of surgical procedures are performed under regional anesthesia, including cervical plexus blocks for neck surgery, brachial plexus blocks for arm and hand procedures, and intercostal blocks for abdominal and thoracic wall surgeries.
- Epidural anesthesia: Epidural or peridural anesthesia is produced by injecting the local anesthetic into the space surrounding the dura mater of the spinal cord. Epidural anesthesia may be maintained by placement of a catheter into the proper anatomic location. Caudal anesthesia is produced by injecting the anesthetic into the sacral canal. Applications for this type of anesthesia include obstetric, perineal, and lower extremity procedures.
- Spinal anesthesia: Also known as *intrathecal* or *subarachnoid block,* spinal anesthesia is mediated by injection of the local anesthetic into the cerebrospinal fluid (CSF) of the spinal subarachnoid space. Inhibition of the spinal nerve roots and the dorsal root ganglia precipitate a sympathetic block, loss of sensation, and skeletal muscle relaxation.
- Infiltration anesthesia: Direct injection of a local anesthetic into skin or deeper structures to block the pain that accompanies superficial procedures such as su-

turing of wounds, skin or breast biopsy, arterial punctures, and insertion of central lines is called infiltration anesthesia.

Contraindications

Contraindications to the use of local anesthetic agents include hypersensitivity to local anesthetics, patients hypersensitive to para-aminobenzoic acid (a metabolite of procaine) or parabens (methylparaben is a preservative found in multiple-dose containers of the amide-type local anesthetics). Do not use preparations containing preservatives for spinal or epidural anesthesia. Large doses of a local anesthetic are contraindicated for patients with heart block. Because prilocaine induces the formation of methemoglobinemia, it is contraindicated for patients with methemoglobinemia. Chloroprocaine is not used for subarachnoid administration.

Precautions

1. Resuscitative equipment and drugs should be immediately available when local anesthetics are used.
2. Use with caution if inflammation or sepsis is present at the proposed injection site.
3. Some of these agents contain sulfites. Sulfite-containing local anesthetics should not be used for patients with hyperreactive airways.
4. Use amide-type local anesthetics cautiously, if at all, for patients with impaired hepatic function.
5. Local anesthetics rapidly cross the placenta and may adversely affect the fetus.
6. Solutions containing a vasopressor (e.g., epinephrine, phenylephrine) should be used with caution for patients with compromised blood supply. Individuals who may exhibit an exaggerated vasopressor response include patients with hypertension, peripheral vascular disease, heart block, or cerebral vascular insufficiency.
7. For infiltration or regional anesthesia: the local anesthetic should always be injected slowly, with frequent aspirations. Slow injections with frequent aspirations may also avoid systemic reactions as well as prevent intravascular injections.

Adverse Reactions

Most adverse reactions are dose-related and result from rapid absorption from the injection site.

CNS: Restlessness, anxiety, dizziness, tinnitus, blurred vision, nausea, vomiting, chills, pupil constriction.

Cardiovascular: Peripheral vasodilation, myocardial depression, hypotension (with spinal anesthesia), or hypertension, decreased cardiac output, heart block, bradycardia, ventricular arrhythmias, cardiac arrest.

Allergic: Urticaria, pruritus, erythema, sneezing, syncope, anaphylactoid symptoms (including hypotension).
Respiratory: Respiratory impairment, respiratory arrest.

Overdosage

High plasma levels as well as unintentional subarachnoid injection may precipitate convulsions and apnea. Maintaining a patent airway and assisted ventilation are of primary concern. If convulsions persist, small increments of thiopental or thiamylal (ultrashort-acting barbiturates) or diazepam (benzodiazepine) may be given.

Dosage and Administration

The local anesthetics are summarized in Table 15.10.

Table 15.10.
Injectable Local Anesthetic Agents

Anesthetic	Dosage	Onset (min)	Duration (hours)
Esters:			
Chloroprocaine hydrochloride (Nesacaine, Nesacaine-MPF)	***For most procedures:*** 1% to 2% solution. ***For infiltration, peripheral, epidural, or caudal block:*** 2% to 3% solution (without preservatives).	6–12	0.25–0.5
Procaine hydrochloride (Novocain)	***For infiltration anesthesia:*** 0.25% to 0.5% solution. ***For peripheral nerve block:*** 0.5% to 2% solution. ***For spinal anesthesia:*** 10% solution.	2–5	0.25–0.5
Tetracaine hydrochloride (Ponocaine HCl)	***For spinal anesthesia:*** 0.2% to 0.3% solution. ***For prolonged spinal anesthesia (2–3 hours):*** 1% solution.	up to 15	2–3
Amides:			
Bupivacaine hydrochloride (Marcaine HCl, Sensorcaine)	***For local infiltration:*** 0.25% solution. ***For lumbar epidural:*** 0.25%, 0.5%, or 0.75% solution. ***For subarachnoid block:*** 0.75% solution. ***For caudal block:*** 0.25% and 0.5% solutions. ***For peripheral nerve block:*** 0.25% and 0.5% solutions. ***For sympathetic block:*** 0.25% solution.	5	2–4
Etidocaine hydrochloride (Duranest HCl)	***For peripheral or epidural nerve block:*** 1% and 1.5% solutions	3–5	2–3
Lidocaine hydrochloride (Xylocaine HCl, Caine-1, Dilocaine, L-Caine, Lidoject-1, Nervocaine, Nulicaine)	***For percutaneous infiltration:*** 0.5% or 1% solution ***For IV regional infiltration:*** 0.5% solution ***For peripheral or sympathetic nerve block:*** 1% or 1.5% solution ***For central neural blocks:*** 1%, 1.5%, or 2% solution ***For spinal anesthesia:*** 5% solution with glucose ***For transtracheal injection:*** 4% solution	0.5–1	0.5–1
Mepivacaine hydrochloride (Carbocaine, Polocaine, Isocaine HCl)	***For peripheral nerve block:*** 1% or 2% solution ***For epidural or caudal blocks:*** 1%, 1.5%, or 2% solution ***For infiltration:*** 1% solution	3–5	0.75–1.5
Prilocaine hydrochloride (Citanest HCl)	***For local anesthesia by nerve block or infiltration:*** 4% solution	1–2	0.5–1.5

VI
Psychotherapeutic Agents

Three primary classes of drugs comprise the psychotherapeutic agents:

- Antianxiety agents
- Antipsychotic agents
- Antidepressants

ANTIANXIETY AGENTS

Anxiety is an extremely unpleasant sensation associated with various medical conditions. The individual experiences helplessness, apprehension, uneasiness, and distress during an anxiety attack. Other symptoms may include headache, pain, sweating, tachypnea, tachycardia, nausea, and palpitations. The symptoms may be mild in nature or quite severe, leading to interruption of normal functioning, lifestyle, work, and interpersonal relationships. The anxiety can become so counterproductive that it is psychologically paralyzing. At these times, the patient may require medication with an antianxiety or *anxiolytic* drug.

Drugs used to treat anxiety are CNS depressants employed for their sedative effect. The benzodiazepine derivatives are currently the most important drugs of choice for the management of anxiety disorders (see *Section IV*). Other agents include the carbamate derivatives (meprobamate), buspirone, and the piperazine antihistamine hydroxyzine.

Meprobamate (Equanil, Miltown, Neuramate, Meprospan) is the prototype for the propanediol carbamate antianxiety agents that exhibit selective effects at various sites in the CNS, including the thalamus and limbic system. It also seems to inhibit multineuronal spinal reflexes. Meprobamate is not commonly used as an antianxiety agent owing to the tendency of causing psychological and physical dependence as well as producing withdrawal symptoms (anorexia, anxiety, insomnia, muscle spasms, tremors) upon discontinuation of the drug. Additionally, meprobamate may precipitate seizures in epileptic patients. Meprobamate is available as tablets and sustained-release capsules. The usual oral adult dose is 1.2 to 1.6 g/day in three to four divided doses or 400 to 800 mg (sustained-release capsules) in the morning and at bedtime. As with all sedatives, the patient is cautioned to avoid alcohol and other CNS depressants while taking this drug.

Buspirone (BuSpar) is a member of a new series of antianxiety drugs that is not chemically related to the barbiturates, benzodiazepines, or other sedative-hypnotic agents. Its mechanism of action is unknown; however, in vitro, buspirone demonstrates a high affinity for serotonin receptors and a moderate affinity for brain D_2-dopaminergic receptors. It does not interact or affect GABA receptors. Buspirone does not seem to cause tolerance or psychological or physical dependence. Although buspirone is an effective antianxiety agent, it lacks the anticonvulsant and muscle relaxant effects of the benzodiazepines. Its most common adverse effects include dizziness, nausea, headache, nervousness, lightheadedness, and excitement. Buspirone is available as an oral preparation. The usual adult dose is 15 mg daily (5 mg three times a day). The patient is cautioned not to exceed 60 mg/day when titrating the optimal dose.

Hydroxyzine (Anxanil, Atarax, Rezine) possesses antihistaminic, antiemetic, and sedative properties. It seems to exert its sedative effects at subcortical areas of the CNS. As well as use as an antianxiety agent, hydroxyzine has been shown to be effective in the management of motion sickness, as a preanesthetic medication, for alcohol addiction, and for allergic reactions. The normal oral adult dose for symptomatic relief of anxiety is 50 to 100 mg four times per day.

ANTIPSYCHOTIC AGENTS

Mechanism of Action and Indications for Use

The term *psychosis* refers to a variety of mental disorders. Schizophrenia, in particular, is a type of psychosis that is manifest by a clear sensorium but distorted thought processes. The pathogenesis of schizophrenia is unknown; however, current views suggest that excessive CNS dopaminergic activity in the limbic system underlies the disorder. This is because drugs that act as CNS dopaminergic agonists, such as levodopa, amphetamines, and apomorphine, aggravate schizophrenia. The antipsychotic drugs are primarily employed in the treatment and management of schizophrenic patients. Other clinical uses of the antipsychotic drugs include the treatment and management of senile dementia of the Alzheimer type.

Generally, the antipsychotic agents target the limbic area of the brain to inhibit D_2-dopaminergic receptor transmission. By this mechanism, extreme emotions such as rage, fear, and aggression are blocked. Neuroleptic is a term synonymous with antipsychotic agents, which refers to the effects these agents have that differ from classical CNS depressants. Most of the neuroleptics have little efficacy as sedatives; they primarily act to diminish conditional behavioral responses and dampen neurophysiologic effects of stimuli on the forebrain. These agents cause a lack of initiative, emotion, and interest in the surrounding environment.

The antipsychotic agents produce a variety of effects owing to their activity at other dopaminergic receptor sites in the brain, including the basal ganglia, the CTZ of the medulla, and the hypothalamus. Blockade of dopamine receptors in the basal ganglia causes extrapyramidal syndrome symptoms such as tremors and muscle rigidity. The antipsychotic agents produce antiemetic effects owing to the blockade of dopamine receptors in the CTZ of the medulla. Thus, these agents are therapeutically useful in the treatment and management of nausea and vomiting. Hypothalamic dopamine blockade results in a reduced release of pituitary hormones, including growth hormone.

The side effects precipitated from the antipsychotic agents relate to their blocking activity at cholinergic receptor sites and at peripheral α-adrenoceptors. The anticholinergic action of these agents lead to tachycardia, urinary retention, blurred vision, and constipation, as well as a decrease in glandular secretion resulting in dry mouth and potential mucus plugging in the respiratory tract. Blockade of α-adrenoceptors mediate orthostatic hypotension and reflexive tachycardia caused by diffuse peripheral vasodilation.

Various groups of drugs have antipsychotic activity and are classified according to their chemical structures. Antipsychotic drugs include the phenothiazines, butyrophenones, thioxanthines, dihydroindolones, dibenzoxazepines, dibenzodiazepines, benzisoxazoles, and diphenylbutylpiperidines. Lithium (Eskalith, Lithonate, Lithobid) is a mood-stabilizing agent usually used in combination with other antipsychotic agents for the treatment of manic episodes of manic-depressive illness.

Contraindications

Contraindications to the use of antipsychotic agents include coma or severe depression, hypersensitivity to any antipsychotic component, bone marrow depression, subcortical brain damage, liver damage, coronary artery disease, and severe hypo- or hypertension.

Precautions

1. The antipsychotic agents may impair mental or physical abilities, especially during the first few days of therapy.
2. Potential of aspiration is possible owing to the suppression of the cough reflex by these agents.
3. Pneumonias may develop in patients using phenothiazine derivatives. Use with caution for patients with acute or chronic respiratory disorders such as asthma or emphysema.
4. Some of these agents have significant anticholinergic effects; use with caution for patients with glaucoma. An increase in side effects may be noted in patients who are receiving anticholinergics in addition to antipsychotic drugs.
5. Administer cautiously for patients with renal or hepatic dysfunction as well as patients with cardiovascular disease or mitral insufficiency.
6. Some antipsychotic agents contain sulfites that may cause allergic-type symptoms in patients with asthma.
7. Antipsychotic agents potentiate the effects of other CNS depressants (alcohol, barbiturates, opioid analgesics, general anesthetics, antianxiety agents).
8. Because of the inhibition of dopamine neurotransmission and suppression of the extrapyramidal system, these agents may produce Parkinsonism-type side effects (involuntary muscle movements, tremors).

Adverse Reactions

CNS: Cerebral edema, headache, weakness, tremor, staggering, twitching, jitteriness, ataxia, fatigue, insomnia, vertigo, drowsiness, tardive dyskinesia.

Cardiovascular: Hypotension, postural hypotension, hypertension, tachycardia (especially noted with rapid administration or a rapid increase in dosage), bradycardia, cardiac arrest, circulatory collapse. The phenothiazine derivatives are direct myocardial depressants and may produce cardiomegaly, congestive heart failure, or refractory arrhythmias.

Respiratory: Laryngospasm, bronchospasm, dyspnea, increased depth of ventilation, thickening of secretions.

Autonomic: Dry mouth, nasal congestion, nausea, vomiting, paresthesia, salivation, perspiration, constipation, diarrhea, polyuria.

Extrapyramidal: Pseudo-Parkinsonism, including drooling, tremors, shuffling gait, shaking, uncontrollable and involuntary muscle movements and contractions.

Hematologic: Eosinophilia, leukopenia, leukocytosis, anemia, thrombocytopenia, granulocytopenia, aplastic anemia, hemolytic anemia, agranulocytosis.

Adverse Behavioral Effects: Exacerbation of psychotic symptoms including hallucinations, catatonic-like states, lethargy, restlessness, hyperactivity, agitation, nocturnal confusion, bizarre dreams, depression, euphoria, excitement, paranoid reactions.

Allergic: Pruritis, angioneurotic edema, dry skin, jaundice, erythema, eczema, asthma, laryngeal edema, photosensitivity, anaphylactoid reactions, hair loss. Contact dermatitis may result from exposure to phenothiazine liquids.

Other: Blurred vision, neuroleptic malignant syndrome (fever, tachycardia, tachypnea, profuse diaphoresis).

Overdosage

Symptoms of antipsychotic drug overdose include CNS depression leading to somnolence, deep sleep, coma. Other overdose symptoms include restlessness, convulsions, fever, ECG changes, and cardiac arrhythmias. Treatment includes the usual supportive measures, ensuring a patent airway and adequate ventilation. IV phenytoin, 1 mg/kg, may be used for ventricular arrhythmias. Control convulsions with pentobarbital or diazepam. Do not use epinephrine for hypotension if the patient has been on chlorpromazine because this agent decreases the pressor effect of epinephrine and sometimes reverses its action. Norepinephrine or phenylephrine may be used instead.

Dosage and Administration

Select pharmacologic parameters of the antipsychotic drugs as well as their daily dosage ranges are listed in Table 15.11.

Table 15.11.
Antipsychotic Agents

Antipsychotic	Adult Daily Dosage Range (mg/day)	Anticholinergic Effects	Sedative Effects	Hypotensive Effects	Extrapyramidal Symptoms
Benzisoxazole:					
Risperidone (Risperdal)	4–16	+	+	+	±
Butyrophenone:					
Haloperidol (Haldol)	1–15 (up to 100 if necessary)	+	+	+	+++
Dibenzodiazepine:					
Clozapine (Clozaril)	300–900	+++	+++	+++	+
Dibenzoxazepine:					
Loxapine (Loxitane)	20–250	+	++	++	+++
Dihydroindolone:					
Molindone (Moban)	15–225	+	+	+	+++
Diphenylbutylpiperidine:					
Pimozide (Orap)	1–10	++	++	+	+++
Phenothiazines, Aliphatic:					
Chlorpromazine (Thorazine)	30–800	++	+++	+++	++
Promazine (Sparine)	40–1200	+++	++	++	++
Triflupromazine (Vesprin)	60–150	+++	+++	++	++
Phenothiazines, Piperdine:					
Mesoridazine (Serentil)	30–400	+++	+++	++	+
Thioridazine (Mellaril)	150–800	+++	+++	+++	+
Phenothiazines, Piperazine:					
Acetophenazine (Tindal)	60–120	+	++	+	+++
Fluphenazine (Prolixin, Permitil)	0.5–40	+	+	+	+++
Perphenazine (Trilafon)	12–64	+	+	+	+++
Prochlorperazine (Compazine)	15–150	+	++	+	+++
Trifluoperazine (Stelazine)	2–40	+	+	+	+++
Thioxanthenes:					
Chlorprothixene (Taractan)	75–600	++	+++	++	++
Thiothixene (Navane)	8–30	+	+	+	+++

+, infrequent incidence of side effects.
++, occasional incidence of side effects.
+++, frequent incidence of side effects.

ANTIDEPRESSANT AGENTS

Depression, one of the most common psychiatric disorders, is a condition that is manifested by a significantly lowered mood or mental outlook for a prolonged period of time (longer than 2 weeks) that prevents an individual from functioning normally. The mood disturbance is usually accompanied by other symptoms, such as insomnia, changes in appetite, psychomotor changes, loss of interest in the surrounding environment or pleasure, feelings of worthlessness or guilt, and thoughts leaning toward suicide or death.

There are three primary types of depression. Reactive or secondary depression is a condition that is precipitated by some traumatic event, such as the stress caused by the death of a child or news of terminal cancer. Reactive depression is the most common type of depression. Major or unipolar depression is a result of an endogenous biological change caused by a genetic disturbance. Major depressive disorder is also known as a primary depressive disorder because it originates from some biological change occurring within the body. Bipolar depression, also known as "manic depression," is characterized by alternating high and low mood swings.

The onset and duration of depression are believed to be associated with a deficiency of the CNS neurotransmitters norepinephrine and serotonin. Antidepressant agents ultimately lead to an increase in the activity and duration of these neurotransmitters and are classified according to their primary mechanism of action: they either block neurotransmitter uptake (norepinephrine and/or serotonin [5-HT]) or they are inhibitors of MAO.

Agents that Block Neurotransmitter Uptake

Mechanism of Action and Indications for Use

The tricyclic antidepressants (TCAs)—so called because they have a characteristic three-ring nucleus—are the largest group of drugs that have specific blocking action on the neuronal uptake of norepinephrine and serotonin, thus prolonging the duration and activity of these neurotransmitters. These agents also seem to antagonize the effects of norepinephrine at presynaptic α_2-adrenoceptor sites, causing an enhanced release of norepinephrine at adrenergic nerve terminals (see Fig. 2.10). Maximal antidepressive effects usually occur after 2 to 3 weeks of continuous therapy with these agents. The reason for this seems to be the subsequent down-regulation of β-adrenoceptors and serotonin receptors that occurs from chronic neuronal uptake blockade.

The relative potencies of these agents vary according to their ability to block norepinephrine versus serotonin uptake. Most tricyclic compounds have sedative and antihistaminic effects in addition to their antidepressant effects. These agents also have both central and peripheral anticholinergic activity as well as peripheral α-adrenoceptor antagonistic activity and can produce orthostatic hypotension, especially in elderly patients.

The tricyclic antidepressants have occasionally been used as hypnotics owing to their sedative property. These agents, especially the imipramine-like drugs, reduce the number of awakenings by suppressing the total time spent in rapid-eye-movement (REM) sleep.

Although the tricyclic antidepressants are effective and relatively inexpensive, the antimuscarinic, antihistaminic, and α-adrenoceptor blocking actions of these agents contribute to their toxicity. A series of second-generation antidepressants with diverse structures have been developed that have a lower incidence of undesirable side effects because they lack significant antagonistic activity at muscarinic, adrenergic, and histaminic receptors. Such agents include amoxapine, bupropion, maprotiline, trazodone, and venlafaxine. Serotonin selective reuptake inhibitors (SSRIs) have also been introduced for clinical use as antidepressant agents. Fluoxetine (Prozac), the prototypic SSRI, does not adversely affect the autonomic and cardiovascular systems as does the tricyclic antidepressants. The pharmacologic activity of these agents are summarized in Table 15.12.

Current clinical uses of the antidepressants that block neurotransmitter uptake include the relief of symptoms associated with depression (especially endogenous type), the management and control of acute episodes of anxiety associated with panic attacks, treatment of obsessive-compulsive disorder (clomipramine), and treatment of manic-depressive disorders. Investigational uses of these agents include control of acute pain (in combination with narcotic analgesics), prevention of migraine and cluster headaches (amitriptyline), treatment of obstructive sleep apnea (protriptyline, see *Section I*), symptomatic management and treatment of peptic ulcers (doxepin, trimipramine), and treatment of attention-deficit disorders (desipramine).

Contraindications

Contraindications include severe renal or hepatic impairment, simultaneous use of MAO inhibitors, narrow-angle glaucoma, acute recovery phase of myocardial infarction, and history of seizure activity.

Precautions

1. Coadministration of TCAs with electroconvulsive therapy may increase the hazards of these agents.
2. Coadministration of TCAs with anticholinergics may potentiate the side effects of these agents.
3. Coadministration of TCAs with barbiturates may produce additive central and ventilatory depressant effects.
4. In high doses, TCAs may precipitate cardiac arrhythmias and sinus tachycardia and prolong conduction time. Use with extreme caution for patients with cardiovascular disorders.

Table 15.12.
Pharmacologic Properties and Dosages of Antidepressants that Block Neurotransmitter Uptake

Antidepressant	Usual Adult Daily Dosage Range (mg/day)	NE Blocking Activity	Serotonin (5-HT) Blocking Activity	Anticholinergic Effects	Sedative Effects	Hypotensive Effects
Tricyclics—Tertiary Amines:						
Amitriptyline (Elavil)	50–300	++	++++	++++	++++	++
Clomipramine (Anafranil)	25–250	++	+++++	+++	+++	++
Doxepin (Sinequan, Adapin)	25–300	+	++	++	+++	++
Imipramine (Tofranil)	30–300	++	++++	++	++	+++
Trimipramine (Surmontil)	50–300	+	+	++	+++	++
Tricyclics—Secondary Amines:						
Amoxapine[a] (Asendin)	50–600	+++	++	+++	++	+
Desipramine (Norpramin, Pertofrane)	25–300	++++	++	+	+	+
Nortriptyline (Aventyl, Pamelor)	30–100	++	+++	++	++	+
Proriptyline (Vivactil)	15–60	++++	++	+++	+	+
Tetracyclic:						
Maprotiline (Ludiomil)	50–225	+++	±	++	++	+
Serotonin Selective:						
Fluoxetine (Prozac)	20–80	±	+++++	±	±	±
Paroxetine (Paxil)	10–50	±	+++++	—	±	—
Sertraline (Zoloft)	50–200	±	+++++	—	±	—
Other:						
Bupropion[b] (Wellbutrin)	200–450	±	±	++	++	+
Trazodone (Desyrel)	150–600	—	+++	+	++	++
Venlafaxine (Effexor)	75–375	+++	+++	—	—	—

[a]Also blocks dopamine receptors.
[b]Inhibits dopamine uptake.
— = No effect.
± = Little to no effect.
+ = Slight effect.
++ = Moderate effect.
+++ = High effect.
++++ = Very high effect.
+++++ = Highest effect.

5. Patients should observe caution when performing tasks that require mental alertness, coordination, and dexterity owing to the potential mental or physical impairment that the TCAs produce.

Adverse Reactions

Most Common: Sedation, anticholinergic effects (blurred vision, dry mouth, tachycardia, constipation, urinary retention), headache, muscle twitching, weight gain.

CNS: Anxiety, restlessness, agitation, fever, insomnia, nightmares, irritability, dizziness, hallucinations, tremors, extrapyramidal symptoms, paresthesia, seizures.

Cardiovascular: Orthostatic hypotension, arrhythmias, palpitations, congestive heart failure, infarction, heart block, ECG changes.

GI: Nausea, anorexia, vomiting, diarrhea, cramping, epigastric distress, stomatitis.

Hematologic: Eosinophilia, leukopenia, thrombocytopenia, agranulocytosis, bone marrow depression.

Allergic: Skin rash, pruritis, urticaria, photosensitization, edema, fever.

Miscellaneous: Altered liver function (including jaundice), parotid gland enlargement, flushing, sweating, nasal congestion, lacrimation.

Overdosage

Overdose causes CNS symptoms, including confusion, agitation, hyperreflexia, seizures, hallucinations, and autonomic effects such as dilated pupils, flushing, and hyperpyrexia. Cardiovascular complications include tachycardia, arrhythmias, pulmonary edema, hypotension, and possibly ventricular fibrillation.

Treatment consists of supportive care: ensure an adequate airway, oxygenation, and ventilation, as well as monitoring cardiac rhythm and vital signs. No specific antidotes are known.

Dosage and Administration

The antidepressants that block neuronal uptake of norepinephrine and/or serotonin are listed in Table 15.12.

MAO Inhibitors

Mechanism of Action and Indications for Use

MAO is an enzyme that is widely distributed throughout the body and is responsible for the degradation (inactivation) of the biologic amines, including norepinephrine, epinephrine, and serotonin. Drugs that block MAO activity cause an increase in the concentration of these amines, which is the basis for their antidepressant activity.

MAO inhibitors are indicated for patients with atypical (exogenous) depression and for some patients who are unresponsive to other antidepressant therapy. These drugs are rarely used owing to their potential severe adverse effects and high toxicity (see below).

Contraindications

Contraindications to MAO inhibitors include hypersensitivity to these agents, pheochromocytoma, congestive heart failure, cardiovascular disease, and a history of liver disease or impairment of renal function.

Precautions

1. Use MAO inhibitors with caution for patients with epilepsy, diabetes, depression accompanying drug or alcohol addiction, chronic brain syndrome, history of anginal attacks, and pregnancy and lactation.
2. Effects of sympathomimetic drugs may be potentiated, resulting in severe hypertension, headache, and possibly cerebrovascular hemorrhage.
3. Hypertensive reactions may occur in patients taking MAO inhibitors who ingest certain types of foods containing tyramine, a pressor substance. Such foods include sour cream, beer and ale, red wines, cheeses, chicken livers, aged meats, yeasts, overripe avocados, yogurt, fermented sausages, bananas, raisins, as well as caffeine, chocolate, and licorice.
4. Concurrent use of MAO inhibitors and certain tricyclic antidepressants (or within 10 days of each other) may cause severe adverse reactions such as severe hypertension, convulsions, fever, circulatory collapse, delirium, tremor, and coma.
5. Coadministration of MAO inhibitors with antihypertensive drugs may potentiate orthostatic hypotension.
6. Coadministration of MAO inhibitors with CNS depressants (alcohol, anesthetics, narcotics, and sedative-hypnotics) may result in respiratory arrest, hypotension, shock, and coma.
7. MAO inhibitors may reduce the efficacy of antiepileptic drugs.
8. The most serious reactions with use of these agents involves changes in blood pressure that may precipitate a hypertensive crisis. These drugs should be used with extreme caution for elderly or debilitated patients and for patients with hypertension and cardiovascular or cerebrovascular disease. The first symptom of a hypertensive crisis may be a headache.
9. MAO inhibitors may mask anginal pain that would otherwise serve as a warning of myocardial ischemia. This is due to their peripheral vasodilatory, hypotensive actions.

Adverse Reactions

Most Common: Orthostatic hypotension, dizziness, weakness, fatigue, jitteriness, hyperactivity, insomnia, GI disturbances, headache, palpitations, dry mouth, blurred vision, and hyperhidrosis.

CNS: Vertigo, tremors, hypomania, euphoria, confusion, memory impairment, ataxia, excessive sweating, drowsiness, delirium, convulsions, hallucinations.

Cardiovascular: Palpitations, tachycardia.

Hematologic: Leukopenia, hypochromic anemia, agranulocytosis, thrombocytopenia.

Allergic: Skin rash, photosensitivity.

Ophthalmic: Glaucoma, nystagmus.

GU: Incontinence, dysuria, urinary retention.

GI: Constipation, nausea, diarrhea, abdominal pain.

Miscellaneous: Black tongue, sweating, hypernatremia, hypermetabolic syndrome, sexual disturbances, edema of the glottis.

Overdosage

Symptoms of overdose include restlessness, tachycardia, ventilatory depression, hypotension, confusion, incoherence, convulsions, and shock. Treatment includes emesis or gastric lavage. Protect the airway from possible aspiration; use oxygenation and mechanical ventilation as required.

Dosage and Administration

The dosages of the MAO inhibitors are listed in Table 15.13.

VII
Anticonvulsant Agents

The second most common neurologic disorder, after stroke, is epilepsy. Between 0.5% and 1.5% of the population of the USA has epilepsy. Epilepsy is a chronic

Table 15.13.
MAO Inhibitor Antidepressants

Antidepressant	Usual Dosage Range
Isocarboxazid (Marplan)	*Initially:* 30 mg/day. Maintenance doses range between 10 and 20 mg/day. Reduce to maintenance levels as soon as possible.
Pheneizine (Nardil)	*Initially:* 15 mg t.i.d. Reduce slowly to maintenance levels, usually 15 mg every 1–2 days.
Tranylcypromine (Parnate)	*Initially:* 20–30 mg/day. Reduce to 10–20 mg/day as needed.

CNS disorder characterized by recurrent seizures that unexpectantly occur as a result of abnormal neuronal discharges in the CNS. The causes of epilepsy are quite diverse and include neurological diseases, infection, head injury, and genetic disturbances. *Status epilepticus* is a condition in which there is a series of rapid, repetitive seizures. Status epilepticus may be fatal unless terminated quickly.

Seizures are broadly classified as being partial or generalized. Partial, or focal seizures are those in which there is a localized onset in the brain. Partial seizures are of three primary types: simple, complex, and partial becoming generalized. The primary difference between simple and complex partial seizures is that in simple seizures, the individual remains alert and conscious and can remember the attack in detail, whereas in complex seizures, the individual has no recollection of the attack and usually exhibits confused behavior during the attack or may lose consciousness. The last type of partial seizures are those that immediately precede a generalized tonic-clonic (grand mal) seizure, as described below.

Generalized seizures are those in which there is bilateral involvement of both cerebral hemispheres. Types of generalized seizures include the following:

- Tonic seizures, which produce muscle rigidity and loss of consciousness.
- Clonic seizures, which consist of alternating relaxation and contraction of skeletal muscles with loss of consciousness.
- Tonic-clonic (grand mal) seizures. This type of generalized seizure is quite dramatic and is characterized by tonic rigidity of all extremities. Tongue and cheek biting may occur with the initial jaw closure. Urinary and fecal incontinence may also occur. The tonic phase usually lasts 20 to 40 seconds and is followed by the clonic phase, in which there is alternating relaxation with stiffening of the skeletal muscles for an additional 20 to 40 seconds.
- Absence (petit mal) seizures. Absence seizures usually begin in childhood (within the first decade of life) and may occur up to hundreds of times per day. These seizures are characterized by sudden onset and rapid cessation with a duration of 5 to 30 seconds. During the attack, the individual briefly lapses into unconsciousness. Absence seizures may be accompanied by clonic jerking of the eyelids, head, or extremities. After the seizure, the individual is alert and usually able to resume normal activity.

Mechanism of Action and Indications for Use

Total seizure control may require a combination of two or even three types of anticonvulsant drugs. Anticonvulsant agents do not cure the affliction that precipitated the seizure attack but do allow the epileptic or seizure patient to function normally.

Various classes of drugs have therapeutic usefulness as anticonvulsant agents.

The barbiturates mephobarbital, phenobarbital, and thiopental as well as certain benzodiazepines (e.g., diazepam, clonazepam, clorazepate) have demonstrated efficacy as anticonvulsant agents (see *Section IV* of this chapter). Other anticonvulsant agents include the hydantoins (ethotoin, mephenytoin, phenytoin), the oxazolidinediones (paramethadione, trimethadione), and the succinimides (ethosuximide, methsuximide, phensuximide). The remaining anticonvulsant agents include primidone, acetazolamide, carbamazepine, felbamate, gabapentin, magnesium sulfate, phenacemide, and valproic acid.

The anticonvulsant agents all possess the ability to depress abnormal neuronal discharges in the CNS, thus inhibiting seizure activity. The primary site of action of many of these agents seems to be the motor cortex, in which they either promote the efflux of sodium ions from neurons or decrease the influx of sodium ions across cell membranes. By this mechanism, anticonvulsant agents depress nerve transmission at the motor cortex and stabilize the threshold against hyperexcitability caused by excessive stimulation. Some anticonvulsant agents also have significant influence on GABA-mediated transmission within the CNS in which they enhance the inhibitory action of GABA.

Magnesium and acetazolamide are two drugs that have unusual mechanisms of action in reference to their anticonvulsant activity. Magnesium controls seizures by blocking neuromuscular transmission and decreasing the amount of acetylcholine liberated at the motor endplate. With IV use, magnesium's onset of anticonvulsant activity is immediate and usually lasts for about 30 minutes. Magnesium also has a CNS depressant effect. Acetazolamide is a diuretic that is classified as a carbonic anhydrase inhibitor (see also Chapter 17). Inhibition of carbonic anhydrase in the CNS seems to reduce abnormal, paradoxical, excessive discharge from CNS neurons. Acetazolamide's anticonvulsant action may also be due in part to acidosis produced by acetazolamide therapy.

Anticonvulsant agents, also known as antiepileptic drugs, are effective in controlling seizures occurring in patients with epilepsy or seizures that occur as a result from some type of acute CNS disturbance (such as that which occurs from trauma, hyperthermia, infection, or drug overdose).

Contraindications

Contraindications to the use of anticonvulsant agents include hypersensitivity to these agents, hepatic abnormalities, hematologic disorders, heart block, and porphyria. Phenytoin is contraindicated for patients with sinus bradycardia, sinoatrial block, second- and third-degree AV block and in patients with Adams-Stokes syndrome (phenytoin depresses spontaneous depolarization in ventricular tissues). Carbamazepine is contraindicated for patients with a history of bone marrow depression. See *Section IV* for contraindications of using barbiturate and benzodiazepine preparations.

Precautions

1. Abrupt withdrawal of some of these agents may precipitate absence (petit mal) seizures or status epilepticus.
2. Hydantoins are not indicated in seizures due to hypoglycemia or other metabolic causes.
3. Use these agents with caution for patients with hypotension and severe myocardial insufficiency.
4. Generally, the anticonvulsant agents that control grand mal seizures are not effective for petit mal seizures. If both conditions are present, combined drug therapy may be required.
5. Succinimides may increase the frequency of grand mal seizures in some patients.
6. Some of these agents, especially the oxazolidinediones and primidone, may produce drowsiness or blurred vision. Patients should be advised to observe caution when driving or performing tasks that require mental alertness.
7. Myasthenia gravis-like symptoms have been associated with the chronic use of the oxazolidinediones.
8. Carbamazepine has mild anticholinergic activity; use cautiously for patients with glaucoma.
9. The safety and efficacy of many of these agents have not been established for children younger than 6 years of age, pregnancy, and lactation.
10. Phenacemide can produce serious side effects as well as direct organ toxicity. Do not use this agent unless other anticonvulsants are ineffective in controlling seizures.
11. Because magnesium is primarily excreted by the kidneys, parenteral use of magnesium should be avoided for patients with renal insufficiency.

For barbiturate and benzodiazepine precautions and adverse reactions, refer to *Section IV* of this chapter.

Adverse Reactions

Most Common: Sluggishness, ataxia, confusion, slurred speech, drowsiness, GI distress (nausea, upset, cramping pain, diarrhea), abnormal behavior, fatigue.

CNS: Ataxia, insomnia, motor twitching, transient nervousness, tremor, lethargy, headache.

Cardiovascular: Cardiovascular collapse CNS depression, hypotension (through rapid IV administration).

GI: Nausea, vomiting, diarrhea, constipation.

Hematologic: Thrombocytopenia, leukopenia, granulocytopenia, agranulocytosis, pancytopenia.

Miscellaneous: Rash, photosensitivity.

Table 15.14. Nonbarbiturate Nonbenzodiazepine Anticonvulsant Agents

Anticonvulsant	Labeled Indications	Usual Dosage Range
Hydantoins:		
Ethotoin (Peganone)	Tonic-clonic Psychomotor	*Adults:* 250 mg q.i.d. (maximum: 3 g/day) *Children:* 750 mg/day (maximum: 1000 mg/day, based on age and weight)
Mephenytoin (Mesantoin)	Tonic-clonic Psychomotor Focal	*Adults:* 50–100 mg/day (maximum: 600 mg/day) *Children:* 100–400 mg/day
Phenytoin (Dilantin)	Tonic-clonic Psychomotor	*Adults:* PO: 100 mg t.i.d. (maximum: 400 mg/day) IV: for status epilepticus: 150–250 mg, repeat in 30 minutes if required. *Children:* 5 mg/kg/day in two to three divided doses (maximum: 8 mg/kg/day in children <6 years old)
Oxazolidinediones:		
Paramethadione (Paradione)	Absence	*Adults:* 300–600 mg t.i.d., q.i.d. *Children:* 300–900 mg/day in three to four divided doses
Trimethadione (Tridione)	Absence	*Adults:* 300 mg t.i.d. *Children:* 300–900 mg/day in three to four divided doses
Succinimides:		
Ethosuximide (Zarontin)	Absence	*Adults:* 500 mg/day (maximum: 1500 mg/day) *Children:* 250 mg/day
Methsuximide (Celontin)	Absence	*Adults:* 300 mg/day (maximum: 1200 mg/day)
Phensuximide (Milontin)	Absence	*Adults:* 500–1000 mg b.i.d., t.i.d. (maximum: 3 g/day) *Children:* 600–1200 mg b.i.d., t.i.d.
Miscellaneous:		
Acetazolamide (Diamox)	As an adjunct in the control of petit mal seizures or other absence seizures	*Adults:* 250 mg/day (maximum: 1000 mg/day—usually administered in combination with another anticonvulsant agent)
Carbamazepine (Epitol, Tegretol)	Grand mal seizures (with phenytoin) Psychomotor (alone or with primidone or phenytoin) Mixed seizures or complex partial seizures	*Adults and children >12 yr:* 200 mg b.i.d. (maximum: 1200 mg/day) *Children 6–12 yr:* 100 mg b.i.d. (maximum: 800 mg/day)
Felbamate (Felbatol)	Partial (adults) Partial/generalized associated with Lennox-Gastaut syndrome (children)	*Adults:* 1200 mg/day in three to four divided doses (maximum: 3600 mg/day) *Children:* add at a rate of 15 mg/kg/day in divided doses while reducing the dose of other anticonvulsant(s) (maximum: 45 mg/kg/day)
Gabapentin (Neurontin)	Partial seizures, with or without generalized seizures	*Adults:* 900–1800 mg/day in three divided doses (maximum: 3600 mg/day)
Magnesium sulfate	Seizures caused by toxemia of pregnancy and other conditions of abnormally low levels of plasma magnesium	*Adults:* IV: 1–4 g of 10% or 20% solution IM: 1–5 g of 25% or 50% solution
Phenacemide (Phenurone)	Severe mixed psychomotor	*Adults:* 250–500 mg t.i.d. (maximum: 3 g/day) *Children:* 50% of the adult dose
Primidone (Mysoline)	Tonic-clonic Psychomotor Focal	*Adults:* 100–125 mg/day (maintenance range: 250 mg t.i.d., q.i.d.) *Children:* 50 mg/day (maintenance range: 125–250 mg t.i.d.)
Valproic acid (Depakene, Depakote)	Simple and complex absence seizures, including petit mal. Adjunct in the treatment of multiple-seizure types.	*Adults:* 15 mg/kg/day (maximum, 60 mg/kg/day)

Overdosage

Symptoms of overdose include confusion, sleepiness, and unsteadiness; CNS depression including coma with ventilatory depression may follow massive overdosage. Treatment includes general supportive care. An adequate airway must be maintained, and oxygenation and ventilation must be ensured as required.

Dosage and Administration

The nonbarbiturate nonbenzodiazepine anticonvulsant agents with their dosages and specific indications for use are listed in Table 15.14. For the anticonvulsant dose of the barbiturates and benzodiazepines, refer to Tables 15.4 and 15.5, respectively.

REFERENCES/RECOMMENDED READING

Akil H, et al. Endogenous opioids: biology and function. Annu Rev Neurosci 7:233, 1984.

Ananth J, Johnson K. Psychotropic and medical drug interactions. Psychother Psychosom 58:178, 1992.

Baden JM, Rice SA. Metabolism and toxicity of inhaled anesthetics. In: Miller RD, ed. Anesthesia. 4th ed. New York: Churchill Livingstone, 1994.

Bairam A, et al. Doxapram for the initial treatment of idiopathic apnea of prematurity. Biol Neonate 61:209, 1992.

Balant-Gorgia AE, Balant LP, Andreoli A. Pharmacokinetic optimisation of the treatment of psychosis. Clin Pharmacokinet 25(3):217, 1993.

Beaver WT. Impact of non-narcotic analgesics on pain management. Am J Med 84(Suppl 5A):3, 1988.

Brodie MJ, et al. New and potential anticonvulsants. Lancet 336:425, 1990.

Carpenter RL, et al. Extent of metabolism of inhaled anesthetics in humans. Anesthesiology 65:201, 1986.

Covino BG. Pharmacology of local anaesthetic agents. Br J Anaesth 58:701, 1986.

Davis PJ, Cook DR. Clinical pharmacokinetics of the newer intravenous anesthetic agents. Clin Pharmacokinet 11:18, 1986.

Drug Facts and Comparisons. 49th ed. St. Louis: Facts and Comparisons, 1995.

Gerner RH. Treatment of acute mania. Psychiatr Clin North Am 16:443, 1993.

Greenblatt DJ. Basic pharmacokinetic principles and their application to psychotropic drugs. J Clin Psychiatry 54(Suppl 9):8, 1993.

Herregods L, et al. Propofol combined with nitrous oxide-oxygen for induction and maintenance of anesthesia. Anaesthesia 42:360, 1987.

Gilman AG, Goodman LS, Rall TW, Murad F. Goodman and Gilman's The Pharmacological Basis of Therapeutics. 8th ed. New York: McGraw Hill, Inc., 1993.

Glod C. Psychopharmacology and clinical practice. Nurs Clin North Am 26(2):375, 1991.

Katzung BG. Basic and Clinical Pharmacology. 6th ed. Norwalk: Appleton & Lange, 1995.

Levinson DF. Pharmacologic treatment of schizophrenia. Clin Ther 13:326, 1991.
Meldrum BS. GABAergic mechanisms in the pathogenesis and treatment of epilepsy. Br J Pharmacol 27:3S, 1989.
Miller RD. Anesthesia. 3rd ed. New York: Churchill Livingstone, 1990.
Pasternak GW. Pharmacological mechanisms of opioid analgesics. Clin Neuropharmacol 16(1):1, 1993.
Physicians' Desk Reference. 49th ed. Montvale, NJ: Medical Economics, 1995.
Porter RJ, Theodore WH. Recognizing and classifying epileptic seizures and epileptic syndromes. In: Neurologic Clinics: Epilepsy. Philadelphia: WB Saunders, 1986.
Reves JG, et al. Midazolam: pharmacology and uses. Anesthesiology 62:310, 1985.
Schwartz JT, Brotman AW. A clinical guide to antipsychotic drugs. Drugs 44(6):981, 1992.
Scholtes FB, Renier WO, Meinardi H. Generalized convulsive status epilepticus: pathophysiology and treatment. Pharm World Sci 15:17, 1993.
Shantz D, Spitz M. What you need to know about seizures. Nursing 23(11):34, 1993.
Sheikh JI. Anxiety disorders and their treatment. Clin Geriatr Med 8:411, 1992.
Simonds WF. The molecular basis of opioid receptor function. Endocr Rev 9:200, 1988.
Stein C. Peripheral mechanisms of opioid analgesia. Anesth Analg 76:182, 1993.
Thomson AH, Brodie MJ. Pharmacokinetic optimisation of anticonvulsant therapy. Clin Pharmacokinet 23:216, 1992.
Tucker GT. Pharmacokinetics of local anaesthetics. Br J Anaesth 58:717, 1986.
VanValkenburg C, Kluznik JC, Merrill R. New uses of anticonvulsant drugs in psychosis. Drugs 44:326, 1992.
Vissering T. Pharmacologic agents for pain management. Crit Care Nurs Clin North Am 3(1):17, 1991.
Vitale R. Pharmacology of conscious sedation. Images 12(1):7, 1993.
Volpicelli JR, et al. Naltrexone in the treatment of alcohol dependence. Arch Gen Psychiatry 49:876, 1992.
Votey SR, et al. Flumazenil: a new benzodiazepine antagonist. Ann Emerg Med 20:181, 1991.
Waugaman W, Foster S. New advances in anesthesia. Nurs Clin North Am 26(2):451, 1991.

ANTI-INFECTIVE AGENTS 16

In this chapter, the broad range of anti-infective agents are subdivided into five major categories: 1) the antibacterial (antibiotic) agents, 2) the antimycobacterial agents, 3) the antifungal agents, 4) the antiviral agents, and 5) the anti-infective agents specific for *Pneumocystis carinii*. Because of the wide variety of anti-infective agents that are currently available, the primary purpose of this chapter is to focus on the most commonly used anti-infective agents that are indicated for use in respiratory tract infections and those agents used for infections in critically ill patients. Table 16.1 summarizes some important dates in the history of microbiology and antibiotic development. Table 16.2 summarizes some of the various anti-infective agents used for specific infections.

CLASSIFICATION OF ANTI-INFECTIVE AGENTS

Several methods are used to classify and group the antimicrobial agents, many of which are based on the agent's chemical structure or mechanism of action. The following summarizes some of the more common methods used to classify these agents:

CATEGORY I: Agents that have the ability to inhibit the synthesis of the bacterial cell wall or to activate certain enzymes that disrupt the bacterial cell wall. Agents within this group include the penicillins, cephalosporins, vancomycin, and the antifungal agents such as ketoconazole and miconazole.

CATEGORY II: Agents that act directly on the microbe's cell membrane, causing leakage of the intracellular components. Agents within this group include amphotericin B, nystatin, and the detergents polymyxin and colistimethate.

CATEGORY III: Agents that disrupt the functions of the bacterial ribosomes, causing the inhibition of protein synthesis. Agents within this group include chloramphenicol, clindamycin, erythromycin (macrolides), and the tetracyclines.

Table 16.1.
Some Important Dates in the History of Microbiology and Antibiotic Development

Year	Accomplishment
1546	Girolamo Fracastoro of Verona suggested that a mysterious contagion could be passed from person to person through the air or by objects touched by people. Little attention was paid to these remarks. Disease, after all, was associated with magic and mysticism.
1676	Anton van Leeuwenhoek developed a crude lens system that magnified objects about 200 times. During the course of his work, he discovered tiny microbes, which he called "wee beasties." During a 50-year period, van Leeuwenhoek wrote more than 200 letters describing the structure of thread-like fungi, several forms of bacteria and their movement, and the structure of the protozoa known today as the *paramecium* and *amoeba*. Even with these discoveries, microorganisms were just idle curiosities, and nothing more. Van Leeuwenhoek invited no one to work with him and showed no one the construction of his microscopes. By these actions, the development of microbiology was delayed almost 100 years until the instrumentation and the method of associating microbes with disease came together.
1859	Successful publication of Darwin's *On the Origin of Species* showed that the human body was susceptible to the laws of nature. It followed then that disease was a biological phenomenon apart from magic and mysticism and the involvement of microbes was a possibility that bore consideration.
1860 to 1885	Louis Pasteur disproved the theory of spontaneous generation, discovered that fermentation is caused by living yeasts, discovered immunization techniques, and developed the rabies vaccine.
	Robert Koch isolated the tubercle and cholera bacilli, developed pure culture techniques for microorganisms, and presented the germ theory of disease (proved that bacteria could be isolated and shown to cause disease).
	Christian Gram discovered and developed the Gram stain technique.
1870 to 1914	The "Golden Age of Microbiology." Most agents of bacterial disease were identified and cultivated.
1908	Salvarsan (the first chemotherapeutic agent) was developed by Paul Ehrlich.
1928	Sir Alexander Fleming isolated and identified penicillin.
1935	Sulfanilamide was discovered and developed. Sulfanilamide quickly became the principal agent for the treatment of war-related infections.
1945	Sir Alexander Fleming, Ernst Boris Chain, and Sir Howard W. Florey received the Nobel Prize for discovery and development of penicillin. The discovery of the chemotherapeutic effects of sulfanilamide led to a renewed interest in penicillin. Penicillin was reisolated and made available for war-related infections. Since the 1940s, penicillin has remained the most important of the antibiotics due to its low cost and the broad use of the thousands of penicillin derivatives.
1949	The first broad-spectrum antibiotic, chloramphenicol, was introduced.
1950s	The β-lactam nucleus of the penicillin molecule was identified and synthesized, thereby creating new penicillins.
1952	Selman Waksman received the Nobel Prize for the discovery and development of streptomycin. Erythromycin was also discovered and developed at this time and was later shown to be a valuable antibiotic during outbreaks of atypical pneumonia in the 1970s.
1953	Tetracycline, a broad-spectrum antibiotic, was discovered and developed.
1954	John F. Enders, Thomas H. Weller, and Frederick C. Robbins received the Nobel Prize for cultivation of the polio viruses.
1957	Amphotericin B, the drug of choice for serious systemic fungal infections, was introduced.
1958	Vancomycin, especially useful for severe staphylococcal diseases in which penicillin allergy or resistance exists, was introduced.
1963	Ampicillin, a valuable agent against certain Gram-negative rods and organisms of gonorrhea and meningococcal meningitis, was introduced.
1964	Nalidixic acid, the prototype of the quinolone group of drugs, was synthesized by Lesher et al. (1962) and introduced into clinical use.
1966	Gentamicin, one of the most popular of the aminoglycosides, was introduced.
1970	Clindamycin, an alternative agent used where penicillin resistance is found, was discovered and developed.
1971	Rifampin, a semisynthetic drug prescribed for tuberculosis and leprosy, was introduced.
1972	Spectinomycin, similar to streptomycin, was developed and introduced.
1980s	The newer second-generation quinolone drugs (ciprofloxacin, norfloxacin) were developed for clinical use. These second–generation quinolones have an expanded antibacterial spectrum that is active against most Gram-negative bacteria.

Table 16.2.
Recommended Antimicrobial Therapy for Infections[a,b]

Infecting Organism	Disease	Antibiotic of Choice	Alternative Drugs
Acinetobacter	Various nosocomial infections	An aminoglycoside, imipenem	Amikacin, gentamicin
Aspergillus, Candida	Pneumonia	Amphotericin B	Fluconazole
Bacteroides fragilis	Lung abscess Empyema Bacteremia Endocarditis Brain abscess	Clindamycin, metronidazole	Cefoxitin, or moxalactam
Bacteroides species (oral, pharyngeal)	Lung abscess Brain abscess Sinusitis	Penicillin G, clindamycin	Metronidazole, cefotoxitin, or moxalactam
Clostridium perfringens	Gas gangrene	Penicillin G	Chloramphenicol, clindamycin
Corynebacterium diphtheriae	Pneumonia Pharyngitis Laryngotracheitis	Erythromycin	Penicillin G, G1 cephalosporin[c]
Escherichia coli, Proteus, or *Enterobacter*	Pneumonia	G3 cephalosporin	Ciprofloxacin
Francisella tularensis, Yersinia pestis	Pneumonia	Streptomycin	Chloramphenicol
Haemophilus influenzae	Bronchitis Sinusitis Epiglottitis Pneumonia	Cefotaxime, ceftriaxone, trimethoprim-sulfamethoxazole	Cefactor, amoxicillin or ampicillin
Histoplasma capsulatum	Pneumonia Meningitis	Amphotericin B or ketoconazole	Itraconazole
Influenza A	Influenza	Amantadine (prophylaxis)	
Klebsiella penumoniae	Pneumonia	Cefazolin + gentamicin	Trimethoprim-sulfamethoxazole
Legionella pneumophila	Legionnaires' disease	Erythromycin with or without rifampin	Trimethoprim-sulfamethoxazole
Mycobacterium tuberculosis	Pulmonary	Isoniazid + rifampin	Ethambutol, streptomycin, ethionamide
Mycoplasma pneumoniae	Atypical viral pneumonia	Erythromycin tetracycline	Clarithromycin
Pneumocystis carinii	Pneumonia in immunologically compromised patients	Trimethoprim-sulfamethoxazole	Pentamidine, dapsone
Pseudomonas aeruginosa	Pneumonia Bacteremia	Ciprofloxacin or piperacillin + tobramycin	Other β-lactum antibiotic + an aminoglycoside
Serratia marcescens	Pneumonia	Cefotaxime, ceftizoxime	Trimethoprim-sulfamethoxazole
Staphylococcus aureus	Pneumonia Bacteremia Endocarditis	Penicillin G, nafcillin, or oxacillin	Vancomycin, G1 cephalosporin[c]
Streptococcus pneumoniae	Pneumonia Endocarditis	Penicillin G or V	G1 cephalosporin,[c] erythromycin
Streptococcus pyogenes	Pharyngitis Pneumonia Bacteremia	Penicillin G or V	G1 cephalosporin,[c] erythromycin

[a]Adapted from Gilman AG, Goodman LS, Rall TW, Nies AS, Taylor P. Goodman and Gilman's The Pharmacological Basis of Therapeutics. 8th ed. New York: McGraw-Hill, Inc., 1993; and Pratt W. The Antimicrobial Drugs. Oxford, UK: Oxford University Press, 1986.
[b]This table focuses primarily on respiratory infections and a few other selected serious infections.
[c]G1, G3: first- or third-generation cephalosporin.

CATEGORY IV: Agents that bind to the 30S ribosomal subunit, thereby disrupting protein synthesis. The aminoglycosides comprise this group.

CATEGORY V: Agents that alter the synthesis and metabolism of nucleic acid. Agents within this group include rifampin, the quinolone nalidixic acid and its derivatives, and metronidazole.

CATEGORY VI: Agents that have the ability to inhibit certain metabolic processes that are fundamental to the microorganism. Agents within this group include trimethoprim and the sulfonamides.

CATEGORY VII: Agents that inhibit viral replication by binding to the viral enzymes necessary for deoxyribonucleic acid (DNA) synthesis. Vidarabine and acyclovir comprise this group.

STAINING TECHNIQUES

The most important and simplest diagnostic tools available to determine the microorganism responsible for an infection are the Gram stain technique and the acid-fast staining technique.

The Gram stain technique is a differential diagnostic tool that allows the technician to separate bacteria into two groups. A small amount of bacteria (from samples such as sputum, urinary sediment, cerebrospinal fluid, or purulent drainage from the site of infection) is placed on a glass slide and allowed to air dry. Next, the slide is passed through a flame (heat-fixing), which bonds the cells to the slide and kills most of the organisms to prepare them for the staining technique.

After heat-fixing, the slide is stained with crystal violet dye for 1 minute and then with Gram's iodine solution for another minute. All bacteria on the slide are then stained blue-purple. Next, the slide is rinsed with a decolorizer (such as 95% alcohol). During this process, some bacteria completely lose all color and become transparent (Gram-negative bacteria), whereas other bacteria retain the blue-purple color (Gram-positive bacteria).

The last step in the Gram stain technique involves safranin, which is a red dye. When safranin is applied to the slide, the Gram-negative bacteria absorb the stain and turn red-orange. At the conclusion of the procedure, all Gram-positive bacteria are blue-purple and all Gram-negative bacteria are red-orange.

The acid-fast staining technique is a diagnostic tool that determines the presence of bacteria of the genus *Mycobacterium*. These bacteria are very difficult to stain by conventional methods because of the waxy cell wall structure. Heat must be applied to force the dye molecules through to the bacteria's cytoplasm. After these organisms are stained, they are not easily decolorized by acids (hence, they are acid-resistant or acid-fast).

A sample of respiratory secretions is placed on a glass slide and allowed to air dry, and then the slide is heat fixed. Next, a Ziehl-Neelsen carbol-fuchsin stain is applied to the slide as it is heated. During this process, all of the cells on the slide turn bright red in color. The smear is then rinsed with an acid alcohol decolorizer;

all acid-fast bacteria retain the red color (confirming the presence of *Mycobacterium*), whereas all other bacteria lose color and become transparent. A positive acid-fast test aids the physician in the diagnosis of tuberculosis.

SPECIFIC ANTIBACTERIAL AGENTS

β-LACTAM ANTIBIOTICS

The β-lactam antibiotics are so called because they contain a four-membered β-lactam ring connected to a second ring. These antibiotics are bactericidal and act against bacteria by interfering with the synthesis of the bacterial cell wall. Specifically, these agents attach to drug receptors on bacteria known as penicillin-binding proteins (PBPs). By this mechanism, formation of peptidoglycan, a mucopeptide necessary for cell wall strength and stability, is blocked, and thus, the unstable bacterial cell dies. Four primary groups of drugs contain the β-lactam ring and are thus known as β-lactam antibiotics: the penicillins, the cephalosporins, the carbapenems, and the monobactams.

β-lactamase, also known as penicillinase, is an enzyme produced by a number of Gram-positive bacteria and most Gram-negative enteric rods, including most strains of *Staphylococcus aureus, Bacillus* species, *Enterobacter aerogenes, Pseudomonas aeruginosa, Mycobacterium tuberculosis, Proteus* species, *Escherichia coli,* and some strains of *Haemophilus influenzae*. β-lactamase brings about bacterial resistance to the β-lactam antibiotics through its mechanism of destroying the β-lactam ring of the antibiotic. Because an intact β-lactam ring is necessary for the antibiotic's bactericidal activity, the drug is inactivated and unable to inhibit bacterial growth when β-lactamase acts on its β-lactam ring.

PENCILILLINS

Mechanism of Action

The penicillins are bactericidal antibiotics that effectively kill bacteria by inhibiting the synthesis of the bacterial cell wall. The penicillins bind to penicillin-binding proteins, which then prevents the synthesis of peptidoglycan, a mucopeptide that gives the cell wall its strength and stability. Without the cell wall, lysis of the bacterial cell membrane occurs, and death follows. Penicillins are most effective during the active bacterial replication of young microorganisms. Penicillins have little or no effect on mature, dormant bacteria or bacteria that lack cell walls.

An intact β-lactam ring accounts for the penicillin's biological bactericidal activity. The side chain of the penicillin structure primarily determines the antibacterial spectrum. Narrow-spectrum penicillins act primarily on Gram-positive organisms. Broad-spectrum penicillins are effective not only on Gram-positive organisms but also on many Gram-negative bacilli.

The emergence of resistant strains of bacilli, either through mutations of the original infectious agent or through the ability of the bacilli to release enzymes (e.g., β-lactamase-penicillinase) that can destroy the antibacterial drug, is a factor necessary to consider when administering these drugs.

The first penicillin in clinical use that is still considered a first-line drug against most Gram-positive bacteria (except penicillinase-producing staphylococci) when given by injection (IM, IV) is the natural penicillin—penicillin G. This penicillin is an essentially safe antibiotic because it is virtually nontoxic to human cells, even when administered in large amounts.

The semisynthetic penicillin derivatives include penicillin V; the penicillinase-resistant penicillins (cloxacillin, dicloxacillin, methicillin, nafcillin, oxacillin) used in the treatment of infections caused by penicillinase-producing *Staphylococcus aureus* and other penicillinase-producing bacteria; the aminopenicillins (broad-spectrum agents: amoxicillin, ampicillin, bacampicillin); and the extended-spectrum penicillins (antipseudomonal agents: carbenicillin, mezlocillin, piperacillin, ticarcillin).

Indications for Use

The penicillins have remained for more than 5 decades as the most popular class of antibiotics in nonallergic patients. Modifications of the basic penicillin structure not only enable an enhanced activity against most Gram-positive and Gram-negative organisms but also enable certain penicillins (e.g., cloxacillin, dicloxacillin, methicillin, nafcillin, and oxacillin) to resist enzymes (penicillinases) that convert penicillin to inactive penicilloic acid.

Figures 16.1 to 16.3 summarize the organisms that are generally susceptible to the penicillins.

Contraindications

Contraindications to penicillin include hypersensitivity to the drug.

Precautions

1. Use with caution for patients with asthma, hay fever, history of any allergy, or renal impairment.
2. Do not use oral penicillin to treat severe pneumonia, empyema, bacteremia, meningitis, pericarditis, or purulent or septic arthritis during the acute stage.
3. Use with caution for neonates owing to an incompletely developed renal system.
4. Therapy must be of sufficient duration (at least 10 days and up to 4 weeks for severe infections) to completely eradicate the organism; otherwise, endocarditis or rheumatic fever may develop.
5. Superinfection (secondary infection) may occur with the use of antibiotics due to bacterial or fungal overgrowth of nonsusceptible organisms.

Gram-positive organisms			Penicillinase-resistant					Aminopenicillins			Extended spectrum			
	Penicillin G	Penicillin V	Methicillin	Nafcillin	Oxacillin	Cloxacillin	Dicloxacillin	Ampicillin	Bacampicillin	Amoxicillin	Carbenicillin	Ticarcillin	Mezlocillin	Piperacillin
Staphylococci	●1	●1	●	●	●	●	●	●1	●1	●1	●1	●1		●1
Staphylococcus aureus	●1	●1	●	●	●	●	●				●1	●1	●1	●1
Streptococci	●	●	●					●						
Streptococcus pneumoniae	●	●	●	●	●	●	●	●	●	●	●	●	●	●
Beta-hemolytic streptococci	●	●	●	●				●	●	●	●	●	●	●
Streptococcus faecalis	●	●						●	●	●	●	●	●	●
Streptococcus viridans	●	●		●				●		●				●
Corynebacterium diphtheriae	●	●												
Bacillus anthracis	●	●						●						
Listeria monocytogenes	●	●						●						

[1] Nonpenicillinase-producing.

Figure 16.1. Gram-positive organisms that are susceptible to the penicillins. (Adapted from Drug Facts and Comparisons. 49th ed. St. Louis: Facts and Comparisons, 1995; and Gilman AG, Goodman LS, Rall TW, Nies AS, Taylor P. Goodman and Gilman's The Pharmacological Basis of Therapeutics. 8th ed. New York: McGraw-Hill, Inc., 1993.)

6. Avoid concurrent use of other antibiotics (e.g., erythromycin, tetracycline). These agents may diminish the effectiveness of penicillin.
7. These drugs should be taken on an empty stomach 1 hour before meals or 2 hours after meals.

Adverse Reactions

Most Common: Allergic reactions (skin rash, urticaria, itching).

Other Allergic Reactions: Erythema, contact dermatitis, hives, wheezing, anaphylaxis, fever, eosinophilia, bronchospasm, laryngospasm, hypotension, vascular collapse.

CNS: Penicillin, carbenicillin, ampicillin, and ticarcillin have caused neurotoxicity when given in large IV doses and to patients with renal failure. Symptoms include lethargy, hallucinations, convulsions, seizures, and neuromuscular irritability.

GI: Diarrhea, abdominal cramps, nausea, vomiting, increased thirst.

Renal: Hematuria, pyuria, albuminuria, oliguria.

Miscellaneous: Superinfection, swelling of face and ankles, labored breathing, weakness, ecchymoses, hematomas.

Overdosage

Overdose may result in neuromuscular hyperexcitability or convulsive seizures. For severe allergic or anaphylactic reactions, administer epinephrine (0.3 to 0.5

Gram-negative organisms			Penicillinase-resistant					Aminopenicillins			Extended spectrum			
	Penicillin G	Penicillin V	Methicillin	Nafcillin	Oxacillin	Cloxacillin	Dicloxacillin	Ampicillin	Bacampicillin	Amoxicillin	Carbenicillin	Ticarcillin	Mezlocillin	Piperacillin
Escherichia coli	•							•	•	•	•	•	•	•
Hemophilus influenzae								•	•	•	•	•	•	•[2]
Klebsiella species													•	•
Neisseria gonorrhoeae	•[1]	•						•	•	•	•	•	•	•
Neisseria meningitidis	•							•				•		•
Proteus mirabilis	•							•	•	•	•	•	•	•
Salmonella species	•							•			•	•	•	•
Shigella species	•							•					•	•
Morganella morganii											•	•	•	•
Proteus vulgaris											•	•	•	•
Providencia species														
Providencia rettgeri											•	•	•	•
Providencia stuartii													•	
Enterobacter species	•										•	•	•	•
Citrobacter species											•	•	•	•
Pseudomonas aeruginosa											•	•	•	•
Serratia species											•	•	•	•
Acinetobacter species													•	•
Streptobacillus moniliformis	•	•												

[1] Nonpenicillinase-producing.
[2] Non-beta-lactamase-producing.

Figure 16.2. Gram-negative organisms that are susceptible to the penicillins. (Adapted from Drug Facts and Comparisons. 49th ed. St. Louis: Facts and Comparisons, 1995; and Gilman AG, Goodman LS, Rall TW, Nies AS, Taylor P. Goodman and Gilman's The Pharmacological Basis of Therapeutics. 8th ed. New York: McGraw-Hill, Inc., 1993.)

ml of 1:1000 solution SC or IM or 0.2 to 0.3 ml diluted with 10 ml saline given slowly by IV). Allergic reactions are more likely to occur in patients with asthma, hay fever, or urticaria. Severe or fatal potassium poisoning has occurred in patients receiving continuous IV therapy with potassium penicillin G in high dosage (10 to 100 million units per day).

Narrow-Spectrum Penicillins

Dosage

Penicillin G potassium*—For moderate to severe systemic infections:* **PO:** 1.6 to 3.2 million units/day, given every 6 hours in divided doses. **IM, IV:** 1.2 to 24 million units/day, given every 4 hours in divided doses. *Children:* **PO:** 25,000 to 100,000 units/kg/day, given every 6 hours in divided doses. **IM, IV:** 25,000 to 300,000 units/kg/day, given every 4 hours in divided doses.

			Penicillinase-resistant					Aminopenicillins			Extended spectrum			
Anaerobic organisms	Penicillin G	Penicillin V	Methicillin	Nafcillin	Oxacillin	Cloxacillin	Dicloxacillin	Ampicillin	Bacampicillin	Amoxicillin	Carbenicillin	Ticarcillin	Mezlocillin	Piperacillin
Clostridium species	●	●						●		●	●	●	●	●
Peptococcus species	●	●						●		●	●	●	●	●
Peptostreptococcus species	●	●								●	●	●	●	●
Bacteroides species	●[1]										●	●	●	●
Fusobacterium species	●										●	●	●	●
Eubacterium species	●											●	●	●
Treponema pallidum	●	●												
Actinomyces bovis	●	●												
Veillonella species													●	●

[1] *B. fragilis* is resistant.

Figure 16.3. Anaerobic organisms that are susceptible to the penicillins. (Adapted from Drug Facts and Comparisons. 49th ed. St. Louis: Facts and Comparisons, 1995; and Gilman AG, Goodman LS, Rall TW, Nies AS, Taylor P. Goodman and Gilman's The Pharmacological Basis of Therapeutics. 8th ed. New York: McGraw-Hill, Inc., 1993.)

Penicillin G procaine*—For moderate to severe systemic infections:* **IM:** 600,000 to 1.2 million units/day, given as single dose. *Children:* **IM:** 300,000 units/day, given as single dose.

Penicillin G sodium*—For moderate to severe systemic infections:* **IM, IV:** 1.2 to 24 million units/day, given every 4 hours in divided doses. *Children:* **IM, IV:** 25,000 to 300,000 units/kg/day, given every 4 hours in divided doses.

Penicillin V*—For moderate to severe systemic infections:* **PO:** 400,000 to 800,000 units (250 to 500 mg) every 6 hours. *Children:* **PO:** 25,000 to 90,000 units/kg/day (15 to 50 mg/kg), given every 6 to 8 hours in divided doses.

Aminopenicillins: Broad-Spectrum Penicillins

Dosage

Amoxicillin trihydrate (Amoxil, Polymox, Trimox)—**PO:** 750 mg to 1.5 g/day, given every 8 hours in divided doses. *Children:* **PO:** 20 to 40 mg/day, given every 8 hours in divided doses.

Ampicillin (Amcill, Omnipen, Ampicin, Principen)—**PO:** 1 to 4 g/day, given every 6 hours in divided doses. **IM, IV:** 2 to 12 g/day, given every 6 hours in divided doses. *Children:* **PO:** 50 to 100 mg/kg/day, given every 6 hours in divided doses.

Bacampicillin (Penglobe, Spectrobid)—*For adults and children weighing more than 25 kg:* **PO:** 400 to 800 mg every 12 hours.

Penicillinase-Resistant (Antistaphylococcal) Penicillins

Dosage

Cloxacillin sodium (Cloxapen, Tegopen)—**PO:** 2 to 4 g/day, divided into doses given every 6 hours. *Children:* **PO:** 50 to 100 mg/kg/day, given every 6 hours in divided doses.

Dicloxacillin sodium (Dycill, Dynapen, Pathocil)—**PO:** 1 to 2 g/day, divided into doses given every 6 hours. *Children:* **PO, IM:** 25 to 50 mg/kg/day, given every 6 hours in divided doses.

Methicillin sodium (Staphcillin)—**IM, IV:** 4 to 12 g/day, given every 4 to 6 hours in divided doses. *Children:* **IM, IV:** 100 to 300 mg/kg/day, given every 4 to 6 hours in divided doses.

Nafcillin sodium (Nafcil, Unipen)—**PO:** 2 to 4 g/day, given every 6 hours in divided doses. **IM, IV:** 2 to 12 g/day, given every 4 to 6 hours in divided doses. *Children:* **PO:** 50 to 100 mg/kg/day, given every 4 to 6 hours in divided doses. **IM, IV:** 100 to 200 mg/kg/day, given every 4 to 6 hours in divided doses.

Oxacillin sodium (Bactocill, Prostaphlin)—**PO:** 2 to 4 g/day, given every 6 hours in divided doses. **IM, IV:** 2 to 12 g/day, given every 4 to 6 hours in divided doses. *Children:* **PO:** 50 to 100 mg/kg/day, given every 6 hours in divided doses. **IM, IV:** 100 to 200 mg/kg/day, given every 4 to 6 hours in divided doses.

Extended-Spectrum Penicillins

Dosage

Carbenicillin disodium (Geocillin, Geopen)—**PO:** 382 to 764 mg q.i.d.

Ticarcillin disodium (Ticar)—**IM, IV:** 18 g/day divided into doses given every 4 to 6 hours. *Children:* **IV, IM:** 200 to 300 mg/kg/day, given every 4 to 6 hours in divided doses.

Mexlocillin sodium (Mezlin)—**IV:** 200 to 300 mg/kg/day given in four to six divided doses (usual dose: 3 g every 4 hours or 4 g every 6 hours). *Children aged 12 years or younger:* **IV:** 50 mg/kg every 4 hours.

Piperacillin sodium (Pipracil)—**IV:** 100 to 300 mg/kg/day divided into equal doses given every 4 to 6 hours (dose depends on severity of infection).

CEPHALOSPORINS AND CEPHAMYCINS

Mechanism of Action

Cephalosporins are structurally and pharmacologically similar to the penicillins. These agents are the semisynthetic derivatives of *Cephalosporium acremonium.* Cephamycins are included because of their similarity to the cephalosporins. Cephalosporins inhibit the synthesis of the bacterial cell wall by attaching to penicillin-binding proteins and thus interfering with mucopeptide biosynthesis, the final step in the formation of the cell wall. The unstable bacterial cell membrane disintegrates and the microorganism dies. Cephalosporins are more effective against rapidly growing microbes forming cell walls than against mature, dormant bacteria or those that lack cell walls.

Indications for Use

The cephalosporins and cephamycins are indicated for use in a variety of mild to severe infections caused by both Gram-positive and Gram-negative bacteria. These agents are subclassified into first, second, or third generation according to their broad or narrow antibacterial spectrum. The first-generation cephalosporins have a narrower antibacterial spectrum compared to the other generations of cephalosporins and are primarily effective against Gram-positive organisms, although they do exhibit some biological activity against a few Gram-negative species. The second-generation cephalosporins exhibit more activity against Gram-negative and some anaerobic bacteria than the first-generation cephalosporins. The third-generation cephalosporins have a broader antibacterial spectrum against aerobic Gram-negative bacilli, resistant organisms, and some anaerobic organisms than the first- and second-generation cephalosporins; however, the third-generation cephalosporins may be less effective against Gram-positive bacteria than first-generation cephalosporins. All cephalosporins are ineffective against enterococci and methicillin-resistant staphylococci. Figure 16.4 summarizes the organisms that are generally susceptible to the cephalosporins.

Contraindications

Contraindications to cephalosporins and cephamycins include hypersensitivity to these agents.

Precautions

1. Use with caution for patients with impaired renal or hepatic function owing to cephalosporin elimination by the kidneys. In most cases, the dosage must be adjusted according to the degree of renal impairment.
2. Use of these antibiotics may result in bacterial or fungal superinfection.
3. Avoid concurrent administration with other bacteriostatic agents; they may diminish the effectiveness of cephalosporins.

Adverse Reactions

Most Common: Hypersensitivity and unwanted GI activity. Hypersensitivity is noted in patients with a history of asthma, allergy, hay fever, or urticaria. Hypersensitivity reactions range from mild to life-threatening and include urticaria, rashes, pruritus, fever, chills, erythema, angioedema, and anaphylaxis.

GI: Nausea, vomiting, diarrhea, abdominal cramps, dyspepsia, heartburn.

FIRST-GENERATION CEPHALOSPORINS (also covered by second- and third-generation cephalosporins)

- Staphylococci†
- *Streptococcus pneumoniae*
- Beta-hemolytic streptococci
- *Escherichia coli*
- *Hemophilus influenzae*
- *Klebsiella* species
- *Proteus mirabilis*

SECOND-GENERATION CEPHALOSPORINS (also covered by third-generation cephalosporins)

- *Morganella morganii*
- *Providencia rettgeri*
- *Enterobacter* species†
- *Clostridium* species
- *Peptococcus* species
- *Peptostreptococcus* species
- *Fusobacterium* species
- *Proteus vulgaris*
- *Providencia* species
- *Neisseria gonorrhoeae*
- *Bacteroides* species

THIRD-GENERATION CEPHALOSPORINS

- *Neisseria meningitidis*
- *Salmonella* species*
- *Shigella* species*
- *Eubacterium* species*
- *Clostridium difficile**
- *Citrobacter* species
- *Serratia* species
- *Salmonella typhi**
- *Bacteroides fragilis*
- *Pseudomonas aeruginosa*†
- *Acinetobacter* species

* Some strains are resistant.
† Demonstrated in vitro activity.
Organisms may not exhibit susceptibility to each cephalosporin in a particular generation.

Figure 16.4. Summary of the organisms that are generally susceptible to the cephalosporins.

CNS: Headache, dizziness, lethargy, paresthesia, seizures.
Miscellaneous: Hypotension, fever, dyspnea, interstitial pneumonitis.

First-Generation Cephalosporins

Uses

First-generation cephalosporins are indicated for respiratory tract infections caused by *Streptococcus pneumoniae, Klebsiella* species, staphylococci, Group A β-hemolytic streptococci, *Haemophilus influenzae, Staphylococcus aureus;* meningitis caused by *S. pneumoniae,* Group A β-hemolytic streptococci and staphylococci; septicemia, endocarditis caused by *S. pneumoniae,* staphylococci, *Streptococcus viridans, Escherichia coli, Proteus mirabilis, Klebsiella* species, Group A β-hemolytic streptococci; and genitourinary infections caused by *E. coli, P. mirabilis, Klebsiella* species. These agents are also used for bone and joint infections caused by staphylococci, *S. aureus,* and for skin and soft tissue infections caused by staphylococci, *E. coli, P. mirabilis, Klebsiella* species, and Group A β-hemolytic streptococci.

Dosage

Cefadroxil monohydrate (Duricef, Ultracef)—**PO:** 500 mg to 2 g/day in a single dose or two divided doses. *Children:* 30 mg/kg/day. *For pharyngitis and tonsillitis:* 500 mg every 12 hours for 10 days.

Cefazolin sodium (Ancef, Kefzol)—**IM, IV:** 250 to 500 mg every 8 hours up to 1 g every 6 hours for severe infections. *Life-threatening infections (septicemia, endocarditis):* up to 8 g daily given by IV. *Children:* 25 to 100 mg/kg/day, not to exceed 100 mg/kg/day.

Cephalexin monohydrate (Keflex, Keftab, Keflet)—**PO:** 1 to 4 g/day in divided doses given every 6 hours. Usual dose: 250 mg every 6 hours. *Children:* **PO:** 25 to 50 mg/kg/day; for severe infections, may double the dose.

Cephalothin sodium (Keflin, Seffin)—**IV, IM:** 500 mg to 1 g every 4 to 6 hours, or 4 to 12 g daily in divided doses (reserve higher doses for life-threatening conditions). *Children:* **IV:** 100 mg/kg/day in divided doses given every 4 to 6 hours.

Cephapirin sodium (Cefadyl)—**IM, IV:** 500 mg to 1 g every 4 to 6 hours, up to 12 g daily. *Children:* 40 to 80 mg/kg in four equally divided doses.

Cephradine (Anspor, Velosef)—**PO:** 250 to 500 mg every 6 hours or 1 g every 12 hours. **IV, IM:** up to 8 g daily. *Children:* **PO:** 25 to 100 mg/kg/day. Not to exceed 4 g total daily dose. **IM, IV:** 2 to 4 g daily.

Second-Generation Cephalosporins

Uses

Second-generation cephalosporins have the same antibacterial spectrum as first-generation cephalosporins, in addition to lower respiratory tract infections, including pneumonia caused by *S. pneumoniae,* and *H. influenzae.* Second-generation cephalosporins are also used for upper respiratory tract infections caused by *S. pyogenes,* peritonitis caused by *E. coli* and *Enterobacter* species, and intra-abdominal infections caused by *E. coli, Klebsiella* species, some *Bacteroides* species, and *Clostridium* species.

Dosage

Cefaclor (Ceclor)—**PO:** 250 to 500 mg every 8 hours, up to a maximum of 4 g daily. *Children:* 20 to 40 mg/kg/day, up to 1 g/day.

Cefamandole naftate (Mandol)—**IM, IV:** 500 mg to 1 g every 4 to 8 hours, up to 2 g every 4 hours for life-threatening infections. *Children:* 50 to 100 mg/kg/day, up to 150 mg/kg/day (not to exceed maximum adult daily dose).

Cefmetazole (Zefazone)—**IV, IM:** 1 to 8 g/day in equally divided doses given every 6 to 12 hours.

Cefoxitin sodium (Mefoxin)—**IM, IV:** 1 to 2 g every 6 to 8 hours, up to 12 g/day. For serious infections: 6 to 8 g/day. For life-threatening infections: 12 g/day. *Children:* 80 to 160 mg/kg/day in four to six divided doses.

Cefonicid sodium (Monocid)—**IM, IV:** 0.5 to 2 g once daily.

Ceforanide (Precef)—**IM, IV:** 0.5 to 1 g every 12 hours. *Children:* 20 to 40 mg/kg/day.

Cefotetan (Cefotan)—**IV, IM:** 1 to 2 g every 12 hours for 5 to 10 days.

Cefprozil (Ceftin, Zinacef, Kefurox)—**PO:** 250 to 500 mg every 12 to 24 hours. *Children:* 7.5 mg/kg every 12 hours for pharyngitis or tonsillitis. *Infants:* 15 mg/kg every 12 hours for otitis media.

Cefuroxime (Lorabid)—**PO:** 125 to 500 mg every 12 hours.

Loracarbef (Lorabid)—**PO:** 200 to 400 mg every 12 hours. *Children:* 7.5 to 15 mg/kg every 12 hours.

Third-Generation Cephalosporins

Uses

Third-generation cephalosporins are generally less active against Gram-positive cocci than first- or second-generation cephalosporins. Third-generation cephalosporins are primarily indicated for infections caused by *Neisseria meningitidis, H. influenzae, Citrobacter, Enterobacter, E. coli, Klebsiella* species, *N. gonorrhoeae, Proteus, Morganella, Providencia, Serratia, Pseudomonas aeruginosa,* and *Bacteroides fragilis.*

Dosage

Cefixime (Suprax)—**PO:** 400 mg/day as a single dose or two equally divided doses. *Children:* 4 mg/kg every 12 hours.

Cefoperazone sodium (Cefobid)—**IM, IV:** 2 to 4 g/day, up to 16 g/day for severe infections.

Cefotaxime sodium (Claforan)—**IM, IV:** 1 g/day, up to 12 g for life-threatening infections. *Children:* 50 to 180 mg/kg/day. **Additional uses:** CNS infections (meningitis and ventriculitis) caused by *N. meningitidis, H. influenzae, S. pneumoniae, Klebsiella pneumoniae,* and *E. coli.*

Cefpodoxime proxetil (Vantin)—**PO:** 100 to 400 mg every 12 hours. *Children:* 5 mg/kg every 12 hours.

Ceftizoxime sodium (Cefizox)—**IM, IV:** 1 or 2 g every 8 to 12 hours, up to 12 g/day for life-threatening infections. *Children:* 50 mg/kg every 6 to 8 hours, up to 200 mg/kg/day.

Ceftriaxone sodium (Rocephin)—**IM, IV:** 1 to 2 g once a day, not to exceed a total daily dose of 4 g. *Children:* 50 to 75 mg/kg/day, not to exceed 2 g/day. For meningitis: 100 mg/kg/day, not to exceed 4 g/day.

Cefotetan disodium (Cefotan)—**IM, IV:** 1 to 4 g daily, up to 6 g for life-threatening infections.

Ceftazidime (Fortaz, Tazicef, Tazidime)—**IM, IV:** 250 mg every 12 hours, up to 2 g every 8 hours for serious infections. *Children:* 30 to 50 mg/kg every 8 hours, up to 6 g/day.

Moxalactam disodium (Moxam)—**IM, IV:** 2 to 6 g daily, up to 12 g/day. *Children:* 50 mg/kg every 6 to 8 hours, up to 200 mg/kg/day (not to exceed the adult daily dose).

Carbapenems: Imipenem-Cilastatin (Primaxin)

Imipenem (Primaxin) is a relatively new antibiotic that is structurally related to the β-lactam antibiotics. Imipenem exhibits the same pharmacologic activity as other β-lactam antibiotics in that it interferes with bacterial cell wall synthesis by binding to penicillin-binding proteins and blocking the formation of peptidoglycan.

Imipenem has a broad-spectrum activity against a wide variety of pathogens, including many organisms that are resistant to the penicillins, cephalosporins, and aminoglycosides. The notable exceptions to imipenem use include infections caused by *Pseudomonas maltophilia, Streptococcus faecium,* groups A, C, and G streptococci, and methicillin-resistant staphylococci. Imipenem is usually reserved for serious infections.

The most common adverse effects of imipenem include nausea, vomiting, diarrhea, skin rash, and reactions at the injection site. Allergic reactions have occurred in patients who are also allergic to the penicillins. Excessive doses in patients with renal failure may lead to seizures.

The usual dose of imipenem is 0.5 to 1 g given IV every 6 hours.

Monobactams: Aztreonam (Azactam)

Aztreonam (Azactam) is a synthetic bactericidal antibiotic that is the first of a new class of antibiotics designated as monobactams owing to a monocyclic β-lactam nucleus rather than a bicyclic β-lactam nucleus. The bactericidal activity of aztreonam results from the inhibition of bacterial cell wall synthesis.

Aztreonam exhibits a fairly wide spectrum of activity against Gram-negative organisms but little to no efficacy against Gram-positive or anaerobic organisms.

Aztreonam has demonstrated effectiveness against infections caused by Gram-negative aerobic organisms such as *Pseudomonas aeruginosa, E. coli, Enterobacter, Klebsiella, Proteus mirabilis, Serratia,* and *Haemophilus.*

Common side effects include swelling at the injection site, nausea, vomiting, diarrhea, and mild skin rash. Penicillin-allergic patients usually tolerate aztreonam without reaction.

The usual dose of aztreonam is 1 to 2 g given IV every 8 hours.

AMINOGLYCOSIDES

Mechanism of Action

The aminoglycosides irreversibly bind to the bacterial intracellular ribosomal 30S subunit. This action causes the inhibition of ribosomal protein synthesis and subsequent alteration of the genetic code. The ribosomal unit separates from messenger ribonucleic acid (RNA); cell death follows.

Indications for Use

The aminoglycosides are broad-spectrum antibiotics indicated for a variety of severe, complicated, Gram-negative infections caused by *Pseudomonas, E. coli, Proteus, Klebsiella* species, *Serratia* species, *Providencia* species, *Acinetobacter* species, and *Enterobacter* species. The aminoglycosides are used concomitantly with other anti-infective agents to combat certain Gram-positive microorganisms such as *Staphylococcus aureus, Streptococcus faecalis,* and certain other streptococcus species and staphylococcus species. These drugs are not indicated for trivial infections or for infections that can be eliminated with less toxic antibacterial agents because of their ototoxic and nephrotoxic potential. Figure 16.5 lists a summary of the organisms generally susceptible to the aminoglycosides.

Contraindications

Contraindications to the use of aminoglycosides include hypersensitivity to the agents. Aminoglycosides are not indicated for long-term therapy (except for streptomycin, which is used for tuberculosis) because of the ototoxic and nephrotoxic hazards.

Precautions

1. Use with caution for patients with neuromuscular disorders; aminoglycosides may increase muscle weakness because of a potential curare-like effect at the neuromuscular junction.
2. If these agents are used concurrently with penicillins or cephalosporins, a synergistic effect may be noted.
3. Patients should be monitored for the occurrence of superinfection.

	Microorganisms	Streptomycin	Kanamycin	Gentamicin	Tobramycin	Amikacin	Netilmicin
Gram-positive	*Mycobacterium tuberculosis*	●[1]				●	
	Staphylococcus species			●[2]	●	●[2]	●[2]
	Staphylococcus aureus		●[2]	●	●	●	●[2]
	Staphylococcus epidermidis		●			●	●
	Streptococcus species	●[1]					
	Streptococcus faecalis	●[1]		●[1]	●[1]		●[1]
Gram-negative	*Acinetobacter* species		●			●	●
	Brucella species	●					
	Citrobacter species	●	●	●	●	●	●
	Enterobacter species	●	●	●	●	●	●
	Escherichia coli	●	●	●	●	●	●
	Hemophilus influenzae	●[1]	●			●	
	Hemophilus ducreyi	●					
	Klebsiella species	●[1]	●	●	●	●	●
	Morganella morganii				●		
	Neisseria species	●	●			●	●
	Proteus species	●	●[3]	●[3]	●[3]	●[3]	●
	Proteus mirabilis				●		●
	Proteus vulgaris				●		
	Providencia species	●	●	●	●	●	●
	Pseudomonas species					●	●
	Pseudomonas aeruginosa	●		●[1]	●	●	●
	Salmonella species	●	●	●	●	●	●
	Serratia species	●	●	●			●
	Shigella species	●	●	●	●	●	●
	Yersinia pestis	●	●	●	●	●	●

[1] Usually used concomitantly with other anti-infective agents.

[2] Penicillinase-producing and nonpenicillinase-producing.

[3] Indole-positive and indole-negative.

Figure 16.5. Organisms that are generally susceptible to the aminoglycosides. (Adapted from Drug Facts and Comparisons. 49th ed. St. Louis: Facts and Comparisons, 1995; and Gilman AG, Goodman LS, Rall TW, Nies AS, Taylor P. Goodman and Gilman's The Pharmacological Basis of Therapeutics. 8th ed. New York: McGraw-Hill, Inc., 1993.)

4. Use with caution for renally impaired patients and for neonates and premature infants. Aminoglycosides are excreted primarily through glomerular filtration.

Adverse Reactions

CNS: Confusion, disorientation, depression, lethargy, respiratory depression, headache, fever, acute organic brain syndrome, nystagmus, visual disturbances.

GI: Nausea, vomiting, anorexia, stomatitis.

Nephrotoxic: Proteinuria, hematuria, granular casts, azotemia, oliguria, rising blood urea nitrogen (BUN).

Ototoxic: Tinnitus, dizziness, vertigo, roaring in the ears.

Neurotoxic: Numbness, skin tingling, tremor, muscle twitching, neuromuscular blockade.

Miscellaneous: Myocarditis, palpitations, hypotension, hypertension, pulmonary fibrosis, hyperkalemia.

Overdosage

To reduce excess serum levels, hemodialysis may be necessary.

Dosage

Amikacin sulfate (Amikin)—**IM, IV:** 15 mg/kg/day, given every 8 to 12 hours in divided doses. *Newborns:* loading dose of 10 mg/kg, then 7.5 mg/kg every 12 hours.

Gentamicin sulfate (Garamycin)—**IM, IV:** 3 to 5 mg/kg/day, given every 6 to 8 hours in divided doses. *Children:* 6 to 7.5 mg/kg/day (2 to 2.5 mg/kg every 8 hours). *Infants and neonates:* 7.5 mg/kg/day in three divided doses.

Kanamycin sulfate (Kantrex, Klebcil)—**IM, IV:** 15 mg/kg/day, up to 1.5 g/day, given every 8 to 12 hours in divided doses. **PO:** For hepatic coma: 8 to 12 g daily. Intestinal bacteria suppression preoperatively: 1 g every hour for 4 hours, then 1 g every 6 hours for 36 to 72 hours. **Inhalation:** 250 mg in saline nebulized b.i.d. or q.i.d. **Additional uses:** Primarily used orally for a number of aerobic bacteria in the GI tract preoperatively. This agent has also been used as an aerosol for respiratory tract infections.

Netilmicin sulfate (Netromycin)—**IM, IV:** 4 to 6.5 mg/kg/day, given every 8 to 12 hours in divided doses. *Children:* 5.5 to 8 mg/kg/day. **Additional uses:** Netilmicin has been effective in the treatment of serious infections caused by some organisms resistant to other aminoglycosides. Also, in combination with carbenicillin or ticarcillin for the treatment of life-threatening infections caused by *Pseudomonas aeruginosa.*

Streptomycin sulfate—**IM:** 1 to 2 g/day, given every 12 hours in divided doses. *Children:* 20 to 40 mg/kg/day. For tuberculosis: 1 g daily in combination with an antituberculous drug. *Children:* 20 to 40 mg/kg/ day. For tularemia: 1 to 2 g daily. For plague: 2 to 4 g daily. For bacterial endocarditis: 1 g twice daily for 1 week, then 0.5 g twice daily for the second week; use in conjunction with penicillin. **Additional uses:** Used in combination with antituberculous drugs to combat *Mycobacterium tuberculosis.* Also effective against a variety of serious infections in which less hazardous therapeutic agents are ineffective or contraindicated.

Tobramycin sulfate (Nebcin, Tobrex)—**IM, IV:** 3 to 5 mg/kg/day, given every 6 to 8 hours in divided doses. *Children:* 6 to 7.5 mg/kg/day in three to four equally divided doses. *Neonates:* up to 4 mg/kg/day in two equal doses every 12 hours.

ERYTHROMYCINS (MACROLIDES)

Mechanism of Action

Erythromycins bind to the bacterial ribosomal 50S subunit, thereby suppressing protein synthesis and the transmission of genetic information. Erythromycins are effective against rapidly growing, reproducing microorganisms. The bacterial activity of erythromycins may be bactericidal or bacteriostatic, depending on susceptible organisms and drug concentration.

Indications for Use

Erythromycins are the drug of choice for respiratory infections caused by *Mycoplasma pneumoniae,* for Legionnaires' disease caused by *Legionella pneumophila,* and for upper respiratory tract infections (otitis media) caused by *H. influenzae* when used in conjunction with sulfonamides. Also, erythromycins are effective against *Corynebacterium diphtheriae, Corynebacterium minutissimum,* and *Bordetella pertussis.* Erythromycins are also used as alternative drugs when penicillin or tetracycline is contraindicated or not tolerated or when the patient exhibits hypersensitivity. Alternative uses include upper and lower respiratory infections (including pneumonia and bronchitis) caused by *Streptococcus pyogenes* and *S. pneumoniae* and skin and soft tissue infections caused by *S. pyogenes* and *S. aureus.* Erythromycins are also indicated for pharyngitis, scarlet fever, cellulitis, and erysipelas caused by Group A *S. pyogenes.*

Contraindications

Contraindications to the use of erythromycins include hypersensitivity to the drug and preexisting liver disease (erythromycin estolate and ethylsuccinate).

Precautions

1. Use with extreme caution for patients with impaired hepatic function; these agents are excreted principally by the liver.
2. Monitor patient for superinfection.

3. Synergistic activity against *H. influenzae* has been noted with concomitant use with sulfonamide.
4. Coadministered erythromycin with penicillin may decrease the effectiveness of penicillin; these drugs are rarely used together.

Adverse Reactions

Allergic: Skin rashes, urticaria, eczema, anaphylaxis (rare).
GI: Oral dose-related side effects: abdominal cramps, anorexia, nausea, vomiting, diarrhea.
Miscellaneous: Superinfection.

Dosage (stated as erythromycin base)

Erythromycin base (E-mycin)
Erythromycin estolate (Ilosone)
Erythromycin ethylsuccinate (E.E.S., Erythrocin, Pediamycin, Wyamycin E, Eryped)
Erythromycin gluceptate (Ilotycin)
Erythromycin lactobionate (Erythrocin)—**PO:** 250 mg every 6 hours or 500 mg every 12 hours; for severe infections, may give up to 4 grams daily. *Children:* 30 to 50 mg/kg/day; for severe infections, may double the dose. **IV:** 15 to 20 mg/kg/day; for very severe infections, may give up to 4 grams daily.

TETRACYCLINES

Mechanism of Action

The tetracyclines are bacteriostatic antibiotics that inhibit protein synthesis by binding to the 30S ribosomal subunit.

Indications for Use

Tetracyclines are used for a variety of Gram-positive, Gram-negative, aerobic, and anaerobic organisms and especially for infections caused by *Rickettsiae* (Rocky Mountain spotted fever, typhus fever, every fever, rickettsialpox, tick fevers), *Chlamydia,* and *Mycoplasma pneumoniae*. Tetracyclines are not usually the drug of first choice for any staphylococcal infections or for infections that respond to penicillin; however, they are indicated for patients who are hypersensitive to penicillins and other antibiotics or when bacteriologic testing demonstrates susceptibility of the organism to tetracycline.

Contraindications

Contraindications to tetracyclines include hypersensitivity to any of these agents.

Precautions

1. Tetracyclines are not generally used for children younger than 8 years of age, unless other drugs are contraindicated or less effective. Tetracyclines cause permanent discoloration of teeth during the formative tooth development period.
2. Use with caution for patients with renal impairment. Excessive systemic accumulation may occur.
3. Use of antibiotics may lead to bacterial or fungal overgrowth; secondary infection may occur.
4. Theophylline coadministered with tetracycline may increase the incidence of unwanted GI side effects.

Adverse Reactions

CNS: Lightheadedness, dizziness, vertigo.

GI: Anorexia, nausea, vomiting, diarrhea, stomatitis, sore throat, dysphagia, hoarseness.

Renal: Increase in BUN.

Hepatic: Liver damage, pancreatitis.

Bones and Teeth: Permanent discoloration of teeth in children younger than 8 years of age. Temporary depressed bone growth in children and fetuses.

Dosage

Tetracycline HCl (Achromycin V, Cyclinex, Tetra-C, Tetram, Cyclopar 500, Sumycin, Nor-Tet, Robitet)—**PO:** 250 to 500 mg every 6 hours. *Children older than 8 years of age:* 25 to 50 mg/kg/day in four divided doses. **IM:** 250 mg/day given in a single dose. *Children older than 8 years of age weighing less than 40 kg:* 15 to 25 mg/kg/day in divided doses at 8- to 12-hour intervals. **IV:** 250 to 500 mg b.i.d. at 12-hour intervals. *Children older than 8 years of age:* 20 to 30 mg/kg/day in divided doses at 8- to 12-hour intervals.

Oxytetracycline HCl (Dilimycin, Oxlopar, Terramycin)—**PO:** 1 to 2 g/day, given in two to four divided doses; do not exceed 500 mg every 6 hours. *Children older than 8 years of age:* 25 to 50 mg/kg/day in four divided doses. **IM:** 100 mg every 8 to 12 hours. *Children older than 8 years of age:* 15 to 25 mg/kg/day up to a maximum of 250 mg in a single daily dose. **IV:** 500 mg to 1 g daily in two doses. *Children older than 8 years of age:* 10 to 20 mg/kg/day in two divided doses.

Demeclocycline HCl (Declomycin)—**PO:** 600 mg/day in two to four divided doses. *Children older than 8 years of age:* 6 to 12 mg/kg/day in two to four divided doses.

Methacycline HCl (Rondomycin)—**PO:** 600 mg daily in two to four divided doses. *Children older than 8 years of age:* 10 mg/kg/day given in divided doses every 6 to 12 hours.

Doxycycline (Vibramycin, Doxychel, Vivox, Doryx)—**PO:** 100 mg given at 12-hour intervals for two doses, followed by 100 mg given once daily. *Children older than 8 years of age and weighing less than 45 kg:* 4.4 mg/kg/day at 12-hour intervals for two doses and then 2.2 mg/kg once daily.

Minocycline HCl (Minocin)—**PO:** Initially 200 mg and then 100 mg every 12 hours. *Children 8 to 12 years of age:* 4 mg/kg/day in divided doses every 12 hours. **IV:** *Adults:* same as PO. *Children older than 8 years of age:* Initially 4 mg/kg and then 2 mg/kg every 12 hours.

MISCELLANEOUS ANTIBACTERIAL AGENTS

CHLORAMPHENICOL

CHLOROMYCETIN

Mechanism of Action

Chloramphenicol binds to the bacterial 50S ribosomal subunit, thereby inhibiting genetic transmission and protein synthesis.

Indications for Use

Chloramphenicol is the treatment of choice for typhoid fever caused by *Salmonella typhi* and serious infections caused by *Salmonella* (e.g., bacteremia), *Rickettsia* (when tetracyclines are contraindicated), and *Chlamydia.* This agent is also indicated for epiglottitis and cellulitis caused by *H. influenzae,* which is resistant to ampicillin.

Contraindications

Contraindications to the use of chloramphenicol include hypersensitivity to the agent. Chloramphenicol is not to be used for trivial infections or as prophylaxis for bacterial infections. This agent is indicated for serious infections in which less dangerous drugs are ineffective or contraindicated.

Precautions

1. Use with caution for patients with impaired renal and hepatic functions.
2. Monitor patient for superinfection.

Adverse Reactions

Most Serious: Blood dyscrasias (aplastic anemia, hypoplastic anemia, thrombocytopenia, and granulocytopenia).

CNS: Headache, depression, confusion, delirium.

GI: Nausea, vomiting, glossitis, stomatitis, diarrhea.

Dosage

PO: 50 to 100 mg/kg/day in divided doses every 6 or 8 hours. Higher doses are reserved for exceptional infections (e.g., meningitis, brain abscess).

IV: Administer as a 10% solution injected over at least 1 minute. Substitute oral dosage as soon as feasible.

LINCOMYCINS: CLINDAMYCIN
CLEOCIN HYDROCHLORIDE, CLEOCIN PHOSPHATE

Mechanism of Action

Clindamycin has the ability to prevent bacterial protein synthesis by binding to the 50S subunit of bacterial ribosomes.

Indications for Use

Clindamycin is effective against and indicated for serious respiratory tract infections (such as empyema, anaerobic pneumonitis, and lung abscess) and also for serious skin and soft tissue infections. Clindamycin is effective against Gram-positive organisms such as *S. aureus, Staphylococcus epidermidis, Staphylococcus pyogenes, S. pneumoniae,* β-hemolytic streptococci, *S. viridans, C. diphtheriae,* and *Nocardia asteroides*. Clindamycin is also indicated for infections caused by anaerobic organisms such as *Fusobacterium, Bacteroides, Clostridium perfringens, Eubacterium, Actinomyces* species, *Peptococcus, Peptostreptococcus,* microaerophilic streptococci, *Clostridium tetani,* and *Veillonella*. For anaerobic infections, clindamycin is initially given parenterally and then may be followed by oral therapy.

Contraindications

Contraindications to the use of clindamycin include hypersensitivity to the agent. Clindamycin is not to be used for minor bacterial or viral infections owing to its serious adverse side effects.

Precautions

1. Use with caution for patients with history of asthma or allergies because of possible hypersensitivity reactions.
2. Use with extreme caution for patients with history of GI disease, especially colitis (clindamycin may cause severe or fatal colitis). Patients should be instructed to report diarrhea and not to treat such diarrhea themselves.
3. Renal, hepatic, and hematopoietic functions should be monitored during prolonged therapy.
4. Erythromycin should not be used concurrently with clindamycin; erythromycin may block clindamycin's ability to inhibit bacterial protein synthesis.

5. Appropriate measures should be taken if superinfection occurs.
6. Clindamycin may enhance the actions of neuromuscular blocking agents; use cautiously.
7. Each oral dose of clindamycin should be taken with a full glass of water to avoid esophageal irritation.

Adverse Reactions

Cardiovascular: Hypotension, cardiopulmonary arrest (following too rapid IV administration—rare occurrence).

GI: Nausea, vomiting, diarrhea, pseudomembranous colitis, abdominal pain, esophagitis, anorexia.

Miscellaneous: Neutropenia, leukopenia, jaundice, skin rashes, urticaria.

Dosage

PO: 150 to 450 mg every 6 hours. **IM, IV:** 600 to 1200 mg/day up to 2.7 g/day (for more severe infections) in two to four divided doses. Life-threatening occurrences: up to 4.8 g/day given IV. *Children:* 8 to 25 mg/kg PO daily; or 15 to 40 mg/kg IM or IV given daily in three to four equal doses.

VANCOMYCIN HYDROCHLORIDE
VANCOCIN HYDROCHLORIDE

Mechanism of Action

Vancomycin is a bactericidal glycopeptide antibiotic that inhibits bacterial cell wall biosynthesis by binding to the cell walls of reproducing microorganisms and inhibiting mucopeptide formation. By this mechanism, the bacterial cell becomes susceptible to lysis. Vancomycin also acts to disrupt cell membrane function and RNA synthesis.

Indications for Use

Vancomycin is indicated for serious life-threatening infections (including methicillin-resistant staphylococci) caused by Gram-positive cocci (*S. pyogenes, S. pneumoniae*) and is the most potent antibiotic available for infections caused by *S. aureus* and *S. epidermidis*. Vancomycin is also effective, alone or in combination with an aminoglycoside, for endocarditis caused by *S. viridans* or *Streptococcus bovis*.

Contraindications

Contraindications to the use of vancomycin include hypersensitivity to the agent. Because of this drug's serious adverse effects, vancomycin is reserved for potentially life-threatening infections that are not treatable with other less toxic antibiotics, including the penicillins and cephalosporins.

Precautions

1. Avoid rapid IV bolus administration, which may cause serious hypotension, cardiac arrest.
2. Use cautiously for renally impaired patients because of the drug's nephrotoxicity.
3. Use cautiously for patients with previous hearing loss owing to the drug's potential ototoxicity.
4. As with all antibiotics, monitor the patient for superinfection.

Adverse Reactions

Most Serious: Ototoxicity, nephrotoxicity.
Other: Nausea, urticaria, macular rashes, chills, eosinophilia, anaphylactic reactions.

Dosage

PO: 500 mg every 6 hours or 1 g every 12 hours. **IV:** Same dose as oral. *Children:* 40 mg/kg/day in four divided doses, not to exceed 2 g/day. **IV:** Same dose as oral.

QUINOLONES AND FLUOROQUINOLONES

The quinolones and fluoroquinolones are a group of structurally similar anti-infectives that are potent inhibitors of bacterial nucleic acid synthesis and have demonstrated efficacy for a variety of many different microorganisms. The older quinolone derivatives (nalidixic acid and cinoxacin) are selectively used for urinary tract infections caused by common Gram-negative pathogens, whereas the newer fluorinated derivatives (fluoroquinolones: ciprofloxacin, enoxacin, lomefloxacin, norfloxacin, and ofloxacin) exhibit a broad spectrum of action and are used in treating various systemic infections. The following section presents the fluoroquinolones.

Mechanism of Action

The fluoroquinolones interfere with the enzyme DNA gyrase, which is needed for bacterial DNA synthesis. The increased bacterial susceptibility to these newer quinolones, as compared to older quinolones, such as nalidixic acid, may be related to their superior capability to penetrate the bacterial outer membrane.

Indications for Use

These broad-spectrum agents are especially useful for lower respiratory tract infections caused by *E. coli, K. pneumoniae, Enterobacter cloacae, P. mirabilis, P.*

aeruginosa, H. influenzae, Haemophilus parainfluenzae, and *S. pneumoniae.* Also, infections caused by *S. aureus* (including those that are methicillin susceptible and methicillin resistant), *S. pyogenes,* and *S. pneumoniae.* The fluoroquinolones usually do not exhibit activity against anaerobic organisms.

Ciprofloxacin is the most active and thus widely used fluoroquinolone and is especially useful against infections caused by *P. aeruginosa.* Ciprofloxacin and ofloxacin are also active against infections caused by *Chlamydia trachomatis* and *Mycobacterium tuberculosis.*

Contraindications

Contraindications to the use of quinolones and fluoroquinolones include hypersensitivity to these agents. These agents are generally contraindicated for prepubertal children because of the emergence of arthropathy in immature animals.

Precautions

1. Additive effects may be noted when these agents are used with other agents such as β-lactams or aminoglycosides.
2. Prolonged or repeated use may result in superinfection.
3. These agents should be used with caution for patients with renal or hepatic dysfunction as well as for nursing mothers.
4. Avoid concurrent use of antacids. Antacids may inhibit the absorption of these agents.
5. Concurrent use with theophylline may result in increased theophylline-related adverse reactions.
6. These agents may be taken with or without meals; however, the preferred time is 2 hours after a meal. Liberal use of fluids is recommended.
7. Use caution when performing tasks that require alertness; ciprofloxacin may cause drowsiness and dizziness.

Adverse Reactions

Most Frequent: Nausea, diarrhea, vomiting, abdominal discomfort, headache, restlessness, dizziness, skin rash.

CNS: Headache, photophobia, insomnia, nervousness, tremors, confusion, mania, convulsions, tingling sensation, tinnitus, toxic psychosis.

Cardiovascular: Palpitations, hypertension, angina, ventricular ectopy.

GI: Dysphagia, intestinal bleeding, oral candidiasis.

GU: Dysuria, polyuria, urinary retention, vaginitis.

Respiratory: Epistaxis, laryngeal edema, hiccoughs, dyspnea, bronchospasm.

Miscellaneous: Altered BUN, serum creatinine, alkaline phosphatase, as well as joint or back pain, pruritus, edema, photosensitivity, hyperpigmentation.

Dosage

Ciprofloxacin (Ciloxin, Cipro)—**PO:** Mild to moderate infections: 500 to 750 mg every 12 hours. Severe or complicated infections: up to 750 mg every 12 hours. **IV infusion:** 400 mg every 12 hours. For patients with impaired renal function, the recommended dose is half that of the usual dose; however, serum drug levels indicate the most reliable method for dosage adjustment.

Enoxacin (Penetrex)—**PO:** 200 to 400 mg every 12 hours for 7 to 14 days.

Lomefloxacin (Maxaquin)—**PO:** 400 mg once daily for 10 days.

Norfloxacin (Chibroxin, Noroxin)—**PO:** 400 mg every 12 hours for 3 to 10 days.

Ofloxacin (Ocuflox, Floxin)—**PO:** 400 mg every 12 hours for 10 days. **IV infusion:** 200 to 400 mg every 12 hours.

Antimycobacterial Agents

Tuberculosis (TB), an infection resulting from the organism *Mycobacterium tuberculosis,* is a disease that is usually confined to the lungs. Tuberculosis may be symptomatic or asymptomatic but typically is a chronic disease. Clinically active TB presents with severe inflammation, tissue necrosis, and the development of scarring and open cavities in the lungs. All of these factors lead to an impairment in pulmonary function. If the pathogen gains entry to the bloodstream or lymph system, other organs may become infected.

The most common mode of transmission of the disease is through inhalation of cough-expelled droplets from infected people. Other modes of transmission, although uncommon, include punctures of the skin by a contaminated object, consumption of contaminated milk, and contact with infected animals. The acid-fast staining technique is the diagnostic tool for determining the presence of *Mycobacterium* species (see *Staining Techniques* presented earlier in this chapter). Obtaining a sputum sample to determine whether acid-fast bacilli (AFB) are present is usually performed early in the morning for 3 consecutive days.

The increasing numbers of people being infected with TB, especially of the drug-resistant type, is a concern not only in the USA but also worldwide. Increases in the incidence of the disease are concentrated in specific epidemiologic groups, including racial and ethnic minority populations, foreign-born immigrants (especially from Southeast Asia and Central and South America), people with human immunodeficiency virus (HIV) infection, homeless people, and prison inmates. The greatest risk factor for TB is people infected with HIV. TB is often the initial manifestation of HIV infection and, consequently, testing for HIV infection is highly recommended for all patients with TB.

ANTITUBERCULOUS DRUGS

Mechanism of Action

Antituberculous agents are categorized as first-line drugs (primary) and second-line drugs (secondary or retreatment agents). The primary agents (such as isoniazid, INH) are bactericidal and act against actively growing tubercle bacilli by inhibiting lipid, protein, and nucleic acid biosynthesis in the growing organism. The second-line drugs are generally bacteriostatic (inhibits or retards bacterial growth rather than kills the organism) and indicated for use only in combination with the first-line drugs in which drug-resistant mycobacteria are present. Second-line drugs are generally not as effective and are far more toxic than first-line drugs.

First-line drugs:
Isoniazid (INH)
Rifampin
Ethambutal
Streptomycin
Pyrazinamide
Second-line drugs:
Capreomycin
Cycloserine
Ethionamide
Para-aminosalicylate sodium (PAS)
Kanamycin

Indications for Use

Antituberculous drugs are indicated for all forms of tuberculosis and as preventive therapy. Many of these agents are used in combination with each other for effective control of tuberculosis. The most recent recommended regimen consists of isoniazid (INH) 300 mg and rifampin 600 mg, both administered in single daily doses (or twice weekly with an increased isoniazid dose) for a total of 6 months, with pyrazinamide 30 mg/kg/day added during the first 8 weeks of therapy. Ethambutol should be added to this regimen if resistance is suspected. Sputum conversion (failure of growth of *M. tuberculosis* in sputum cultures) usually occurs within 1 month.

The American Thoracic Society and the Tuberculosis Control Division of the Centers for Disease Control and Prevention have endorsed a 9-month regimen of isoniazid-rifampin as an alternative for adults who have had previously untreated, uncomplicated pulmonary tuberculosis. After 2 weeks to 2 months of daily therapy, treatment may be continued with twice-weekly supervised doses of isoniazid (15 mg/kg) and rifampin (600 mg). Ethambutol should be added to this regimen if resistance is suspected. It is currently recommended that patients with HIV who develop tuberculosis be treated with the standard 9-month antituberculosis regimen. In some cases, the treatment period may need to be extended.

Retreatment regimens usually consist of two or more agents that were not previously administered. However, isoniazid is always included as part of the retreatment regimen unless there is resistance to the drug. Patients resistant to isoniazid are treated with rifampin 600 mg/day in combination with ethambutol and streptomycin. Pyrazinamide may be used in place of ethambutol. Patients resistant to streptomycin may be given capreomycin (preferred) or kanamycin. Ethionamide, para-aminosalicylate sodium (PAS), and cycloserine are usually not required as part of the retreatment regimen. For complete control of TB, continuous therapy for 18 to 24 months may be necessary. The most toxic agents are usually eliminated from the course of therapy as soon as feasible. Patients with drug-resistant disease should be treated with regimens customized to their situation.

Contraindications

Contraindications to the use of antituberculosis drugs include hypersensitivity to any of these agents, hepatic injury or acute liver disease (isoniazid, pyrazinamide, ethionamide), known optic neuritis (ethambutol), Epilepsy, depression, severe anxiety or psychosis, and severe renal insufficiency (cycloserine).

Precautions

1. Patients with active chronic liver disease or severe renal dysfunction should be carefully monitored. Assessment of renal, hepatic, or hematopoietic systems should be performed periodically during long-term treatment.
2. Concomitant administration of isoniazid and continuous or chronic alcohol ingestion may lead to an increased incidence of isoniazid-induced hepatitis.
3. Urine, feces, saliva, sputum, sweat, and tears may be colored red-orange when using rifampin. Additionally, soft contact lenses may become permanently stained. Patients should be forewarned of this occurrence.
4. Pyrazinamide and ethionamide should be used with caution for patients with a history of diabetes mellitus, because management of the diabetes may be more difficult.
5. PAS should be used with caution for patients with congestive heart failure (CHF) or patients for whom excess sodium is a potential hazard.

6. Serum potassium levels should be monitored frequently when administering capreomycin, because hypokalemia may occur during therapy.

Adverse Reactions

Serious toxic effects are usually dose related; the most common effects affect the nervous system, the liver, and/or the renal system. The most common adverse reactions of these agents include the following:

Nervous System: Peripheral neuropathy (isoniazid, ethionamide). Other neurotoxic effects include convulsions, optic neuritis, memory impairment, and toxic psychosis.
CNS: Headache, drowsiness, confusion, inability to concentrate, possible hallucinations.
GI: Nausea, vomiting, diarrhea, epigastric distress.
Other: Mild hepatic dysfunction, paresthesias.

Dosage:

	Adult Daily Dose	Pediatric Daily Dose	Activity
	mg/kg/day	*mg/kg*	
PRIMARY AGENTS			
Isoniazid (INH)	5–10 as single dose (15 mg/kg twice weekly) Usual daily dose: 300 mg	10–20 (20–40 twice weekly)	Bactericidal
Rifampin	10 as single dose (10 mg/kg twice weekly) Usual daily dose: 600 mg	10–20 (10–20 twice weekly)	Bactericidal
Ethambutol	15–25 as single dose (50 twice weekly) Usual daily dose: 800–1600 mg	15–25 (50 twice weekly)	Bacteriostatic
Pyrazinamide	15–30 as single dose (50–70 twice weekly) Usual daily dose: 1–2 g	15–30 (50–70 twice weekly)	Bactericidal
Streptomycin[a]	7–15 as single dose (25–30 twice weekly) Usual daily dose: 0.75–1 g	20–40 (25–30 twice weekly)	Bactericidal
SECONDARY OR RETREATMENT AGENTS			
Capreomycin[a]	15 as single dose Usual daily dose: 1 g	15	Bactericidal
Cycloserine	10–15 (four divided doses every 6 hr) Usual daily dose: 0.75–1 g	10–20	Bacteriostatic
Ethionamide	7–15 (four divided doses every 6 hr) Usual daily dose: 0.75–1 g	15–20 max: 750 mg/day	Bacteriostatic
Para-aminosalicylate sodium (PAS)	200 (four divided doses every 6 hr) Usual daily dose: 12–16 g	150–200	Bacteriostatic
Kanamycin[a]	15 as single dose Usual daily dose: 0.5–1 g	7.5–15	Bactericidal

[a]IM route only; all other drugs are given orally.

ANTIFUNGAL AGENTS

Fungal infections are of three types:

1. Dermatophytic—Infections that involve the hair, skin, and nails. These infections are treated topically with preparations such as Desenex, Aftate, Halotex, Lotrimin, or Monistat-Derm, depending on the causative organism. Causative organisms include *Epidermophyton, Trichophyton,* and *Microsporum.*
2. Mucocutaneous—These infections include only candidiasis. Moist skin and mucous membranes are the areas infected. Causative organisms include *Candida albicans* (most common), *Candida tropicalis,* and *Candida parapsilosis.*
3. Systemic—These infections are classified as deep or subcutaneous. Organisms causing deep systemic mycoses generally enter the body through inhalation and spread to other organs. Infections such as aspergillosis, blastomycosis, coccidioidomycosis, cryptococcosis, histoplasmosis, mucormycosis, and paracoccidioidomycosis are generally deep mycoses. Some subcutaneous mycoses include chromomycosis, mycetoma, and sporotrichosis. Subcutaneous infections usually enter the body through the skin and then spread to adjacent tissues.

This section concentrates on the more serious, potentially life-threatening systemic fungal infections and the antifungal drugs used to treat these infections.

AMPHOTERICIN B
FUNGIZONE
Mechanism of Action

Amphotericin B is a fungicidal (or fungistatic, depending on organism and drug concentration) antibiotic that has the ability to bind to the fungal cell membrane and alter the cellular permeability, thereby inhibiting growth and reproduction of the organism. Amphotericin B is selective in that it exerts its influence only on fungal cell membranes (due to the presence of sterol in the cellular membrane). Bacteria and viruses do not contain the component sterol in their cellular membranes; therefore, amphotericin B is ineffective against these organisms.

Indications for Use

Amphotericin B is the drug of choice for severe progressive and potentially fatal systemic fungal infections and is specifically intended to treat blastomycosis, candidiasis, cryptococcosis, histoplasmosis, and paracoccidioidomycosis. Mucormycosis, aspergillosis, and sporotrichosis infections also respond to amphotericin B. Because of amphotericin B's serious toxicity, it should not be used to treat trivial or clinically insignificant fungal infections.

Contraindications

Contraindications to the use of amphotericin B include hypersensitivity, unless the infection is life-threatening and responsive only to amphotericin B.

Precautions

1. Monitor patient for signs of renal damage, which is the most important toxic adverse effect of amphotericin B therapy.
2. Potentiation of effects is noted with coadministered digitalis and skeletal muscle relaxants.
3. Extended treatment time is usually necessary. Adverse reactions are common and can be potentially dangerous. Amphotericin B should only be administered to hospitalized patients who are under close supervision.
4. Cautious use is recommended for patients with renal impairment, blood dyscrasias, neurologic disorders, and peptic ulcers as well as for pregnant women.

Adverse Reactions

Most Common: Fever, headache, chills, anorexia, muscle and joint pain, nausea, vomiting, diarrhea.

Cardiovascular: Arrhythmias, ventricular fibrillation, cardiac arrest, hypertension, hypotension.

Renal: Hypokalemia, azotemia, hyposthenuria, renal tubular acidosis.

Pulmonary: Acute dyspnea, hypoxemia, interstitial infiltrates in neutropenic patients.

GI: Melena or hemorrhagic gastroenteritis, acute liver failure.

Hematologic: Coagulation abnormalities, thrombocytopenia, leukopenia, agranulocytosis, eosinophilia, leukocytosis.

Miscellaneous: Weight loss, anaphylactoid reactions, flushing.

Dosage

IV: Individualized dosage depending on the severity of the disease. Do not exceed a total daily dose of 1.5 mg/kg. Total dose may range from 1.5 to 4 g (reserved for life-threatening infections). Several months (9 to 12) of therapy are usually necessary.

FLUCONAZOLE

DIFLUCAN

Mechanism of Action

Fluconazole, a synthetic broad-spectrum bis-triazole antifungal agent, selectively inhibits fungal cytochrome P-450 enzymes required for the synthesis of ergosterol, the chief sterol in fungal cell membranes. This action results in increased membrane permeability by which leakage of cellular contents occurs.

Indications for Use

Fluconazole is useful for the treatment of meningitis caused by *Cryptococcus neoformans* and in the treatment of oropharyngeal and esophageal candidiasis, as well as serious systemic candidal fungal infections such as peritonitis, pneumonia, and urinary tract infections.

Contraindications

Contraindications to fluconazole include hypersensitivity to the agent.

Precautions

1. Cautious use is recommended for patients who are hypersensitive to azoles.
2. Concomitant use with oral contraceptives may decrease the effectiveness of oral contraceptives.
3. Injection sites and veins should be monitored for signs of phlebitis.
4. Fluconazole should be discontinued if signs of renal toxicity occur.
5. Frequent, small meals are encouraged if GI upset occurs.

Adverse Reactions

Most Common: Skin rash, nausea, headache.
CNS: Delirium, coma, psychiatric disturbances, dizziness.
GI: Vomiting, diarrhea, abdominal pain.
Hepatic: Increased liver enzymes and bilirubin.
Miscellaneous: Fever, hypotension, edema, oliguria, arthralgia, myalgia, diffuse rash, pruritus, exfoliative skin disorders.

Dosage

PO: 200 to 400 mg on the first day of therapy, followed by 100 to 200 mg once daily for 2 to 12 weeks. **IV infusion:** 200 mg/hr as constant infusion for up to 14 days.

FLUCYTOSINE
ANCOBON
Mechanism of Action

The exact mode of action of flucytosine, a synthetic pyrimidine, is unknown; however, it is metabolized to 5-fluorouracil within the fungal cell and is known to produce synergistic activity when coadministered with amphotericin B.

Indications for Use

For the treatment of serious infections (septicemia, endocarditis, meningitis, and pulmonary infections) caused by strains of *Candida* and *Cryptococcus*. Flucytosine is usually used in conjunction with amphotericin B because of the emergence of resistant strains of *Candida*.

Contraindications

Contraindications to the use of flucytosine include hypersensitivity to the agent.

Precautions

1. Monitor patients frequently for renal status; drug accumulation may occur in renally impaired patients.
2. Use cautiously for bone marrow depressed patients; this drug may potentiate bone marrow depression.
3. Although coadministration of amphotericin B is usually therapeutic, it also increases the incidence of toxicity.

Adverse Reactions

Most Frequent: Nausea, vomiting, diarrhea, rash, anemia, leukopenia, thrombopenia.

Less Frequent: Confusion, hallucinations, headache, drowsiness, vertigo.

Dosage

PO: 50 to 150 mg/kg/day in divided doses given at 6-hour intervals. With amphotericin B (0.3 mg/kg/day): 150 mg/kg/day in four divided doses.

ITRACONAZOLE

SPORANOX

Mechanism of Action

Itraconazole is a triazole derivative that is structurally related to fluconazole and has a similar mechanism of action as fluconazole. It inhibits fungal cytochrome P-450 enzymes required for ergosterol synthesis and cell membrane strength and stability.

Indications for Use

Itraconazole is especially useful for treating blastomycosis (pulmonary and extrapulmonary), histoplasmosis (including chronic cavitary pulmonary disease), and aspergillosis (pulmonary and extrapulmonary) in both immunocompromised and nonimmunocompromised patients. Investigational uses include treatment of systemic mycoses involving candidiasis, cryptococcal infections, coccidioidomycosis, and paracoccidioidomycosis.

Contraindications

Contraindications to the use of intraconazole include hypersensitivity to the agent. Coadministration of terfenadine with itraconazole has been documented to cause serious cardiovascular adverse events, including death or ventricular tachycardia.

Precautions

1. Itraconazole is extensively metabolized by the liver; therefore, carefully monitor hepatic enzymes in patients with preexisting hepatic dysfunction. Additionally, patients should report any signs and symptoms (such as fatigue, anorexia, nausea, vomiting, jaundice, dark urine) that may suggest liver dysfunction.
2. Absorption is increased by food; therefore, administration with meals is highly recommended.
3. The long-term effect of itraconazole in children is unknown; however, itraconazole, when administered to rats, has been shown to produce bone toxicity.

Adverse Reactions

Most Common: Nausea, headache, rash.

Other: Diarrhea, fever, pruritus, dizziness, psychiatric disturbances, abdominal pain, edema, hypertension, hepatic dysfunction, hypokalemia.

Dosage

PO: 200 to 400 mg once daily taken with food. **Severe infections:** 200 mg t.i.d. for the first 3 days of therapy.

KETOCONAZOLE
NIZORAL
Mechanism of Action

Ketoconazole is an imidazole broad-spectrum antifungal agent that alters the fungal plasma membrane by interfering with the cytochrome P-450 enzymes responsible for the biosynthesis of ergosterol. This action causes the leakage of cellular components, promoting the death of the fungal cell.

Indications for Use

Ketoconazole is indicated for and effective against both mucocutaneous and systemic fungal infections of candidiasis, chronic mucocutaneous candidiasis, oral thrush, candiduria, blastomycosis, coccidioidomycosis, histoplasmosis, chromomycosis, and paracoccidioidomycosis. High doses (800 to 1200 mg/day) of ketoconazole have been effective against CNS fungal infections. Ketoconazole (800 to 1200 mg/day) has also been effective for treatment of Cushing's syndrome owing to its ability to inhibit adrenal steroidogenesis. Finally, ketoconazole (400 mg every 8 hours) has also been used in the treatment of advanced prostrate cancer.

Contraindications

Contraindications to the use of ketoconazole include hypersensitivity to the agent. Ketoconazole should not be used for treatment of fungal meningitis because of the poor penetration of the drug into the cerebral spinal fluid.

Precautions

1. Do not use this drug in direct conjunction with antacids, anticholinergics, or H_2 blockers. These agents may block the effect of ketoconazole because of their alkaline environment. Dissolution and absorption of the drug may be impaired.
2. This agent should be taken with food to alleviate GI distress.
3. Ketoconazole undergoes extensive metabolism in the liver; therefore, patients should report any signs or symptoms (see above, under *Itraconazole*) that suggest liver dysfunction or if abdominal pain, fever, or diarrhea become pronounced.
4. Renal impairment does not alter dosing requirements.
5. Ketoconazole may produce dizziness, headache, drowsiness: patients should observe caution when performing tasks that require mental alertness.

Adverse Reactions

Most Common: Nausea, vomiting, GI upset, pruritus.
CNS: Headache, dizziness, somnolence, photophobia.
GI: Nausea, vomiting, abdominal pain, diarrhea.
Neuropsychiatric: Suicidal tendencies.
Miscellaneous: Pruritus, fever, chills, impotence, thrombocytopenia, leukopenia, hemolytic anemia, urticaria.

Dosage

PO: 200 mg given in a single daily dose, up to 400 mg daily for serious infections. *Children older than 2 years of age:* 3.3 to 6.6 mg/kg/day as a single daily dose. Treatment times: 1 to 2 weeks for candidiasis, 4 weeks for recalcitrant dermatophytal infections, and 6 months for other systemic mycotic infections.

MICONAZOLE
MONISTAT IV
Mechanism of Action
Miconazole, an imidazole derivative, is a broad-spectrum antifungal agent that alters the permeability of the fungal plasma membrane by inhibiting the synthesis of ergosterol, resulting in the leakage of cellular components and ultimately causing cell death.

Indications for Use
Miconazole is effective in the treatment of severe fungal infections such as coccidioidomycosis, candidiasis, cryptococcosis, petriellidiosis, paracoccidioidomycosis, and chronic mucocutaneous candidiasis. Miconazole is not indicated in the treatment of trivial fungal diseases. Miconazole is an alternative drug to amphotericin B for patients with renal impairment or those who do not tolerate amphotericin B therapy.

Contraindications
Contraindications to the use of miconazole include hypersensitivity to the agent.

Precautions
1. Administer drug by slow IV infusion; rapid infusion may cause transient tachycardia, arrhythmia, or even cardiac arrest.
2. Amphotericin B and miconazole have been noted to have antagonistic properties; that is, when these drugs are given concurrently, the effects produced are less than when they are given alone.
3. Inadequate treatment may result in recurrence of the infection.

Adverse Reactions
Most Common: IV use: phlebitis, pruritus, nausea, vomiting, fever, rash.
GI: Nausea, vomiting, diarrhea, anorexia.
Other: Fever, drowsiness, flushes, decrease in serum sodium levels, decreased hematocrit, thrombocytopenia, arrhythmias (with too rapid IV administration).

Dosage:
IV injection, total daily dosage range:

For coccidioidomycosis: 1800 to 3600 mg
For cryptococcosis: 1200 to 2400 mg
For petriellidiosis: 600 to 3000 mg

For candidiasis: 600 to 1800 mg
For paracoccidioidomycosis: 200 to 1200 mg
Children: 20 to 40 mg/kg/day, not to exceed 15 mg/kg per infusion.
Duration of therapy usually is a minimum of 3 to 4 weeks.

ANTIVIRAL AGENTS

Classification of Viruses

Viruses are initially classified according to the viral genome (hereditary factors), which may contain either RNA or DNA but never both. The following list includes some of the more common RNA and DNA viruses and the infectious diseases they cause.

RNA Virus	Diseases
Coronaviridae	Coronaviruses (respiratory infections)
Orthomyxoviridae	Influenza viruses
Paramyxoviridae	Parainfluenza viruses (croup, pneumonia, bronchitis), measles virus, respiratory syncytial virus (bronchiolitis, pneumonia)
Picornaviridae	Polioviruses, coxsackieviruses, echoviruses (aseptic meningitis), rhinoviruses, hepatitis infections
Reoviridae	Rotaviruses (diarrhea), Colorado tick fever, respiratory infections
Retroviridae	Retroviruses (primary agent of acquired immune deficiency syndrome [AIDS], also known as the human immunodeficiency virus [HIV]
Rhabdoviridae	Rabies virus
Togaviridae	Encephalitis viruses (mosquito borne), yellow fever viruses, rubella virus

DNA Virus	Diseases
Adenoviridae	Adenoviruses (acute respiratory diseases)
Herpesviridae	Herpes simplex types 1 and 2, varicella-zoster (chickenpox, shingles), cytomegalovirus, Epstein-Barr virus (mononucleosis)
Papovaviridae	Papilloma viruses (warts)
Poxviridae	Variola virus (smallpox)

SPECIFIC ANTIVIRAL DRUGS

AMANTADINE HYDROCHLORIDE

SYMMETREL

Mechanism of Action

Amantadine acts to uncoat the RNA virus, thereby blocking the transfer of viral nucleic acid into the host cell.

Indications for Use

Amantadine is specific for the prevention and treatment of respiratory tract infections caused by influenza A virus strains. Early immunization is the treatment of choice, especially for high-risk patients with underlying disease states.

Contraindications

Contraindications to the use of amantadine include hypersensitivity to the agent.

Precautions

1. Use with caution for patients with liver disease, CHF, and renal impairment and for elderly individuals. Dosage may need to be reduced or adjusted.
2. CNS effects include blurred vision. Patients should use with caution while driving or performing other similar tasks.
3. Monitor patient carefully if CNS stimulants are administered concurrently.

Adverse Reactions

Most Frequent: CNS side effects, including confusion, hallucinations, anxiety, insomnia, lightheadedness, and depression of mental alertness.

Less Frequent: Vomiting, headache, dyspnea, fatigue.

Dosage

PO: 200 mg as a single dose or 100 mg b.i.d. *Children 9 to 12 years of age:* 100 mg b.i.d. *Children 1 to 9 years of age:* 4.4 mg/kg to 8.8 mg/kg daily in two to three divided doses, not to exceed 150 mg/day.

RIBAVIRIN
VIRAZOLE

Mechanism of Action

Ribavirin is an antiviral agent with selective inhibitory activity against respiratory syncytial virus (RSV), influenza A and B viruses, and herpes simplex virus. The mechanism of action of ribavirin is unknown; it appears to inhibit guanidine monophosphate synthesis and subsequent nucleic acid formation in viral particles.

Indications for Use

Ribavirin aerosol is indicated for infants and young children with severe lower respiratory tract infections caused by RSV. Ribavirin aerosol is not indicated for RSV infections not accompanied by severe lower respiratory tract infections; therefore, the decision to treat patients with RSV infections is based on the severity of the RSV infection. This drug should not be administered without documentation of RSV because of its serious adverse effects.

Investigational uses include aerosol administration for the treatment of influenza A and B virus infection, and oral therapy (600 mg to 1800 mg/day for 10 to 14 days) for the treatment of acute and chronic hepatitis virus, measles, and Lassa fever.

Contraindications

Contraindications to the use of ribavirin include pregnancy, known or suspected. Ribavirin has been found to be teratogenic.

Precautions

1. The presence of prematurity or existing cardiopulmonary disease in infants and young children may increase the severity of the RSV infection.
2. Ribavirin aerosol is generally not indicated for patients requiring assisted ventilation (not approved by the Food and Drug Administration). Precipitation of the drug may occur, hindering safe and effective ventilation.
3. Worsening of respiratory status with the use of ribavirin has been noted in infants and in adults with chronic obstructive lung disease or asthma.
4. Careful monitoring of respiratory and fluid status is required for patients with severe lower respiratory tract infections caused by RSV.
5. Ribavirin administered by aerosol is absorbed systemically. Plasma half-life is 8 to 10 hours. Ribavirin and its metabolites accumulate in red blood cells, with a corresponding half-life of approximately 40 days.
6. Aerosolized ribavirin may escape into the air around the patient; therefore, both visitors and staff may be exposed to the drug. Because of the serious adverse reactions that ribavirin may cause to visitors and staff, as with other potentially hazardous drugs, pregnant women should avoid exposure to the drug.

Adverse Reactions

Cardiovascular: Cardiac arrest (rare), hypotension, digitalis toxicity.

Pulmonary: Deteriorating respiratory function, bacterial pneumonia, pneumothorax, apnea, ventilator dependence.

Pregnancy: Teratogenic effects.

Miscellaneous: Rash, conjunctivitis, reticulocytosis.

Dosage

Ribavirin aerosol may be administered only through a Small Particle Aerosol Generator (SPAG). Complete familiarity with this system is essential before use (refer to Viratek SPAG-2 Operator's Manual for operating instructions). Treatment is usually effective if initiated within 3 days after the onset of RSV lower respiratory tract infection and is carried out for 12 to 18 hours per day for 3 to 7 days. Use of the SPAG-2 aerosol generator requires an infant oxygen hood, face mask, or oxygen tent.

Ribavirin aerosol is not to be coadministered with any other aerosolized medications or other aerosol generating device other than that mentioned above. Additionally, ribavirin should not be used for patients requiring assisted mechanical ventilation because of obstruction and subsequent inadequate ventilation and/or precipitate or fluid accumulation in tubing. If using simultaneously with assisted ventilation, check equipment, including the endotracheal tube, frequently.

Ribavirin aerosol is supplied in 100-ml vials as 6 grams of lyophilized drug. To administer, solubilize the drug with sterile USP water for injection or inhalation in the 100-ml vial. Transfer the solution to the 500-ml wide-mouthed Erlenmeyer flask (SPAG-2 reservoir). Add sterile USP water for injection or inhalation to obtain a total volume of 300 ml. The final concentration is 20 mg/ml when reconstituted with 300 ml sterile water. **Warning:** The sterile USP water for injection or inhalation should not have any antimicrobial agent or other additives. Store powder at 15° to 25°C (59° to 78°F). Reconstituted solutions may be stored at room temperature for up to 24 hours. Discard used solution every 24 hours and before adding newly reconstituted solution. Inspect solution before using. Discard if discolored or cloudy.

ZIDOVUDINE (AZT)
RETROVIR
Mechanism of Action

Zidovudine inhibits the viral replication of some retroviruses, including HIV, by interfering with the HIV viral RNA-dependent DNA polymerase (reverse transcriptase).

Indications for Use

Oral therapy for adults: Management of patients with HIV infection who have evidence of impaired immunity (CD4 cell count of $\leq 500/mm^3$) before therapy is initiated.

Oral therapy for children: HIV-infected children older than 3 months of age who have HIV-related symptoms or who are asymptomatic and also have abnormal laboratory values indicating HIV-related immunosuppression.

IV therapy for adults: Management of adult patients with symptomatic HIV infection (AIDS and advanced ARC) who have a cytologically confirmed *Pneumocystis carinii* pneumonia (PCP, see following section) or an absolute CD4 (T4 helper/inducer) lymphocyte count of $<200/mm^3$.

Contraindications

Zidovudine is contraindicated for patients who exhibit life-threatening allergic reactions to any of the agent's components.

Precautions

1. Coadministered acetaminophen may increase the toxicity of zidovudine.
2. Zidovudine has not been shown to reduce the risk of HIV transmission.
3. Oral zidovudine must be taken every 4 hours around the clock.
4. Patients may continue to have illnesses associated with AIDS or ARC.
5. Coadministration with drugs that are nephrotoxic or cytotoxic (e.g., amphotericin B, flucytosine, dapsone, pentamidine) may increase the risk of toxicity during zidovudine administration.

Adverse Reactions

Most Frequent: Granulocytopenia and anemia. Also, headache, nausea, insomnia, myalgia.

Other: Anorexia, diarrhea, vomiting, dysphagia, edema of the tongue, dizziness, paresthesias, somnolence, anxiety, confusion, nervousness, syncope, depression, dyspnea, nosebleed, sinusitis, hoarseness, rhinitis, polyuria, dysuria, urinary frequency, muscle spasm, tremor.

Dosage

PO: initially, 200 mg every 4 hours around the clock. After 1 month of therapy, dosage may be reduced to 100 mg every 4 hours. If anemia or significant granulocytopenia occurs, reduce dose or discontinue the drug. *Children older than 3 months:* **PO:** 180 mg/m^2 every 6 hours, not to exceed 200 mg every 6 hours. **IV infusion:** *Adults:* 1 to 2 mg/kg infused over 1 hour every 4 hours around the clock.

AGENTS USED TO TREAT *PNEUMOCYSTIS CARINII* PNEUMONIA

This section identifies the specific anti-infective agents used to treat *Pneumocystis carinii* pneumonia.

PENTAMIDINE ISETHIONATE
PENTAM 300, NEBUPENT

Mechanism of Action

Pentamidine is an antimicrobial agent, the mode of action of which is not fully known; however, studies indicate that pentamidine interferes with nuclear metabolism and inhibits the synthesis of DNA, RNA, phospholipids, and protein synthesis.

Indications for Use

Pentamidine is indicated for the treatment of *Pneumocystis carinii* pneumonia (PCP). Additionally, aerosol pentamidine is used extensively for the prevention of PCP in high-risk, HIV-infected patients (such as patients with a history of one or more episodes of PCP or those patients with a peripheral CD4+ (T4 helper/inducer) lymphocyte count $\leq$200 mm^3.

Contraindications

There are no contraindications to the use of pentamidine after the diagnosis of PCP has been established. Contraindications to prophylactic aerosol administration of the agent include history of anaphylactic reaction to inhaled or parenteral pentamidine.

Precautions

1. Use with caution for patients with renal disease (accumulation may occur), hypertension, hypotension, hypoglycemia, hyperglycemia, leukopenia, thrombocytopenia, anemia, or hepatic impairment.
2. Monitor patient carefully for sudden, severe hypotension, hypoglycemia, cardiac arrhythmias, or other serious adverse effects.
3. Strict isolation techniques (gown, cap, gloves, mask, goggles) should be used by health care providers to protect themselves when administering aerosolized medications to AIDS patients.

Adverse Reactions

Most Serious: Leukopenia, hypoglycemia, thrombocytopenia, hypotension, acute renal failure, hypocalcemia, ventricular tachycardia, Stevens-Johnson syndrome; death due to severe hypotension, hypoglycemia, cardiac arrhythmias.

Aerosol Administration: Bronchospasm, fatigue, severe cough (usually in patients with asthma or smoking), unpleasant taste, burning sensation in back of throat. mild hypoglycemia. Systemic side effects have not been noted with aerosol administration.

Dosage

IM, IV: 4 mg/kg/day in a single dose for 14 days. Dosage must be reduced for patients with renal failure.

Aerosol administration for prevention of PCP: 300 mg once every 4 weeks administered via the Respirgard II nebulizer by Marquest or other specialized filter-designed nebulizer. To administer, dissolve 300 mg (one vial) of lyophilized pentamidine with 6 ml of sterile water for injection, USP (do not use saline solution because it will cause the drug to precipitate). Place solution in a specialized jet nebulizer and administer therapy until nebulizer chamber is empty (approximately 30 to 45 minutes). Do not coadminister or mix pentamidine with any other medications. If bronchospasm occurs, reduce flow rate or administer a bronchodilator before or during pentamidine use (preferred).

Use only freshly prepared solutions. Store dry product at controlled room temperature 15° to 30°C (50° to 86°F). Reconstituted solutions are generally stable for 48 hours if stored in the original vial at room temperature and protected from light.

TRIMETHOPRIM AND SULFAMETHOXAZOLE (TMP-SMZ)
BACTRIM, SEPTRA

Mechanism of Action

The combination of trimethoprim and sulfamethoxazole (TMP-SMZ) effectively interferes with bacterial biosynthesis of essential nucleic acids and proteins.

Indications for Use

TMP-SMZ is the drug of choice for the treatment of pneumonia caused by *P. carinii* in children and adults immunosuppressed by cancer chemotherapy or other immunosuppressive therapy or suffering from AIDS. Other uses include acute exacerbations of chronic bronchitis, acute otitis media caused by *H. influenzae* and *S. pneumoniae,* and shigellosis enteritis caused by *Shigella flexneri* and *Shigella sonnei.*

Contraindications

Contraindications to the use of the TMP-SMZ combination include hypersensitivity to either agent, in addition to infants younger than 2 months of age, pregnancy and lactation, and megaloblastic anemia caused by folate deficiency.

Precautions

1. This agent is not indicated for treatment of streptococcal pharyngitis.
2. Use with caution for elderly individuals and patients with renal or hepatic impairment; increased adverse reactions may occur.
3. For patients with AIDS, an increased incidence of side effects is noted, such as rash, fever, and leukopenia.
4. Monitor patients for the occurrence of superinfection.

Adverse Reactions

Most Common: Nausea, vomiting, anorexia, allergic skin rashes.

CNS: Headache, convulsions, hallucinations, vertigo, nervousness, apathy, mental depression.

GI: Nausea, vomiting, anorexia, stomatitis, abdominal pain, diarrhea, hepatitis, jaundice, pancreatitis.

Dosage

For *Pneumocystis carinii* pneumonitis in adults and children: 20 mg TMP/kg/day and 100 mg SMZ/kg/day, orally or by IV infusion in equally divided doses every 6 hours for 14 days. When administering by IV infusion, give slowly over 60 to 90 minutes. TMP-SMZ is not to be given by IM route.

DAPSONE

Dapsone (DDS: 4,4-diaminodiphenylsulphone) is a leprostatic agent that is bactericidal as well as bacteriostatic against *Mycobacterium leprae*. The mechanism of action of dapsone has not been clearly defined; it seems to inhibit folate synthesis. The reason for its inclusion in this section is its investigational use in conjunction with trimethoprim for treatment of PCP and for prophylaxis of PCP. Dapsone (Avlosulfon in Canada) is available in 25- and 100-mg tablets.

REFERENCES/RECOMMENDED READING

Alderson T. New directions for the anti-retroviral chemotherapy of AIDS—a basis for a pharmacological approach to treatment. Biol Rev 68:265, 1993.

American Thoracic Society. Treatment of tuberculosis and tuberculosis infection in adults and children. Am Rev Respir Dis 134:355, 1986.

Chopra I, Hawkey PM, Hinton M. Tetracyclines, molecular and clinical aspects. J Antimicrob Chemother 29:245, 1992.

Donowitz GR, Mandell GL. Drug therapy: beta-lactam antibiotics. N Engl J Med 318:490, 1988.

Drug Facts and Comparisons. 49th ed. St. Louis: Facts and Comparisons, 1995.

Edson RS, Terrell CL. The aminoglycosides: streptomycin, kanamycin, gentamycin, tobramycin, amikacin, netilmicin, and sisomicin. Mayo Clin Proc 62:916, 1987.

Gallis HA, Drew RH, Pickard WW. Amphotericin B: thirty years of clinical experience. Rev Infect Dis 12:308, 1990.

Hussar D. New drugs. Nursing 23(5):57, 1993.

Lee BL, et al. Dapsone, trimethoprim-sulfamethoxazole plasma levels during treatment of Pneumocystis pneumonia in patients with AIDS. Ann Intern Med 110:606, 1989.

Neu HC. New antibiotics: areas of appropriate use. J Infect Dis 155:403, 1987.

Physicians' Desk Reference, 49th ed. Montvale, NJ: Medical Economics, 1995.

Remington J. Current clinical management of infections: use of third generation cephalosporins, Part 1. Hosp Pract 26(Suppl 4):5, 1991.

Agents Affecting Renal Function and Electrolyte Balance 17

Of vital importance in maintaining body homeostasis is the regulation of fluid and electrolyte balance by the renal system. The basic objective of renal therapy is to restore the volume and composition of the body fluids to a normal state. Diuretic agents are one of the most widely used, useful groups of drugs that can significantly alter renal function.

Because the kidneys regulate the retention and excretion of several electrolytes and the diuretics can profoundly affect the distribution of these electrolytes, the first section of this chapter presents the major body electrolytes, their normal values, and clinical implications of abnormal values. A clear understanding of renal physiology, presented in the second section of this chapter, will lead the practitioner to a comprehensible working knowledge of how the diuretics pharmacologically control the activity of the kidneys. The third section of this chapter details the diuretic agents themselves. Some of the diuretics also have other therapeutic applications, as listed under indications for use.

Major Body Electrolytes

Electrolytes are substances that dissociate into ions when dissolved in the blood and are capable of carrying an electric charge. Acids, bases, and salts are common electrolytes. *Cations* are electrolytes that carry a positive charge, whereas *anions* are electrolytes that carry a negative charge. Electroneutrality exists when the cations balance the anions, which is a state that is vital to normal body homeostasis.

Cations: Na^{+} (sodium), K^{+} (potassium), Ca^{+2} (calcium), Mg^{+2} (magnesium)

Anions: Cl^{-} (chloride), HCO_3^{-} (bicarbonate), HPO_4^{-2} (phosphate), SO_4^{-2} (sulfate), protein, organic acids

Electrolytes are essential for normal bodily function and have a variety of intrinsic purposes. In general, electrolytes:

- Help regulate acid-base balance. Hydrogen is exchanged for potassium or sodium in the kidneys to maintain a proper blood pH. The kidneys may also cause bicarbonate or chloride ions to be absorbed or excreted in response to blood pH.
- Help regulate neuromuscular activity.
- Help maintain osmotic equilibrium between the intracellular fluid (ICF) and extracellular fluid (ECF). Primary intracellular electrolytes: potassium, magnesium, phosphate. Primary extracellular electrolytes: sodium, calcium, chloride, bicarbonate.
- Sustain proper conditions for chemical reactions within the body.

Electrolyte imbalance may reflect fluid, acid-base, kidney, neuromuscular, endocrine, or skeletal disorders. Severe electrolyte imbalance may precipitate life-threatening cardiac arrhythmias.

Serum Calcium (Ca^{+2})

Most body calcium is stored in the skeleton and teeth, which are primary reserve sources for maintaining calcium blood levels. Approximately 50% of the blood calcium is ionized and the rest is protein bound. Only the ionized blood calcium is able to be used in bodily processes such as muscular contraction, cardiac contraction, transmission of nerve impulses, and blood coagulation. In acidemia, the ratio of ionized calcium will be higher (fewer calcium ions are bound to protein), whereas in alkalemia, the ionized concentration of calcium will be lower (more calcium ions are bound to protein).

Specifically, calcium's role in body homeostasis includes:

- Participation in the transmission of nerve impulses.
- Initiation of muscular contraction (calcium is an essential component of neuromuscular and cardiac contractility).
- Essential for normal blood coagulation (blood will not clot if deprived of calcium).
- Gives firmness and rigidity to bones and teeth.
- Acid-base regulation.

Parathyroid hormone, vitamin D, and, to a lesser extent, calcitonin and adrenal steroids regulate calcium blood levels. Serum calcium is measured to aid diagnosis of neuromuscular, skeletal, and endocrine disorders as well as acid-base imbalances, blood-clotting deficiencies, or cardiac dysrhythmias.

Normal range:
Total: 8.5 to 10.5 mg/dl, 2.1 to 2.6 mmol/L, or 4.5 to 5.5 mEq/L
Ionized: 4.4 to 5.4 mg/dl, or 1.09 to 1.33 mmol/L

Clinical implications:

Critical values include a calcium level less than 7.0 mg/dl (associated with tetany, convulsions), and greater than 13.5 mg/dl (associated with hypercalcemic coma and metastatic cancer)

Hypercalcemia:

Increased serum calcium concentration.

ETIOL: Cancer, primary hyperparathyroidism, hyperthyroidism, adrenal insufficiency, excessive intake of vitamin D, prolonged immobilization, multiple fractures, acute renal disease, excessive calcium supplements or antacids (calcium carbonate), acidosis (fewer calcium ions are bound to protein).

ECG CHANGES: Serum calcium level greater than 16 mg/dl: shortened QT interval and ST duration, inverted T waves, ventricular dysrhythmias.

SIGNS AND SYMPTOMS: Cardiac arrhythmias, muscle weakness, neuromuscular paralysis, anorexia, nausea, vomiting, peptic ulcer, abdominal pain, stupor, coma, cardiac arrest.

TX: Correct underlying cause, rectify acidemia; correct dehydration; diuretic therapy to induce excretion of calcium ions; administer phosphate to allow movement of calcium into the bone; steroid therapy to decrease intestinal absorption of calcium ions.

Hypocalcemia:

Decreased serum calcium concentration.

ETIOL: Acute pancreatitis, hypoparathyroidism, peritonitis, vitamin D deficiency, diarrhea, osteomalacia, renal failure, rickets, alkalosis (more calcium ions become bound to protein).

ECG CHANGES: Serum calcium level less than 6.1 mg/dl: prolonged QT interval and ST duration, flattened or inverted T waves.

SIGNS AND SYMPTOMS: Numbness, paresthesia, muscle cramping, seizure activity, tetany, cardiac arrhythmias.

TX: Correct underlying cause, administer vitamin D; administer calcium gluconate or calcium chloride.

Serum Sodium (Na^+)

Sodium comprises approximately 90% of the electrolyte fluid, is the chief base of the blood, and is the principal cation found in extracellular fluid. Sodium functions to:

- Chemically maintain osmotic pressure of extracellular fluid.
- Regulate water excretion. Extracellular sodium concentration helps the kidney regulate water balance (low sodium levels promote water excretion and high sodium levels promote water retention); therefore, sodium concentration must

be evaluated in relation to the amount of water in the body (the patient's state of hydration). Results of water imbalance include: hypervolemia—water and electrolyte retention, increased extracellular fluid volume; hypovolemia—water and electrolyte loss, decreased extracellular fluid volume.

- Help regulate acid-base balance.
- Aid in the transmission of nerve impulses.

Serum sodium is measured to evaluate fluid-electrolyte and acid-base balance. Also, related neuromuscular, renal, and adrenal functions.

Normal range:
135 to 145 mEq/L or 135 to 145 mmol/L

Clinical implications
Critical values include a sodium level less than 120 (cardiac failure) or greater than 160 (vascular collapse).

Hypernatremia:
Increased serum sodium concentration.
ETIOL: Essential water loss (through sweating, fever, burns, high ambient temperatures, renal impairment, diabetes insipidus, hypothalamic disorders), dehydration and insufficient water intake, excessive hypertonic NaCl intake or $NaHCO_3$, Cushing's syndrome, primary aldosteronism, excessive sodium intake.
SIGNS AND SYMPTOMS: Thirst, restlessness, dry mucous membranes, oliguria, lethargy, muscle weakness, twitching, seizures, coma.
TX: Correct underlying cause, administer water.

Hyponatremia:
Decreased serum sodium concentration.
ETIOL: Inadequate sodium intake, severe burns, severe diarrhea, vomiting, diabetic acidosis, renal failure, hepatic insufficiency, adrenal insufficiency, profuse sweating, diuretic therapy.
SIGNS AND SYMPTOMS: [Na^+] below 120 mEq/L: headache, muscle cramps, nausea, thirst, anorexia, apathy, lethargy. [Na^+] below 110 mEq/L: drowsiness, coma, convulsions.
TX: Correct underlying cause, administer sodium and fluid volume replacement.

Serum Chloride (Cl^-)

Chloride exists primarily in the extracellular spaces; a small portion is found in the intravascular spaces and in the cell itself. Common compounds of chloride include sodium chloride and hydrochloric acid. Chloride has a primary effect on osmotic pressure, thereby helping to regulate cellular integrity. Because chloride closely interacts with sodium (counterbalances the positive ionic charge of sodium to help maintain electrolyte neutrality), chloride is also significant in monitoring acid-base balance and water balance. Serum chloride is measured to detect acid-base imbalance, fluid status, and extracellular cation-anion balance.

Normal range:
95 to 105 mEq/L or 95 to 105 mmol/L

Clinical implications:
Critical value includes a chloride level less than 70 or greater than 120 (similar to sodium response).

Hyperchloremia:
Increased serum chloride concentration.
ETIOL: Dehydration, Cushing's syndrome, decreased renal excretion, decreased HCO_3 (this electrolyte concentration is inversely proportional to Cl^- owing to the exchange of Cl^- and HCO_3^- by the kidney), respiratory alkalosis (hyperventilation).
SIGNS AND SYMPTOMS: Rapid deep breathing, stupor, weakness, coma.
TX: Correct underlying cause, administer water.

Hypochloremia:
Decreased serum chloride concentration.
ETIOL: Severe vomiting, severe diarrhea, severe burns, increased renal excretion, diabetic acidosis, aldosteronism, HCO_3^- retention (such as occurs in metabolic alkalosis or chronic obstructive pulmonary disease [COPD]).
SIGNS AND SYMPTOMS: Irritability of muscles, tetany, depressed respirations.
TX: Correct underlying cause, administer NaCl.

Serum Potassium (K^+)

Approximately 90% of potassium is located within the cell; the rest is located in bone and blood. As the primary cation of intracellular fluid, potassium is the chief buffer within the cell itself. Potassium functions to help regulate enzyme activity, acid-base balance, osmotic pressure, nerve impulse conduction (helps maintain electrical conduction within the cardiac and skeletal muscles), and muscle function. Most potassium is excreted daily in the urine; the remainder is eliminated through sweating and in the stool. Serum potassium aids in evaluating the origin of cardiac dysrhythmias, renal function, acid-base balance, glucose metabolism, and neuromuscular and endocrine disorders.

Normal range:
3.5 to 5.0 mEq/L or 3.5 to 5.0 mmol/L

Clinical implications:
Critical values of potassium include less than 2.5 or greater than 6.5; serious life-threatening arrhythmias and cardiotoxicity may occur.

Hyperkalemia:
Increased serum potassium concentration.
ETIOL: Conditions in which excessive cellular potassium enters the blood (burn patients, crushing injuries, diabetic ketoacidosis, myocardial infarction), renal failure, Addison's disease, internal hemorrhage, uncontrolled diabetes, selective hypoaldosteronism, acidosis (drives potassium from the cells), excessive intake.
ECG CHANGES: Prolonged PR interval, wide QRS complex, tall, tented T wave; or ST depression.
SIGNS AND SYMPTOMS: Metabolic acidosis, muscle weakness, malaise, nausea, vomiting, diarrhea, confusion, paresthesia. Cardiac arrhythmias may occur with high potassium levels: sinus bradycardia, sinus arrest, ventricular tachycardia, ventricular fibrillation, ventricular arrest, first-degree atrioventricular block, nodal rhythm, idioventricular rhythm.
TX: Correct underlying cause, administer diuretic therapy, administer IV glucose and insulin (increases the uptake of potassium into cells), administer calcium chloride or calcium gluconate to impede the cardiotoxic effects.

Hypokalemia:
Decreased serum potassium concentration.
ETIOL: Diarrhea, starvation, malabsorption, severe vomiting, excessive nasogastric suctioning, steroid therapy, renal tubular acidosis, diuretic therapy, liver failure, cirrhosis, primary aldosteronism, insulin-induced hypoglycemia, alkalosis.
ECG CHANGES: Flattened T wave, ST depression, prominent U wave, PVCs.
SIGNS and SYMPTOMS: Metabolic alkalosis, muscle weakness, fatigue, confusion, hypotension, irregular pulse, loss of tendon reflexes. Severe hypokalemia—respiratory paralysis and cardiac arrest. Cardiac arrhythmias that may occur with low potassium levels: premature ventricular beats, atrial tachycardia, nodal tachycardia, ventricular tachycardia, ventricular fibrillation.
TX: Correct underlying problem, administer potassium.

Serum Phosphates (P), Inorganic Phosphorous (PO_4)

Most (approximately 85%) of the body's phosphorous content is located in the bone in combination with calcium; the remainder is located within the cell itself.

Because phosphate is closely linked with calcium (an excess of serum levels of one causes the kidneys to excrete the other), both are always evaluated in relation to each other. Many of the causative factors of high calcium levels are also the causative factors of lowered phosphate levels and vice versa. Phosphate is required in the generation of bony tissue, in the metabolism of glucose and lipids, and in the regulation of acid-base balance.

Serum phosphates are measured to aid diagnosis of renal disorders, acid-base imbalance, and endocrine, skeletal, and calcium disorders.

Normal range:
2.7 to 4.5 mg/dl, 0.87 to 1.45 mmol/L, or 1.8 to 2.6 mEq/L

Clinical implications:
Critical values of high phosphate levels (greater than 4.5) must be monitored in relation to reduction in calcium levels—arrhythmias and/or muscle twitching may occur.

Hyperphosphatemia:
Increased serum phosphorus concentration.
ETIOL: Hypoparathyroidism, renal failure, excessive intake of vitamin D, bone tumors, Addison's disease, hypocalcemia, acromegaly, severe catabolic state, acidosis.
SIGNS and SYMPTOMS: Renal osteodystrophy, ectopic calcification, secondary hyperparathyroidism.
TX: Correct underlying cause, renal dialysis may be necessary, administer aluminum hydroxide (decreases absorption of phosphates).

Hypophosphatemia:
Decreased serum phosphorus concentration.
ETIOL: Rickets, malnutrition, osteomalacia, diabetic coma, chronic alcoholism, septicemia, vitamin D deficiency, glucose and insulin administration, steroid therapy, primary hyperparathyroidism, alkalosis.
SIGNS and SYMPTOMS: Muscle weakness, paresthesia, seizures, impaired metabolism, decreased reabsorption of HCO_3, coma.
TX: Correct underlying cause, administer oral phosphate or IV $K_2\ HPO_4$.

Serum Magnesium (Mg^{+2})

Most magnesium is located within the bones and intracellular fluid; a small amount is found in extracellular fluid. Magnesium is associated with regulation of body temperature, neuromuscular contraction, and synthesis of protein. Magnesium is required to stimulate enzymes that catalyze the reactions between phosphate ions and adenosine triphosphate (ATP). Magnesium also helps transport sodium and potassium across cell membranes.

Serum magnesium analysis helps evaluate acid-base balance, in addition to neuromuscular and renal function.

Normal range:
1.7 to 2.1 mg/dl, 0.8 to 1.3 mmol/L, or 1.5 to 2.5 mEq/L

Clinical implications:
Critical values for serum magnesium are less than 0.5 (tetany) or greater than 3.0 (acts as a sedative—respiratory depression).

Hypermagnesemia:
Increased serum magnesium concentration.
ETIOL: Renal failure, uncontrolled diabetes mellitus, metabolic acidosis, excessive intake of magnesium (e.g., Milk of Magnesia), dehydration, Addison's disease, adrenalectomy, hypothyroidism.
SIGNS and SYMPTOMS: Sedative effects; bradycardia, hypotension, drowsiness, lethargy, slurred speech, respiratory depression, weak or absent deep tendon reflexes.
TX: Correct underlying cause, diuretic therapy, renal dialysis for renal failure.

Hypomagnesemia:
Decreased serum magnesium concentration.
ETIOL: Chronic diarrhea, hemodialysis, chronic renal disease, cirrhosis, diuretic therapy, hyperaldosteronism, chronic alcoholism, GI disturbances (excessive gastric drainage).
SIGNS and SYMPTOMS: Muscle tremors, leg and foot cramps, twitching, tetany, tachycardia, central nervous system depression, irritability.
TX: Correct underlying problem, administer magnesium sulfate.

Serum Osmolality

A measurement of the fluid and electrolyte balance in the blood. Serum osmolality is especially helpful in evaluating and monitoring hydration status and antidiuretic hormone (ADH) production or suppression. Overhydration will decrease serum osmolality whereas dehydration will increase it.

Normal range:
280 to 295 mOsm/kg or 280 to 295 mmol/kg

Clinical implications:
Critical values of serum osmolality are less than 240 (severe overhydration) or

greater than 321 (385 is associated with stupor in hyperglycemia, 400 may generate grand mal seizures, values greater than 420 may result in death).

Hyperosmolality:
Increased serum osmolality concentration.
ETIOL: Water loss (dehydration), hypercalcemia, diabetes insipidus, diabetes mellitus caused by increased glucose, brain trauma with impaired release of ADH.

Hypo-osmolality:
Decreased serum osmolality concentration.
ETIOL: Loss of sodium with diuretics or low sodium diet, Addison's disease, adrenogenital syndrome, inappropriate secretions of ADH (as noted in trauma or lung cancer), excessive water replacement (overhydration).

RENAL PHYSIOLOGY—AN OVERVIEW

The unit of structure and function in the kidney is known as the *nephron.* There are approximately 1 million nephrons in each human kidney. Each nephron unit contains a renal corpuscle and a long, convoluted renal tubule, as illustrated in Figure 17.1. A renal corpuscle consists of a glomerulus and an enclosing epithelial-lined capsule, known as the capsule of Bowman. The capsule of Bowman is considered the beginning of a renal tubule. Other components of a renal tubule include the proximal convoluted tubule, the loop of Henle, and the distal convoluted tubule, which is the end of a nephron unit. The contents of the distal tubule empty into the collecting duct, which subsequently empties into the ureter to be stored in the bladder. The corpuscles of the nephrons lie in the cortex, whereas the collecting tubules begin in the cortex and unite with one another to form a series of larger tubes that descend into the medulla.

Reabsorption and *secretion* are common terms employed in describing the activity of the renal tubules. Reabsorption is the process by which the renal tubule returns vital nutrients and other substances to the bloodstream, whereas secretion is the process that transfers substances from the bloodstream into the renal tubule for subsequent elimination by the body.

Juxtaglomerular Cells

Just before the afferent arteriole gives rise to the glomerulus, there are a cluster of cells known as *juxtaglomerular (JG) cells.* These cells are involved in the production of a chemical substance known as renin. Renin is secreted from the JG cells in response to such conditions as reduced renal blood flow, hypotension, hyponatremia, hypovolemia, and β-adrenoceptor stimulation.

Upon entering the bloodstream, renin interacts with the plasma protein an-

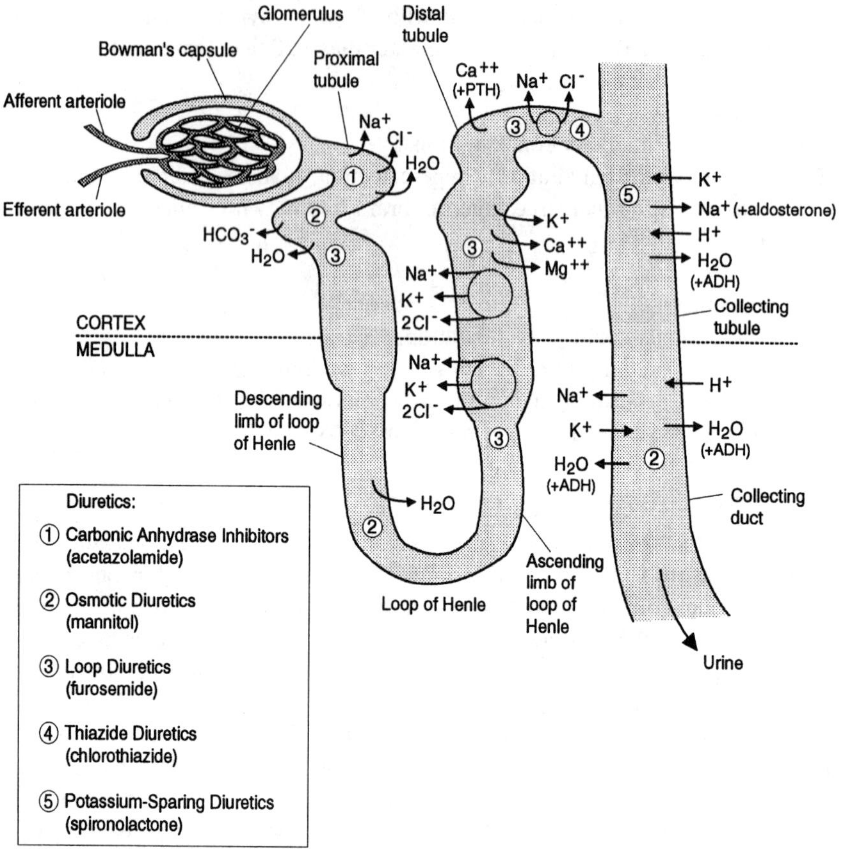

Figure 17.1. Schematic representation of nephron unit showing sites of electrolyte and water reabsorption as well as sites of action of diuretics.

giotension to form *angiotension I*. In the lungs, angiotension I is further metabolized by angiotension-converting enzymes to the vasoactive compound *angiotension II*. Angiotension II is a potent vasoconstrictor that promotes intense peripheral vasoconstriction and increased peripheral resistance, leading to an elevation of the blood pressure. By this mechanism, there is an increase in blood flow through the vital organs, including the kidney. Angiotension II also enhances the secretion of aldosterone by the adrenal cortex. Aldosterone acts on the sodium pumps in the renal tubule to increase the reabsorption of sodium. The increased sodium retention correspondingly causes increased water retention, which then leads to an increased blood volume, which also will elevate the blood pressure.

This renin-angiotension-aldosterone system can be affected by drugs such as angiotension-converting enzyme (ACE) inhibitors and drugs that decrease renin secretion, such as the β-adrenoceptor blockers. The therapeutic usefulness of such drugs lies in the treatment of hypertensive states, and, in the case of ACE inhibitors, in the treatment of congestive heart failure (CHF) (see also Chapter 18).

Nephrons

Nephrons have three primary functions: glomerular filtration, renal tubular reabsorption, and renal tubular secretion. The end result of nephron activity is the return of many essential materials to the bloodstream and urine formation for elimination.

Glomerular Filtration

Approximately one-fifth of the plasma flowing through each glomerulus is passively transferred out of the bloodstream and into the capsule of Bowman. This glomerular filtration allows only the passage of small molecules into the capsule of Bowman (see Chapter 3 and Fig. 3.9), whereas larger high-molecular-weight substances, such as red blood cells and plasma proteins, remain in the bloodstream. The average adult glomerular filtration rate is 125 ml/min. This high filtration rate results in a total of approximately 180 L of plasma filtered in 24 hours. The fact that only 1 to 1.5 L of urine is eliminated in a 24-hour period points to a very large reabsorption of fluid during tubular transport.

Renal Tubular Reabsorption

As the glomerular filtrate flows out of the capsule of Bowman and into the component parts of the renal tubule, many substances are reabsorbed into the bloodstream (see Fig. 17.1). Approximately 80% of the reabsorption of water and various solutes occurs in the proximal tubule. Constituents are either reabsorbed via active transport (such as potassium and sodium) or by passive transport (such as water, which is accomplished by the simple process of osmosis).

The efficiency of the renal tubule to reabsorb sodium is such that less than 1% is excreted in the urine. About 80% of the filtered sodium is reabsorbed in association with chloride (NaCl), whereas approximately 20% of the filtered sodium is reabsorbed in combination with bicarbonate ($NaHCO_3$). Tubular reabsorption of sodium is the major driving force for the reabsorption of water and, thus, volume replacement.

The transport system in the thick portion of the ascending limb of Henle's loop is a $Na^+/K^+/2Cl^-$ cotransporter system in which one Na^+, one K^+, and two Cl^- move together in the same direction from the filtrate to the bloodstream. Loop diuretics, such as furosemide, are potent selective inhibitors of the $Na^+/K^+/2Cl^-$ cotransporter system. Inhibition of sodium and chloride reabsorption by loop diuretics in the ascending loop of Henle also lead to an increase in urinary excretion of other cations such as calcium and magnesium.

In the distal convoluted tubule, the Na^+/Cl^- cotransporter system is pharmacologically distinct from the above-mentioned $Na^+/K^+/2Cl^-$ cotransporter system. The Na^+/Cl^- cotransporter system is blocked by diuretics of the thiazide class, such as chlorothiazide. The loop diuretics have a higher maximal efficacy than the thiazide diuretics and are known as high-ceiling diuretics, whereas the less efficacious thiazide agents are known as low-ceiling diuretics.

Osmotic agents, including mannitol, primarily inhibit water reabsorption in those segments of the nephron that are freely permeable to water. Such segments include the proximal tubule and the descending limb of Henle's loop.

Aldosterone stimulates sodium reabsorption and potassium secretion in the late distal and collecting tubules. Aldosterone inhibitors, such as spironolactone, are also known as potassium-sparing diuretics because they prevent the potassium-sodium exchange that occurs in the late distal and collecting tubules, thereby sparing potassium from excretion by the body.

ADH enhances water reabsorption in the collecting tubule and collecting duct. ADH antagonists would correspondingly induce water diuresis; however, such agents are not yet clinically available. Parathyroid hormone (PTH) increases calcium reabsorption in the distal tubule (see Fig. 17.1).

Carbonic anhydrase (CA) is an enzyme present in many nephron sites, including the luminal membrane of the proximal tubule. Carbonic anhydrase's function is to catalyze the union of CO_2 and H_2O to form carbonic acid (H_2CO_3):

$$CO_2 + H_2O \Leftrightarrow^{CA} H_2CO_3 \Leftrightarrow H^+ + HCO_3^-$$

Carbonic acid freely dissociates into H^+ (hydrogen) and HCO_3^- (bicarbonate). Bicarbonate is then available for reabsorption. Inhibitors of carbonic anhydrase, such as acetazolamide, block the formation of carbonic acid, which will ultimately lead to a significant reduction in bicarbonate reabsorption. As more bicarbonate is retained in the tubule and excreted in the urine, blood pH falls as urine pH rises.

Renal Tubular Secretion

Renal tubular secretion involves the movement of substances from the bloodstream into the renal tubule. These secretory activities primarily occur in the distal portion of the renal tubule and are part of the final phase of urine formation. A primary secretory action of the renal tubule is to regulate the amount of potassium in the body. As previously stated, in the late distal tubule and collecting tubule, active secretion of potassium occurs in exchange for sodium (i.e., potassium is transferred from the bloodstream to the tubule, whereas sodium is transferred from the tubule to the bloodstream). By this action, the body not only rids itself of excess potassium but has an additional mechanism for conserving sodium.

Hydrogen ions are also secreted into the lumen of the tubule in exchange for sodium. Sodium, accompanied by bicarbonate, returns to the bloodstream, where it serves as an important buffer system.

Acid Base Regulation

The kidney serves as an important organ in the regulation of acid-base balance. The kidney is designed to excrete a large quantity of acids without losing too much bicarbonate in the urine. By this mechanism, a normal acid-to-base ratio is maintained, resulting in a normal blood pH.

If an electrolyte abnormality exists in which the kidney either retains or excretes excessive amounts of these vital substances, a severe life-threatening condition may ensue. The diuretics are notorious for causing an excessive loss of certain electrolytes, such as sodium, chloride, and potassium as well as bicarbonate. If either hypochloremia (low chloride) or hypokalemia (low potassium) occurs, the kidney will be forced to exchange a large quantity of sodium for hydrogen to maintain electrical neutrality. The resulting loss of H^+ in the blood will lead to metabolic alkalosis. The loss of bicarbonate, primarily due to carbonic anhydrase inhibitors, leads to metabolic acidosis.

DIURETIC AGENTS

Diuretic agents have the ability to facilitate urinary output of water and sodium by enhancing the normal function of the kidney. This is done by one of three primary mechanisms:

1. Increased glomerular filtration rate.
2. Decreased sodium reabsorption by the renal tubules.
3. Induction and promotion of the excretion of sodium by the kidney.

Classification of a diuretic agent is based on its primary mechanism of action. An example from each category is given, followed by a listing of related diuretics.

CARBONIC ANHYDRASE INHIBITORS

ACETAZOLAMIDE

DIAMOX

Mechanism of Action

As previously stated, carbonic anhydrase is an enzyme that catalyzes the union of CO_2 and water to form carbonic acid (H_2CO_3), which dissociates into free hydrogen and bicarbonate. Acetazolamide inhibits the action of carbonic anhydrase, thereby preventing hydrogen ion formation and secretion in the renal tubule, which then causes increased excretion of sodium, potassium, bicarbonate, and water. The total diuretic action of acetazolamide is hindered by the development of tolerance because of its promotion of metabolic acidosis through depletion of bicarbonate.

Indications

With the advent of newer diuretic agents, carbonic anhydrase inhibitors are rarely used as primary diuretic agents; however, there are still several specific applications for use:

1. Treatment of glaucoma. Carbonic anhydrase inhibition decreases the rate of aqueous humor formation, thus causing a reduction in intraocular pressure (IOP).
2. Prevention and treatment of symptoms associated with acute mountain sickness. Rapid ascent above 3000 m by mountain climbers can lead to weakness, dizziness, insomnia, headache, and nausea. By decreasing the formation of cerebrospinal fluid and pH of the cerebrospinal fluid and brain, acetazolamide enhances performance status and reduces the symptoms of mountain sickness.
3. Treatment of metabolic alkalosis. In some cases, metabolic alkalosis is a result of a significant reduction in body K^+ and intravascular volume. In these situations, correction of the underlying condition that caused the metabolic alkalosis is desirable. However, in cases in which metabolic alkalosis is caused by excessive use of diuretics and for patients with severe heart failure, acetazolamide may be useful in alleviating the metabolic alkalosis as well as producing a mild diuresis for the correction of heart failure.
4. Adjunctive therapy in the treatment of epilepsy (see Chapter 15).
5. Adjunctive therapy for diuresis in CHF or drug-induced edema.

Contraindications

Contraindications to acetazolamide include hypersensitivity to this drug, decreased sodium or potassium levels, moderate renal and hepatic disease or dysfunction, hyperchloremic acidosis, adrenocortical insufficiency, electrolyte imbalance, patients with severe COPD, and long-term use for chronic noncongestive angle-closure glaucoma.

Precautions

1. Increasing the dosage does not increase diuresis. It may actually act to decrease diuresis.
2. Electrolyte imbalance should be corrected before administration of this drug.
3. Acetazolamide may aggravate acidosis; therefore, use with extreme caution for patients with severe degrees of respiratory acidosis.
4. Because of the potential for the enhanced excretion of potassium, supplemental KCl may be administered simultaneously.

Adverse Reactions

CNS: Convulsions, fatigue, nervousness, sedation, depression, confusion, headache, vertigo, paresthesia of the extremities.
GI: Vomiting, nausea, constipation, anorexia.
Miscellaneous: Weight loss, fever, acidosis (may be corrected by administering bicarbonate), electrolyte imbalance, hepatic insufficiency.

Diuretic Dosage and Administration

For diuresis in CHF or drug-induced edema: 250 to 375 mg (5 mg/kg) once daily for 1 or 2 days.

OTHER CARBONIC ANHYDRASE INHIBITORS

The following are primarily indicated for use in the treatment of glaucoma: dichlorphenamide (Daranide), methazolamide (GlaucTabs, Neptazane).

THIAZIDE DIURETICS

CHLOROTHIAZIDE: DIURIL

Mechanism of Action

Chlorothiazide is a thiazide diuretic that increases the excretion of sodium and chloride (with a corresponding loss of water) by decreasing the rate of sodium and chloride reabsorption by the distal renal tubules. Other effects include increased potassium excretion, uric acid retention, and reduced calcium excretion. Onset of action occurs within 1 to 2 hours with a duration of 6 to 12 hours.

Indications

1. Used in conjunction with other diuretics for patients with edema associated with CHF, patients with hepatic cirrhosis, and patients with edema due to renal impairment (nephrotic syndrome, acute glomerulonephritis, and chronic renal failure) as well as edema associated with corticosteroid and estrogen therapy.
2. Hypertension; this drug may be used alone or with other hypotensive agents to enhance their effectiveness.

Contraindications

Contraindications to the use of chlorothiazide include hypersensitivity to thiazides, anuria, renal decompensation. Excessive administration or overzealous use of any diuretic is unwarranted for patients with hepatic cirrhosis, borderline renal failure, or CHF.

Precautions

1. IV administration is indicated only when oral medication cannot be taken or in acute emergencies. IV administration is not recommended in infants and children.
2. Monitor fluid and electrolyte balance for the precipitation of hepatic coma for patients with hepatic impairment or progressive liver disease.
3. This agent may increase the toxic effects of lithium.
4. Episodes of apnea may occur with concurrent use with nondepolarizing muscle relaxants (possibly due to potentiating effects and hypokalemia).

Adverse Reactions

CNS: Dizziness, vertigo, headache, paresthesia, syncope, anxiety, depression.

Cardiovascular: Orthostatic hypotension, PVCs, palpitations.

Pulmonary: Sore throat, congestion, cough, respiratory distress, possibly with pneumonitis.

GI: Nausea, vomiting, abdominal pain, diarrhea, pancreatitis, cholecystitis, jaundice.

Miscellaneous: Fluid/electrolyte imbalance (especially hyponatremia, hypokalemia), neutropenia, weight loss, hyperglycemia (especially noted in patients with overt diabetic).

Overdosage

Symptoms include electrolyte imbalance, potassium depletion, nausea, vomiting, hypotension, apnea, coma. Treatment consists of gastric lavage (prevent aspiration), monitoring of electrolyte balance, and cardiopulmonary support if necessary.

Dosage and Administration

For edema: 0.5 to 1 g once or twice daily orally or IV. IV route not recommended unless oral medication is not feasible or for emergency situations.

For hypertension: 0.5 to 1 g daily (oral route only). Some patients may require up to 2 g/day in divided doses. As blood pressure falls, a reduced dosage may be necessary.

Other Thiazides and Related Diuretics:	***Usual Daily Oral Dose:***
Bendroflumethiazide (Naturetin)	2.5–10 mg as single dose
Benzthiazide (Exna)	25–100 mg in two divided doses
Chlorthalidone (Hygroton, Thalitone)	50–100 mg as single dose
Hydrochlorothiazide (Esidrix, Oretic)	25–100 mg as single dose
Hydroflumethiazide (Diucardin, Saluron)	25–100 mg in two divided doses
Indapamide (Lozol).	2.5–10 mg as single dose
Methyclothiazide (Enduron, Aquatensen)	2.5–10 mg as single dose

Metolazone (Zaroxolyn, Mykrox)	2.5–10 mg as single dose
Polythiazide (Renese)	1–4 mg as single dose
Quinethazone (Hydromox)	50–100 mg as single dose
Trichlormethiazide (Metahydrin, Naqua, Diurese)	2–8 mg as single dose

LOOP DIURETICS

FUROSEMIDE: LASIX

Mechanism of Action

Loop diuretics are selective inhibitors of the $Na^+/K^+/2Cl^-$ transport system in the thick ascending limb of Henle's loop. Furosemide is a potent diuretic agent that inhibits the reabsorption of sodium and chloride not only in the ascending loop of Henle but also in the proximal and distal tubules. In addition, furosemide promotes the excretion of potassium, magnesium, calcium, and, to a lesser extent, bicarbonate. The onset of action of orally administered furosemide is within 60 minutes with a duration of 6 to 8 hours. The onset of action of intravenously administered furosemide is within 5 minutes with a duration of 2 hours.

Indications

1. Edema associated with CHF, hepatic cirrhosis, and renal disease, including nephrotic syndrome.
2. Used as an adjuvant for acute pulmonary edema.
3. Hypertension (orally administered); alone or in combination with other antihypertensive agents.
4. Acute management of severe hyperkalemia to enhance urinary excretion of K^+.
5. Promotion of calcium diuresis in hypercalcemic states.

Contraindications

Contraindications to the use of furosemide include hypersensitivity to the agent, anuria, hepatic coma, or severe electrolyte depletion.

Precautions

1. IV administration is indicated when a rapid onset of action is preferred (e.g., acute pulmonary edema), when GI absorption is impaired, or when oral administration is not feasible.
2. Monitor patients for signs of dehydration. Rapid and excessive weight loss may potentiate an acute hypotensive crisis.
3. If given in excessive amounts, furosemide may cause electrolyte depletion. Monitor patients for hyponatremia, hypochloremic alkalosis, and hypokalemia.

Many patients receive K^+ or KCl supplemental therapy to restore the loss of these vital electrolytes.

4. Coadministration of aminoglycosides may increase the potential for ototoxicity.

Adverse Reactions

CNS: Paresthesia, restlessness, xanthopsia, headache, vertigo, dizziness.

Cardiovascular: Orthostatic hypotension, thrombophlebitis, chronic aortitis.

GI: Anorexia, nausea, vomiting, cramping, diarrhea, constipation, pancreatitis, jaundice, ischemic hepatitis.

Hematologic: Anemia, leukopenia, purpura, aplastic anemia, thrombocytopenia, agranulocytosis.

Miscellaneous: Glycosuria, muscle spasm, weakness, hyperglycemia, hyperuricemia, urinary bladder spasm.

Overdosage

Profound water loss and electrolyte depletion, dehydration, circulatory collapse. Treatment consists of supportive measures and replacement of fluid and electrolyte loss.

Dosage and Administration

Edema: Oral dose ranges from 20 to 80 mg/day up to 600 mg/day for patients with severe edema. **IM, IV:** 20 to 40 mg up to 80 mg for acute pulmonary edema.

Hypertension: Oral administration only, 40 mg twice daily. As blood pressure falls, reduce dosage or discontinue other antihypertensive agents.

Other Loop Diuretics:	***Usual Daily Oral Dose:***
Bumetanide (Bumex)	0.5–2 mg
Ethacrynic acid (Edecrin)	50–200 mg
Torsemide (Demadex)	2.5–20 mg

OSMOTIC DIURETICS
MANNITOL
OSMITROL
Mechanism of Action

Mannitol is an osmotic diuretic that promotes water diuresis by inhibiting the reabsorption of sodium and water in the proximal tubules, the loop of Henle, and the collecting duct. This effect is brought about by mannitol's ability to elevate the osmotic pressure of the glomerular filtrate, thereby impeding the reabsorption of water in the renal tubules. By this action, the excretion not only of water but also sodium and chloride, is increased. The onset of intravenously administered mannitol is within 60 minutes with a duration of 6 to 8 hours.

Indications

1. Treatment or prevention of acute renal failure.
2. Reduction of intracranial pressure and cerebral edema.
3. Reduction of intraocular pressure.
4. As a diagnostic tool to measure the glomerular filtration rate.
5. To promote urinary excretion of toxic substances.

Contraindications

Contraindications to the use of mannitol include severe pulmonary congestion, severe dehydration, and anuria caused by severe renal disease.

Precautions

1. Serious electrolyte imbalance may occur with excessive use.
2. Patient's cardiovascular system must be carefully monitored before rapid administration of mannitol because of the prompt expansion of extracellular fluid and the potential of developing fulminating congestive heart failure and pulmonary edema.
3. Sustained diuresis may precipitate hypovolemia.

Adverse Reactions

CNS: Headache, convulsions, dizziness, blurred vision.

Cardiovascular: Hypotension, hypertension, edema, tachycardia, angina-like chest pains, CHF.

Pulmonary: Pulmonary congestion, edema.

GI: Nausea, vomiting, diarrhea.

Metabolic: Fluid/electrolyte imbalance, acidosis, dehydration.

Overdosage

Symptoms of mannitol overdose consist of orthostatic hypotension, tachycardia, polyuria, stupor, convulsions, and hyponatremia. Treatment includes supportive care to correct fluid and electrolyte imbalance, discontinuing the drug, and hemodialysis if necessary to clear mannitol.

Dosage and Administration

IV: Usual adult dose, 20 to 200 g/day (administration rate is adjusted to maintain a urine flow of at least 30 to 50 ml/hr).

To reduce intracranial pressure: 1.5 to 2 g/kg of a 15%, 20%, or 25% solution given slowly over 30 to 60 minutes.
Prevention of acute renal failure: 50 to 100 g as a 5% to 25% solution given during cardiovascular or other types of surgery.

Other Osmotic Diuretics:	***Usual Daily Dose:***
Glycerin (Glyrol, Osmoglyn)	1–2 g/kg
Isosorbide (Ismotic)	1–3 g/kg b.i.d., t.i.d.
Urea (Ureaphil)	1–1.5 g/kg

POTASSIUM-SPARING DIURETICS
SPIRONOLACTONE
ALDACTONE
Mechanism of Action
Spironolactone blocks sodium reabsorption in the distal tubule by competitively inhibiting the actions of the aldosterone receptors. Owing to this mechanism of action, agents in this group of diuretics are known as aldosterone inhibitors. Potassium is normally exchanged for sodium in the distal tubule and then secreted into the urine. By preventing the potassium-sodium exchange, potassium is spared from secretion.

Indications
1. Essential hypertension (in combination with other drugs).
2. Hypokalemia and the prophylaxis of hypokalemia for patients taking digitalis.
3. Management of edema and sodium retention, alone or in combination with thiazide or loop diuretics, for patients with CHF.
4. Cirrhosis of the liver when accompanied by edema or ascites.
5. Primary hyperaldosteronism.

Contraindications
Contraindications to the use of spironolactone include anuria, acute renal failure, and hyperkalemia.

Precautions
1. Patients must be carefully monitored for possible fluid and electrolyte imbalances.
2. Spironolactone may induce or aggravate hyponatremia, especially when administered in combination with other diuretics.
3. Coadministered potassium preparations may result in hyperkalemia, resulting in an increased risk of cardiac arrhythmias or cardiac arrest.

4. The absorption rate of spironolactone is increased when administered with food.
5. May produce drowsiness; observe caution when driving or operating machinery that requires alertness.
6. Potassium-sparing diuretics are used generally in combination with thiazides and loop diuretics to enhance these drugs' actions and effects and to overcome the kaliuretic effect produced by these agents.

Adverse Reactions

GI: Cramping, diarrhea, gastric bleeding, ulceration, gastritis, vomiting.
CNS: Drowsiness, lethargy, headache, mental confusion, ataxia.
Miscellaneous: Drug fever, thirst, skin rash, hyperchloremic metabolic acidosis in decompensated hepatic cirrhosis, agranulocytosis.

Dosage and Administration

Edema: range, 25 to 200 mg/day.
Essential hypertension: Initially, 50 to 100 mg/day.
Hypokalemia: 25 to 100 mg/day.

Other Potassium-Sparing Diuretics:	***Usual Daily Dose:***
Amiloride (Midamor)	5–10 mg
Triamterene (Dyrenium)	100 mg b.i.d.

Note: These agents are not aldosterone inhibitors, as is spironolactone, but act directly on the distal tubule to inhibit sodium reabsorption.

REFERENCES/RECOMMENDED READING

Beermann B, Groschinsky-Grind M. Clinical pharmacokinetics of diuretics. Clin Pharmacokinet 5:221, 1980.
Brenner BM, Rector FC Jr. The Kidney. 4th ed. Philadelphia: WB Saunders, 1990.
Drug Facts and Comparisons. 49th ed. St. Louis: Facts and Comparisons, 1995.
Gifford RW Jr. Role of diuretics in treatment of hypertension. Am J Med 77:102, 1984.
Katzung BG. Basic and Clinical Pharmacology. 6th ed. Norwalk: Appleton & Lange, 1995.
Physicians' Desk Reference. 49th ed. Montvale, NJ: Medical Economics, 1995.
Rose BD. Diuretics. Kidney Int 39:336, 1991.
Sonnenblick M, et al. Diuretic induced severe hyponatremia. Chest 103:601, 1993.
Stanton BA. Cellular actions of thiazide diuretics in the distal tubule. J Am Soc Nephrol 1:832, 1990.
Welling PG. Pharmacokinetics of the thiazide diuretics. Biopharm Drug Dispos 7:501, 1986.

CARDIOVASCULAR AGENTS 18

This chapter presents the various agents used to treat cardiovascular disorders:

- Antianginal Agents and Vasodilators
- Antiarrhythmic Agents
- Antihypertensive Agents
- Cardiotonic Agents Used in Congestive Heart Failure
- Vasopressors Used in Shock
- Agents Used in Disorders of Coagulation

To comprehensively understand the mechanisms by which the cardiovascular agents affect the heart and vascular system, it is helpful to have a sound foundation in the normal functioning of the cardiovascular system, the terminology associated with cardiovascular drugs, and normal hemodynamic parameters. Therefore, these topics will be presented before the individual agents.

THE CARDIOVASCULAR SYSTEM—AN OVERVIEW

Figure 18.1 depicts the route by which blood flows throughout the body. The blood from all body parts (as well as blood from the vessels of the heart itself) empties into the right atrium of the heart. As the right atrium contracts, blood flows from the right atrium, through the tricuspid valve, and into the right ventricle. During right ventricular contraction, blood flows from the right ventricle, through the pulmonic valve, into the pulmonary trunk, into the right and left pulmonary arteries and their branches, and then into the pulmonary capillary bed, where it picks up a fresh load of inspired oxygen and unloads carbon dioxide for eventual exhalation to the atmosphere. The oxygenated blood then flows through

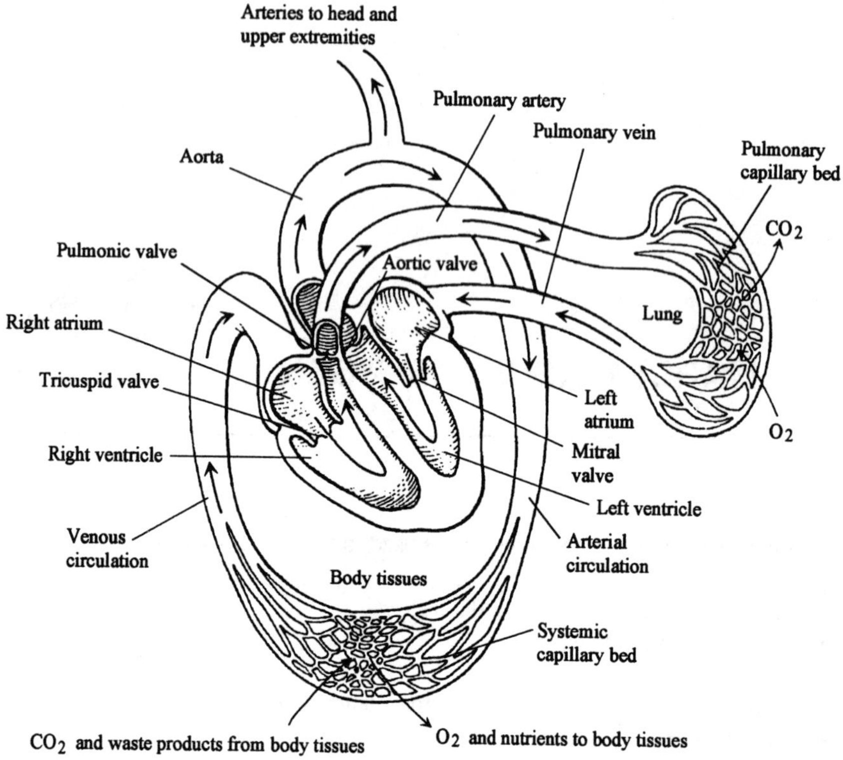

Figure 18.1. The heart and circulatory system (see text for explanation).

the pulmonary veins and into the left atrium. The above-described circulatory blood flow is called the pulmonary circulation, and its vessels comprise the pulmonary vascular system.

As the left atrium contracts, blood flows from the left atrium through the mitral valve and into the left ventricle. During left ventricular contraction, the blood flows from the left ventricle through the aortic valve and into the aorta. The blood is then distributed to all of the systemic arteries and systemic capillaries, where oxygen and nutrients are delivered to the tissues and carbon dioxide and other waste products are picked up. From the systemic capillaries, the blood passes to the veins and ultimately returns to the right atrium to begin its circuit all over again. The above-described circulatory blood flow is called the systemic circulation, and its vessels comprise the systemic vascular system.

Cardiac Conduction

Figure 18.2 depicts the sequence in which the heart is electrically stimulated. Normal conduction of the electrical signal arises spontaneously at the sinoatrial node (SA node, 1 in Fig. 18.2). The SA node is the main cardiac pacemaker and initiates, at rest, 60 to 100 impulses per minute. After stimulation of the SA node, wave-like impulses are sent through the atria (2 in Fig. 18.2) causing contraction of first the right and then the left atrium. Contraction, or depolarization, of the atria is noted as a P wave on an ECG tracing (Fig. 18.2).

The impulse slows as it reaches the atrioventricular node (AV node, 4 in Fig. 18.2), thus allowing time for the atria to completely contract and for the ventricles, which are resting (diastole), to fill with blood from the atria. The P-R interval on an ECG tracing reflects this pause in electrical transmission. If the main pacemaker of the heart, the SA node, is dysfunctional or fails to initiate impulses, the AV node may take over as the primary pacemaker and transmit impulses at a rate of 40 to 60 per minute. Excessive prolongation of the impulse at the AV node results in heart block.

After the brief delay at the AV node, the wave of excitation then spreads to the bundle of His (5 in Fig. 18.2), the right and left bundle branches (6, 7 in Fig. 18.2), and the Purkinje fibers (8 in Fig. 18.2), which terminate in the ventricles. This sequence of events causes ventricular depolarization and contraction, which are seen as the QRS complex on an ECG tracing. The T wave corresponds to ventricular repolarization (relaxation). The Purkinje fibers have an inherent pacing rate that ranges between 20 to 40 impulses per minute in the event that the SA node or AV node fails to initiate impulses.

One complete cardiac cycle consists of one complete heartbeat and includes contraction (systole) and relaxation (diastole) of both the atria and ventricles. This mechanical work of the heart occurs in response to electrical stimulation. A dis-

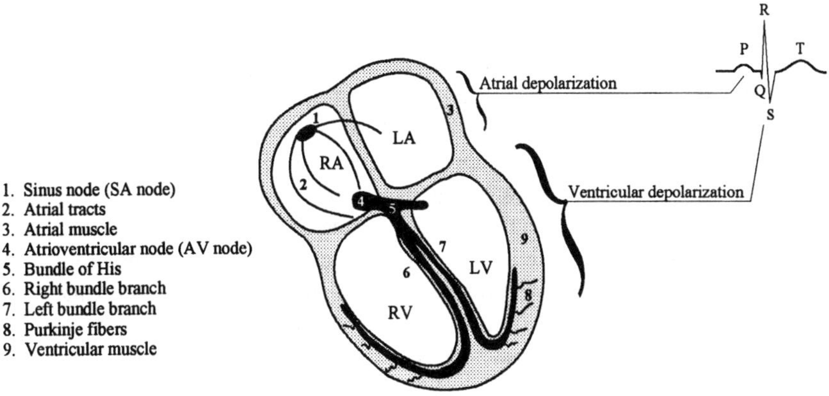

Figure 18.2. Route of cardiac conduction (see text for explanation). RA = right atrium; RV = right ventricle; LA = left atrium; LV = left ventricle.

turbance in any of the processes of the cardiac cycle will result in a change in the electrical forces needed to maintain normal, rhythmic heartbeats and may produce an arrhythmia. Electrical stimulation without mechanical activity is a life-threatening condition known as electromechanical dissociation (EMD), or what is currently known as pulseless electrical activity (PEA). The prognosis for a patient experiencing PEA is very poor owing to the fact that there is no pulse, or cardiac output.

Electrophysiology of the Heart

Each muscle cell in the heart is stimulated to contract by going through an electrical process known as the action potential (Fig. 18.3). The action potential is composed of five phases (0, 1, 2, 3, 4). During their resting stage (phase 4 of the action potential), the myocardial cells are said to be polarized, meaning an equal number of positive charges are on the outside of the cell with an equal number of negative charges on the inside of the cell. During this polarized state, the cations sodium (Na) and calcium (Ca), located on the outside of the cell, are unable to cross the cell membrane. The cation potassium (K), located primarily on the inside of the cell, leaks slowly across the cell membrane to the outside. This slow loss of potassium causes the inside of the cell to be negative (−) relative to the outside, which is positive (+).

The initiation of an electrical stimulus changes the membrane permeability of the cell to ion flow; resulting in the inside of the cell suddenly becoming positive (+) and the outside negative (−). This change, phase 0 of the action potential, is brought about by the rapid influx of sodium ions into the cell. Sodium gains entry to the cell through pathways known as *fast channels,* which open in response to the change in membrane permeability. Subsequently, another set of pathways, called *slow channels,* open to calcium, allowing the slow influx of calcium into the cell. This change in polarity during phase 0 is called depolarization, during which the myocardial cells contract. Contraction of the atria during phase 0 of the action potential is recorded as a P wave on the ECG, whereas contraction of the ventricles during phase 0 is recorded as a QRS complex on the ECG tracing.

Phases 1, 2, and 3 of the action potential represent repolarization, or recovery, of the cells. During recovery, the inside of the cell changes from positive (+) back to its original resting negative (−) charge. During phase 1, the fast sodium channels close while the slow calcium channels remain open. Phase 2 represents the plateau phase, in which the continued flow of calcium into the cell is counterbalanced by the flow of potassium to the outside of the cell. This phase correlates with the ST segment on the ECG. During phase 3, the calcium channels close, but potassium continues to leak to the outsize. Phase 3 correlates with the T wave on the ECG. When the repolarization process is complete, the cell returns to its fully polarized state (phase 4) and is ready to be activated or depolarized again.

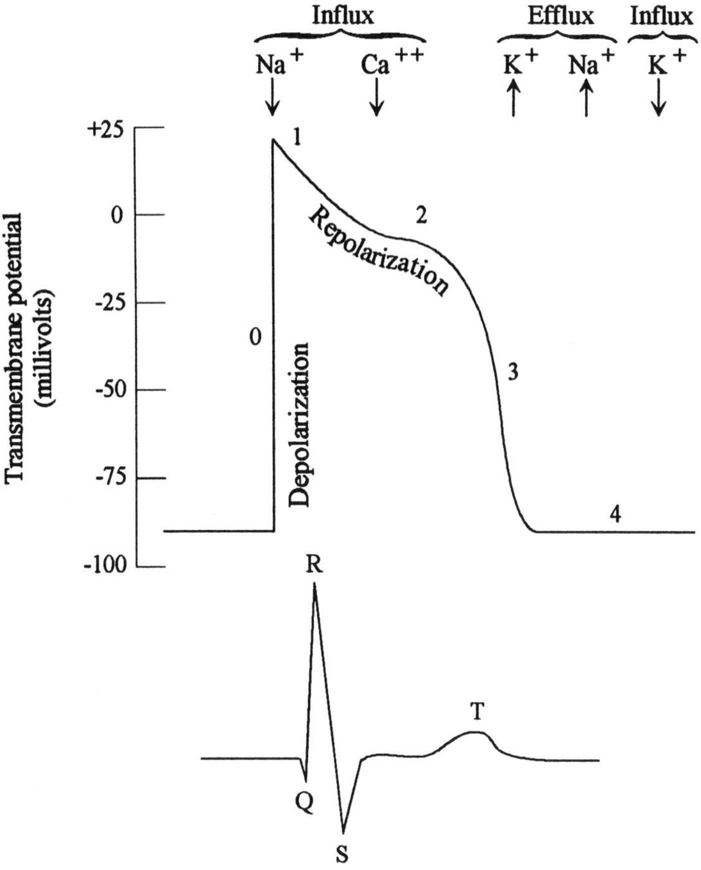

Figure 18.3. The action potential of myocardial cells. The phases of the action potential (0, 1, 2, 3, 4) correlate with waveforms recorded on the ECG. Phase 0 represents depolarization, whereas phases 1, 2, and 3 of the action potential represent repolarization, or recovery, of the cells. Phase 4 reflects the action potential while the myocardial cells are at rest.

In contrast to muscle cells, which require a stimulus to depolarize, pacemaker cells (such as the SA node) are automatic and initiate depolarization spontaneously. During phase 4 of the action potential of pacemaker cells, there is a slow leak of potassium from the inside to the outside of the cell; however, unlike muscle cells, sodium also gradually leaks into the cell at the same time that potassium leaks out. As sodium continues to leak into the pacemaker cell, a critical voltage threshold is reached, which then causes phase 0 of the action potential (depolarization) to begin. Depolarization of the pacemaker cell is primarily precipitated by the influx of calcium through slow channels, not by sodium entry by fast channels as in muscle cells. Thus, pacemaker cells are described as *slow cells,* whereas muscle cells are referred to as *fast cells.* Phases 1, 2, and 3 (repolarization, or recovery phase) in pacemaker cells are similar to those that occur in muscle cells.

The clinical importance of the action potential lies with the treatment of specific arrhythmias, as described in later sections of this chapter. Many of the drugs used to treat or prevent arrhythmias alter one or more phases of the action potential, which will then bring about changes in depolarization or repolarization.

TERMINOLOGY ASSOCIATED WITH CARDIOVASCULAR DRUGS

Afterload—The stress or tension that develops in the ventricular wall during systole: the sum of the forces opposing ventricular ejection. Afterload reflects the level of work that must be performed by the ventricles in ejecting their content. High afterload conditions make it more difficult for the ventricles to eject blood, whereas low afterload conditions make it easier for the ventricles to eject their contents. The parameters that assess afterload are the pulmonary vascular resistance (PVR, right ventricle afterload) and systemic vascular resistance (SVR, left ventricle afterload). The integrity of the pulmonary and systemic vascular systems, the integrity of the pulmonary and aortic valves, and blood viscosity all act together in determining afterload.

AGENTS USED TO IMPROVE AFTERLOAD: Abnormally low afterload, as evidenced by a reduced SVR and/or PVR, occurs when there is minimal resistance to blood flow into and through the systemic or pulmonary circulatory systems. To counteract the loss of resistance, vasopressors (α-adrenoceptor stimulators) are used. These agents induce vasoconstriction secondary to stimulation of α-adrenoceptors in vascular smooth muscle. As a result of the systemic vasoconstriction, the SVR increases as well as the arterial blood pressure.

AGENTS USED TO REDUCE AFTERLOAD: High afterload pressures, as evidenced by an elevated SVR and/or PVR, can significantly increase the ventricular work of ejecting volume. Generally, afterload is inversely related to cardiac output or stroke volume and directly related to myocardial oxygen consumption—as afterload (impedance to blood flow) increases, the cardiac output and stroke volume fall while myocardial oxygen consumption increases. Pharmacologic afterload-reducing agents are used primarily to improve stroke volume while reducing myocardial oxygen consumption. These agents include a variety of arterial vasodilators that act to reduce SVR and arterial blood pressure by either causing direct vasodilation of the systemic vasculature or by preventing vasoconstriction of the systemic vasculature.

The following drug groups are used as afterload-reducing agents:

Vascular smooth muscle relaxants (vasodilators)
Calcium channel blockers

α-adrenoceptor inhibitors
Angiotension-converting enzyme (ACE) inhibitors

Chronotropic—Influencing the rate of cardiac contraction (heartbeat). Positive chronotropic agents will increase the heart rate, whereas negative chronotropic agents will decrease the heart rate.

AGENTS USED TO INCREASE HEART RATE (POSITIVE CHRONOTROPIC AGENTS): Bradycardia with heart rates < 50 beats/min can significantly reduce cardiac output, which then leads to inadequate tissue perfusion and oxygenation. Treating low heart rates relies on the underlying cause of the bradycardia. Vasovagal inhibition is managed with parasympatholytic agents (e.g., atropine), whereas β_1-adrenoceptor stimulators are employed for their direct chronotropic property (e.g., isoproterenol). A pacemaker may be necessary if heart block is present.

AGENTS USED TO DECREASE HEART RATE (NEGATIVE CHRONOTROPIC AGENTS): Heart rates between 100 and 120 beats/min may increase cardiac output ($CO = SV \times HR$); however, tachycardia manifested by heart rates > 120 beats/min may significantly decrease stroke volume and cardiac output owing to the loss of adequate filling volumes from shortened diastolic filling time (i.e., the high rate of ventricular ejection caused by the increased heart rate does not allow enough time for the ventricles to fill with blood during diastole). Pharmacologic agents used to decrease heart rate include those with negative chronotropic effects (β_1-adrenoceptor blockers) and those that decrease myocardial conduction (calcium channel blockers).

Hemodynamics—The study of the forces involved in circulating blood throughout the body (see the following section, *Normal Hemodynamic Parameters*).

Inotropic—Influencing the force of myocardial contractility. Positive inotropic agents increase myocardial contractility, whereas negative inotropic agents decrease myocardial contractility (see below, *Myocardial contractility*).

Myocardial contractility—The force by which the myocardial fibers contract or shorten during systole: the force necessary to eject the heart's contents.

DRUGS USED TO IMPROVE CONTRACTILITY (POSITIVE INOTROPIC AGENTS): Improvement in myocardial contractility involves the use of positive inotropic agents. These drugs act on the heart by increasing the amount of calcium available for myocardial contraction. The resulting increased force of contraction improves stroke volume, cardiac output, and blood pressure. The most commonly used inotropes are the sympathomimetic amines with β_1-adrenoceptor stimulation. Other types of inotropes include myocardial phosphodiesterase inhibitors and cardiac glycosides.

DRUGS USED TO DECREASE CONTRACTILITY (NEGATIVE INOTROPIC AGENTS): Because of the increase in oxygen demands that accompanies increased myocardial contractility, some patients (e.g., those with myocardial ischemia) may benefit from reductions in contractility. Negative inotropic agents, such as β_1-adrenoceptor blockers and calcium channel blockers, effectively reduce the force of myocardial muscle contraction by inhibiting or reducing the amount of calcium ion influx across cardiac cells. The overall effects of these agents include reductions in contractility, cardiac output, blood pressure, and heart rate.

Preload—The load or tension placed on the myocardial fibers just before systole. Preload is a direct reflection of ventricular end-diastolic volume (the amount of blood in the ventricles just before contraction). The concept of preload is based on Frank Starling's law, which states: *the strength (or force) of contraction is directly related to the amount of stretch placed on the myocardial fibers just prior to contraction* (i.e., the greater the amount of blood in the ventricles just prior to contraction, the greater the myocardial fibers stretch, the greater the preload will be, and thus, the force of contraction [myocardial fiber shortening] increases, thereby ejecting more blood from the ventricles). The parameters that assess preload include the central venous pressure (CVP: right ventricle preload) and the pulmonary artery wedge pressure (PAWP: left ventricle preload).

AGENTS USED TO IMPROVE PRELOAD: Adequate end-diastolic filling volume (i.e., preload) is essential in maintaining cardiac output and blood pressure. As stated previously, preload is indirectly assessed by noting the CVP (right heart preload) and the PAWP (left heart preload). Low preload pressures, as evidenced by abnormally low CVP and PAWP, are best corrected by adding fluid to the circulatory system with the use of agents known as volume expanders. This is most commonly achieved with IV fluid challenges of either a crystalloid or a colloid solution. Most often, 100 to 250 cc of crystalloid solution is injected over 10 minutes or until evidence of improved perfusion occurs.

Volume Expanders: Crystalloids—normal saline, lactated Ringer's, dextrose in water (D_5W). Colloids—albumin, hetastarch (Hespan), whole blood.

AGENTS USED TO REDUCE PRELOAD: High preload pressures correspond to elevated right ventricular end-diastolic filling pressure (CVP) and left ventricular end-diastolic filling pressure (PAWP). Reductions in preload pressures are best achieved by either reducing vascular volume with the use of diuretics (see Chapter 17) or by reducing venous return to the heart with the use of venous vasodilators.

NORMAL HEMODYNAMIC PARAMETERS

Heart Rate (HR)—60 to 100 beats/min. The HR is usually measured by counting the number of pulses occurring in 1 minute.

Systemic Arterial Blood Pressure (BP)—90 to 140 mmHg systolic; 60 to 90 mmHg diastolic. The BP can be measured by either a blood pressure cuff or an arterial line.

Mean Arterial Blood Pressure (MAP)—70 to 100 mmHg. The MAP is used in calculating the SVR and is a useful parameter in assessing the body's response to vasoactive drug therapy. MAP is calculated by the following formula:

$$MAP = (\text{systolic pressure}) - (\text{diastolic pressure} \times 2)/3$$

Pulse Pressure (systemic)—40 mmHg. The pulse pressure is useful in assessing the degree of blood flow. Pulse pressure is the difference between systolic and diastolic pressures:

$$\text{Pulse Pressure} = \text{systolic} - \text{diastolic}$$

Stroke Volume (SV)—60 to 130 ml/beat. The SV is affected by preload, afterload, and contractility and can be estimated by the following formula:

$$SV = CO/HR$$

Stroke Index (SI)—30 to 65 ml/m^2. The stroke index is calculated by one of two methods:

$$SI = CI/HR \text{ or } SI = SV/BSA$$

Cardiac Output (CO)—4 to 8 L/min. The CO is the product of SV and HR and can be measured by one of three ways; thermodilution, dye dilution, or the Fick equation.

Thermodilution technique—requires the use of a PA (Swan-Ganz) thermodilution catheter. A bolus (usually 10 cc) of iced (usually 0°C) or room temperature (22° to 24°C) fluid (usually 5% dextrose in water or normal saline) is injected into the right atrium through the proximal port of the PA catheter. The resulting blood temperature change is recorded by the thermistor located at the distal catheter tip, which resides in the pulmonary artery. The change in blood temperature is plotted on a graph against time and converted to the cardiac output by the following equation:

$$CO = (V) \times (Tb - Ts)/(\text{mean } Tb) \times (t)$$

where:

V = volume of the injected solution
Tb = temperature of the blood
Ts = temperature of the injected solution
mean Tb = mean change in the temperature of the blood
t = time from the onset of the temperature change at the sampling site to the return of the base line temperature

Dye dilution technique (also known as the indicator dilution method)—a nontoxic indicator dye (usually indocyanine green) is injected into the right atrium or pulmonary artery. The dye solution passes a systemic arterial (such as the brachial artery) sampling site, which is further downstream in the circulation. Arterial blood samples are repetitively withdrawn at specified intervals. The concentration of the dye solution is measured by spectrophotometry and plotted on a time/concentration curve. The cardiac output is then calculated by the following formula:

$$CO = (Do)/(\text{mean } Dc) \times (t)$$

where:

Do = amount of dye injected
mean Dc = mean concentration of dye
t = time from onset of dye at the sampling site to the disappearance of the dye at the sampling site

Fick equation—by measuring the amount of oxygen consumed by the tissues and the arterial-venous oxygen content difference, the cardiac output can be calculated:

$$CO = \dot{V}O_2/CaO_2 - CvO_2$$

where:

$\dot{V}O_2$ = total tissue extraction of oxygen per minute (normal value = 250 ml/minute)
CaO_2 = arterial content of oxygen (normal value = 20 vol%)
CvO_2 = venous oxygen content (normal value = 15 vol%)

Cardiac Index (CI): 2.5 to 4 L/min/m^2. The CI assesses overall cardiac performance (eliminates body size as a variable). The CI is calculated by the following formula:

$$CI = CO/BSA$$

Central Venous Pressure (CVP)—1 to 6 mmHg. The CVP is directly measured from a CVP catheter or from the proximal lumen of the PA catheter. The CVP estimates right ventricular preload.

Right Ventricular Pressure (RVP)—15 to 30 mmHg systolic; 0 to 8 mmHg diastolic. The RVP is generally only measured during catheter insertion, when the distal tip of the PA catheter passes through the right ventricle.

Pulmonary Artery Pressure (PAP)—15 to 30 mmHg systolic; 5 to 15 mmHg diastolic. The PAP is measured from the distal tip of the PA catheter (balloon deflated).

Mean Pulmonary Artery Pressure (MPAP)—10 to 20 mmHg. The MPAP is useful in assessing the pulmonary vascular system and in calculating the pulmonary vascular resistance. Mean PAP is calculated by:

$$\text{MPAP} = (\text{PA systolic}) + (\text{PA diastolic} \times 2)/3$$

Pulmonary Artery Wedge Pressure (PAWP, PCWP, or PAOP)—4 to 12 mmHg. The PAWP is measured from the distal tip of the PA catheter (balloon inflated). The PAWP estimates left ventricular filling and preload. PCWP = pulmonary capillary wedge pressure; PAOP = pulmonary artery occluding pressure.

Partial Pressure of Mixed Venous Oxygen (PvO_2)—40 mmHg. To measure the PvO_2, a mixed venous blood sample is withdrawn from the distal tip of the PA catheter and analyzed for its oxygen tension. The PvO_2 is an important parameter for assessing the overall function of the cardiopulmonary system.

Venous Oxygen Saturation of Hemoglobin (SvO_2)—60% to 80%. The SvO_2 is measured from the distal tip of the PA catheter. The SvO_2 reflects the overall use of oxygen by the tissues.

Partial Pressure of Arterial Oxygen (PaO_2)—80 to 100 mmHg. The PaO_2 is measured from a systemic artery. The PaO_2 reflects the adequacy of arterial oxygenation.

Arterial Oxygen Saturation of Hemoglobin (SaO_2)—96% to 99%. The SaO_2 is either measured from a systemic artery or by pulse oximetry (SpO_2). The SaO_2 reflects the availability of oxygen delivered to the tissues.

Systemic Vascular Resistance (SVR)—15 to 20 units (mmHg/L/min) or 900 to 1400 dynes/sec/cm^5. The SVR is a useful parameter in assessing left ventricular afterload because it reflects the resistance facing the left ventricle during contraction. In addition, the SVR has a greater influence of controlling BP than does CO. An elevation of SVR increases myocardial work and myocardial oxygen consumption (MVO_2). SVR is calculated by:

$$\text{SVR (units)} = (\text{MAP} - \text{CVP})/\text{CO}$$

$$\text{SVR (dynes/sec/cm}^5\text{)} = (\text{MAP} - \text{CVP})/\text{CO} \times 80$$

Systemic Vascular Resistance Index (SVRI)—1900 to 2400 dynes/sec/cm^5/m^2. The SVRI uses the CI instead of the CO:

$$\text{SVRI} = (\text{MAP} - \text{CVP})/\text{CI} \times 80$$

Pulmonary Vascular Resistance (PVR)—1 to 3 units (mmHg/L/min) or 150 to 250 dynes/sec/cm^5. The PVR is a useful parameter in assessing right ventricular afterload as it reflects the resistance facing the right ventricle during contraction. An elevated PVR indicates that there is a high degree of resistance in the pulmonary vascular bed (i.e., pulmonary hypertension). PVR is calculated by:

$$\text{PVR (units)} = (\text{MPAP} - \text{PAWP})/\text{CO}$$

$$\text{PVR (dynes/sec/cm}^5) = (\text{MPAP} - \text{PAWP})/\text{CO} \times 80$$

Pulmonary Vascular Resistance Index (PVRI)—225 to 315 dynes/sec/cm^5/m^2. The PVRI utilizes the CI instead of the CO:

$$\text{PVRI} = (\text{MPAP} - \text{PAWP})/\text{CI} \times 80$$

Ejection Fraction (EF) — 65—75%. The EF represents the percentage of the total blood volume that is ejected from the ventricle with each contraction. As cardiac function deteriorates, the EF falls, which results in a reduced CO. The EF is usually measured directly.

Ventricular Stroke Work Index—ventricular work is defined as the energy required to eject blood from the ventricle. Elevated aortic and pulmonary pressures increase the energy required of each ventricle (left and right) to eject its contents, whereas reduced aortic and pulmonary pressures decrease the work of each ventricle. The force required to eject blood from the left ventricle is described as the left ventricular stroke work index (LVSWI). The force required to eject blood from the right ventricle is described as the right ventricular stroke work index (RVSWI). Ventricular work can be calculated from the following formulas:

$$\text{LVSWI} = \text{SI} \times (\text{MAP} - \text{PAWP}) \times 0.0136^* = 43 - 61 \text{ g} \times \text{m/m}^2$$

$$\text{RVSWI} = \text{SI} \times (\text{MPAP} - \text{CVP}) \times 0.0136^* = 7 - 12 \text{ g} \times \text{m/m}^2$$

*0.0136 is a conversion factor that converts ml/mmHg to g × m/m^2.

Arterial Oxygen Content (CaO_2)—20 ml of oxygen per 100 ml of blood (20 vol%). The CaO_2 determines the total content of oxygen in arterial blood. The CaO_2 represents the amount of oxygen that is available for tissue use and is calculated by the following formula:

$$CaO_2 = \text{Bound } O_2 + \text{Dissolved } O_2 = (\text{Hb} \times 1.34 \times SaO_2) + (PaO_2 \times 0.003)$$

Mixed Venous Oxygen Content (CvO_2)—15 ml of oxygen per 100 ml of blood (15 vol%). The CvO_2 determines the total content of oxygen in mixed venous blood. The CvO_2 represents the amount of oxygen returning to the right heart and is calculated by the following formula:

$$CvO_2 = \text{Bound } O_2 + \text{Dissolved } O_2 = (\text{Hb} \times 1.34 \times SvO_2) + (PvO_2 \times 0.003)$$

Arterial-to-Venous Oxygen Content Difference ($avDO_2$ or $Ca\text{-}vO_2$)—3 to 5 ml of oxygen per 100 ml of blood (3 to 5 vol%). The $avDO_2$ reflects the amount of oxygen used by the tissues and is calculated by the following formula:

$$avDO_2 = CaO_2 - CvO_2$$

Oxygen Delivery (DO_2)—1000 ml of oxygen per minute. The DO_2 represents not only the amount of oxygen delivered to the tissues (CaO_2) but also the rate at which this occurs (CO).

$$DO_2 = CaO_2 \times CO \times 10$$

Oxygen Consumption ($\dot{V}O_2$): 250 ml of oxygen per minute. The $\dot{V}O_2$ represents the amount of oxygen extracted from the blood as it flows through peripheral tissues. The $\dot{V}O_2$ may be measured directly by noting the volume of oxygen in exhaled gas and subtracting it from the volume of oxygen inhaled. Alternatively, $\dot{V}O_2$ may be measured indirectly by the following formula:

$$\dot{V}O_2 = CO \times (CaO_2 - CvO_2) \times 10$$

Oxygen Extraction Ratio—25%. The oxygen extraction ratio is a useful indicator of the balance that exists between oxygen delivery and oxygen consumption. Normally, 1000 ml of oxygen is transported to the tissues and 250 ml of this is used by the tissues. The amount of oxygen extracted by the tissues, therefore, is 25%. This leaves a venous reserve of 750 ml, or 75%.

Pulmonary Shunt (Qs/Qt)—3 to 5%. Normally, a small portion of the blood ejected from the right heart bypasses the lungs and returns to the left heart unoxygenated. The portion of shunted blood (Qs) is usually expressed as a percentage of the total cardiac output (Qt).

$$Qs/Qt = (CcO_2{}^{*} - CaO_2)/(CcO_2{}^{*} - CvO_2)$$

*CcO_2 is a reflection of end-capillary (alveolar) oxygen content.

The following formula is used to calculate CcO_2:

$$CcO_2 = (Hb \times 1.34 \times SAO_2) + (PAO_2 \times 0.003)$$

where:

SAO_2 = end-capillary oxygen saturation (normally assumed to be 100% if the PAO_2 is greater than 150 mmHg)

PAO_2 = partial pressure of alveolar oxygen: $PAO_2 = (P_B - P_{H2O})(FIO_2) - PaCO_2\,(1.25)$

SPECIFIC CARDIOVASCULAR AGENTS

ANTIANGINAL AGENTS AND VASODILATORS

Inadequate cardiac oxygenation due to a reduced coronary blood supply or an excessive myocardial oxygen consumption requirement leads to myocardial ischemia and possible necrosis (tissue death) to the region affected. Angina pectoris is the severe chest pain that occurs when there is an imbalance between the oxygen requirements of the heart and the oxygen supplied to it by the coronary vessels. Angina has three primary classifications:

- *Classic, stable angina (also known as angina of effort):* This type of angina occurs when the coronary blood flow rate does not keep pace with the increased oxygen demand placed on the heart during exercise, stress, or physical exertion. The pain is usually promptly relieved by rest or nitroglycerin. The most common cause of classic angina is atherosclerosis or some other form of obstructive artery disease.
- *Unstable angina:* This type of angina occurs even at rest and is usually due to a significantly compromised coronary blood flow. Unstable angina may be an indication of impending myocardial infarction (MI) and should be treated as a medical emergency.
- *Vasospastic (Prinzmetal) angina (also known as variant angina):* This type of angina is unrelated to exercise or an increase in heart rate; it occurs from coronary artery spasm.

The primary therapeutic goal of antianginal agents is to improve the oxygen supply:demand ratio of the heart. This goal is accomplished by increasing the oxygen supply to the heart by improving coronary blood flow and/or by decreasing the oxygen demand (consumption) of the heart, thereby decreasing the work of the heart. Three drug groups are useful as antianginal agents: the nitrates, the calcium channel blocking agents, and the β_1-adrenoceptor blocking agents.

THE NITRATES

Mechanism of Action

The nitrates are antianginal, antihypertensive agents, the primary pharmacologic action of which is to cause the liberation of nitric oxide (NO) in vascular smooth muscle. Nitric oxide activates the enzyme guanyl cyclase, which in turn increases the synthesis of cyclic guanosine monophosphate (cGMP), resulting in general relaxation and dilation of vascular smooth muscle of both arterial and venous vessels (see also Chapters 2 and 8).

The venous dilatory effects of these agents lead to pooling of blood in the great veins, which then leads to a reduced venous return to the right atrium. The corresponding reduction in preload and cardiac output lowers the myocardial oxygen demand (antianginal effect). Relaxation of arteriolar smooth muscle lowers the systemic vascular resistance (SVR), thereby causing a reduction in afterload and improved left ventricular function. Therapeutic doses of these agents reduce systolic, diastolic, and mean arterial blood pressure (antihypertensive effect). Other beneficial effects of these agents include reductions in pulmonary vascular pressures and heart size. Nitroglycerin is considered the prototype of the group.

Indications for Use

1. Nitroglycerin IV: For the control and prevention of hypertensive episodes caused by surgical procedures, cardiovascular procedures, and coronary artery bypass surgery. Also, congestive heart failure (CHF) associated with acute MI.
2. Sublingual, transmucosal, or translingual spray formulations: For the relief of acute anginal periods. To reduce the work of the heart for patients with acute MI or CHF.
3. Topical, oral, transmucosal, or translingual spray formulations: prophylaxis and long-term management of recurrent angina.
4. Nitroglycerin ointment: as adjunctive therapy in the treatment of Raynaud's disease and other peripheral vascular diseases.

Contraindications

Contraindications to the use of nitrates include hypersensitivity to the agents, hypotension, uncorrected hypovolemia, acute or recent MI, severe anemia, and increased intracranial pressure.

Precautions

1. Excessive doses may produce severe headaches because these agents also dilate cerebral blood vessels. Generally, the first indication that the drug is effective is the complaint of a headache by the patient.
2. Additive hypotensive effects may be noted with concurrent use of other antihypertensive agents, β-adrenoceptor blockers, alcohol, narcotics, and tricyclic antidepressants. Severe hypotension and cardiovascular collapse may result with concurrent use of these agents, especially alcohol.
3. Nitrates may potentiate the effects of anticholinergic drugs, antihistamines, and tricyclic antidepressants.
4. These agents may antagonize the pressor effects of sympathomimetic drugs.
5. Monitoring of the pulmonary artery wedge pressure (PAWP) facilitates titration of the drug. A reduction in the PAWP usually precedes the onset of hypotension.
6. Use with caution for patients with severe hepatic or renal disease.

Adverse Reactions

CNS: Headache (may be persistent and severe), dizziness, vertigo, restlessness, weakness.

Cardiovascular: Reflex tachycardia, palpitations, syncope, collapse, orthostatic hypotension, paradoxical bradycardia.

GI: Nausea, vomiting, abdominal pain.

Methemoglobinemia: High doses of nitrates may interfere with the normal conversion of methemoglobin to hemoglobin.

Overdosage

Symptoms include marked responses listed under *Adverse Reactions*. Treatment consists of IV fluids and monitoring of arterial blood gases and methemoglobin. Epinephrine administration is contraindicated in overdosage. The hemodynamic effects of these agents are usually of short duration and no further intervention should be necessary.

Dosage and Administration

Amyl Nitrate (Aspirols, Vaporole)—0.3 ml inhaled as needed. *Onset of action:* 0.5 minute. *Duration of effect:* 3 to 5 minutes.

Erythrityl Tetranitrate (Cardilate)—**Sublingual:** 5 to 10 mg t.i.d. or before stressful episodes or activity. *Onset of action:* 5 minutes. *Duration of effect:* 3 hours. **Oral:** 10 mg t.i.d. *Onset of action:* 15 to 30 minutes. *Duration of effect:* 6 hours.

Isosorbide Dinitrate (Isordil, Sorbitrate)—**Sublingual:** 2.5 to 10 mg as needed for pain or every 2 to 3 hours for prophylaxis. *Onset of action:* 2 to 5 minutes. *Duration of effect:* 1 to 3 hours. **Chewable:** 5 to 10 mg every 2 to 3 hours for prophylaxis. **Oral tablets:** 10 to 40 mg t.i.d. for prophylaxis. *Onset of action:* 20 to 40 minutes. *Duration of effect:* 4 to 6 hours. **Sustained-release tablets:** 40 to 80 mg b.i.d. *Onset of action:* up to 4 hours. *Duration of effect:* 6 to 8 hours.

Isosorbide Mononitrate (Imdur, Ismo, Monoket)—20 mg b.i.d. or 60 mg (Imdur) given once daily. *Onset of action:* 30 to 60 minutes. *Duration of effect:* no data available.

IV Nitroglycerin (Nitro-Bid IV, Tridil)—Dose may be titrated until a response is observed. Start with 5 μg/min and titrate upward in 5 μg/min increments with increases every 3 to 5 minutes up to 20 μg/min. If no response, increments of 10 to 20 μg/min may be given until an effect is noted. *Onset of action:* 1 to 2 minutes. *Duration of effect:* 3 to 5 minutes.

Sublingual Nitroglycerin (Nitrostat)—Dissolve one tablet under the tongue at the first sign of an acute anginal attack. Repeat every 5 minutes until relief is obtained. Do not exceed three tablets in 15 minutes. *Onset of action:* 1 to 3 minutes. *Duration of effect:* 30 to 60 minutes.

Translingual Nitroglycerin (Nitrolingual)—One to two sprays onto oral mucosa. Do not exceed three sprays within 15 minutes. Spray should not be inhaled. *Onset of action:* 2 minutes. *Duration of effect:* 30 to 60 minutes.

Transmucosal Nitroglycerin (Nitrogard)—One tablet placed in buccal pouch every 3 to 5 hours while awake. *Onset of action:* 1 to 2 minutes. *Duration of effect:* 3 to 5 hours.

Topical Ointment Nitroglycerin (Nitro-Bid, Nitrol)—Initially, half-inch strip of ointment every 4 to 8 hours. Usual dose is 1 to 2 inches every 8 hours. Occasionally, 4 to 5 inches have been used every 4 hours. Do not rub ointment into skin, apply by spreading a thin, uniform layer on skin. *Onset of action:* 30 to 60 minutes. *Duration of effect:* 2 to 12 hours.

Sustained-Release Nitroglycerin (Nitro-Bid, others)—Initially, 2.5 mg every 6 to 8 hours; may increase in 2.5-mg increments two to four times per day until side effects limit the dose. *Onset of action:* 20 to 45 minutes. *Duration of effect:* 3 to 8 hours.

Transdermal Nitroglycerin (Deponit, Minitran, Nitrocine, Nitrodisc, Nitro-Dur, Transderm-Nitro)—Apply one patch to nonhairy skin area every 16 to 18 hours. Patch should be removed for 6 to 8 hours overnight. *Onset of action:* 30 to 60 minutes. *Duration of effect:* up to 24 hours.

Pentaerythritol tetranitrate (P.E.T.N.) (Pentylan, Peritrate, Duotrate)—Initially, 10 or 20 mg, t.i.d. or q.i.d. Titrate to 40 mg q.i.d., 30 minutes before meals or 1 hour after meals and at bedtime. Not intended to relieve acute anginal attacks. *Onset of action:* 20 to 60 minutes. *Duration of effect:* approximately 5 hours.

THE CALCIUM CHANNEL BLOCKING AGENTS

Mechanism of Action

These agents are antiarrhythmic, antianginal, antihypertensive calcium channel blocking agents (also referred to as slow channel blockers or calcium antagonists) that have the ability to not only inhibit calcium ion transport across the myocardial cell membrane but also to inhibit calcium entry into arterial smooth muscle. The effect of inhibiting calcium entry across myocardial cells delays impulse transmission through the AV node (antiarrhythmic effect), depresses myocardial contraction (negative inotropic effect), and reduces spontaneous rhythm of sinus node (antiarrhythmic effect). The effect of inhibiting calcium entry into arterial smooth muscle results in arterial vasodilation with a corresponding reduction in systemic vascular resistance and arterial blood pressure (antihypertensive effect). Dilation of coronary arteries and arterioles and preventing coronary artery spasm by inhibiting calcium influx increases coronary blood flow, which in turn, increases oxygen supply to the myocardium (antianginal effect). Some of these agents (e.g., verapamil) also inhibit stimulation of α-adrenoceptors in the peripheral vascular system, resulting in peripheral vasodilation (antihypertensive effect). Verapamil is considered the prototype of the group.

Indications

1. Angina pectoris:
   a. Chronic stable: amlodipine, bepridil, diltiazem, nicardipine, nifedipine, verapamil.
   b. Unstable: oral verapamil.
   c. Vasospastic: amlodipine, diltiazem, nifedipine, verapamil.
2. Essential hypertension: amlodipine, diltiazem, felodipine, isradipine, nicardipine, nifedipine, verapamil. Sustained-release verapamil and diltiazem are only indicated for essential hypertension. See also *Antihypertensive Agents*.
3. Patients with chronic atrial fibrillation or atrial flutter: oral verapamil in conjunction with digitalis has been shown to control ventricular rate at rest and during exercise or stress. Additionally, for prophylactic treatment of paroxysmal supraventricular tachycardia (PSVT).
4. Supraventricular tachyarrhythmias: IV verapamil. Additionally, temporary control of rapid ventricular rates for patients with atrial fibrillation or atrial flutter.
5. Subarachnoid hemorrhage: nimodipine.
6. Unlabeled uses:
   a. Migraine headache: nifedipine, nimodipine, verapamil.
   b. Raynaud's syndrome: diltiazem, nifedipine.
   c. Congestive heart failure: nicardipine, nifedipine.
   d. Cardiomyopathy: nifedipine, verapamil.
   e. Exercise-induced asthma: verapamil.
   f. Recumbent nocturnal leg cramps: verapamil.
   g. To quickly lower blood pressure in hypertensive emergencies: nifedipine.
   h. Treatment of primary pulmonary hypertension, asthma, preterm labor: nifedipine.
   i. To reduce the progression of coronary artery disease (CAD) or CHF.

Contraindications

Contraindications to the use of calcium channel blockers include hypersensitivity to these agents, cardiogenic shock, severe hypotension, sick sinus syndrome (except with a functioning ventricular pacemaker), second- or third-degree AV block, hypotension that exhibits a systolic pressure less than 90 mmHg (bepridil, diltiazem, verapamil), acute MI and pulmonary congestion (diltiazem), advanced aortic stenosis (nicardipine), and severe left ventricular dysfunction (verapamil, diltiazem).

Precautions

1. Abrupt withdrawal of these agents may cause chest pain.
2. Use with caution for patients with impaired renal and hepatic function.
3. Verapamil may increase the effects of nondepolarizing muscle relaxants and those of theophylline.
4. IV verapamil should not be used concomitantly (within a few hours) with β-adrenoceptor blocking agents. Both of these agents depress myocardial contractility and AV conduction and may increase the severity of congestive heart failure or produce severe hypotension. Additionally, concurrent administration of these agents may worsen existing angina.
5. An additive hypotensive effect may be noted when these agents are coadministered with other antihypertensive agents.
6. Coadministration of calcium and vitamin D may reduce the effectiveness of verapamil.

Adverse Reactions

CNS: Dizziness, nervousness, headache, fatigue, tremor, confusion, sleep disturbances.

Cardiovascular: Peripheral and pulmonary edema, tachycardia, palpitations, hypotension, syncope, third-degree AV block, bradycardia, CHF, MI.

GI: Nausea, vomiting, heartburn, diarrhea, constipation, abdominal cramps.

Respiratory: Dyspnea, cough, wheezing, chest congestion, pulmonary edema.

Musculoskeletal: Muscle cramping, joint stiffness, inflammation.

Other: Dermatitis, urticaria, fever, sweating, chills, hair loss, menstrual irregularities, impotence, claudication.

Overdosage

Symptoms of overdose include hypotension, bradycardia, decreased cardiac output, junctional rhythms, and second- or third-degree AV block. Treatment consists of supportive care with IV fluids and Trendelenburg position (with hypotensive effects) and monitoring of cardiac and respiratory functions. β-adrenoceptor agonists and IV calcium may be administered to counteract effects.

Dosage and Administration

Calcium Blockers

Amlodipine (Norvasc)—5 to 10 mg once daily.

Bepridil (Vascor)—200 to 400 mg orally once daily.

Diltiazem (Cardizem)—**PO:** 30 to 80 mg every 6 hours. **IV:** 75 to 150 μg/kg.

Felodipine (Plendil)—5 to 10 mg once daily.

Isradipine (DynaCirc)—2.5 to 10 mg every 12 hours.
Nicardipine (Cardene)—20 to 40 mg every 8 hours orally. **Sustained release:** 30 to 60 mg b.i.d.
Nifedipine (Adalat, Procardia)—**PO:** 20 to 40 mg every 8 hours. **Sustained release:** 30 to 60 mg once daily. **IV:** 3 to 10 μg/kg.
Nimodipine (Nimotop)—60 mg every 4 hours orally.
Verapamil (Calan, Isoptin, Verelan)—**PO:** 240 to 480 mg/day. **IV:** 5 to 10 mg given by slow infusion over 2 minutes. 10 mg may be given additionally, if necessary, in 30 minutes.

THE β_1-ADRENCOCEPTOR BLOCKING AGENTS

Of the various β_1-adrenoceptor blocking agents, only four have been approved for patients with angina pectoris: atenolol, metoprolol, nadolol, and propranolol. Bisoprolol, carteolol, and esmolol are currently undergoing investigation as antianginal agents. This section briefly presents those aspects that pertain to the currently approved β_1-adrenoceptor blocking agents used in the control of angina. Many of the β_1-adrenoceptor blocking agents are also used as antiarrhythmic agents and as antihypertensive agents and will be reviewed in the sections on *Antiarrhythmic Agents* and *Antihypertensive Agents*. For a complete listing (e.g., contraindications, precautions, adverse reactions, overdosage), see *Antihypertensive Agents,* presented later in this chapter.

ATENOLOL (TENORMIN)
METOPROLOL (LOPRESSOR, TOPROL XL)
NADOLOL (CORGARD)
PROPRANOLOL (INDERAL)
Mechanism of Action

Atenolol, metoprolol, nadolol, and propranolol are especially useful in reducing the frequency and severity of anginal episodes because they have the ability to significantly reduce the myocardial oxygen demand at rest and during exercise. This action directly relates to the blockade of cardiac β_1-adrenoceptors by these agents (see also Chapter 2). The overall hemodynamic effects of blocking the cardiac β_1-adrenoceptors include decreased automaticity of the sinus node (antiarrhythmic effect), prolongation of the AV nodal refractory period (antiarrhythmic effect), reduction in blood pressure (antihypertensive effect), and myocardial contractility (negative inotropic effect). The decreased workload placed on the heart effectively reduces myocardial oxygen requirements (antianginal effect). The β_1-adrenoceptor blocking agents are additionally effective in preventing reinfarction after a myocardial infarction (propranolol and timolol only). Generally, combined nitrate-beta blocker therapy is employed in the treatment of angina to offset the deleterious effect of the beta blockers in causing an increase in the end-diastolic volume that accompanies slowing of the heart rate and an increase in ejection time.

The prototypic agent in this group is propranolol, a nonselective β-adrenoceptor blocking agent (i.e., it blocks both β_1- and β_2-adrenoceptors). Nadolol is also a nonselective β-adrenoceptor blocking agent, whereas both atenolol and metoprolol are selective in blocking only β_1-adrenoceptors and are thus safer to use for patients with asthma (at therapeutic doses only β_1-adrenoceptors are blocked; however, higher doses may also block β_2-adrenoceptors).

Dosage and Administration

The antianginal doses of these agents include the following:

Atenolol (Tenormin)—50 to 100 mg once daily.

Metoprolol (Lopressor, Toprol XL)—Initially 50 mg b.i.d. Dosage may be increased gradually at weekly intervals as needed. Usual dose is 100 to 400 mg daily in two divided doses.

Nadolol (Corgard)—Initially 40 mg once daily. May increase dosage at 3- to 7-day intervals until desired response is observed. Usual maintenance dose is 80 to 240 mg/day.

Propranolol (Inderal)—Initially 10 to 20 mg t.i.d., q.i.d. Dosage may be gradually increased at weekly intervals until desired response is observed. Usual maintenance dose is 80 to 160 mg/day. Usually given in combination with nitrates.

ANTIARRHYTHMIC AGENTS

An arrhythmia occurs when there is a significant deviation in the rate of impulse firing from the SA node, in the normal cardiac impulse formation, or in the normal impulse conduction. Sinus tachycardia results when the SA node fires more than 100 times per minute, whereas sinus bradycardia is caused by a slowing of the SA node firing rate (less than 60 times per minute). Normal cardiac impulse formation should begin with the SA node. When ectopic beats (impulses arising from areas of the heart other than the SA node) originate the firing mechanism of the heart, atrial arrhythmias (from atrial ectopic beats) or ventricular arrhythmias (from ventricular ectopic beats) ensue. Heart blocks are a result of an abnormal delay in impulse conduction. For example, characteristic of first-degree heart block is a prolonged P-R interval. This is a direct reflection that the impulse delay at the AV node is abnormally long. Conversely, if there is no impulse delay at the AV node, supraventricular tachycardias (SVTs) occur.

Antiarrhythmic agents have two primary therapeutic goals: to restore the cardiac rhythm to normal sinus rhythm and to prevent the recurrence of the arrhythmia. Owing to the complexity of the antiarrhythmic agents, they have been categorized into four main groups on the basis of their dominant mechanism of action:

- Group I Antiarrhythmic Agents: This is the largest group of antiarrhythmic agents and consists of membrane-stabilizing agents that depress phase 0 of the action potential and those agents that either prolong or shorten the action potential duration. Group I antiarrhythmic agents are subdivided into groups IA, IB, and IC.

Group IA drugs depress phase 0 and lengthen the duration of the action potential. Group IA drugs include quinidine, procainamide, and disopyramide.

Group IB drugs depress phase 0 slightly and shorten the action potential duration and include lidocaine, tocainamide, phenytoin, and mexiletine. As a group, these agents interact rapidly with sodium channels to block sodium influx across the myocardial cell membrane. Phenytoin is not approved specifically as an antiarrhythmic agent but is used for digitalis-induced arrhythmias. The other group IB drugs are primarily used to correct or prevent ventricular arrhythmias.

Group IC drugs cause marked depression of phase 0, decrease impulse conduction (especially His-Purkinje) and prolong the ventricular refractory period. Group IC drugs include flecainide, encainide, propafenone, and moricizine. Encainide has been withdrawn from the market; however, it is available on a limited basis. Moricizine is a group I agent that has properties that can place it in either group IA, IB, or IC. These agents are potent blockers of sodium channels and are usually reserved for life-threatening ventricular arrhythmias owing to their potential for exacerbating arrhythmias.

- Group II Antiarrhythmic Agents: The β_1-adrenoceptor blocking agents, propranolol, esmolol, and acebutolol, comprise the group II agents. By nature of their cardiac β_1-blocking activity, these agents slow AV conduction, prolong the AV nodal refractory period, and decrease the automaticity of the SA node.
- Group III Antiarrhythmic Agents: This group is composed of drugs that prolong phase 3 (repolarization) of the action potential. Agents in this group include bretylium, amiodarone, and sotalol. Sotalol has both group II (beta blocking) and group III properties. Group III properties are noted in doses greater than 160 mg. These agents are usually reserved for life-threatening ventricular arrhythmias that do not respond to other treatment. Bretylium is usually used in a cardiopulmonary resuscitation setting when lidocaine and cardioversion have failed to convert the ventricular arrhythmia (see also Chapter 19).
- Group IV Antiarrhythmic Agents: The calcium channel blocking agents, verapamil and diltiazem, constitute this group of antiarrhythmic agents. Owing to their calcium channel blocking activity, these agents are effective in decreasing AV conduction velocity, in prolonging the AV nodal refractory period, and

in decreasing SA nodal automaticity. Arrhythmias that these agents are indicated for include supraventricular tachyarrhythmias and control of rapid ventricular rates in atrial fibrillation.

A yet unnamed group of antiarrhythmic drugs, potentially group V, because they do not fit into the conventional group I through IV scheme, are currently categorized as miscellaneous antiarrhythmic agents. This group of antiarrhythmic drugs include digitalis and adenosine. These agents act to decrease the automaticity of the SA node, decrease AV conduction velocity, and prolong AV refractory period.

Table 18.1 summarizes some of the more important pharmacokinetic, electrophysiologic, and ECG properties of the various antiarrhythmic agents.

Group IA Antiarrhythmic Agents

QUINIDINE SULFATE (QUINORA)
QUINIDINE GLUCONATE (QUINALAN, QUINAGLUTE)
QUINIDINE POLYGALACTURONATE (CARDIOQUIN)

Mechanism of Action

Quinidine's antiarrhythmic action depresses conduction velocity, excitability, and automaticity. It also increases the heart's refractory time period, thereby increasing the time interval in which the heart may respond to contraction. The antiarrhythmic activity of quinidine results primarily from its ability to bind to and block activated sodium channels. Quinidine also possesses α-adrenoceptor blocking properties that lead to vasodilation and a reflex increase in SA nodal firing and antimuscarinic activity that inhibits parasympathetic (vagal) effects in the heart.

Indications for Use

1. Oral: Premature atrial contractions (PACs), premature ventricular contractions (PVCs), paroxysmal atrial tachycardia (PAT), paroxysmal and chronic A-fib, paroxysmal ventricular tachycardia (those not associated with complete heart block), paroxysmal AV junctional rhythm, A-flutter. Maintenance therapy after electrical conversion of A-fib or A-flutter.
2. Parenteral: Indicated when rapid effect is required or when oral therapy is not feasible.

Contraindications

Contraindications to the use of quinidine include hypersensitivity to the agent. Use with extreme caution for patients with subacute endocarditis, bradycardia, coronary occlusion, or extensive myocardial damage.

Table 18.1.
Pharmacokinetic, Electrophysiologic, and ECG Properties of Antiarrhythmic Drugs

		Pharmacokinetics			*Electrophysiology*									*ECG Changes*			
					Automaticity		*Conduction velocity*			*Refractory period*							
Group	*Drug*	Onset (min)	Duration (hr)	Therapeutic serum levels (μg/ml)	SA node	Ectopic pacemaker	Atrium	AV node	His-Purkinje	Atrium	AV node	His-Purkinje	Ventricle	Heart rate	P-R interval	QRS complex	Q-T interval
IA	Quinidine	30	6–10	2–6	↑↓	↓	↓	↑↓	↓	↑↑	↑	↑↑	↑	↑↓	↑↓	↑	↑
	Procainamide	30	3–5	4–8	↑↓	↓	↓	↑↓	↓	↑	↑	↑↑	↑	↑↓	↑↓	↑	↑
	Disopyramide	30	5–7	2–8	↑↓	↓	↓	↑↓	↓	↑↑	↑	↑↑	↑	↑↓	↑↓	↑	↑
IB	Lidocaine	1–3[a]	0.25	1.5–6	0	↓	—	↑	↑	—	↑↓	↑↓	↑↓	0	0	0	0—↓
	Phenytoin	30–60	24	10–20	↑↓	↓	—	↑	↑	0	↑↓	↑↓	↑↓	↑↓	0—↓	0	↓
	Tocainide	30–60	4–8	4–10	↑↓	↓	0	0	0	↓	↓	↑↓	↓	0	0	0	0—↓
	Mexiletine	30–60	4–8	0.5–2	↓	↓	0	0	0	0	↑↓	↑	↑	—	0	0	0
IC	Flecainide	30–60	8–12	0.2–1	↓	↓	↓↓	↓	↓↓	0	↑↓	↑	↑	0	↑	↑↑	0—↑
	Encainide	30–60	8–12	varies	↑↓	↓	↓↓	↓	↓↓	0—↑	0—↑	↑	↑	0	↑	↑↑	0—↑
	Propafenone	30–60	8	0.6–1	0	↓	0	↓	↓	0	↑	↑	↑	0	↑	↑	0—↑
	Moricizine	120	10–24	n/a	0	↓	0	↓	↓	↑↓	0	0	0—↑	0—↑	↑	↑	0
II	Propranolol	30	3–6	0.5–1	↓	↓	↑↓	↓	↓	↑↓	↑	0	0	↓	0—↑	0	0—↓
	Acebutolol	30	12–16	n/a	↓	↓	↑↓	↓	↓	↑↓	↑	0	0	↓	0—↑	0	0—↓
	Esmolol	1–2	0.1	n/a	↓	↓	↑↓	↓	0	↑↓	↑	0	0	↓	0—↑	0	0—↓
III	Bretylium	1–3[a]	6–8	0.5–1.5	↑	↑	0	0	↑	0	↑↓	↑	↑	0	0	0	0
	Amiodarone	varies	varies	0.5–2.5	↓	↓	↓	↓	↓	↑	↑	↑	↑	↓	↑	↑	↑↑
	Sotalol	varies	8–12	n/a	↓	↓	0	↓	0	↑↑	↑	↑↑	↑↑	↓	↑	0	↑↑
IV	Verapamil	30	6–8	0.8–0.3	↓	↓	0	↓	0	0	↑	0	0	↓	↑	0	0
	Diltiazem	30–60	1–3	0.5–0.2	↓	↓	0	↓	↓	0	↑	0	0	↓	↑	0	0
—	Digitalis	30–120	24+	0.5–2[b]	↓	↑	↑↓	↓	0—↓	↑↓	↑	0	↓	↓	↑	0	↓
—	Adenosine	0.5[a]	0.01	n/a	↓	↓	0	↓	0	0	↑	0	0	↑	↑	0	0

[a]With IV use.
[b]ng/ml.
[c]n/a, not applicable; ↑, increase; ↓, decrease; 0, no significant effect; ↑↓, variable effect.

Precautions

1. Use with caution for patients with myasthenia gravis, acute infections, respiratory distress, and asthma.
2. Monitor plasma quinidine levels frequently when doses of greater than 2 g/day are used.
3. Quinidine may not be effective if cholinergic drugs are used concurrently.
4. Quinidine's effects are diminished in the presence of hypokalemia and enhanced by potassium.
5. Elderly patients and patients with CHF or renal or hepatic impairments may require a reduced dosage.

Adverse Reactions

CNS: Confusion, nervousness, headache, flushing, edema.

Cardiovascular: Bradycardia, heart block (partial or total), syncope, circulatory collapse, shock, widening of the QRS complex, cardiac asystole, ventricular ectopy.

GI: Nausea, vomiting, abdominal pain, diarrhea.

Overdosage

Symptoms include lethargy, coma, respiratory arrest, seizures, tachyarrhythmias. Treatment consists of symptomatic support, respiratory intervention with assisted ventilations if necessary, ECG and blood pressure monitoring, and cardiac pacing if indicated.

Dosage and Administration

Oral:

For premature atrial and ventricular contractions: 200 to 300 mg given up to 4 times daily.

For paroxysmal supraventricular contractions: 400 to 600 mg given every 2 to 3 hours until arrhythmia is suppressed.

Maintenance therapy: 200 to 300 mg given up to four times daily.

Sustained-release forms: 300 to 600 mg every 8 to 12 hours.

Parenteral (rarely used):

For parenteral use, patient must be continuously monitored for ECG changes. Parenteral use has, for the most part, been replaced by lidocaine or procainamide. **IV:** 330 mg or less of quinidine gluconate. May require up to 750 mg. **IM:** 600 mg quinidine gluconate initial dose for episodes of acute tachycardia. Then, 400 mg as often as every 2 hours may be given.

PROCAINAMIDE (PROCAN, PRONESTYL)

Mechanism of Action

The mechanism of action and antiarrhythmic effects of procainamide are essentially identical to quinidine; perhaps the most important difference between the two is that procainamide has less prominent antimuscarinic activity. In addition, procainamide has ganglionic-blocking properties that reduce peripheral vascular resistance and consequently lead to hypotension, especially with IV administration.

Indications for Use

1. Treatment of premature ventricular contractions (PVCs), ventricular tachycardia, paroxysmal atrial tachycardia (PAT), and atrial fibrillation.
2. Drug of second choice (after lidocaine) for patients with sustained ventricular arrhythmias associated with acute myocardial infarction.

Contraindications

Contraindications to the use of procainamide include complete heart block, idiosyncratic hypersensitivity to local anesthetics (procainamide is a derivative of procaine), lupus erythematosus, torsade de pointes, and myasthenia gravis.

Precautions

1. Cardiotoxic effects of procainamide are similar to those of quinidine. Antimuscarinic and direct depressant effects may occur. Use with caution for patients with CHF and patients with acute ischemic heart disease or cardiomyopathy because even a slight depression in myocardial contractility may further compromise the patient by causing a significant life-threatening reduction in cardiac output.
2. Coadministration of procainamide with other group IA antiarrhythmic drugs may precipitate new arrhythmias. Coadministration is usually reserved for serious arrhythmias in which a single drug is ineffective.
3. Frequent monitoring of vital signs and ECG changes are necessary during procainamide administration, as with all antiarrhythmic agents.
4. During long-term therapy of procainamide, serologic abnormalities (e.g., rising serum antinuclear antibodies, ANA) occur in nearly all patients. Approximately one-third of patients receiving procainamide therapy develop lupus erythematosus or related symptoms. A rising titer of serum antinuclear antibody (ANA) may precede clinical symptoms of lupus erythematosus.
5. Procainamide may increase the hypotensive effects of antihypertensives and diuretics.

6. Worsening of muscular weakness occurs in patients with myasthenia gravis owing to procainamide's procaine-like effects on diminishing acetylcholine release at skeletal muscle motor nerve endings.

Adverse Reactions

Most Common: Anorexia, nausea (orally), hypotension (IV administration).

Cardiovascular: Ventricular asystole or fibrillation (IV administration).

CNS: Dizziness, giddiness, weakness, mental depression, psychosis with hallucinations.

GI: Anorexia, nausea, vomiting, abdominal pain, diarrhea.

Hematologic: Neutropenia, thrombocytopenia, hemolytic anemia (rare), agranulocytosis.

Lupus Erythematosus: Lupus-like syndrome including symptoms such as arthralgia, pleural or abdominal pains, arthritis, pleural effusion, pericarditis, fever, chills, myalgia, and skin lesions.

Overdosage

Symptoms of overdose include progressive widening of the QRS complex, prolonged P-R and Q-T intervals, as well as AV block. Ventricular tachycardia or fibrillation may ensue. Treatment includes general supportive measures, close observation, monitoring of vital signs, and possibly IV administration of pressor agents and mechanical ventilatory support. There is no specific antidote for procainamide overdose, and as such, hemodialysis may be necessary.

Dosage and Administration

Oral:

For less urgent arrhythmias: initially, 1 g loading dose, then 50 mg/kg/day in divided doses every 3 hours (every 6 hours for sustained-release formulations).

Parenteral:

IM: initially, 50 mg/kg/day in divided doses every 3 to 6 hours. As soon as feasible, switch to oral therapy. **IV:** 100 mg every 5 minutes by slow IV injection (25 to 50 mg/min) to a maximum of 500 mg. Continuous ECG monitoring is essential.

For life-threatening arrhythmias:

30 mg/min IV until one of the following occurs: suppression of the arrhythmia, onset of hypotension, QRS complex greater than 50% of base line, administration of a total of 17 mg/kg.

DISOPYRAMIDE (NORPACE)

Mechanism of Action

The antiarrhythmic effects of disopyramide are similar to those of quinidine: disopyramide decreases the rate of depolarization (phase 4) in myocardial cells, prolongs the action potential duration and effective refractory period of both the atria and ventricles, and suppresses ectopic pacemaker activity. Disopyramide's antimuscarinic activity is even more pronounced than that of quinidine; therefore, a drug that slows AV conduction time should be coadministered with disopyramide in the treatment of atrial fibrillation or flutter to ensure that drug-induced increases in AV conduction do not result in rapid ventricular rates. Disopyramide's negative inotropic effect (decreased force of contraction) is frequently troublesome for patients with preexisting left heart failure.

Indications for Use

In the USA, disopyramide is approved for use in the treatment of ventricular arrhythmias such as unifocal or multifocal premature ventricular contractions, paired premature ventricular contractions, and episodes of ventricular tachycardia. Disopyramide is more commonly used when quinidine or procainamide has been poorly tolerated or ineffective. An unlabeled use of disopyramide includes the treatment of paroxysmal supraventricular tachycardia (PSVT).

Contraindications

Contraindications to the use of disopyramide include cardiogenic shock, preexisting second- or third-degree heart block, congenital Q-T prolongation, sick sinus syndrome, and hypersensitivity to the agent.

Precautions

1. Use with lesser, nonthreatening arrhythmias is usually not recommended owing to disopyramide's proarrhythmic effects.
2. Disopyramide may cause or aggravate CHF or induce severe hypotension, especially for patients with depressed systolic function. Use cautiously, if at all, for patients with an already compromised left ventricular abnormality.
3. Patients with preexisting atrial fibrillation or flutter should be predigitalized to ensure that enhancement of the AV conduction does not lead to a rapid ventricular rate beyond acceptable limits.
4. If heart blocks occur, reduce or discontinue use.
5. Use with special consideration for patients with myasthenia gravis, urinary retention, and glaucoma owing to disopyramide's anticholinergic activity.
6. Continuous ECG monitoring is necessary.
7. Disopyramide may be ineffective in hypokalemic states, and its toxic effects may be enhanced in hyperkalemic states. Potassium deficits should be corrected before administration.

Adverse Reactions

Most Common: Dry mouth, urinary hesitancy, nausea, bloating, abdominal pain, constipation, blurred vision, fatigue, headache, malaise.
Most Serious: Hypotension and CHF.

Overdosage

Apnea, loss of consciousness, cardiac arrhythmias, and death may result from excessive dosage administration of disopyramide. Toxic levels produce excessive widening of the QRS complex and Q-T interval. Severe anticholinergic effects may also be observed and can be reversed with neostigmine. Treatment consists of emesis, gastric lavage, as well as administration of pressor agents to overcome hypotension. Mechanical ventilation may be necessary.

Dosage and Administration

Oral administration only: initially, 200 to 300 mg loading dose, followed by 150 mg every 6 hours. Sustained-release capsules may be given every 8 hours. Usual dose is 400 to 800 mg/day.

Group IB Antiarrhythmic Agents

LIDOCAINE (LIDOPEN, XYLOCAINE)

Mechanism of Action

Lidocaine is a potent antiarrhythmic agent that suppresses arrhythmias associated with depolarization (e.g., ischemia, digitalis toxicity) and, as such, is highly effective in abolishing arrhythmias that occur in conjunction with myocardial infarction. Lidocaine seems to interact exclusively on blocking sodium channels, both in the activated and inactivated state. By this mechanism, lidocaine increases the electrical stimulation threshold of the ventricle during diastole, suppresses ectopic pacemaker activity, and shortens the effective refractory period. In therapeutic doses, lidocaine has little effect on atrial muscle, AV conduction, absolute refractory period, systolic arterial blood pressure, myocardial contractility, and cardiac output. Lidocaine's local anesthetic properties are presented in Chapter 15.

Indications

1. Treatment of acute ventricular arrhythmias associated with myocardial infarction, cardiac surgery, cardiac catheterization, and digitalis intoxication.
2. Agent of choice for abolishing ventricular tachycardia and fibrillation after cardioversion (see also Chapter 19).

3. Agent of choice for patients with sustained ventricular arrhythmias associated with acute myocardial infarction.

Contraindications

Hypersensitivity to amine local anesthetics, Stokes-Adams syndrome, Wolff-Parkinson-White syndrome, severe SA, AV, or intraventricular block in the absence of an artificial pacemaker.

Precautions

1. Use with caution for patients with CHF, reduced cardiac output, digitalis toxicity accompanied by AV block, for elderly individuals, and for patients with renal or liver impairment.
2. Coadministration of lidocaine with cimetidine or beta blockers may result in toxic serum lidocaine levels.
3. Accelerated cardiodepressant action may occur if lidocaine is coadministered with procainamide or tocainide.
4. Lidocaine may prolong the neuromuscular blocking action of succinylcholine.
5. Constant ECG monitoring is essential when administering lidocaine.
6. Resuscitative equipment should be immediately available to treat significant adverse reactions involving the CNS or cardiopulmonary systems.

Adverse Reactions

Most Common: Drowsiness, lightheadedness, slurred speech, paresthesias, mild tremor, sensations of heat, cold, or numbness.

Cardiovascular: Hypotension, bradycardia, cardiovascular collapse, cardiac arrest.

CNS: Hallucinations, euphoria, tinnitus, blurred or double vision, twitching, convulsions, unconsciousness.

Miscellaneous: Fever, vomiting, respiratory depression and arrest.

Overdosage

Symptoms of overdose range from mild CNS toxicity (drowsiness, dizziness) to an attenuated response as listed under *Adverse Reactions*. Treatment consists of supportive measures such as ensuring a patent airway and adequate ventilation. If circulatory depression occurs, administer vasopressors and, if required, initiate CPR.

Dosage and Administration

Parenteral only: **Injection loading dose:** 1 to 1.5 mg/kg given IV. Maximum total dose is 3 mg/kg. **IV infusion:** 30 to 50 μg/kg/min (2 to 4 mg/min) of a 0.1%

to 0.2% solution. **IM:** 300 mg, may repeat in 60–90 minutes. Use only 10% solution, or LidoPen Auto-Injector (300 mg/3 ml).

PHENYTOIN (DILANTIN, DIPHENYLAN)

Although phenytoin does not have specific approval for use as an antiarrhythmic agent, it has been shown to be effective as a second-line drug for patients experiencing digitalis-induced arrhythmias such as paroxysmal atrial tachycardia and ventricular ectopic rhythms. Phenytoin suppresses ectopic pacemaker activity and improves AV and intraventricular conduction in the digitalis-depressed heart primarily by blocking sodium and, to some extent, calcium current. Phenytoin's primary use is as an anticonvulsant for treatment of grand mal seizures (see Chapter 15 for a detailed presentation of this drug). The usual antiarrhythmic dose is 1000 mg orally given in divided doses the first day, then 500 to 600 mg on the second and third days, followed by a maintenance dose of 100 mg b.i.d., q.i.d. For IV injection: 100 mg every 5 to 10 minutes until the arrhythmia is abolished or toxicity appears.

TOCAINIDE (TONOCARD), MEXILETINE (MEXITIL)

Tocainide and mexiletine are group IB antiarrhythmic agents that are congeners of lidocaine that are unaffected by the first-pass hepatic metabolism and therefore can be taken by the oral route. Both agents have electrophysiologic and antiarrhythmic actions that are similar to lidocaine and, as lidocaine, are indicated for ventricular arrhythmias such as premature ventricular contractions and tachycardia. However, because of the proarrhythmic effects of these agents (especially mexiletine), they are usually reserved for life-threatening ventricular arrhythmias refractory to lidocaine or in which oral therapy is feasible. Adverse effects of these agents are seen frequently at therapeutic doses and are primarily neurologic in nature: tremor, blurred vision, lethargy, confusion, hallucinations, impaired coordination. Nausea is also a common side effect. The usual dose of tocainide is 800 to 2400 mg/day; the usual dose of mexiletine is 600 to 1200 mg/day.

Group IC Antiarrhythmic Agents

FLECAINIDE (TAMBOCOR)
ENCAINIDE (ENKAID)
PROPAFENONE (RYTHMOL)

Mechanism of Action

Flecainide, encainide, and propafenone are potent sodium channel blockers that decrease intracardiac conduction in all parts of the heart, with the greatest effect noted in the His-Purkinje system (especially noted with flecainide and encainide). Ventricular refractory period is prolonged, with little effect noted on the resting heart rate.

Indications for Use

1. Treatment of life-threatening ventricular arrhythmias (e.g., sustained ventricular tachycardia).
2. Propafenone: unlabeled use—treatment of supraventricular tachycardias, including atrial flutter or fibrillation and arrhythmias associated with Wolff-Parkinson-White syndrome.

Contraindications

Bundle branch block, second- or third-degree heart block, cardiogenic shock, sick sinus syndrome.

Precautions

The National Heart, Lung, and Blood Institutes' Cardiac Arrhythmia Suppression Trial (CAST) demonstrated that there is an excessive mortality or nonfatal cardiac arrest rate associated with the use of flecainide and encainide. Whether propafenone exhibits this undesired feature is currently unknown. Encainide has been withdrawn from the market by its manufacturer and is available on a limited basis only. Group IC drugs have potent proarrhythmic effects; therefore, these agents may precipitate new arrhythmias or worsen existing arrhythmias. As such, group IC drugs are *reserved* for documented life-threatening ventricular arrhythmias in which the benefits of using these drugs outweigh the risks.

Adverse Reactions

Most Common: Dizziness, nausea, vomiting, constipation, headache.

Most Serious: Proarrhythmic effects: increased premature ventricular contractions, worsening of ventricular tachycardia, heart block, prolonged QRS interval, cardiac arrest.

Overdosage

Overdose symptoms are usually most severe within 3 hours of ingestion and may include hypotension, somnolence, bradycardia, intra-atrial and intraventricular conduction delays, convulsions, asystole, or high-grade ventricular arrhythmias. Treatment consists of defibrillation and the administration of vasopressors to restore rhythm and blood pressure. Ensure a patent airway and adequate ventilation. Cardiopulmonary resuscitation may be required.

Dosage and Administration

Flecainide—Up to 400 mg/day.

Encainide—Up to 75 mg q.i.d.

Propafenone—Up to 300 mg every 8 hours.

MORICIZNE (ETHMOZINE)

Mechanism of Action

Moricizine exhibits properties of groups IA, IB, and IC. It blocks sodium influx across myocardial cells during depolarization and shortens phase 2 and 3 repolarization (resulting in a decreased action potential duration and effective refractory period). Moricizine usually does not interact with atrial muscle or affect SA nodal firing rate.

Indications for Use

Treatment of documented life-threatening ventricular arrhythmias such as sustained ventricular tachycardia.

Contraindications

Preexisting second- or third-degree heart block, right bundle branch block associated with left hemiblock unless a pacemaker is present, cardiogenic shock, hypersensitivity to the drug.

Precautions

1. Like other potent sodium channel blockers, moricizine may exacerbate arrhythmias and should be reserved for life-threatening arrhythmias.
2. Electrolyte disturbances such as hypokalemia, hyperkalemia, and hypomagnesemia may alter moricizine's response. Correct electrolyte disturbances before use.
3. Use with extreme caution, if at all. for patients with sick sinus syndrome, because moricizine may precipitate sinus arrest.

Adverse Reactions

Most Common: Palpitations, dizziness, headache, fatigue, nausea.

Most Serious: Hypotension, bradycardia, CHF, sustained ventricular tachycardia, apnea, cardiac death.

Overdosage

Symptoms of overdose include vomiting, lethargy, coma, syncope, hypotension, conduction disturbances, exacerbation of CHF, MI, sinus arrest, and arrhythmias. Treatment includes supportive care, including avoiding aspiration, ensuring a patent airway, and adequate ventilation. Patients should be monitored for cardiac, respiratory, and CNS changes.

Dosage and Administration

200 mg orally every 8 hours (usual range is 600 to 900 mg/day).

Group II Antiarrhythmic Agents

THE β-ADRENOCEPTOR BLOCKING AGENTS

Propranolol, acebutolol, and esmolol are the only β-adrenoceptor blocking agents approved for use as group II antiarrhythmic agents. Atenolol, metoprolol, nadolol, tomolol, pindolol, and bisoprolol are currently being investigated for use as antiarrhythmic agents in treating ventricular and supraventricular arrhythmias. Sotalol has antiarrhythmic properties, which place it in group III (see below, *Group III Antiarrhythmic Agents*). For a complete listing (e.g., contraindications, precautions, adverse reactions, overdosage), see *Antihypertensive Agents* presented later in this chapter.

PROPRANOLOL (INDERAL)
ACEBUTOLOL (SECTRAL)
ESMOLOL (BREVIBLOC)

Mechanism of Action

Specifically, propranolol, acebutolol, and esmolol suppress ectopic pacemaker activity and prolong the effective refractory period of the AV node as well as reduce the rate, force of myocardial contraction, irritability, AV conduction velocity, and automaticity of the SA node. The antiarrhythmic effects of these agents are a direct reflection of their cardiac β-adrenoceptor blocking action and direct membrane stabilizing activity (propranolol and acebutolol only). Propranolol is nonselective in its β-blocking activity, whereas both acebutolol and esmolol are β_1-selective (at higher than normal doses, β_2-adrenoceptors may be blocked).

Indications for Use

Propranolol:

1. Dysrhythmias caused by a hyperactive sympathetic nervous system.
2. Catecholamine- or digitalis-induced supraventricular arrhythmias.
3. Premature ventricular contractions.
4. As an adjunct with digitalis therapy to control chronic A-fib or A-flutter.
5. Myocardial infarction; to reduce cardiovascular mortality and the risk of reinfarction.
6. As a hypotensive agent in the treatment of hypertensive (see *Antihypertensive Agents*) and anginal episodes (see *Antianginal Agents*).

Acebutolol:

1. Premature ventricular contractions.
2. As a hypotensive agent in the treatment of hypertension (see *Antihypertensive Agents*).

Esmolol:

1. Noncompensatory sinus tachycardia.
2. Catecholamine- or digitalis-induced supraventricular arrhythmias.
3. Supraventricular tachycardia—for rapid control of ventricular rate in patients with atrial fibrillation or flutter in perioperative, postoperative, or other emergent situations in which a short-acting agent is desired.

Dosage and Administration

***Propranolol*—Oral:** 10 to 30 mg t.i.d., q.i.d. **IV:** 1 to 3 mg at a rate of 1 mg/min (reserve IV propranolol for life-threatening arrhythmias).

***Acebutolol*—Oral:** usual range is 600 to 1200 mg/day.

***Esmolol*—IV:** Initial loading dose of 500 μg/kg/min for 1 minute, followed immediately by a continuous infusion of 50 μg/kg/min for 4 minutes. Repeat loading dose and increase infusion to 100 μg/kg/min if desired response is not achieved with the usual loading and infusion dose. Maximum continuous infusion rate is 300 μg/kg/min.

Group III Antiarrhythmic Agents

BRETYLIUM (BRETYLOL)

Mechanism of Action

First introduced into clinical practice as an antihypertensive agent, bretylium has antiarrhythmic activity that prolongs the ventricular (but not atrial) action potential duration and effective refractory period. Bretylium markedly raises the ventricular fibrillation threshold, thereby abolishing ventricular fibrillatory activity. When first administered, bretylium causes the release of norepinephrine from adrenergic nerve terminals, which may result in ventricular tachyarrhythmias, hypertension, or worsening of the preexisting arrhythmia; these conditions must be closely watched for at the onset of therapy. Subsequently, norepinephrine's neuronal release is reduced in response to repetitive nerve stimulation, although norepinephrine's stores are not depleted.

Indications for Use

Bretylium is reserved for emergent life-threatening ventricular arrhythmias (e.g., ventricular tachycardia and fibrillation) unresponsive to first-line drugs such as lidocaine or procainamide. Additionally, use of this drug is restricted to intensive care facilities in which resuscitation equipment and continuous monitoring of cardiac function are immediately available (see Chapter 19).

Contraindications

No absolute contraindications to the use of bretylium exist when there are documented life-threatening ventricular arrhythmias refractory to lidocaine or procainamide.

Precautions

1. Avoid for patients with severe pulmonary hypertension, patients with severe aortic stenosis, or patients exhibiting fixed cardiac output because severe hypotension may occur from a fall in peripheral resistance without a corresponding compensatory increase in cardiac output. Administer a vasopressor agent promptly if severe hypotension occurs.
2. Bretylium may aggravate digitalis toxicity by causing the release of norepinephrine.
3. Coadministration with catecholamines may enhance the pressor effects of these agents. Blood pressure should be monitored closely.

Adverse Reactions

Most Common: Hypotension, postural hypotension, nausea, vomiting, lightheadedness.

Cardiovascular: Transient hypertension and increased frequency of arrhythmias may occur due to the initial release of norepinephrine from adrenergic nerve terminals.

CNS: Vertigo, dizziness, syncope.

Overdosage

Rapidly injecting the drug may lead to marked hypertension. If toxicity develops, administer nitroprusside or another short-acting IV antihypertensive agent. Always have resuscitative equipment available when using bretylium.

Dosage and Administration

IV bolus for acute ventricular fibrillation: 5 mg/kg (undiluted) administered by rapid injection. May repeat at 10 mg/kg as necessary. Maintenance therapy: 5 to 10 mg/kg (diluted solution) infused slowly over 10 minutes every 4 to 6 hours or by a constant infusion of 0.5 to 2 mg/min.

AMIODARONE (CORDARONE)

Mechanism of Action

Amiodarone is a group III antiarrhythmic agent that is a very potent blocker of sodium channels (in the inactivated state), potassium channels, and calcium channels (weak effect). Additionally, amiodarone exhibits noncompetitive α- and β-adrenoceptor blocking properties. Amiodarone's predominant antiarrhythmic effects include prolongation of the myocardial cell-action potential duration and prolongation of the refractory period. Amiodarone relaxes vascular smooth muscle and reduces peripheral vascular resistance. This action is caused by its α and calcium blocking activity in vascular smooth muscle.

Indications for Use

In the USA, amiodarone has been approved for use as an antiarrhythmic agent in the treatment of documented life-threatening arrhythmias such as recurrent ventricular fibrillation and recurrent hemodynamically unstable ventricular tachycardia. Amiodarone's unlabeled uses include treatment of refractory sustained or paroxysmal atrial fibrillation (low dose), symptomatic atrial flutter, and paroxysmal supraventricular tachycardia.

Contraindications

Contraindications to the use of amiodarone include severe SA nodal dysfunction, second- or third-degree heart block, syncope due to bradycardia, and hypersensitivity to the drug.

Precautions

1. Amiodarone is a highly toxic drug that can cause potentially fatal pulmonary toxicity (hypersensitivity pneumonitis, interstitial/alveolar pneumonitis) as well as significant sinus bradycardia, heart block, and adverse ECG changes in susceptible patients.
2. Amiodarone can cause serious exacerbation of the existing arrhythmia.
3. Use cautiously for patients with hepatic abnormalities, thyroid abnormalities, electrolyte disturbances, and coagulation difficulties and for pregnant and nursing mothers.
4. Amiodarone should be discontinued if the following occur: pulmonary infiltrates or fibrosis, paroxysmal ventricular tachycardia, CHF, or symptoms of hepatic failure.
5. Coadministration of amiodarone with calcium channel blockers or beta blockers may potentiate AV block or bradycardia, which may lead to sinus arrest.

Adverse Effects

Most Common: Nausea, vomiting, photosensitivity, fatigue, tremor, incoordination, paresthesias, corneal microdeposits.

Most Serious: Fatal pulmonary toxicity, sinus bradycardia, heart block, liver disease, CHF, ARDS.

Overdosage

Treatment of overdose includes usual supportive measures. Blood pressure and cardiac rhythm should be monitored. Treat hemodynamically unstable hypotension with positive inotropic or vasopressor agents. If bradycardia occurs, treat with β-adrenoceptor agonist or pacemaker.

Dosage and Administration

Amiodarone is available in 200-mg tablets for oral use only.

For life-threatening recurrent ventricular arrhythmias: Initially, administer a loading dose of 800 to 1600 mg/day for 1 to 3 weeks. When the arrhythmia is controlled, reduce dosage to 600 to 800 mg/day for 1 month and then 400 mg/day.

For paroxysmal atrial fibrillation: Initially, 600 to 800 mg/day for 7 to 10 days and then 200 to 400 mg/day.

SOTALOL (BETAPACE)

Mechanism of Action

Sotalol is a unique nonselective β-adrenoceptor blocking agent that also prolongs myocardial cell-action potential duration and effective refractory period. Its major adverse effects are those associated with beta blockade (see *Antihypertensive Agents*) and with prolongation of repolarization, including torsade de pointes.

Indications for Use

Treatment of life-threatening supraventricular and ventricular arrhythmias.

Dosage and Administration

Initially, 80 mg orally b.i.d. Usual dosage range is 160 to 320 mg/day or 4 to 6 mg/kg/day given in two or three divided doses.

Group IV Antiarrhythmic Agents

VERAPAMIL (CALAN, ISOPTIN, VERELAN)
DILTIAZEM (CARDIZEM)

Mechanism of Action

Verapamil and diltiazem are calcium channel blocking agents that inhibit the influx of calcium through slow channels across myocardial cell membranes. By this mechanism, AV conduction is slowed, the effective refractory period of the AV node is prolonged, and myocardial contractility is reduced. These agents also inhibit the entry of calcium into vascular smooth muscle, thereby inducing vascular smooth muscle dilation and lowering the systemic vascular resistance. The major adverse effects of these agents are those associated with other calcium channel blocking agents (see *Antianginal Agents*).

Indications for Use

As antiarrhythmic agents: treatment of supraventricular tachyarrhythmias and control of excessive ventricular rate for patients with atrial flutter or fibrillation. (See *Antianginal Agents* and *Antihypertensive Agents*.)

Dosage and Administration

For control of supraventricular tachyarrhythmias or excessive ventricular rate in association with atrial flutter or fibrillation:

Verapamil—Initially, 5 to 10 mg given by slow IV injection over 2 to 3 minutes. May repeat with 5 to 10 mg 30 minutes after first dose if first dose does not abolish the arrhythmia. *For continuous IV infusion:* 0.4 μg/kg/min. Effective oral doses range from 120 to 600 mg/day given t.i.d. or q.i.d.

Diltiazem—Initially, 0.25 mg/kg given by slow IV injection over 2 to 3 minutes. May administer 0.35 mg/kg if first dose is inadequate in controlling the arrhythmia. *For continuous IV infusion:* administer 5 to 15 mg/hour.

MISCELLANEOUS ANTIARRHYTHMIC AGENTS

DIGITALIS

Digitalis is an antiarrhythmic agent that produces both direct and indirect inotropic effects on the myocardium. Direct effects include increased myocardial contractility, increased refractory time period of the AV node, and increased peripheral resistance. Indirect actions include depression of the SA node and prolonged conduction to the AV node, which is a result of digitalis' parasympathetic (vagal) actions. Digitalis is indicated for use in arrhythmias associated with congestive heart failure, atrial fibrillation (agent of choice to reduce ventricular rates and abolish the pulse deficit), atrial flutter, and paroxysmal atrial tachycardia. (See *Cardiotonic Agents Used in Congestive Heart Failure*.)

ADENOSINE (ADENOCARD)

Mechanism of Action

Adenosine is a nucleoside that is found naturally in all cells of the body. Adenosine acts to inhibit cAMP-induced calcium influx across myocardial cell membranes and enhance potassium conductance. By this mechanism, adenosine directly slows AV nodal conduction velocity and increases the AV nodal refractory period. Adenosine is antagonized competitively by the methylxanthines such as caffeine and theophylline (see Chapter 10, *Xanthine Bronchodilators*).

Indications for Use

Agent of choice for prompt management of paroxysmal supraventricular tachycardia, including that associated with Wolff-Parkinson-White syndrome, owing to its high efficacy and short duration of action.

Contraindications

Contraindications to the use of adenosine include second- or third-degree heart block, sick sinus syndrome (except for patients with a functioning pacemaker), atrial flutter, atrial fibrillation, and ventricular tachycardia.

Precautions

1. Adenosine *may* produce bronchospasm in patients with asthma.
2. Patients may not respond to the usual dose of adenosine if they are concurrently given adenosine receptor blocking agents such as the methylxanthines caffeine or theophylline.
3. Coadministration of carbamazepine or dipyridamole may potentiate the effects of adenosine.

Adverse Reactions

Most Common: Flushing, lightheadedness, vertigo, headache, shortness of breath, chest pain.

Most Serious: Heart block, asystole, arrhythmias.

Overdosage

Because the half-life of adenosine is very short ($<$10 seconds), adverse effects are generally self-limiting.

Dosage and Administration

For rapid IV bolus use only. Initial dose: 6 mg as a rapid IV injection given over 1 to 2 seconds and followed with a rapid saline flush. If first dose is not effective, may repeat within 1 to 2 minutes with a 12-mg rapid IV bolus dose, again followed by a rapid saline flush. May repeat the 12-mg dose once. Doses $>$ 12 mg are not recommended.

ANTIHYPERTENSIVE AGENTS

Sustained hypertension (systolic blood pressure ≥ 140 mmHg and/or diastolic blood pressure ≥ 90 mmHg) damages blood vessels in the major organs (kidney, heart, brain) and can lead to renal failure, left ventricular hypertrophy, congestive heart failure, and stroke. A small percentage (approximately 15%) of patients with hypertension have an established cause for it. Most patients with hypertension have what is known as essential hypertension, a term used to describe hypertension that has no specific cause. A classification scheme for hypertension has been established that delineates hypertension into stages:

Systolic (mmHg)	Diastolic (mmHg)	Category
<130	<85	Normal blood pressure (BP)
130–139	85–89	High normal BP
140–159	90–99	Stage I (mild hypertension)
160–179	100–109	Stage II (moderate hypertension)
180–209	110–119	Stage III (severe hypertension)
≥210	≥120	Stage IV (very severe hypertension

The first approach in treating hypertension consists of lifestyle modifications such as weight reduction, sodium and alcohol restriction, smoking cessation, regular exercise, and a diet low in saturated fats. If the patient remains hypertensive 3 to 6 months after the initiation of lifestyle modifications, antihypertensive therapy is started. Pharmacologic intervention with antihypertensive agents has been shown to significantly reduce or prevent damage to blood vessels and to decrease cardiovascular mortality and morbidity in patients with hypertension. The vast array of agents used in hypertension are classified according to their primary site of action and include the following:

- Centrally Acting α_2-Adrenoceptor Agonists
- Peripherally Acting α_1-Adrenoceptor Blocking Agents
- β-Adrenoceptor Blocking Agents
- α/β-Adrenoceptor Blocking Agents
- Angiotension Converting Enzyme (ACE) Inhibitors
- Calcium Channel Blocking Agents
- Diuretics
- Vasodilators
- Agents For Pheochromocytoma
- Agents For Hypertensive Emergencies
- Miscellaneous Antihypertensive Agents

The initial pharmacologic selection of an antihypertensive agent usually begins with a diuretic agent or a β-adrenoceptor blocking agent. For Stage I and

Stage II hypertension, monotherapy with one of these agents is preferred. If the diuretic or β-adrenoceptor blocking agent is ineffective or not tolerated, a calcium channel blocking agent, ACE inhibitor, α_1-adrenoceptor blocker, or an α/β-adrenoceptor blocking agent is used. If there is still an inadequate response from the antihypertensive agent selected, its dosage may be increased, another drug may be substituted, or a second antihypertensive agent may be added to the drug regimen. Coadministration of three different types of antihypertensive agents may be required in some cases.

CENTRALLY ACTING α_2-ADRENOCEPTOR AGONISTS

Mechanism of Action

As described in Chapter 2, activation of central α_2-adrenoceptors blocks the interneuronal release of norepinephrine. This mechanism inhibits sympathetic outflow from the vasopressor centers in the brain stem (specifically, the medulla) resulting in a decreased peripheral resistance, renal vascular resistance, heart rate, and blood pressure (see Fig. 2.10). A transient rise in blood pressure may be initially noted owing to the activation of α_1-adrenoceptors in arterioles. Because these drugs bind more tightly to α_2 rather than α_1-adrenoceptors, the initial hypertension is followed by more prolonged hypotension. Currently, there are four centrally acting α_2-adrenoceptor agonists: clonidine, guanabenz, guanfacine, and methyldopa.

Indications for Use

Treatment of mild to moderate degrees of hypertension given alone or in combination with other antihypertensive agents. Methyldopa is commonly coadministered with other antihypertensive agents to control sustained moderate to moderately severe hypertension. Methyldopa has also been used in controlling acute hypertensive crises; however, owing to its slow onset of action, other agents are preferred for rapid reduction of blood pressure. Unlabeled uses for clonidine include prophylaxis of migraine, management of opiate detoxification, treatment of episodes of menopausal flushing, and treatment of Gilles de la Tourette disease.

Contraindications

Contraindications to the use of centrally acting α_2-adrenoceptors include hypersensitivity to any component of the drug and active hepatic disease (methyldopa).

Precautions

1. A positive Coombs test, hemolytic anemia, and liver disorders may occur with methyldopa therapy, which could lead to fatal complications unless properly recognized and treated.

2. Paradoxical pressor response or rebound hypertension has been noted with the use of these agents.
3. Use with caution for patients with severe coronary insufficiency, recent myocardial infarction, cerebrovascular disease, and severe hepatic or renal failure.
4. Some of these agents cause sedation or drowsiness (e.g., guanabenz, guanfacine, methyldopa).

Adverse Reactions

(Not all reactions are noted with all drugs).

Most Common: Dry mouth, drowsiness, sedation, constipation, dizziness, headache, fatigue.

CNS: Nervousness, insomnia, anxiety, depression, nightmares.

Cardiovascular: Palpitations, flushing, congestive heart failure (rare occurrence), Raynaud's syndrome.

GI: Anorexia, nausea, vomiting, parotid pain, liver function abnormalities.

Dermatologic: Skin rash, angioedema, urticaria, hives, hair loss, pruritus.

Other: Hyperglycemia, urinary retention, weight gain, impotence, pallor, nasal mucosal drying.

Overdosage

Management of overdose consists of careful attention to cardiac rate, cardiac output, blood volume, electrolyte balance, urinary function, and cerebral activity. Sympathomimetic drugs (e.g., norepinephrine, epinephrine) may be required in severe cases to restore cardiac output and blood pressure.

Dosage and Administration

Clonidine (Catapres)—Initially, 0.1 mg orally b.i.d. Usual oral dose is 0.2 to 0.8 mg/day. Maximum dose is 2.4 mg/day. **Transdermal patch:** apply one patch to hairless body part once every 7 days. Release rates range from 0.1 mg per 24 hours to 0.3 mg per 24 hours. Unlabeled route of administration: 0.2 to 0.4 mg/day sublingual.

Guanabenz (Wytensin)—Initially, 4 mg b.i.d. Maximum dose is 32 mg/day in two divided doses.

Guanfacine (Tenex)—Initially, 1 mg daily at bedtime. May increase up to 3 mg/day if necessary.

Methyldopa (Aldomet, Amodopa)—Initially, 250 mg orally b.i.d., t.i.d. Usual maintenance dosage is 500 to 2000 mg/day in two to four divided doses. Maximum dose is 3 g/day. **IV infusion:** 250 to 500 mg given at 6-hour intervals. Maximum dosage is 1 g every 6 hours.

PERIPHERALLY ACTING α_1-ADRENOCEPTOR BLOCKING AGENTS

Mechanism of Action

Peripherally acting α_1-adrenoceptor blocking agents selectively block postsynaptic α_1-adrenoceptors of both arterioles (resistance vessels) and veins (capacitance vessels), thus inducing vasodilation leading to a reduction in blood pressure (see also Chapter 2). As can be expected by dilating both resistance and capacitance vessels, blood pressure is reduced more in the upright position than in the supine position. This effect is most pronounced on the diastolic blood pressure. Peripherally acting α_1-adrenoceptor blocking agents are more effective when used in combination with other agents (such as propranolol and a diuretic) than when used alone. Salt and water retention occurs with the use of these agents; therefore, coadministration of a diuretic is recommended. Peripherally acting α_1-adrenoceptor blocking agents include prazosin, terazosin, and doxazosin.

Indications for Use

Treatment of mild to moderate hypertension, preferably in conjunction with a diuretic or other antihypertensive agent. As adjunctive therapy in the treatment of severe, refractory congestive heart failure.

Contraindications

Hypersensitivity to any component of the drug.

Precautions

1. First-dose effect: These agents may cause marked hypotension and syncope with potential loss of consciousness with the first few doses. The first-dose effect may be minimized by limiting the initial dose and then gradually increasing the dose to the normal effective range.
2. Use doxazosin with caution for patients with impaired hepatic function.
3. Coadministration of these agents with beta blockers may potentiate the acute postural hypotensive reaction.

Adverse Reactions

Most Common: Nausea, headache, malaise, drowsiness, dizziness, weakness, palpitations, nasal congestion.

CNS: Vertigo, depression, nervousness, paresthesias.

Cardiovascular: Orthostatic hypotension, angina, syncope, edema, tachycardia.

Other: Skin rash, pruritus, urinary frequency or incontinence, impotence, blurred vision, tinnitus, dry mouth, epistaxis, diaphoresis, leukopenia, arthralgia.

Overdosage

Treatment includes the administration of vasopressors to restore the blood pressure. Patient should be kept supine. Renal function should be monitored and supported.

Dosage and Administration

Caution: do not exceed the initial dose owing to the first-dose effect (see above).

Prazosin (Minipress)—Initially, 1 mg b.i.d., t.i.d. Usual maintenance range is 6 to 15 mg/day in two or three divided doses.

Terazosin (Hytrin)—Initially, 1 mg at bedtime. Usual dosage range is 1 to 5 mg/day. Maximum dose is 20 mg/day.

Doxazosin (Cardura)—Initially, 1 mg daily. Monitor blood pressure between 2 and 6 hours after the first dose (and after each increase in dose) as postural hypotensive effects are more likely to occur in this time period. May titrate to achieve desired effect (up to 16 mg/day).

β-ADRENOCEPTOR BLOCKING AGENTS

Mechanism of Action

Most of the β-adrenoceptor blocking agents have therapeutic efficacy as antihypertensive agents. Initially, these agents cause a reduction in blood pressure primarily as a result of a decrease in cardiac output that occurs when the heart rate decreases. This mechanism is caused by the blockade at myocardial β_1-adrenoceptors. Eventually, the cardiac output returns to a normal level while the blood pressure remains low owing to the decrease in peripheral vascular resistance induced by these agents. These agents also inhibit the renin-angiotension-aldosterone system (see Chapter 17), which also leads to a reduction in blood pressure. Propranolol, nadolol, timolol, penbutolol, carteolol, and pindolol inhibit both the β_1- and β_2-adrenoceptors, whereas metoprolol, acebutolol, bisoprolol, betaxolol, and atenolol are cardioselective and preferentially block the myocardial β_1-adrenoceptors.

Indications for Use

Treatment of mild to moderate hypertension. Used alone as a Step I agent or in combination with other drugs, especially a thiazide diuretic. These agents are not indicated for treatment of hypertensive emergencies. For other indications, see *Antianginal Agents* and *Antiarrhythmic Agents.*

Contraindications

Contraindications to the use of β-adrenergic blocking agents include hypersensitivity to the agents, overt cardiac failure, sinus bradycardia, cardiogenic shock, greater than first-degree heart block, and CHF unless accompanied with a tachyarrhythmia treatable with blockers. Contraindications to nonselective β blockers include severe chronic obstructive pulmonary disease (COPD), asthma, and bronchospasm.

Precautions

1. Use with caution for patients with impaired renal or hepatic function.
2. The effects of succinylcholine and tubocurarine may be enhanced by β-adrenoceptor blockers.
3. Use with caution for patients with cardiac failure; use of β_1-adrenoceptor blockers depresses myocardial contractility and may potentiate more severe cardiac failure.
4. Use with caution for patients with hyperreactive airway disease; use of β-adrenoceptor blockers may cause or aggravate bronchospasm.

Adverse Reactions

Not all reactions are seen with all drugs.

Most Common: Drowsiness, lightheadedness, lethargy, nausea, cramping, bradycardia, paresthesias.

CNS: Dizziness, fatigue, vertigo, mental depression, anxiety, nervousness, behavioral changes.

Cardiovascular: Bradycardia, chest pain, angina, edema, hypotension, tachycardia, arrhythmias, palpitations, syncope, first- and third-degree heart block.

Pulmonary: Bronchospasm, dyspnea, cough, wheezes, rales, rhinitis, pharyngitis, bronchial obstruction.

GI: Nausea, vomiting, anorexia, abdominal cramping, acute pancreatitis.

Overdosage

Treatment of overdose consists of monitoring the blood pressure and ECG. Respiratory support should be implemented if indicated. PVCs should be treated with lidocaine, hypotensive bradycardia should be treated with atropine, and bronchospasm should be treated with a β_2-adrenoceptor agonist or theophylline derivative.

Dosage and Administration

Antihypertensive doses:

Acebutolol (Sectral)—Initially, 400 mg once daily or twice daily. Usual dosage range is 400 to 800 mg/day. Maximum dose is 1220 mg/day.

Atenolol (Ternormin)—Initially, 50 mg once/day. May increase to 100 mg/day to achieve desired clinical response.
Betaxolol (Kerlone)—Initially, 10 mg once/day. May increase to 40 mg once daily.
Bisoprolol (Zebeta)—Initially, 2.5 to 5 mg/day. May increase to a maximum of 20 mg/day if necessary.
Carteolol (Cartrol)—Initially, 2.5 mg/day. Usual dosage range is 2.5 to 5 mg/day. Maximum dose is 10 mg/day.
Metoprolol (Lopressor)—Initially, 100 mg/day. Usual maintenance dosage is 100 to 450 mg/day.
Nadolol (Corgard)—Initially, 40 mg/day. Usual maintenance dosage range is 80 to 320 mg/day.
Penbutolol (Levatol)—Initially, 20 mg/day. May increase to 40 to 80 mg/day if necessary.
Pindolol (Visken)—Initially, 5 mg b.i.d. Maximum dose is 60 mg/day.
Propranolol (Inderal)—Initially 40 mg b.i.d. or 80 mg (sustained-release formulation) once daily. Usual dosage range is 120 to 240 mg/day. Maximum dose is 640 mg/day.
Timolol (Blocadren)—Initially, 10 mg b.i.d. Usual maintenance range is 20 to 40 mg/day. Maximum dose is 60 mg/day.

α/β-ADRENOCEPTOR BLOCKING AGENTS

LABETALOL (NORMODYNE, TRANDATE)

Mechanism of Action

Labetalol is a nonselective β-adrenoceptor blocking agent that also exhibits postsynaptic α_1-adrenoceptor blocking action (3:1 ratio of β:α). The blood pressure is effectively reduced, standing pressure more than supine pressure. Minimal changes are noted in heart rate and cardiac output.

Indications for Use

Owing to labetalol's combined α and β effects, it is useful for treating hypertensive emergencies and hypertension associated with pheochromocytoma (tumor of chromaffin tissue of the adrenal medulla; the symptoms of hypertension reflect the increased production and release of epinephrine and norepinephrine).

Contraindications

Contraindications to the use of labetalol include severe COPD, asthma, bronchospasm, hypersensitivity to the drug, severe bradycardia, second- or third-degree heart block, cardiac failure, and cardiogenic shock.

Precautions

Precautions to the use of labetalol are the same as those that apply to α- and β-adrenoceptor blocking agents.

Adverse Reactions

Adverse reactions to the use of labetalol are the same as those that apply to α- and β-adrenoceptor blocking agents.

Overdosage

Treatment of labetalol overdose is the same as that which applies to α- and β-adrenoceptor blocking agents.

Dosage and Administration

Oral dose ranges from 100 to 400 mg b.i.d. Patients with severe hypertension may require up to 2.4 g/day. For the treatment of hypertensive emergencies: repeated (until desired blood pressure is achieved) IV bolus injections ranging from 20 to 80 mg. Full effect is usually noted 5 minutes after the injections.

ANGIOTENSION CONVERTING ENZYME INHIBITORS

Mechanism of Action

Renin is released from the kidneys' juxtaglomerular cells in response to reduced renal perfusion, hypotension, hyponatremia, hypovolemia, and sympathetic (β-adrenoceptor) stimulation. Released renin acts on a plasma globulin substrate to form angiotension I. Angiotension converting enzyme (ACE) (located primarily in the lungs) interacts with angiotension I to form angiotension II, a potent endogenous vasoconstrictor. Angiotension II elevates the arterial blood pressure by inducing intense peripheral vasoconstriction as well as by stimulating the secretion of aldosterone, a potent sodium-retaining substance.

ACE inhibitors block the production of angiotension II by interfering with the actions of the angiotension converting enzyme. By this mechanism, ACE inhibitors promote a reduction in peripheral vascular resistance leading to a fall in arterial blood pressure. Additionally, inhibition of the angiotension converting enzyme seems to cause a decrease in the inactivation of bradykinin, a potent vasodilator substance. This action may also contribute to the hypotensive effect of ACE inhibitors.

For patients with CHF, ACE inhibitors reduce systemic vascular resistance, which leads to a reduction in afterload and, therefore, pulmonary artery occluding pressure, which correspondingly enhances the cardiac output.

Indications for Use

1. Treatment of all stages of hypertension, administered singly or in combination with other antihypertensive agents, especially thiazide-type diuretics. Blood pressure effects of ACE inhibitors in conjunction with a thiazide diuretic are approximately additive.
2. Treatment of CHF, usually in combination with diuretics and digitalis.
3. Captopril and enalapril: to improve survival after MI in clinically stable patients with left ventricular dysfunction (LVD).
4. Captopril: investigational uses: management of hypertensive crises, rheumatoid arthritis, diagnosis of renal artery stenosis, hypertension related to scleroderma renal crises, diagnosis of primary aldosteronism, idiopathic edema, Raynaud's syndrome.
5. Enalapril: investigational use: diabetic neuropathy.

Contraindications

Contraindications to the use of ACE inhibitors include hypersensitivity to any component and history of angioedema with previous reaction to ACE inhibitors.

Precautions

1. First-dose effect: ACE inhibitors may cause a significant drop in blood pressure after the first dose. The first-dose effect can be minimized by discontinuing the diuretic (if being administered) or increasing salt intake approximately 1 week before the initiation of ACE inhibitor therapy.
2. Cautious use is recommended for patients with severe renal dysfunction, reduced white cell counts, valvular stenosis, systemic lupus-like symptoms, and diabetes mellitus and for pregnant and nursing mothers.
3. ACE inhibitors have been shown to increase the incidence of fetal and neonatal morbidity and death when administered during pregnancy, particularly during the second and third trimesters.

Adverse Reactions

Not all of the listed adverse reactions have been noted with all drugs of this category.

Most Common: Skin rash, pruritus, dizziness, fatigue, headache, chronic nonproductive cough, abdominal distress, lack of taste sensation.
CNS: Headache, insomnia, malaise, memory disturbance, tremor.
Cardiovascular: Palpitations, chest pain, flushing, hypotension, tachycardia, MI (rare occurrence).
GI: Nausea, vomiting, gastric distress, abdominal pain, diarrhea, peptic ulcer.

Hematologic: Neutropenia, agranulocytosis, eosinophilia, hemolytic anemia.
Renal: Polyuria, oliguria, urinary frequency, proteinuria, renal insufficiency.
Miscellaneous: Dry mouth, laryngeal edema, lymphadenopathy, dyspnea, Raynaud's syndrome, elevated liver enzymes.

Overdosage

Hypotension is the most common overdose symptom. Treatment includes supportive care and the administration of volume expanders (preferred) or vasopressor agents to restore the blood pressure.

Dosage and Administration

Benazepril (Lotensin)—Initially, 10 mg/day as a single dose. Usual dosage range is 20–40 mg/day given as a single dose or divided dose.
Captopril (Capoten)—Dosage ranges from 12.5 to 25 mg given b.i.d. or t.i.d. for mild hypertension to 50 to 150 mg b.i.d. or t.i.d. for moderate to severe hypertension. *For congestive heart failure:* Initially, 25 to 50 mg t.i.d. Usual maintenance dosage ranges between 50 and 100 mg given t.i.d.
Enalapril (Vasotec)—Initially, 5 mg orally once daily. Usual oral dosage range is 10 to 40 mg/day. **IV:** 1.25 mg every 6 hours given by slow IV injection (over 5 minutes). *For patients concurrently receiving diuretics:* 0.625 mg given by IV injection over 5 minutes. *For congestive heart failure:* Initially, 2.5 mg once or twice daily. Usual maintenance dosage ranges between 5 and 20 mg/day given in two divided doses.
Fosinopril (Monopril)—Initially, 10 mg/day as a single dose. Usual dosage range is 20–40 mg/day given as a single dose or divided dose.
Lisinopril (Prinivil, Zestril)—Initially, 10 mg once daily. Usual dosage range is 20 to 40 mg/day. *For congestive heart failure:* 5 to 20 mg/day as a single dose.
Quinapril (Accupril)—Initially, 10 mg/day as a single dose. Usual dosage range is 20 to 80 mg/day as a single dose or divided dose.
Ramipril (Altace)—Initially, 1.25 to 2.5 mg/day as a single dose. Usual dosage range is 2.5 to 20 mg/day as a single dose or divided dose.

CALCIUM CHANNEL BLOCKING AGENTS

Mechanism of Action

The antihypertensive effects of calcium channel blocking agents are brought about by their ability to inhibit the influx of calcium into arterial smooth muscle cells. The corresponding dilation of peripheral arterioles leads to a reduction in blood pressure. Some of these agents (e.g., verapamil) also inhibit stimulation of α-adrenoceptors in the peripheral vascular system, resulting in peripheral vasodilation, which adds to the antihypertensive effect.

Indications for Use

Treatment of mild to moderate essential hypertension: amlodipine, diltiazem, felodipine, isradipine, nicardipine, nifedipine, verapamil. Sustained-release verapamil and diltiazem are indicated only for essential hypertension. Investigational use of nifedipine includes the emergency treatment of severe hypertension. For other indications, see *Antianginal Agents* and *Antiarrhythmic Agents*.

Dosage and Administration

The antihypertensive dosages of these agents are the same as the antianginal dosages (see *Antianginal Agents*).

DIURETIC AGENTS

Mechanism of Action

Diuretics are drugs that enhance the excretion of sodium (and water), which then leads to a loss in vascular volume. The corresponding decrease in vascular volume results in a drop in arterial blood pressure. The thiazide diuretics, such as chlorothiazide (Diuril), are preferred for most patients with mild or moderate hypertension. Loop diuretics, such as furosemide (Lasix), are also used occasionally in treating essential hypertension. The potassium-sparing diuretics, such as spironolactone (Aldactone), are administered in combination with the primary diuretic to prevent the depletion of potassium stores. The sites of action within the kidney and the pharmacokinetics of the various diuretic agents are discussed in Chapter 17.

VASODILATORS

This class of antihypertensive agents include the calcium channel blocking agents (previously discussed); the parenteral vasodilators, nitroprusside and diazoxide (see *Agents for Hypertensive Emergencies*); the nitrate, nitroglycerin (see *Antianginal Agents*); and the oral vasodilators, hydralazine and minoxidil. Hydralazine and minoxidil are presented in this section.

Mechanism of Action

Both hydralazine and minoxidil exhibit a peripheral vasodilating effect through a direct relaxation of arteriolar vascular smooth muscle. Hydralazine alters calcium metabolism (thereby interfering with calcium movement within the vascular smooth muscle), whereas minoxidil blocks calcium uptake in arteriolar smooth muscle cells. The peripheral vasodilating effect of these agents results in decreased arterial blood pressure (diastolic more than systolic), decreased peripheral vascular resistance, and an increased heart rate, stroke volume, and cardiac output. These agents have little effect on venous tone; thus, postural hypotension is minimized. Topical application of minoxidil (as Rogaine) seems to enhance hair growth in balding areas; however, the effect lasts only as long as the drug is applied.

Indications for Use

Hydralazine: Oral: for essential hypertension, alone or in combination with other agents. Parenteral: for severe essential hypertension when it is not feasible to administer the oral formulation or when there is a need to rapidly lower the blood pressure. Investigational uses: treatment of hypertensive emergencies, as an adjunct in reducing afterload for patients with CHF and aortic insufficiency and after valve replacement.

Minoxidil: Oral only: for treatment of symptomatic severe hypertension associated with target organ damage and that which is not manageable with maximum therapeutic doses of a diuretic plus two other antihypertensive agents (see *Precautions*).

Contraindications

Contraindications to the use of vasodilators include hypersensitivity to any component of the drug, coronary artery disease, mitral valvular rheumatic heart disease (hydralazine), acute myocardial infarction, and pheochromocytoma (minoxidil).

Precautions

1. Hydralazine may provoke systemic lupus-like symptoms (arthralgia, dermatoses, fever, splenomegaly). Symptoms usually regress after discontinuance of the drug.
2. Use with caution for patients with advanced renal damage.
3. Minoxidil may cause pericardial effusion, occasionally progressing to cardiac tamponade, and it can worsen angina pectoris. Therefore, this agent should be reserved for hypertension refractory to other, safer antihypertensive agents.
4. Rapid changes in blood pressure may precipitate syncope and loss of consciousness.

Adverse Reactions

Most Common: Hydralazine: Headache, nausea, vomiting, diarrhea, sweating, palpitations, tachycardia. Minoxidil: Sweating, headache, temporary edema, hypertrichosis (excessive hair growth).

Most Serious: Hydralazine: Eosinophilia, hepatitis (rare occurrence), paralytic ileus, blood dyscrasias, lupus-like syndrome. Minoxidil: Stevens-Johnson syndrome, pericardial effusion and tamponade, rebound hypotension, reflex tachycardia, temporary decreases in hematocrit, hemoglobin, and erythrocytes.

Overdosage

The most serious symptom of overdosage is exaggerated hypotension. Provide supportive care and administer IV saline to restore blood pressure.

Dosage and Administration

Hydralazine (Alazine, Apresoline)—**Oral:** Initially, 10 mg q.i.d. May increase up to 50 mg q.i.d. if necessary. For resistant patients, 300 mg/day may be required. **IM, IV:** Initially, 5 to 10 mg. Usual dosage range is 20 to 40 mg, repeated as necessary.

Minoxidil (Loniten)—**Oral only:** Initially, 5 mg/day as a single dose. Usual range is 10 to 40 mg/day, up to a maximum of 100 mg/day.

AGENTS FOR PHEOCHROMOCYTOMA

Mechanism of Action

Pheochromocytoma is a chromaffin cell tumor of the sympathoadrenal system that causes the excessive release of the catecholamines norepinephrine and epinephrine. Paradoxical hypertension, pounding headaches, sweating, apprehension, anxiety, palpitations, flushing of the face, nausea, and vomiting are features of this condition. Currently, three antihypertensive agents have shown therapeutic efficacy in treating the hypertension that accompanies pheochromocytoma: phentolamine, phenoxybenzamine, and metyrosine.

Phentolamine and phenoxybenzamine are nonselective α-adrenoceptor blocking agents, whereas metyrosine inhibits tyrosine hydroxylase, the enzyme necessary for the production of 3,4-dihydroxyphenylalanine (DOPA). Because tyrosine is necessary for the eventual biosynthesis of norepinephrine (tyrosine → DOPA → dopamine → norepinephrine), there is a significant depletion of norepinephrine stores.

Indications for Use

Indications for the use of phentolamine and phenoxybenzamine include prevention and control of hypertensive episodes associated with the drug. An investigational use of phentolamine includes the treatment of hypertensive crises occurring secondary to the use of MAO inhibitors.

Contraindications

Contraindications to the use of phentolamine and phenoxybenzamine include hypersensitivity to the drug. Contraindications to phentolamine include myocardial infarction, coronary insufficiency, and angina.

Precautions

1. Tachycardia and arrhythmias may occur with the use of phentolamine.
2. Administer phenoxybenzamine with caution for patients with marked cerebral or coronary arteriosclerosis or renal damage.
3. Use metyrosine with caution for patients with impaired hepatic or renal function.

Adverse Reactions

Phentolamine: Weakness, dizziness, vertigo, flushing, orthostatic hypotension, nasal congestion, nausea, vomiting, diarrhea, tachycardia, cardiac arrhythmias.

Phenoxybenzamine: Orthostatic hypotension, hypotension, miosis, tachycardia, nasal congestion, GI irritation, drowsiness, fatigue.

Metyrosine: Sedation (most common effect), extrapyramidal symptoms (drooling, tremor, slurred speech), diarrhea (may be severe), anxiety and psychic disturbances.

Overdosage

As with all antihypertensive agents, overdose symptoms include marked hypotension. Treatment includes supportive measures and restoration of the blood pressure with volume expanders or IV infusion of vasopressor agents such as epinephrine.

Dosage and Administration

Phentolamine (Regitine)—**Parenteral:** 5 mg, repeat if necessary.

Phenoxybenzamine (Dibenzyline)—**Oral:** Initially, 10 mg b.i.d. The usual dosage range is 20 to 40 mg b.i.d. or t.i.d.

Metyrosine (Demser)—**Oral:** Initially, 250 mg q.i.d. Maximum dosage is 4 g/day given in divided doses.

AGENTS FOR HYPERTENSIVE EMERGENCIES

Hypertensive emergencies are precipitated by a marked or sudden elevation of arterial blood pressure. A hypertensive emergency is a serious threat to life and can occur in such situations as significant hypertension associated with vascular damage (termed malignant hypertension), and hypertension associated with an unstable hemodynamic status such as occurs in cardiac failure, stroke, or dissecting aneurysm. Stupor, coma, and even death may ensue if hypertension is not immediately corrected. Currently, there are three rapidly acting parenteral antihypertensive agents that have demonstrated efficacy in the treatment of hypertensive emergencies: diazoxide, nitroprusside, and trimethaphan. Other parenteral drugs that may be effective include nitroglycerin, captopril, enalapril, hydralazine, labetalol, nicardipine, nifedipine, and phentolamine.

DIAZOXIDE (HYPERSTAT)

Mechanism of Action

Diazoxide is a relatively effective and long-acting antihypertensive agent that has direct-acting vasodilator activity. Diazoxide relaxes peripheral arteriole smooth muscle and reduces blood pressure by opening potassium channels and stabilizing the membrane potential at the resting level. This action causes a reflex increase in heart rate and cardiac output as the blood pressure is reduced. Also, an increase in renal blood flow is noted, after an initial decrease.

Indications for Use

1. Hypertensive emergencies.
2. For patients with hypertensive encephalopathy, malignant hypertension (especially those associated with renal impairment), and when an urgent decrease of diastolic pressure is indicated.

Contraindications

Contraindications to the use of diazoxide include hypersensitivity to the drug and compensatory hypertension.

Precautions

1. Because a rapid reduction in blood pressure is noted, patients must be monitored for ECG changes. Large doses have been associated with angina, myocardial infarction, and cerebral infarction.
2. Repeated use may cause edema, CHF, or electrolyte imbalance (diazoxide causes sodium retention).
3. Diazoxide may cause hypotension; frequent monitoring of the blood pressure is necessary.
4. Coadministered furosemide may be used to prevent sodium and water retention. Furosemide may also enhance the antihypertensive effect of diazoxide.

Adverse Reactions

The most common adverse reactions are hypotension, nausea and vomiting, dizziness, weakness, and sodium and water retention. Larger doses (300 mg) have caused severe hypotension, angina, cerebral ischemia, hemiplegia, and MI.

Overdosage

To treat hypotension, place patient in the Trendelenburg position. If indicated, dopamine or epinephrine may be given to correct hypotension. Hemodialysis may be employed to remove diazoxide from the blood.

Dosage and Administration

IV route only: 1 to 3 mg/kg up to a maximum of 150 mg in a single dose. May be repeated in 5- to 15-minute intervals. Caution: do not give more than 10 days or by IV infusion.

NITROPRUSSIDE SODIUM (NIPRIDE, NITROPRESS)

Mechanism of Action

Nitroprusside is a potent direct-acting hypotensive agent that produces peripheral vasodilation of both arterial and venous vessels. This action is a result of nitroprusside's ability to stimulate guanyl cyclase, either via the release of nitric oxide (NO) in vascular smooth muscle or by direct stimulation of the enzyme. The ultimate effect is the corresponding increase in intracellular cGMP, which relaxes vascular smooth muscle.

For hypertensive or normotensive patients, nitroprusside causes a reduction in the arterial blood pressure, a slight increase in the heart rate, a mild decrease in cardiac output, and a reduction in total peripheral vascular resistance. For patients with left ventricular failure, nitroprusside causes an increase in cardiac output and a reduction in the pulmonary artery wedge pressure (PAWP), in addition to its effect to cause a reduction in blood pressure. Nitroprusside has an immediate onset of action—a reduced blood pressure is noted within 30 to 60 seconds.

Indications for Use

1. Hypertensive emergencies.
2. For controlled hypotension during anesthesia.
3. Severe, refractory, chronic congestive heart failure.
4. Hypertensive and normotensive patients with severe, persistent pump failure associated with a low cardiac output and increased peripheral vascular resistance.

Contraindications

Contraindications to the use of nitroprusside sodium include treatment of compensatory hypertension (e.g., AV shunt or coarctation of the aorta). Not indicated for use to produce or control hypotension for surgery patients with known inadequate cerebral circulation.

Precautions

1. Excessive doses of nitroprusside may cause cyanide toxicity. Nitroprusside is rapidly metabolized to cyanide and thiocyanate by a reaction with hemoglobin. Because metabolic acidosis is the earliest sign of cyanide toxicity, blood pH and acid-base status should be monitored frequently.
2. Use with caution for patients with hepatic and renal insufficiency.
3. Severe hypotensive effects may occur with concurrent use of other antihypertensive agents.
4. Nitroprusside may increase both myocardial and pulmonary arteriovenous shunts because of nitroprusside's action on coronary resistance vessels. Increases in total coronary blood flow are noted, but not necessarily that portion contributing to improved perfusion.
5. Discontinue administration if blood pressure is not reduced in 10 minutes with a dose of 10 mg/kg/min.
6. Like other vasodilators, nitroprusside can cause increases in intracranial pressure by way of dilation of cerebral blood vessels. Use with extreme caution for patients who already have an elevated intracranial pressure.

Adverse Reactions

Most Common Effects (caused by a too-rapid reduction in blood pressure): Nausea, retching, apprehension, palpitations, dizziness, abdominal pain, diaphoresis.

Pulmonary: May worsen the ventilation-perfusion mismatch and produce hypoxemia caused by nitroprusside-induced hypotension.

Other: Thiocyanate accumulation (especially noted for patients with renal impairment) may lead to blurred vision, tinnitus, dyspnea, ataxia, diminished reflexes, delirium, convulsions, mydriasis. Also, hypothyroidism, methemoglobinemia.

Overdosage

Discontinue infusion if profound hypotension or cyanide toxicity occurs. Symptoms of cyanide toxicity include blurred vision, headache, ataxia, dyspnea, delirium, loss of consciousness, absence of reflexes, hypotension, metabolic acidosis. Treatment consists of the administration of amyl nitrite, sodium nitrite, sodium thiosulfate. Patient should be observed for several hours for the possible reemergence of the signs of overdosage.

Dosage and Administration

Continuous IV infusion with sterile 5% dextrose in water: 3 μg/kg/min (range 0.5 to 10 μg/kg/min).

TRIMETHAPHAN (ARFONAD)

Mechanism of Action

Trimethaphan is a short-acting ganglionic blocking agent used for its ability to rapidly lower the blood pressure. Ganglionic blocking agents block transmission in autonomic (both sympathetic and parasympathetic) ganglia. Trimethaphan also exerts a direct peripheral vasodilator effect. Pooling of blood in the capacitance vessels occurs, thus reducing the amount of blood returning to the heart and resulting in a drop in the arterial blood pressure. Trimethaphan also causes the release of histamine.

Indications for Use

1. Hypertensive emergencies.
2. For controlled hypotension during neurosurgery.
3. In the emergency treatment of pulmonary edema for patients with pulmonary hypertension associated with systemic hypertension.

Contraindications

Contraindications to the use of trimethaphan include hypersensitivity to the drug, uncorrected anemia, hypovolemia, shock states, and uncorrected respiratory insufficiency.

Precautions

1. Use with caution for elderly individuals and debilitated patients.
2. Use with caution for allergic individuals, such as patients with asthma, owing to the release of histamine.
3. Excessive doses may result in respiratory arrest.
4. Trimethaphan may potentiate the effects of neuromuscular blocking agents.

Adverse Reactions

Significant adverse reactions are caused by overdose and may cause excessive hypotension, tachycardia, cyanosis, angina, vascular collapse, and respiratory arrest.

Overdosage

Treatment consists of the administration of vasopressors to restore blood pressure.

Dosage and Administration

Only by IV infusion: 500 mg (10 ml) diluted to 500 ml in 5% dextrose. IV drip may range between 0.3 and 6 ml/min.

MISCELLANEOUS ANTIHYPERTENSIVE AGENTS

MECAMYLAMINE (INVERSINE)

Mecamylamine is a potent, oral ganglionic blocking agent indicated for use in moderately severe to severe essential hypertension and uncomplicated malignant hypertension untreatable by other drugs. Mecamylamine is not commonly the agent of choice in treating hypertension because it readily penetrates the CNS and may produce tremors, mental aberrations, and convulsions. Other significant adverse effects include interstitial pulmonary edema, fibrosis, syncope, and postural hypotension. Administration and dosage: Initially, 2.5 mg b.i.d. Usual dose is 25 mg/day in two to four divided doses.

TOLAZOLINE (PRISCOLINE)

Tolazoline is a competitive α-adrenoceptor blocking agent primarily indicated for persistent pulmonary hypertension of the newborn (persistent fetal circulation) when systemic arterial oxygenation cannot be adequately maintained by usual supportive care (supplemental oxygen therapy and mechanical ventilation). Tolazoline decreases peripheral vascular resistance and increases venous capacitance, thereby resulting in reduced arterial blood pressure. It has both sympathomimetic and parasympathomimetic actions that cause cardiostimulation and GI tract stimulation, respectively. Tolazoline also exhibits histamine-like effects. Tolazoline's adverse reactions include hypotension, tachycardia, cardiac arrhythmias, pulmonary hemorrhage, nausea, vomiting, diarrhea, hepatitis, thrombocytopenia, and leukopenia. Administration and dosage: Initially, 1 to 2 mg/kg, via scalp vein over 10 minutes. The initial dose is followed by an infusion of 1 to 2 mg/kg/hour until an increase in arterial oxygen is noted. A response should be noted within 30 minutes after the initial dose.

GUANADREL (HYLOREL)
GUANETHIDINE (ISMELIN)

Guanadrel and guanethidine are peripherally acting antihypertensive agents that accumulate in adrenergic nerve terminals and inhibit norepinephrine's release from neuronal storage sites in response to nerve stimulation. Depletion of norepinephrine induces a relaxation of peripheral vascular smooth muscle, which decreases peripheral resistance, venous return, and blood pressure. The hypotensive effect of these agents is more noticeable in the standing position than in the supine position. For optimum control of blood pressure, these agents are usually coadministered with a diuretic. Adverse effects of these agents include fatigue, headache, nausea, vomiting, paresthesias, tremor, depression, cardiac irregularities, chest pain, nasal congestion, palpitations, and fluid retention. Dosage and administration: Guanadrel: Initially, 10 mg/day (may give 5 mg b.i.d.), usual dosage range is 20 to 75 mg/day. Guanethidine: Usual dose is 10 to 50 mg/day.

RESERPINE (SERPALAN, SERPASIL)

Reserpine, one of the first effective antihypertensive agents marketed, is an alkaloid extracted from the roots of the Indian plant *Rauwolfia serpentina*. Reserpine exerts its antihypertensive effect by depleting the tissue stores of catecholamines (norepinephrine and epinephrine). This mechanism results in depression of sympathetic function leading to a reduced heart rate and blood pressure. Reserpine is indicated for use in controlling mild hypertension and as adjunctive therapy with other antihypertensive agents for treatment of severe hypertension. At low doses, reserpine does not induce postural hypotension; most of its untoward actions result from its effect on the brain and GI tract. Reserpine has a tendency to cause sedation, nightmares, and severe mental depression as well as diarrhea and gastrointestinal cramps. Reserpine also increases gastric acid secretion and should not be administered to patients with peptic ulcers. The usual dose is less than 1 mg (usually, 0.25 mg) administered orally as a single dose. Other rauwolfia derivatives include deserpidine (Harmonyl), rescinnamine (Moderil), and alseroxylon (Rauwiloid).

CARDIOTONIC AGENTS USED IN CONGESTIVE HEART FAILURE

If the left ventricle is unable to pump the blood returning from the lungs into the systemic circulation, a backflow of blood and pressure occurs within the pulmonary vascular system. As volume and pressure continue to increase in the vasculature, fluid will leak into the pulmonary interstitial space, alveoli, and eventually, the terminal airways. When the amount of fluid entering the lungs is greater than the lymphatic system's capacity to remove it, pulmonary edema develops. The most common reason for this volume/pressure overload of the pulmonary vascular system is left ventricular failure. If the mean PAP exceeds 35 to 45 mmHg, the right heart pressures will be affected because the right ventricle will fail to keep pace with the increased demand of ejecting blood against high pressures. When the right ventricle fails, blood backs up in the systemic vessels and the major body organs become congested with venous blood. This results in congestive heart failure (CHF).

The various agents used to treat CHF include:

- Diuretics (presented in Chapter 17)
- Vasodilators (see *Antihypertensive and Antianginal Agents*)
- ACE Inhibitors (see *Antihypertensive Agents*)
- β-Adrenoceptor Stimulators (see *Vasopressors* after this section)
- Cardioactive (Digitalis) Glycosides (presented in this section)
- Phosphodiesterase Inhibitors (presented in this section)

Optimal therapy in treating CHF often includes two or more drugs from the above drug categories. Drugs that have a cardiotonic effect, and thus are known as positive inotropic agents, are of primary importance in controlling CHF. These agents improve the functioning capability of the heart by increasing the force of myocardial contraction. Agents in this category include the cardiac glycosides, myocardial phosphodiesterase inhibitors, and the β-adrenoceptor stimulators.

On the other hand, drugs without positive inotropic effects have been quite successful in treating heart failure. These agents are often included in the CHF drug regimen in conjunction with the cardiotonic agents and include certain vasodilators and diuretics. By reducing vascular tone, the vasodilators unload some of the stress placed on the heart. The same holds true for the diuretics, which reduce vascular volume.

CARDIOACTIVE (DIGITALIS) GLYCOSIDES

Mechanism of Action

The cardiac glycosides are agents that have the ability to enhance cardiac performance by increasing cardiac output (positive inotropic effect) and alter the specialized conduction system of the heart (antiarrhythmic effect). The cardiac glycosides are collectively known as the digitalis glycosides because digitalis, the dried leaf of the foxglove plant, is the primary source of these agents. The cardiac glycosides include digitoxin (derived from *Digitalis purpurea,* the foxglove plant) and deslanoside and digoxin (derived from *Digitalis lanata,* a foxglove species). Of these, digoxin is the prototype and most commonly used preparation.

The influence these agents have on the heart is primarily dose-related and includes both a direct action on myocardial muscle cells and the specialized conduction system as well as indirect actions on the cardiovascular system. The indirect actions of these agents are mediated by a parasympathomimetic (vagomimetic) action and, in higher doses, a sympathomimetic action. The parasympathomimetic actions of the cardiac glycosides are responsible for the depression of the SA node, the prolonged AV conduction, and the increase in the AV refractory period. By this mechanism, the digitalis glycosides are especially useful for atrial arrhythmias in which ventricular rate is elevated. In higher doses, these agents increase sympathetic outflow from the CNS, which may potentiate the toxic effects of these drugs.

The direct actions these agents have on myocardial muscle cells bring about an increase in the force and velocity of myocardial contraction, which leads to an increase in cardiac output. The corresponding improved cardiac performance results in an overall increase in efficiency, especially in the work of the failing heart. The mechanism by which these agents exert their positive inotropic effect is to make more intracellular calcium available for myocardial contraction. The more calcium that is available for contraction, the greater the force and strength of contraction. The cardiac glycosides have the unique ability to inhibit the enzyme Na^+, K^+-ATPase (sodium, potassium-adenosine triphosphatase), also known as the sodium pump. Inactivation of the sodium pump leads to an accumulation of intracellular sodium. By way of the sodium-calcium exchanger (a transporter in the cell membrane), the excess intracellular sodium is exchanged for extracellular calcium, thereby increasing intracellular calcium.

Indications for Use

1. Treatment of CHF, especially low-output states associated with left ventricular failure.
2. Arrhythmias associated with CHF.
3. Treatment of atrial fibrillation, atrial flutter, and paroxysmal atrial tachycardia (PAT) in which there is a rapid ventricular rate.
4. Treatment of cardiogenic shock accompanied by pulmonary edema.

Contraindications

Contraindications to the use of cardiac glycosides include V-fib, V-tach, digitalis toxicity states, and beriberi heart disease.

Precautions

1. Dosage must be adjusted for patients with renal insufficiency.
2. Existing conditions that may precipitate digitalis toxicity include hypokalemia, hypercalcemia, hypothyroidism, hypomagnesemia, alkalosis, and hypoxia. These conditions should be corrected before giving digitalis.
3. Do not administer IV calcium to patients receiving digitalis, because the effects of calcium on the myocardium are similar to those of digitalis and may potentiate the adverse effects of these agents.
4. All dosages are highly individualized.

Adverse Reactions—Digitalis Toxicity

CNS: Headache, weakness, apathy, blurred vision, confusion, disorientation, delirium, seizures.

GI: Anorexia, nausea, vomiting, abdominal pain.

Cardiac Reactions: Multifocal ventricular premature complexes, nonparoxysmal AV junctional tachycardia, sinus irregularities, and other dysrhythmias.

Overdosage

Treatment of toxicity consists of discontinuing the drug, assessing serum potassium levels, and if necessary, administering potassium chloride and/or an antiarrhythmic drug. Digoxin immune Fab, a digoxin antidote, is used to treat potentially life-threatening digoxin (or digitoxin) poisoning.

Dosage and Administration

Digoxin (Lanoxin, Lanoxicaps)—*For rapid oral digitalization:* 0.5 to 0.75 mg initially, followed by 0.25 to 0.5 mg given every 6 to 8 hours. *For slow oral digitalization:* 0.125 to 0.25 mg/day for 7 days. **IV:** 0.25 to 0.5 mg initially, followed by 0.25 mg given every 4 to 6 hours to a total of 1 mg. Oral/IV maintenance dose: 0.125 to 0.5 mg/day.

Digitoxin (Crystodigin)—*For rapid oral digitalization:* 0.6 mg initially, followed by 0.4 mg and then 0.2 mg given every 4 to 6 hours. *For slow oral digitalization:* 0.2 mg b.i.d. for 4 days. The usual maintenance dose ranges between 0.05 and 0.3 mg/day.

Deslanoside (Cedilanid-D)—*Loading dose for rapid digitalization:* 1.6 mg IV or IM.

PHOSPHODIESTERASE INHIBITORS

Mechanism of Action

The phosphodiesterase inhibitors are inotropic agents that block the activity of myocardial cell phosphodiesterase, the enzyme responsible for deactivating cAMP (see also Chapter 2). Inhibition of this enzyme leads to an increase in cellular levels of cAMP, which facilitates myocardial contractility and increases cardiac output. These agents also enhance calcium influx across myocardial cells, which has been postulated as a contributory mechanism to their positive inotropic effects. In addition to their positive inotropic effects, the phosphodiesterase inhibitors also induce peripheral vasodilation, thereby reducing both preload and afterload. Amrinone and milrinone are currently the only approved phosphodiesterase inhibitors used in the treatment of CHF.

Indications for Use

Short-term management of CHF for patients not responding to conventional drug regimens such as digitalis glycosides, diuretics, and vasodilators.

Contraindications

Contraindications to the use of phosphodiesterase inhibitors include hypersensitivity to the drug.

Precautions

1. Fluid, electrolyte, and renal function should be carefully monitored during therapy, especially when coadministered with a diuretic.
2. Amrinone's inotropic effects are additive to those of digitalis. Monitor for untoward reactions.

3. Cautious use is recommended for patients with aortic or pulmonic valvular disease, hypertrophic subaortic stenosis, preexisting arrhythmias, thrombocytopenia, after an acute myocardial infarction, vigorous diuretic therapy, or preexisting hypotension.

Adverse Reactions

Amrinone: Nausea, vomiting, anorexia, abdominal pain, chest pain, hypotension, cardiac arrhythmias, thrombocytopenia, asymptomatic platelet count reductions (to $<150{,}000/mm^3$).

Milrinone: Headache, hypokalemia, tremor, thrombocytopenia, chest pain, ventricular arrhythmias, hypotension.

Overdosage

Most overdoses of these drugs lead to hypotension because of their vasodilator effects. Treatment includes supportive care and general measures for circulatory support.

Dosage and Administration

Amrinone (Inocor)—Initially, 0.75 mg/kg by IV bolus administered slowly over 2 to 3 minutes. Maintenance infusion: 5 to 10 μg/kg/min.

Milrinone (Primacor)—Initially, 50 μg/kg administered slowly over 10 minutes. Maintenance infusion: 0.375 to 0.75 μg/kg/min. Dosage must be adjusted for patients with renal dysfunction.

VASOPRESSORS USED IN SHOCK (THE SYMPATHOMIMETIC AMINES)

Shock is a complex acute cardiovascular syndrome in which blood flow to vital tissues is inadequate to sustain life. It can be caused by, or can cause, a decreased supply of oxygen to the tissues or an increased demand by the tissues for oxygen and nutrients.

There are several causes for shock:

Anaphylactic shock is a medical emergency triggered by an exaggerated reaction to an allergen. Chemical mediators of inflammation (histamine, serotonin, prostaglandins, leukotrienes, etc.) are released that may induce profound third-space fluid losses, massive vasodilatation (with subsequent decrease in SVR), and severe bronchoconstriction (with subsequent loss of ventilation and decrease in PaO_2).

Cardiogenic shock is the most severe form of heart failure, in which the heart is unable to maintain an adequate blood flow to major organs and peripheral tissues.

Cardiogenic shock is commonly seen in end-stage heart failure and carries a mortality rate of 80% or more. In the intermediate and late stages of cardiogenic shock, systemic vasoconstriction occurs as a compensatory mechanism to maintain mean arterial pressure.

Hypovolemic shock occurs when there is a severe reduction in circulating intravascular volume. Hypovolemia leads to inadequate tissue perfusion and ischemic hypoxia. An intravascular volume deficit is usually a result of blood loss, third-space fluid shifts, or dehydration. The loss in intravascular volume reduces the venous return to the heart, which then results in reduced filling volumes. To maintain arterial pressure, extracellular fluid shifts from the tissues to the intravascular space. Because of the fluid shift into the vascular system, the SVR increases.

Neurogenic shock is a shock state caused by injury to or malfunction of the sympathetic nervous system at the level of T-6 or higher. High spinal cord damage or pharmacologic blockade (spinal anesthesia) of the sympathetic system may elicit neurogenic shock. The loss of sympathetic control of arterioles creates a massive vasodilator reaction in which there is venous pooling of blood in the periphery with a concomitant decrease in venous return to the heart. Hypotension and a decreased cardiac output ensue.

Septic shock is a shock condition precipitated by an infectious disease. Shock associated with septicemia (the presence and growth of pathogens in the blood) is classified into hyperdynamic (early shock) and hypodynamic (late shock) phases. The early phase septic shock is characterized by an increased CO with a decreased SVR. This is because the body's initial response to shock is systemic vasodilation. As the duration of shock continues (late shock), the heart has difficulty in maintaining an increased CO to compensate for the vasodilator reaction. As the CO decreases, the arterial pressure decreases. To maintain an adequate arterial pressure, systemic vasoconstriction occurs, which then results in an increased SVR.

The signs and symptoms of shock are variable and nonspecific, in that the degree to which a patient exhibits a response depends on the underlying disease condition, drug therapy, and the patient's age. Some of the clinical manifestations of shock include:

- *CNS:* Agitation, confusion, disorientation, coma.
- *Cardiovascular:* Hypotension, cardiac arrhythmias, tachycardia, wide pulse pressure.
- *Skin:* Pallor, cyanosis, cold and clammy skin, sweating.
- *Pulmonary:* Dyspnea, tachypnea, pulmonary edema.
- *Renal:* Oliguria.
- *Other:* Metabolic acidosis, hypoglycemia or hyperglycemia.

Treatment of shock is aimed at supporting the circulation and restoring the blood pressure. Various inotropic and pressor agents are used for this purpose. All agents used in the treatment of shock are sympathomimetic amines with primary α and/or β_1 activity. This section details the three primary drug groups used in the treatment of shock:

- The endogenous catecholamines (epinephrine, norepinephrine, dopamine)
- The synthetic catecholamines (dobutamine, isoproterenol)
- Vasopressor amines (mephentermine, metaraminol, methoxamine, phenylephrine)

The Endogenous Catecholamines (see also Chapter 2)

EPINEPHRINE (ADRENALIN)

Mechanism of Action

Epinephrine is a potent stimulator of both α-adrenoceptors and β-adrenoceptors of the sympathetic system. At normal doses, epinephrine has predominant activity: it activates the β_1-adrenoceptors of the heart (resulting in an increased rate and force of contraction) as well as the β_2-adrenoceptors of the vasculature and other smooth muscle (resulting in vasodilation and smooth muscle relaxation, especially of the bronchi). At higher doses, epinephrine's α-adrenoceptor effects predominate, resulting in vasoconstriction and a rise in the blood pressure. Epinephrine is also a physiologic antagonist of histamine, which makes it therapeutically useful in the treatment of hypersensitivity reactions.

Indications for Use

1. Acute hypotensive states.
2. For resuscitation and restoration of normal cardiac rhythm during cardiac arrest (see Chapter 19).
3. Bronchodilation (see Chapter 10).
4. Nasal decongestion (see Chapter 9).
5. Agent of choice for the relief of anaphylactic, allergic, and other hypersensitivity reactions.
6. For topical hemostasis in controlling superficial bleeding. Epinephrine is especially useful in controlling bleeding associated with certain surgical procedures, bronchoscopy, and epistaxis (nosebleed).
7. For prolonging the action of local anesthetics (see Chapter 15).
8. Ocular decongestion and production of mydriasis.

Contraindications

Contraindications to the use of epinephrine include hypersensitivity to the drug, severe hypertension, coronary artery disease, shock (nonanaphylactic), narrow-angle glaucoma, organic brain damage, labor (delays the second stage), and general anesthesia with halogenated hydrocarbons or cyclopropane (increases the risk of arrhythmias).

Precautions

1. Epinephrine should be used with caution for patients with cardiovascular disease, hypertension, diabetes, and/or hyperthyroidism and in elderly individuals.
2. Pulmonary edema may occur as a result of the peripheral constriction and cardiac stimulation that epinephrine produces.
3. Tolerance may occur with repeated and prolonged use.
4. Syncope has occurred after the administration of epinephrine to children with asthma.
5. Parenterally administered epinephrine may initially decrease urine formation caused by constriction of renal blood vessels.
6. A sharp and significant rise in arterial blood pressure may produce angina pectoris, cerebrovascular hemorrhage, or aortic rupture (especially noted in patients with coronary insufficiency).
7. Potentiation of epinephrine's effects leading to toxic effects may occur when epinephrine is used in combination with digitalis, general anesthetics, isoproterenol, or propranolol.
8. With IV use, blood pressure and pulse should be frequently checked.
9. Avoid exposing solution to heat, light, or air (see Chapter 10).
10. The effects of epinephrine may be potentiated when coadministered with tricyclic antidepressants, MAO inhibitors, other sympathomimetic drugs, β-adrenoceptor blocking agents, antihistamines, guanethidine, and methyldopa.

Adverse Reactions

Most Common: Nervousness, anxiety, nausea, palpitations, headache, insomnia, sweating, pallor, mucosal drying, sneezing, rebound nasal congestion.

Significant Systemic Reactions: Cerebral hemorrhage, hemiplegia, subarachnoid hemorrhage, hypertension, urinary retention, pulmonary edema, tachycardia, arrhythmias, tremor, dizziness, dyspnea, syncope in children.

Overdosage

Fatalities have occurred with overdose, especially if the 1:100 inhalational solution is injected inadvertently or is mistaken for the 1:1000 solution designed for parenteral administration. In cases of excessive hypertension, a rapidly acting α-adrenoceptor blocking agent or vasodilator may used. Treat cardiac arrhythmias with a β-adrenoceptor blocking agent (e.g., propranolol). Ensure adequate ventilation and oxygenation.

Dosage and Administration

Parenteral:

Cardiac arrest: **IV:** 0.5 to 1 mg (5 to 10 ml of 1:10,000 solution). May be repeated at 5-minute intervals as necessary.
Intracardiac: 0.3 to 0.5 mg (3 to 5 ml of 1:10,000 solution).
Intraspinal: 0.2 to 0.4 ml of 1:1000 solution added to anesthetic solution.
Bronchospasm: **SC or IM:** 0.3 to 0.5 ml of 1:1000 solution. May repeat every 20 minutes up to 4 hours. Or, 0.1 to 0.3 ml 1:200 suspension SC.

Endotracheal tube administration if IV access is not available during cardiopulmonary resuscitation: 1 to 2 mg in 10 ml distilled water.
Inhalational: see Chapter 10.
Nasal decongestion: see Chapter 9.
Control of superficial bleeding: 1:1000 to 1:10,000 applied locally.

NOREPINEPHRINE (LEVARTERENOL, LEVOPHED)

Mechanism of Action

Norepinephrine, like epinephrine, is an endogenous neurotransmitter and modulator of the sympathetic nervous system. Both agents are direct agonists on adrenergic nerves and only differ in the ratio of their effectiveness in stimulating α- and β_2-adrenoceptors: norepinephrine exhibits little action on β_2-adrenoceptors and is somewhat less potent than epinephrine on α-adrenoceptors. However, both agents are approximately equipotent in stimulating the cardiac β_1-adrenoceptors.

Indications for Use

1. Restoration of blood pressure in acute hypotensive states.
2. As an adjunct in the treatment of cardiac arrest and profound hypotension.

Contraindications

Contraindications to the use of norepinephrine include hypersensitivity to the drug. Do not give to patients who are hypotensive because of a blood volume deficit, who have mesenteric or peripheral vascular thrombosis, or who have extreme hypoxia or hypercapnia (may result in life-threatening cardiac arrhythmias). Additionally, do not administer during general anesthesia when halogenated hydrocarbons (e.g., halothane) are used.

Precautions

1. The following conditions require cautious use of norepinephrine: hypertension, hyperthyroidism, cardiovascular disease, elderly patients.

2. Administer IV infusions into a large vein (preferably an antecubital vein) to minimize necrosis and prevent extravasation (escape of fluid from the blood vessel into the surrounding tissue). The infusion site should be monitored closely for free flow.
3. The effects of norepinephrine may be potentiated when coadministered with tricyclic antidepressants, MAO inhibitors, other sympathomimetic drugs, β-adrenoceptor blocking agents, antihistamines, guanethidine, and methyldopa.
4. Severe hypertension may occur if norepinephrine is coadministered with oxytocic agents.
5. Diuretics may reduce arterial responsiveness to norepinephrine.

Adverse Reactions

Most Common: Reflex bradycardia, nervousness, palpitations, headache.

Significant Systemic Reactions: Hypertension, respiratory distress, arrhythmias, tremor, cerebral hemorrhage, convulsions.

Overdosage

Overdosage may result in severe hypertension, reflex bradycardia, increased peripheral resistance, and decreased cardiac output. Treatment consists of appropriate fluid and electrolyte replacement therapy and ensuring a patent airway with adequate ventilation and oxygenation.

Dosage and Administration

IV infusion: Initially, 8 to 12 μg/min (2 to 3 ml/min) of a 4-μg/ml dilution (4 mg norepinephrine/1000 ml 5% dextrose). Maintenance dose: 2 to 4 μg/min (0.5 to 1 ml/min).

DOPAMINE (DOPASTAT, INTROPIN)

Mechanism of Action

Dopamine exerts its positive inotropic effect directly on cardiac β_1-adrenoceptors and indirectly by causing the release of norepinephrine from its storage sites. Dopamine is an endogenous catecholamine and a precursor of norepinephrine that has the ability to enhance cardiac output by increasing myocardial contractility and stroke volume. An increase in renal blood flow and sodium excretion is noted owing to dopamine's ability to activate dopaminergic receptors. Large doses of dopamine stimulate α-adrenoceptor activation (which then overrides dopaminergic effects), leading to vasoconstriction, a diminished systemic vascular resistance (SVR), and correction of hypotension. Dopamine has an onset of action within 5 minutes with a duration of less than 10 minutes.

Indications for Use

1. Shock caused by MI, trauma, septicemia, open heart surgery, renal failure, and congestive heart failure.
2. Hemodynamically significant hypotension.

Contraindications

Contraindications to the use of dopamine include pheochromocytoma and uncorrected tachyarrhythmias or ventricular fibrillation.

Precautions

1. Hypoxia, hypercapnia, and acidosis may decrease dopamine's effectiveness or increase side effects. These conditions should be corrected before administration of dopamine.
2. Dopamine does not replace volume loss. Hypovolemia should be corrected before administration of dopamine.
3. Dopamine has the ability to reverse the effects of β-adrenoceptor blocking agents.
4. Frequent monitoring of the urine output, cardiac output, ECG and blood pressure should be performed and observed for significant changes.
5. IV infusion should be administered into a large vein to prevent extravasation.
6. Use with caution for patients with occlusive vascular disease and for elderly individuals.
7. Dopamine is inactivated in an alkaline environment; do not add dopamine to any alkaline diluent solution.
8. The effects of dopamine may be potentiated when coadministered with tricyclic antidepressants, MAO inhibitors, other sympathomimetic drugs, and oxytocics.
9. Coadministration of dopamine with diuretics may have an additive effect.
10. Arrhythmias may occur if dopamine is used in conjunction with halogenated hydrocarbon anesthetics.

Adverse Reactions

Most Common: Ventricular ectopy, tachycardia, anginal pain, palpitations, hypotension, vasoconstriction, dyspnea, headache, nausea, and vomiting.

Significant Systemic Reactions: Usually occurs with higher than normal doses: hypertension, AV conduction abnormalities, ventricular arrhythmias, bradycardia, azotemia.

Overdosage

Symptoms include a marked elevation of the blood pressure and decreased urinary output. If this occurs, reduce dosage or discontinue the drug. Because the duration of dopamine's action is short, no other measures should be necessary.

Dosage and Administration

IV infusion: 2 to 5 μg/kg/min up to a rate of 20 to 50 μg/kg/min as needed for seriously ill patients. Frequent urine output checks are needed for doses in excess of 50 μg/kg/min.

The Synthetic Catecholamines

DOBUTAMINE (DOBUTREX)

Mechanism of Action

Dobutamine is a direct-acting inotropic agent, the primary site of action of which is on cardiac β_1-adrenoceptors, with little activity on β_2 and α-adrenoceptors. Hemodynamic responses to dobutamine include an increase in myocardial contractility, an increase in cardiac output, and a reduction in total peripheral resistance. Large doses of dobutamine may increase heart rate and blood pressure. Dobutamine is chemically related to dopamine; however, it does not cause the release of norepinephrine as does dopamine. Dobutamine and dopamine have been used together in moderate doses. The combination of these drugs maintains arterial pressure but with less increase in pulmonary artery occlusive pressure and less pulmonary congestion than dopamine alone.

Indications for Use

Dobutamine is indicated for short-term inotropic support for patients with cardiac decompensation (acute heart failure) caused by depressed contractility (e.g., patients with pulmonary congestion and low cardiac output) and for patients with hypotension with pulmonary congestion and left ventricular failure who cannot tolerate vasodilators.

Contraindications

Contraindications to the use of dobutamine include hypersensitivity to the drug and idiopathic hypertrophic subaortic stenosis (IHSS).

Precautions

1. Monitor patient's blood pressure and heart rate frequently. Dobutamine may markedly increase heart rate and blood pressure, especially systolic pressure. Reduce dosage if indicated.
2. Dobutamine may increase ventricular ectopy; however, it rarely produces ventricular tachycardia.
3. Concurrent or previous use of a blocking agent may render dobutamine ineffective.
4. Hypovolemia should be corrected with appropriate volume expanders before initiating dobutamine therapy.

5. The effects of dopamine may be potentiated when coadministered with tricyclic antidepressants, MAO inhibitors, other sympathomimetic drugs, and oxytocics.
6. Arrhythmias may occur if dobutamine is used in conjunction with halogenated hydrocarbon anesthetics.

Adverse Reactions

Most Common: Increased heart rate, mild hypertension, palpitations.

Significant Systemic Reactions: Marked hypertension, anginal pain, ventricular ectopic activity, pronounced tachycardia, headache, dyspnea.

Overdosage

Symptoms of overdose include marked changes in blood pressure or tachycardia. Treatment consists of a reduction in dosage or temporary discontinuation of the drug.

Dosage and Administration

2.5 to 10 μg/kg/min by IV infusion. On rare occasions, up to 40 μg/kg/min may be required.

ISOPROTERENOL (ISUPREL)

Mechanism of Action

Isoproterenol is an extremely potent β-adrenoceptor stimulator that equally activates both β_1- and β_2-adrenoceptors. Isoproterenol has no α activity. The positive inotropic and chronotropic actions of isoproterenol lead to an enhanced myocardial contractility, an increase in cardiac output, and an increase in the heart rate. Isoproterenol markedly increases myocardial oxygen demand and may induce or exacerbate myocardial ischemia. Newer inotropic agents, such as dobutamine and amrinone, have generally replaced isoproterenol in most clinical settings.

Isoproterenol's β_2 properties cause dilation of resistance vessels of skeletal muscles and relaxation of bronchial smooth muscle. It also causes reduced peripheral vascular resistance, which may cause a drop in blood pressure (due from peripheral vasodilation and venous pooling). Onset of action is rapid; however, duration (as with all catecholamines) is brief (less than 60 minutes, rapidly metabolized by COMT).

Indications for Use

1. As adjunct therapy in the management of shock states, cardiac arrest, Adams-Stokes syndrome, AV block, and carotid sinus hypersensitivity.

2. Temporary control of hemodynamically significant bradycardia in the patient with a pulse. Because isoproterenol may exacerbate ischemia or hypotension, atropine, pacing, dopamine, and epinephrine should be used before isoproterenol in the treatment of symptomatic bradycardia.
3. Bronchodilation (see Chapter 10).

Contraindications

Contraindications to the use of isoproterenol include tachycardia, tachyarrhythmias, heart block caused by digitalis toxicity, or concurrent administration of epinephrine (may lead to life-threatening arrhythmias).

Precautions

1. Do not coadminister epinephrine and isoproterenol; potential adverse effects include serious arrhythmias.
2. Correct hypovolemia before administering isoproterenol.
3. Do not administer to patients with ischemic heart disease. Isoproterenol increases myocardial oxygen demand.
4. Isoproterenol may exacerbate tachyarrhythmias caused by digitalis toxicity and hypokalemia.
5. Isoproterenol may reverse the effects of β-adrenoceptor blocking agents.
6. Use with caution for patients with hypertension, coronary artery disease, hyperthyroidism, and/or diabetes.
7. Coadministration of isoproterenol and halogenated hydrocarbon anesthetics may precipitate arrhythmias.
8. During administration, if the heart rate exceeds 110 beats/minute, consider decreasing the infusion rate or discontinuing the drug.

Adverse Reactions

Most Common: Nervousness, anxiety, tremor, headache, palpitations, dizziness, flushing, nausea.
Cardiac: Tachycardia, palpitations, cardiac arrest.
CNS: Headache, dizziness, nervousness, tremors.
Pulmonary: Pulmonary edema (rare).
GI: Nausea, vomiting.

Overdosage

Overdosage leads to cardiac excitability and distress. Treatment consists of discontinuing the drug and monitoring the blood pressure, heart rate, respirations, and ECG.

Dosage and Administration

Parenteral:

For management of shock: 0.25 to 2.5 ml/min of 1:500,000 dilution in dextrose 5% by IV infusion (0.5 to 5 μg/min).

For cardiac arrest: **IV injection:** 1 to 3 ml of a 1:50,000 dilution (0.02 to 0.06 mg). **IV infusion:** 1.25 ml of 1:250,000 dilution per minute (5 μg/min). **SC, IM:** 1 ml of 1:5000 solution undiluted (0.2 mg). **Intracardiac:** 0.1 ml of 1:5000 solution undiluted (0.02 mg).

Bronchospasm (during anesthesia): 0.01 to 0.02 mg IV of a 1:50,000 dilution in saline or dextrose 5%.

Sublingual:

Heart block: Initially, 10 mg (range 5 to 50 mg); maintenance therapy only.

Bronchospasm: 10 to 20 mg t.i.d., q.i.d.

Inhalation: see Chapter 10.

Vasopressor Amines

MEPHENTERMINE (WYAMINE)

METARAMINOL (ARAMINE)

METHOXAMINE (VASOXYL)

PHENYLEPHRINE (NEO-SYNEPHRINE)

Mechanism of Action

The vasopressor amines mephentermine, metaraminol, methoxamine, and phenylephrine are sympathomimetic agents that exhibit both direct and indirect adrenergic activity. Their predominant direct effect is to elicit systemic vasoconstriction via activation of vascular α-adrenoceptors. Their indirect action is to cause the release of norepinephrine from adrenergic nerve terminals, thereby potentiating their pressor effect. The vasopressor amines are potent vasoconstricting agents and should be used with extreme care.

Indications for Use

Mephentermine:

1. Treatment of hypotension secondary to ganglionic blockade and that associated with spinal anesthesia.
2. Short-term emergency measure to restore the blood pressure until blood or blood substitutes become available.

Metaraminol:

1. As adjunct therapy in the treatment of hypotension caused by cardiogenic shock, septicemia, brain tumor, hemorrhage, surgery, or drug reactions.
2. Acute hypotensive states associated with spinal anesthesia.

Methoxamine:

1. Support, restoration, or maintenance of blood pressure during anesthesia.
2. Abolish paroxysmal supraventricular tachycardia.

Phenylephrine:

1. Maintenance of an adequate blood pressure during spinal and inhalational anesthesia.
2. Treatment of vascular failure in shock, shocklike states, hypersensitivity, or drug-induced hypotension.
3. Abolish paroxysmal supraventricular tachycardia.

Contraindications

Contraindications to the use of vasopressor amines include hypersensitivity to the drug, MAO inhibitor therapy, and severe hypertension or ventricular tachycardia.

Precautions

1. Use with caution for patients with cardiovascular disease, partial heart block, myocardial disease, and/or hyperthyroidism or for patients receiving cyclopropane or halogenated hydrocarbon anesthesia as well as for elderly individuals. Additionally, use with care for patients with bradycardia because these agents may potentiate the condition by causing reflex brady-cardia.
2. The use of these agents is not appropriate in maintaining blood pressure in hypovolemic states. Blood, plasma, or fluids should be administered before the use of these agents.
3. Avoid a sharp or excessive rise in blood pressure. Rapidly induced hypertension may result in pulmonary edema, arrhythmias, or cardiac arrest.
4. The pressor effects of these agents may be potentiated by MAO inhibitors, tricyclic antidepressants, sympathomimetic amines, and oxytocic drugs.

Adverse Reactions

Most Common: Reflex bradycardia, palpitations, lightheadedness.

Significant Systemic Reactions: Reflex bradycardia, sustained hypertension, arrhythmias, tremors, tachycardia.

Overdosage

The most common overdose symptom is severe or sustained hypertension. Treatment consists of administering an α-adrenoceptor blocking agent such as phentolamine. If the patient experiences excessive or sustained bradycardia, IV atropine should be administered.

Dosage and Administration

Mephentermine—**IV, IM:** 30 to 45 mg as a single injection. **IV infusion:** 0.1% (1 mg/ml) in 5% dextrose by continuous infusion administered at a rate of 1 mg/min.

Metaraminol—**IV:** 0.5 to 5 mg as a single injection followed by infusion of 15 to 100 mg in 500 ml 5% dextrose. **IV infusion (preferred administration in shock states):** 15 to 100 mg/500 ml 5% dextrose. Adjust rate to maintain a desired blood pressure. **IM, SC:** 2 to 10 mg for the prevention of hypotension.

Methoxamine—*For hypotension:* **IV:** 3 to 5 mg by slow IV injection. **IM:** 10 to 15 mg before anesthesia, may repeat in 15 minutes. *For paroxysmal supraventricular tachycardia:* **IV:** 10 mg by slow IV injection.

Phenylephrine—*For hypotension:* **IV:** 0.1 to 0.5 mg of a 0.1% solution as a single injection. May repeat in 15 minutes. **IV infusion:** 100 to 200 drops/minute of a 1:50,000 solution until stabilization of the blood pressure. Maintenance infusion: 40 to 60 drops/minute. **IM, SC:** 2 to 5 mg of a 1% solution. *To prolong spinal anesthesia:* 2 to 5 mg added to anesthetic solution. *For paroxysmal supraventricular tachycardia:* 0.5 mg by IV injection given over 20 to 30 seconds. May increase by 0.1-mg increments as necessary.

AGENTS USED IN DISORDERS OF COAGULATION

Thrombolytic Agents

ALTEPLASE, RECOMBINANT ACTIVASE
ANISTREPLASE (EMINASE)
STREPTOKINASE (KABIKINASE, STREPTASE)
UROKINASE (ABBOKINASE)

Mechanism of Action

Thrombolytic agents, also known as fibrinolytic agents, rapidly destroy thrombi (blood clots that obstruct blood vessels) by converting plasminogen (an inactive plasma protein) to plasmin (an active, fibrinolytic enzyme). Plasmin is directly responsible for dissolving formed fibrin clots.

The four primary thrombolytic agents are alteplase (recombinant activase), anistreplase, streptokinase, and urokinase. Alteplase is a tissue plasminogen activator (TPA) created by recombinant DNA that indirectly initiates local fibrinolysis by binding to fibrin in a thrombus and converting the entrapped plasminogen to plasmin. Anistreplase is an enzyme that consists of a streptokinase-plasminogen activator complex that cleaves peptide bonds on plasminogen, which then causes the formation of plasmin. Streptokinase is an enzyme derived from beta-hemolytic streptococci that indirectly converts plasminogen to plasmin by first producing an activator complex (in which streptokinase combines with plasminogen to produce a structural alteration in plasminogen). This active form of plasminogen is then converted to plasmin streptokinase, from which streptokinase is detached and fragmented to form lower molecular weight products. Urokinase is an enzyme synthesized from human kidney cells that has the ability to directly convert plasminogen to plasmin.

Indications for Use

1. Lysis of acute, multiple pulmonary emboli that are not massive enough to require surgical intervention (alteplase, urokinase).
2. Lysis of acute, central deep vein thromboses (DVTs) (streptokinase).
3. Management of acute myocardial infarction (AMI). Coronary occlusion caused by a thrombus exists in the infarct-related coronary artery in most patients experiencing transmural myocardial infarction. Lysis of thrombi in the obstructed coronary vessel, reperfusion of the obstructed coronary vessel, and improved left ventricular function are noted after infusion of a thrombolytic agent. For the most effective therapy, treatment must be initiated as soon as possible (within 2 to 4 hours) after AMI symptoms.
4. To restore patency to occluded arteriovenous cannula (streptokinase).
5. To restore patency to occluded IV and central venous catheters that are obstructed by blood clots (urokinase).

Contraindications

Owing to the thrombolytic actions of these agents, an increased incidence of bleeding is noted. Thus, these agents are contraindicated for patients with a high risk of internal bleeding, patients with active internal bleeding, patients with a history of cerebrovascular accident, intracranial or intraspinal surgery patients (within 2 months), and for patients with intracranial neoplasm, arteriovenous malformation or aneurysm, bleeding diathesis, or severe uncontrolled hypertension. Relative contraindications include major surgery, delivery of a child, organ biopsy, serious gastrointestinal bleeding, and serious trauma within the previous 10 days.

Precautions

1. Carefully monitor patients for bleeding (especially patients with IV sites, venous cutdowns, arterial puncture sites, etc.)
2. Arrhythmias have been noted after the infusion of alteplase (sinus bradycardia, ventricular irritability). Have antiarrhythmic therapy available.
3. Concomitant use of heparin may contribute to the incidence of bleeding. Use cautiously.

4. Spontaneous bleeding from internal sites may occur in patients with abnormal platelet count, prothrombin time, partial thromboplastin time, or bleeding time. These patients should be assessed carefully before initiating therapy.
5. Miscellaneous precautions include recent cardiopulmonary resuscitation, subacute bacterial endocarditis, mitral disease with atrial fibrillation, pregnancy, prior severe allergic reaction, advanced age (older than 75 years).

Adverse Reactions

The most frequent adverse reaction to thrombolytic therapy is bleeding, which can be subdivided into two groups: 1) internal bleeding (GI tract, GU tract, retroperitoneal, or intracranial sites) and 2) superficial or surface bleeding from various puncture sites. If serious bleeding occurs, therapy must be discontinued, as well as any concomitant anticoagulant therapy.

Other reactions include nausea, vomiting, hypotension, fever, urticaria, allergic reactions, and bruising.

Dosage and Administration

Alteplase, recombinant (Activase)—*For acute myocardial infarction:* Given by IV infusion only and initiated as soon as possible after the onset of symptoms. Recommended dose: first hour, 60 mg (34.8 million IU). 6 to 10 mg is given as a bolus within the first 1 to 2 minutes. Second hour, 20 mg (11.6 million IU). Third hour, 20 mg (11.6 million IU). An increased incidence of intracranial bleeding is noted with a dose of 150 mg. Recommended maximum dose is 100 mg given over a 3-hour period, or for smaller patients (<65 kg), 1.25 mg/kg given over 3 hours, as described above. *For pulmonary embolism:* 100 mg by IV infusion given over 2 hours.

Anistreplase (Eminase)—*For myocardial infarction:* 30 units by IV injection given over 2 to 5 minutes.

Streptokinase (Kabikinase, Streptase)—*For myocardial infarction:* 1,500,000 U in a single IV infusion given over 1 hour or 20,000 U by bolus intracoronary, followed by 2000 U/min for 1 hour. *For deep venous thrombosis and pulmonary or arterial embolism:* Initially, 250,000 U given IV over 30 minutes, followed by 100,000 U/hour given over 72 hours for venous thrombosis or 100,000 U/hour given over 24 to 72 hours for pulmonary or arterial thrombosis. *For AV cannula occlusion:* 250,000 U/2 ml IV solution given over 30 minutes into each occluded limb of the cannula.

Urokinase (Abbokinase)—Initial loading dose: 2000 units/lb (4400 units/kg) as an admixture with 0.9% sodium chloride injection or 5% dextrose injection given at a rate of 90 ml/hr over 10 minutes. Follow with 2000 units/lb/hr (4400 units/kg/hr) given at a rate of 15 ml/hr for 12 hours. *For lysis of coronary artery thrombi:* After a single bolus dose of heparin (2500 to 10,000 U), administer urokinase into an occluded artery at a rate of 4 ml/min (6000 U/min) for up to 2 hours. Continue therapy until artery is fully patent.

Anticoagulant Agents

HEPARIN (LIQUAEMIN, CALCIPARINE)
ENOXAPARIN (LOVENOX)
DICUMAROL (DICUMAROL)
WARFARIN (COUMADIN, PANWARFIN, SOFARIN)
ANISINDIONE (MIRADON)

Mechanism of Action

Hemostasis is the prevention of loss of blood from the blood vessels, whereas coagulation is the process that occurs to transform liquid blood or plasma into a semisolid gel: the clot. Platelets, enzymes, and the protein fibrinogen are the primary components of the coagulation system, which involves, in various steps, the transformation of soluble fibrinogen into insoluble fibrin. The coagulation process as well as the blood tests used in determining clotting times are detailed further in Appendix B, Section V, *Hemostasis*.

Agents that prevent the formation of blood clots are termed anticoagulants. These agents are capable of altering one or more steps of the coagulation process, thus blocking the conversion of fibrinogen to fibrin. The parenteral anticoagulant agents include heparin and enoxaparin. The orally administered anticoagulant agents include dicumarol, warfarin, and anisindione.

Indications for Use

1. Prophylaxis and treatment of deep venous thromboses, cerebral thrombosis, pulmonary embolism, peripheral venous thrombosis associated with acute MI, and atrial fibrillation associated with embolization.
2. Diagnosis and treatment of acute and chronic consumption coagulopathies (disseminated intravascular coagulation [DIC]).

Contraindications

Contraindications to the use of anticoagulant agents include hypersensitivity to the drug or pork products, active bleeding, or significant bleeding tendencies.

Precautions

1. Use with extreme caution for patients who exhibit an increased risk for hemorrhage. Bleeding may occur at any site during therapy.
2. Periodic complete blood counts, including platelet count, should be performed during the course of therapy.

3. Use heparin with caution for patients with diabetes or renal insufficiency because hyperkalemia may develop.
4. Combined use of anticoagulant agents with thrombolytics may increase the incidence of internal bleeding.

Adverse Reactions

Spontaneous bleeding and hemorrhage are the principal adverse effects of these agents. Other adverse effects include nausea, vomiting, urticaria, and thrombocytopenia.

Overdosage

The antidote and treatment of choice for heparin overdose is protamine sulfate; for overdose of oral anticoagulants, phytonadione is indicated.

Dosage and Administration

Maintenance doses are usually based on prothrombin time (PT).

Anisindione (Miradon)—Initially, 300 mg on the first day, 200 mg on the second day, and 100 mg on the third day; thereafter, 25 to 250 mg/day.

Dicumarol—Initially, 200 to 300 mg first day; thereafter, 25 to 200 mg/day.

Enoxaparin (Lovenox)—Administer by SC injection only: 30 mg b.i.d. First dose should be given as soon after surgery as possible and continued for 7 to 14 days or until the risk of deep vein thrombosis has diminished.

Heparin Sodium (Liquaemin), ***Heparin Calcium*** (Calciparine)—*Guidelines for average-size patients: For anticoagulation:* **IV:** Initially, 10,000 U administered as a single IV injection, then 5000 to 10,000 U every 4 to 6 hours. IV infusion: 20,000 to 40,000 U/day (precede by a 5000 U IV loading dose). **SC:** Initially, 10,000 to 20,000 U, then 8000 to 10,000 U every 8 hours or 15,000 to 20,000 U every 12 hours. *For postoperative prophylaxis:* **SC:** 5000 U 2 hours before surgery, and then 5000 U every 8 to 12 hours for 7 days after surgery. *For heart/blood vessel surgery:* **IV:** 150 to 400 U/kg.

Warfarin (Coumadin, Panwarfin, Sofarin)—Initially, 10 mg daily for 2 to 4 days; thereafter, 2 to 10 mg/day.

REFERENCES/RECOMMENDED REARDING

Burnier M, Waeber B, Brunner HR. First-line pharmacological treatment of hypertension. Ann Intern Med 232:381, 1992.

Calhoun DA, Oparil S. Treatment of hypertensive crisis. N Engl J Med 323:1177, 1990.
Cardiac Arrhythmia Suppression Trial (CAST) Investigators. Preliminary report: effect of encainide and flecainide on mortality in a randomized trial of arrhythmia suppression after myocardial infarction. N Engl J Med 321:406, 1989.
Cooper GS, et al. Cardiac arrhythmias: recent therapeutic changes. Drug Ther 22:15, 1992.
Cross J. Pharmacologic management of heart failure: positive inotropic agents, Crit Care Nurs Clin North Am 5:589, 1993.
Doherty JE. Clinical use of digitalis glycosides. Cardiology 72:225, 1985.
Drug Facts and Comparisons. 49th ed. St. Louis: Facts and Comparisons, 1995.
Eckman MH, Levine HJ, Pauker SG. Effect of laboratory variation in the prothrombin-time ratio on the results of oral anticoagulant therapy. N Engl J Med 329:696, 1993.
Hansson L. Review of state-of-the-art beta-blocker therapy. Am J Cardiol 67:43B, 1991.
Harrison DG, Bates JN. The nitrovasodilators. New ideas about old drugs. Circulation 87:1461, 1993.
Harper KJ, Forker AD. Antihypertensive therapy: current issues and challenges. Postgrad Med J 91:163, 1992.
Hockenberry B. Multiple drug therapy in the treatment of essential hypertension. Nurs Clin North Am 26:417, 1991.
Latini R, Maggioni AP, Cavalli A. Therapeutic drug monitoring of antiarrhythmic drugs: rationale and current status. Clin Pharmacokinet 18:91, 1990.
Mason JW. A comparison of seven antiarrhythmic drugs in patients with ventricular tachyarrhythmias. N Engl J Med 329:452, 1993.
Moncada S, Palmer RMJ, Higgs EA. Nitric oxide: physiology, pathophysiology, and pharmacology. Pharmacol Rev 43:109, 1991.
Om A, Hess ML. Inotropic therapy of the failing myocardium. Clin Cardiol 16:5, 1993.
Physicians' Desk Reference. 49th ed. Montvale, NJ: Medical Economics, 1995.
Prisant LM, Carr AA, Hawkins DW. Treating hypertensive emergencies: controlled reduction of blood pressure and protection of target organs. Postgrad Med J 93:92, 1993.
Poller L. Therapeutic ranges for oral anticoagulation in different thromboembolic disorders. Ann Hematol 64:52, 1992.
Powers ER, Bergin JD. Recent advances in evaluating and managing congestive heart failure. Mod Med 60:54, 1992.
Rinde-Hoffman D, Glaser SP, Arnett DK. Update on nitrate therapy. J Clin Pharmacol 31:697, 1991.
Shammas NW, Zeitler R, Fitzpatrick P. Intravenous thrombolytic therapy in myocardial infarction: an analytical review. Clin Cardiol 16:282, 1993.
Stringer KA, Lindenfeld J. Hirudins: antithrombin anticoagulants. Ann Pharmacother 26:1535, 1992.
Triggle DJ. Calcium-channel antagonists: mechanism of action, vascular selectivities, and clinical relevance. Cleve Clin J Med 5:617, 1992.
Weiner B. Thrombolytic agents in critical care. Crit Care Nurs Clin North Am 5:355, 1993.
Weiner DA. Calcium channel blockers. Med Clin North Am 72:83, 1988.

Resuscitation Pharmacology and the American Heart Association's Advanced Cardiac Life Support Guidelines 19

This chapter focuses on the primary drugs commonly used during cardiopulmonary resuscitation (CPR). To use CPR drugs accurately and effectively, the American Heart Association (AHA) recommends that participants know the following.

- Why an agent is used (actions)
- When to use an agent (indications)
- How to use an agent (dosing)
- What to watch out for (precautions)

The goals of these pharmacologic agents are:

1. Correction of hypoxemia and acidosis.
2. Improvement of hemodynamics.
3. Suppression of significant arrhythmias, especially ventricular tachycardia (V-tach) and ventricular fibrillation (V-fib).
4. Maintenance of coronary and cerebral perfusion to ultimately reestablish spontaneous circulation at an adequate blood pressure.
5. Optimization of cardiac function.

To enhance the learner's comprehension of the factors that interact with the primary resuscitation drugs, the basic arrhythmias with associated drug of choice used to correct the arrhythmia, a flow chart on understanding arterial blood gas analysis, and advanced cardiac life support (ACLS) algorithms (V-fib/Pulseless

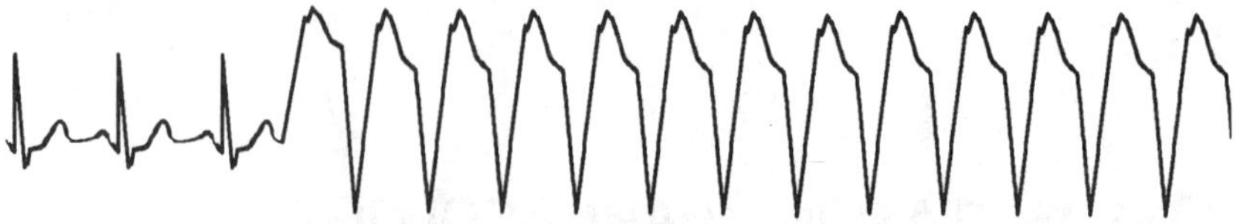

Figure 19.1. Ventricular tachycardia. Ventricular rate ranges from 50 (slow ventricular tachycardia) to 220 (rapid ventricular tachycardia). P waves, ST segments, and T waves are obscured by the QRS complexes, which are wide and bizarre. R-R interval is usually regular. Treatment includes lidocaine, and if the onset of V-tach is witnessed, a precordial thump is given. Direct-current shock (up to 360 joules) is applied if the patient is rapidly deteriorating.

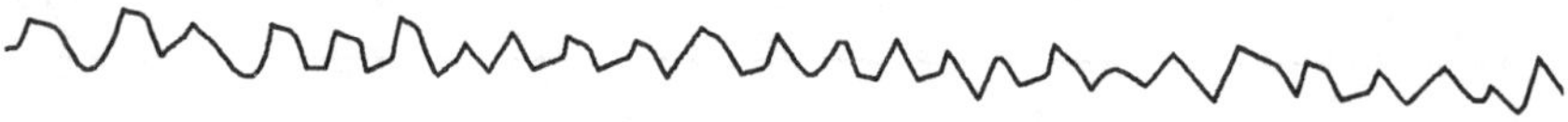

Figure 19.2. Ventricular fibrillation. Ventricular rate is rapid and chaotic, lacking a pattern. Cardiac output is inadequate. Treatment includes immediate direct-current shock (up to 360 joules), lidocaine, and the initiation of CPR if defibrillation is not effective.

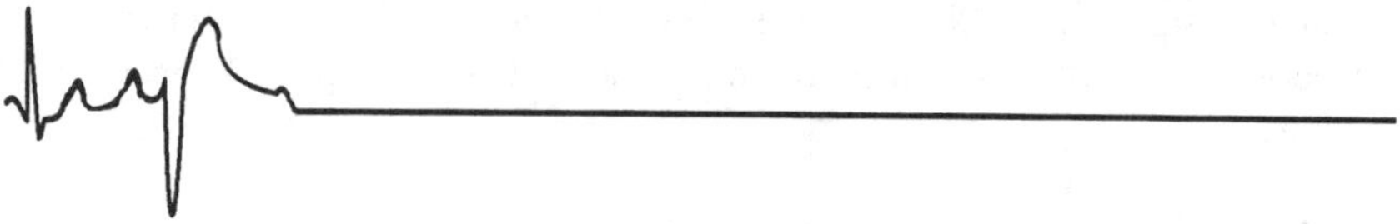

Figure 19.3. Cardiac arrest or asystole. It is caused by complete, acute heart failure. Treatment consists of CPR: intubation, ventilation, closed chest compressions, and epinephrine.

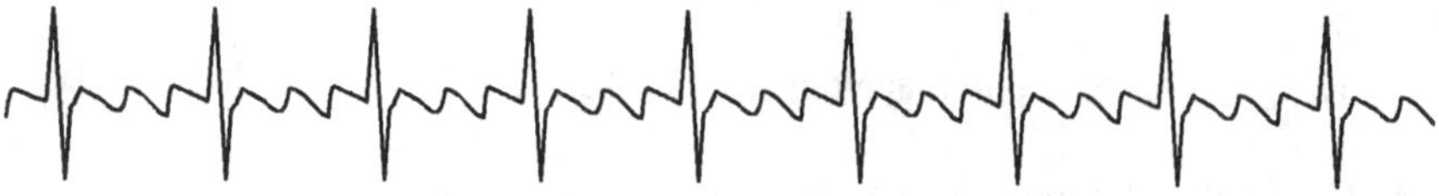

Figure 19.4. Atrial flutter. Atrial rate ranges from 250 to 350 beats per minute. QRS complexes are usually narrow. P waves are superimposed upon T waves (forming F waves) and resemble a "sawtooth" or "picket fence" pattern. Treatment includes digitalis or quinidine, elective cardioversion (20 to 50 w/sec), or a temporary pacemaker.

V-Tach, Pulseless Electrical Activity [PEA], and Asystole) have been included in this chapter (Figs. 19.1 to 19.10).

The first priority of CPR is early intervention, which consists of defibrillation in adults and ventilatory support in infants. Chest compression, assisted ventilation, and pharmacologic intervention are implemented to facilitate circulatory and ventilatory function, with the primary goal being to reestablish spontaneous

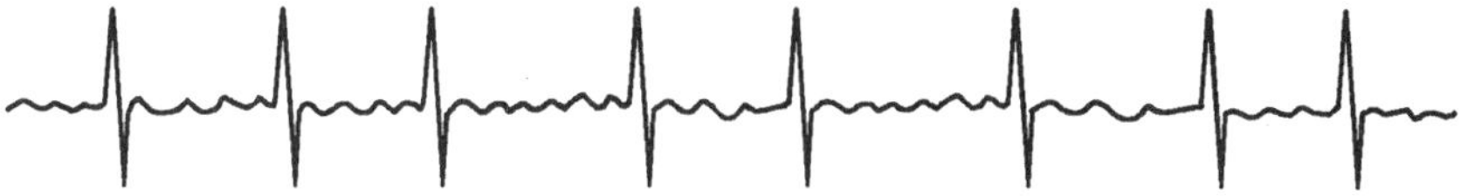

Figure 19.5. Atrial fibrillation. Atrial rate ranges from 350 to 500 beats per minute (but may reach as high as 700 beats per minute). The fibrillatory (or f) waves cause a varying, constantly changing atrial rate. ST segments and T waves will vary. Treatment includes digitalis or quinidine and elective cardioversion or a temporary pacemaker (for low ventricular rates caused by block).

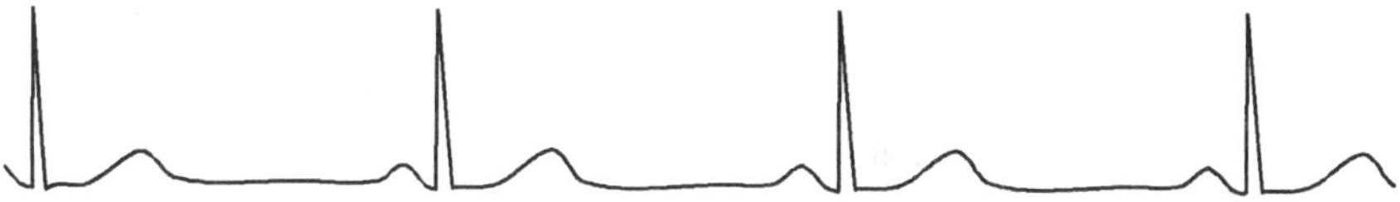

Figure 19.6. Sinus bradycardia. Rate < 60 beats per minute. When accompanied with hypotension, poor cardiac output, or heart failure, may treat with atropine or temporary pacemaker (for low output rates).

cardiopulmonary dynamics. Once a stable rhythm and ventilatory pattern (with mechanical ventilation if necessary) have been established, pressors (such as catecholamines) are used to maintain circulation.

Of essential importance during CPR (along with endotracheal intubation) is the accessibility for drug administration. Intravenous drug administration is the preferred route; the brachial vein is the site of choice for the placement of the IV line. If the intravenous route is not immediately accessible, endotracheal administration of certain drugs (e.g., atropine, lidocaine, and epinephrine [ALE]) may be used; however, the upper range of the IV dose must be given to elicit the same pharmacologic response as that of the IV route. Other drugs, such as bretylium, may also be administered endotracheally, but hopefully an IV route has been established by the time these drugs are necessary, because they are not generally used during the first sequence of CPR.

PRIMARY RESUSCITATION DRUGS

Note: Many of the agents presented in this chapter have been previously detailed in other chapters of this book; therefore, this chapter concentrates on those aspects that are specific to the use of these agents during cardiac arrest and the resuscitation effort. For additional indications or contraindications, precautions, adverse reactions, etc., of the agents listed in this chapter, refer to the chapters cross-referenced under *Actions*.

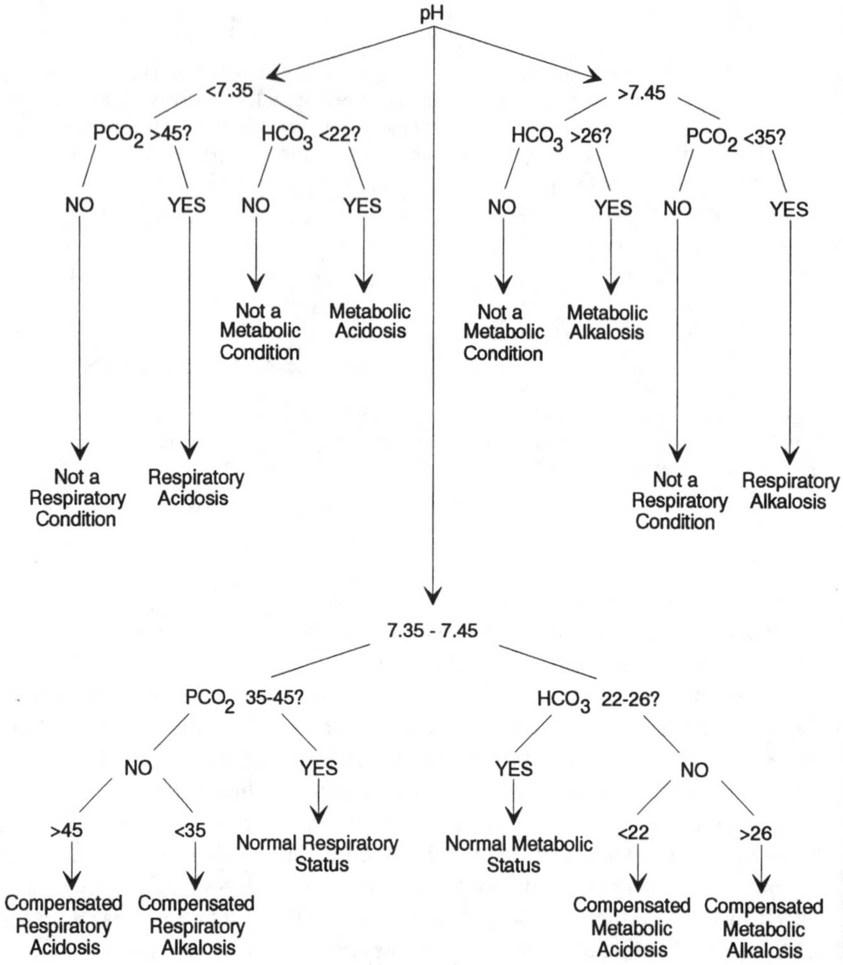

CLASSIFICATION OF HYPOXEMIA

Mild	Moderate	Severe
PaO_2 60-79 mmHg	PaO_2 40-59 mmHg	PaO_2 <40 mmHg

Figure 19.7. Understanding arterial blood gases.

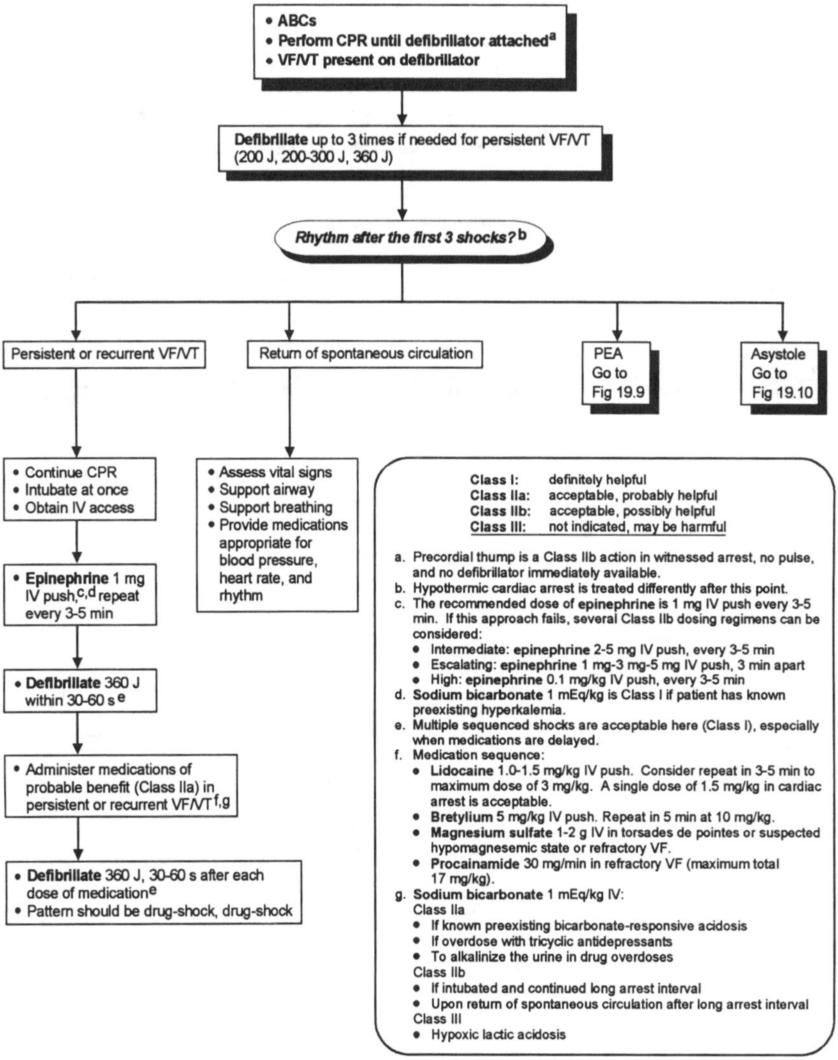
• ABCs
• Perform CPR until defibrillator attached[a]
• VF/VT present on defibrillator
Defibrillate up to 3 times if needed for persistent VF/VT (200 J, 200-300 J, 360 J)
Rhythm after the first 3 shocks? [b]
Persistent or recurrent VF/VT
Return of spontaneous circulation
PEA Go to Fig 19.9
Asystole Go to Fig 19.10
• Continue CPR
• Intubate at once
• Obtain IV access
• Epinephrine 1 mg IV push,[c,d] repeat every 3-5 min
• Defibrillate 360 J within 30-60 s [e]
• Administer medications of probable benefit (Class IIa) in persistent or recurrent VF/VT [f,g]
• Defibrillate 360 J, 30-60 s after each dose of medication[e]
• Pattern should be drug-shock, drug-shock
• Assess vital signs
• Support airway
• Support breathing
• Provide medications appropriate for blood pressure, heart rate, and rhythm
Class I: definitely helpful
Class IIa: acceptable, probably helpful
Class IIb: acceptable, possibly helpful
Class III: not indicated, may be harmful
a. Precordial thump is a Class IIb action in witnessed arrest, no pulse, and no defibrillator immediately available.
b. Hypothermic cardiac arrest is treated differently after this point.
c. The recommended dose of epinephrine is 1 mg IV push every 3-5 min. If this approach fails, several Class IIb dosing regimens can be considered:
• Intermediate: epinephrine 2-5 mg IV push, every 3-5 min
• Escalating: epinephrine 1 mg-3 mg-5 mg IV push, 3 min apart
• High: epinephrine 0.1 mg/kg IV push, every 3-5 min
d. Sodium bicarbonate 1 mEq/kg is Class I if patient has known preexisting hyperkalemia.
e. Multiple sequenced shocks are acceptable here (Class I), especially when medications are delayed.
f. Medication sequence:
• Lidocaine 1.0-1.5 mg/kg IV push. Consider repeat in 3-5 min to maximum dose of 3 mg/kg. A single dose of 1.5 mg/kg in cardiac arrest is acceptable.
• Bretylium 5 mg/kg IV push. Repeat in 5 min at 10 mg/kg.
• Magnesium sulfate 1-2 g IV in torsades de pointes or suspected hypomagnesemic state or refractory VF.
• Procainamide 30 mg/min in refractory VF (maximum total 17 mg/kg).
g. Sodium bicarbonate 1 mEq/kg IV:
Class IIa
• If known preexisting bicarbonate-responsive acidosis
• If overdose with tricyclic antidepressants
• To alkalinize the urine in drug overdoses
Class IIb
• If intubated and continued long arrest interval
• Upon return of spontaneous circulation after long arrest interval
Class III
• Hypoxic lactic acidosis

Figure 19.8. Ventricular fibrillation/pulseless ventricular tachycardia (VF/VT) algorithm. (Reproduced with permission from Textbook of Advanced Cardiac Life Support. Copyright 1994, American Heart Association.)

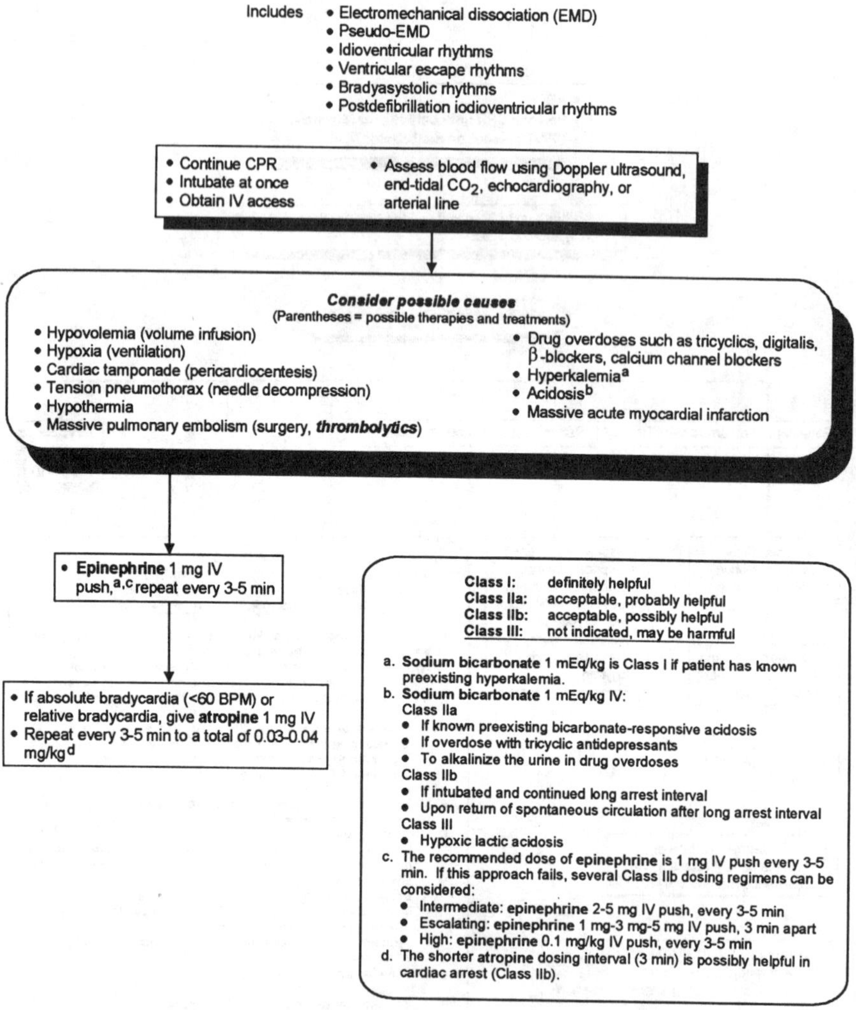
Includes
• Electromechanical dissociation (EMD)
• Pseudo-EMD
• Idioventricular rhythms
• Ventricular escape rhythms
• Bradyasystolic rhythms
• Postdefibrillation iodioventricular rhythms
• Continue CPR
• Intubate at once
• Obtain IV access
• Assess blood flow using Doppler ultrasound, end-tidal CO_2, echocardiography, or arterial line
Consider possible causes
(Parentheses = possible therapies and treatments)
• Hypovolemia (volume infusion)
• Hypoxia (ventilation)
• Cardiac tamponade (pericardiocentesis)
• Tension pneumothorax (needle decompression)
• Hypothermia
• Massive pulmonary embolism (surgery, thrombolytics)
• Drug overdoses such as tricyclics, digitalis, β-blockers, calcium channel blockers
• Hyperkalemia[a]
• Acidosis[b]
• Massive acute myocardial infarction
• Epinephrine 1 mg IV push,[a,c] repeat every 3-5 min
• If absolute bradycardia (<60 BPM) or relative bradycardia, give atropine 1 mg IV
• Repeat every 3-5 min to a total of 0.03-0.04 mg/kg[d]
Class I: definitely helpful
Class IIa: acceptable, probably helpful
Class IIb: acceptable, possibly helpful
Class III: not indicated, may be harmful
a. Sodium bicarbonate 1 mEq/kg is Class I if patient has known preexisting hyperkalemia.
b. Sodium bicarbonate 1 mEq/kg IV:
Class IIa
• If known preexisting bicarbonate-responsive acidosis
• If overdose with tricyclic antidepressants
• To alkalinize the urine in drug overdoses
Class IIb
• If intubated and continued long arrest interval
• Upon return of spontaneous circulation after long arrest interval
Class III
• Hypoxic lactic acidosis
c. The recommended dose of epinephrine is 1 mg IV push every 3-5 min. If this approach fails, several Class IIb dosing regimens can be considered:
• Intermediate: epinephrine 2-5 mg IV push, every 3-5 min
• Escalating: epinephrine 1 mg-3 mg-5 mg IV push, 3 min apart
• High: epinephrine 0.1 mg/kg IV push, every 3-5 min
d. The shorter atropine dosing interval (3 min) is possibly helpful in cardiac arrest (Class IIb).

Figure 19.9. Pulseless electrical activity (PEA) algorithm (electromechanical dissociation [EMD]). (Reproduced with permission from Textbook of Advanced Cardiac Life Support. Copyright 1994, American Heart Association.)

OXYGEN

Actions

Supplemental oxygen is an essential drug during CPR. Oxygen delivery to organs and tissues is highly compromised during cardiopulmonary arrest. Severe hypoxemia in the compromised patient leads to anaerobic metabolism, lactic acid accumulation, and acidosis. Even with properly performed chest compressions, only

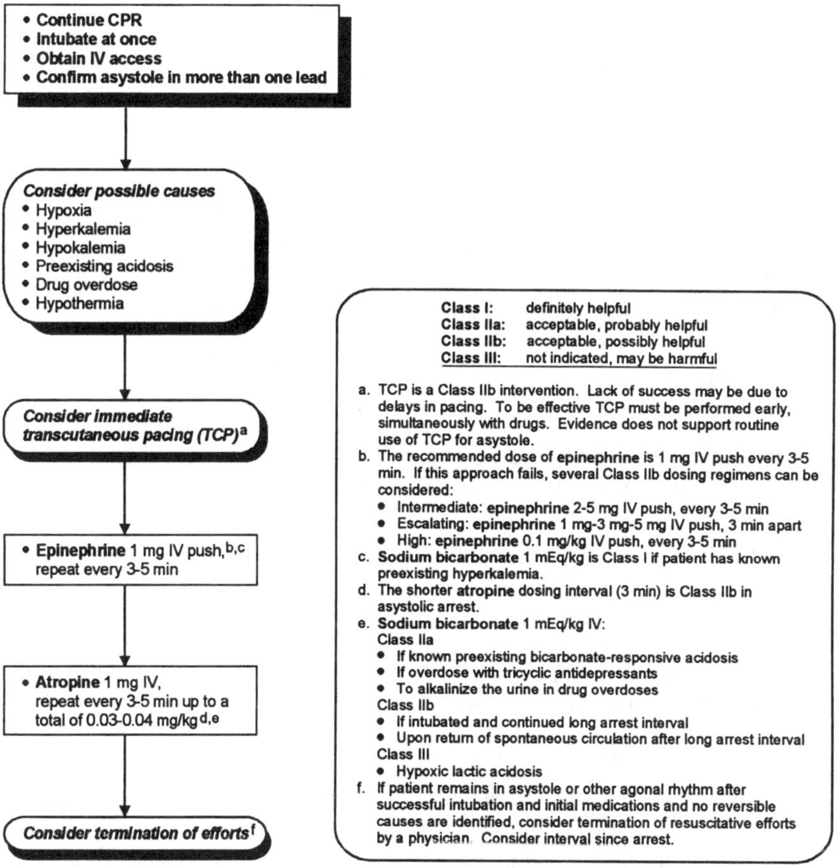
• Continue CPR
• Intubate at once
• Obtain IV access
• Confirm asystole in more than one lead
Consider possible causes
• Hypoxia
• Hyperkalemia
• Hypokalemia
• Preexisting acidosis
• Drug overdose
• Hypothermia
Consider immediate transcutaneous pacing (TCP)[a]
• Epinephrine 1 mg IV push,[b,c] repeat every 3-5 min
• Atropine 1 mg IV, repeat every 3-5 min up to a total of 0.03-0.04 mg/kg[d,e]
Consider termination of efforts[f]
Class I: definitely helpful
Class IIa: acceptable, probably helpful
Class IIb: acceptable, possibly helpful
Class III: not indicated, may be harmful
a. TCP is a Class IIb intervention. Lack of success may be due to delays in pacing. To be effective TCP must be performed early, simultaneously with drugs. Evidence does not support routine use of TCP for asystole.
b. The recommended dose of epinephrine is 1 mg IV push every 3-5 min. If this approach fails, several Class IIb dosing regimens can be considered:
• Intermediate: epinephrine 2-5 mg IV push, every 3-5 min
• Escalating: epinephrine 1 mg-3 mg-5 mg IV push, 3 min apart
• High: epinephrine 0.1 mg/kg IV push, every 3-5 min
c. Sodium bicarbonate 1 mEq/kg is Class I if patient has known preexisting hyperkalemia.
d. The shorter atropine dosing interval (3 min) is Class IIb in asystolic arrest.
e. Sodium bicarbonate 1 mEq/kg IV:
Class IIa
• If known preexisting bicarbonate-responsive acidosis
• If overdose with tricyclic antidepressants
• To alkalinize the urine in drug overdoses
Class IIb
• If intubated and continued long arrest interval
• Upon return of spontaneous circulation after long arrest interval
Class III
• Hypoxic lactic acidosis
f. If patient remains in asystole or other agonal rhythm after successful intubation and initial medications and no reversible causes are identified, consider termination of resuscitative efforts by a physician. Consider interval since arrest.

Figure 19.10. Asystole treatment algorithm. (Reproduced with permission from Guidelines for Cardiopulmonary Resuscitation and Emergency Cardiac Care. American Medical Association, 1992; 268:2171–2295.)

25 to 35% of the normal cardiac output is maintained. Therefore, oxygen delivery to the tissues is severely impaired. Irreversible cell death may occur if supplemental oxygen is not provided immediately. Oxygen administration elevates and maintains alveolar and arterial oxygen tension and content, thereby facilitating maximal tissue oxygenation (see Chapter 8).

Indications

1. Cardiopulmonary arrest.
2. Shock states.

3. Cardiac or pulmonary impaired patients when hypoxemia or hypoxia is present.
4. Poisoning or toxic states in which respiratory depression, acidosis, or decreased levels of consciousness are present.
5. Sickle cell anemia crisis.

Dosage

When available, 100% oxygen (via manual resuscitator) is given to all patients during cardiac arrest. After an endotracheal tube has been established, oxygen may be more effectively delivered directly to the lungs. There are no contraindications to 100% oxygen delivery in the short time required for resuscitation.

EPINEPHRINE

Actions

Epinephrine's potent pharmacologic action produces both α- and β-adrenoceptor responses. Epinephrine's sympathomimetic effects increase:

Myocardial automaticity (heart rate)
Myocardial contractile force
Myocardial oxygen consumption
Myocardial tone (e.g., converts fine V-fib to coarse V-fib).
Systemic vascular resistance
Systolic and diastolic blood pressures
Coronary and cerebral blood flow

The rise in systolic blood pressure after epinephrine administration is partly caused by its positive inotropic and chronotropic actions on the heart (predominantly β_1-adrenoceptors) and partly by the vasoconstriction induced in various vascular beds (α-adrenoceptors). The potent arterial and peripheral vasoconstricting effects of epinephrine via α stimulation increases aortic diastolic pressure as well, which facilitates coronary and cerebral perfusion pressure and ultimately coronary and cerebral blood flow. Epinephrine is the drug of first choice during CPR rather than pure α-adrenoceptor drugs because pure α-adrenoceptor drugs do not enhance and support cerebral blood flow to the same extent as epinephrine (see Chapters 10 and 18).

Indications

1. Primary, first-line drug of choice for anaphylactic shock and cardiac arrest.
2. For use during the resuscitation effort.
3. Antidote of choice for histamine overdose and allergic reactions.
4. Stokes-Adams syndrome.
5. Profound symptomatic bradycardia.

Dosage

For cardiac arrest: 0.5 to 1 mg (5 to 10 ml of 1:10,000 solution) given by IV push.

During resuscitation effort: 0.5 mg to 1 mg (5 to 10 ml of 1:10,000 solution) given by IV push, repeated every 5 minutes as needed. If the patient fails to respond to the standard 1 mg IV dose, one of the following dosing regimens should be considered:

- Intermediate: 2 to 5 mg IV push, given every 3 to 5 minutes.
- Escalating: 1 mg–3 mg–5 mg IV push, given 3 minutes apart.
- High: 0.1 mg/kg IV push, given every 3 to 5 minutes.

Epinephrine may also be administered via endotracheal tube (1 to 2 mg in 10 ml distilled water) if an IV route has not been established. Chest compressions must be stopped; epinephrine is instilled into the endotracheal tube. During the resuscitation effort, epinephrine may also be administered by intracardiac injection into the left ventricular chamber. The intracardiac dose usually ranges from 0.3 to 0.5 mg (3 to 5 ml of 1:10,000 solution). Pediatric: 0.01 mg/kg of 1:10,000 solution (0.1 ml/kg) given IV, ET, or IC.

ATROPINE

Actions

Atropine is a parasympatholytic drug that acts to accelerate the rate of sinus node discharge, improve atrioventricular (AV) conduction by inhibiting vagal tone, and possibly restore cardiac rhythm by initiating electrical activity during asystolic cardiac arrest (see Chapter 10).

Indications

1. Sinus bradycardia with accompanied hemodynamic compromised hypotension, ventricular ectopy, and/or myocardial ischemia.
2. Ventricular asystole.
3. Heart block.

Dosage

For patients with bradyasystolic cardiac arrest: 1 mg IV, repeated every 3 to 5 minutes if asystole persists, up to a total dose of 0.03 to 0.04 mg/kg.

Endotracheal administration: 1 to 2 mg diluted with 10 ml sterile water or normal saline.

For symptomatic bradycardia: Range; 0.5 to 1.0 mg, repeated at 5-minute intervals as needed, up to a maximum dose of 2–3 mg for patients with coronary artery disease (0.03 to 0.04 mg/kg). Lower doses (<0.5 mg) may cause rebound vagotonic effects (e.g., paradoxical bradycardia), which may precipitate ventricular fibrillation.

Pediatric: 0.02 mg/kg IV or ET. Minimum dose 0.1 mg; maximum dose 1.0 mg. May be repeated in 5 minutes.

LIDOCAINE

Actions

Lidocaine is the antiarrhythmic drug of choice for ventricular ectopy. Lidocaine suppresses ventricular arrhythmias (V-tach, V-fib) by elevating the ventricular threshold and also terminates reentrant arrhythmias by suppressing myocardial conduction (see Chapters 15 and 18).

Indications

1. Primary, first-line drug for suppression of ventricular ectopy, including ventricular tachycardia and fibrillation.
2. For suppression of premature ventricular complexes (PVCs) for critically ill patients and patients in whom PVCs are associated with myocardial ischemia or infarction.
3. Prophylaxis against V-fib.
4. Drug of choice for wide-complex tachycardias of unknown origin.

Dosage

For pulseless V-tach or refractory V-fib: 1 to 1.5 mg/kg given by IV push. After administration, defibrillation should be reattempted. Lidocaine may be repeated every 3 to 5 minutes to a maximum dose of 3 mg/kg.

Endotracheal administration: 2 to 2.5 times the IV dose.

Pediatric: 1 to 1.5 mg/kg/dose IV bolus.

For primary prophylaxis against V-fib: Initial bolus of 1 to 1.5 mg/kg followed by continuous infusion at 2 to 4 mg/min (30 to 50 μg/kg/min). Reduce dose by 50% for patients with impaired hepatic blood flow (acute myocardial infarction, congestive heart failure, or shock).

PROCAINAMIDE

Actions

Procainamide suppresses ventricular ectopy and effectively terminates reentrant dysrhythmias by slowing ventricular conduction and prolonging the refractory period of ventricular tissue (see Chapter 18).

Indications

1. For persistent cardiac arrest caused by V-fib.
2. Suppression of PVCs, recurrent V-tach not controlled by lidocaine.
3. Convert or prevent supraventricular arrhythmias.

Dosage

For refractory V-fib: 30 mg/min until one of the following occurs:

- Hypotension
- Widening of the QRS complex by 50%
- Suppression of the arrhythmia
- Administration of a total of 17 mg/kg.

Maintenance IV infusion ranges from 1 to 4 mg/min.

BRETYLIUM

Actions

Bretylium is an antiarrhythmic agent that has both adrenergic and direct myocardial effects. When first administered, bretylium causes the early release of norepinephrine from the adrenergic postganglionic nerve terminals. Subsequently, bretylium inhibits norepinephrine release from peripheral adrenergic sites. Initially, hypertension, tachycardia, and, in some, an increase in the cardiac output is noted; then, orthostatic hypotension occurs from these effects. Bretylium also prevents the reuptake of norepinephrine, thereby potentiating the effects of exogenously administered catecholamines.

Bretylium produces a positive inotropic effect on the myocardium. It elevates the ventricular fibrillation threshold and also increases the action potential duration and effective refractory period in the heart, which may act to terminate reentrant dysrhythmias (see Chapter 18).

Indications

Bretylium is indicated for V-tach or V-fib that is refractory to lidocaine, procainamide, or repeated shocks. Bretylium is not indicated as first-line treatment during CPR efforts.

Dosage

For V-fib: 5 mg/kg undiluted bretylium, given by IV push.
For persistent V-fib: Increase dosage to 10 mg/kg and repeat as necessary.

MAGNESIUM

Actions

Magnesium is an essential body electrolyte that helps regulate body temperature, neuromuscular contraction, and synthesis of protein. Magnesium is required to stimulate enzymes that catalyze the reactions between phosphate ions and adenosine triphosphate (ATP). Magnesium also helps regulate the activities of the enzyme Na^+, K^+-ATPase mentioned in Chapter 18 as well as ion flow across sodium channels, certain potassium channels, and calcium channels. Hypomagnesemia can lead to arrhythmias, cardiac insufficiency, and even cardiac arrest. It can also precipitate refractory ventricular fibrillation and hinder the replenishment of intracellular potassium (see Chapter 17).

Indications

1. To reduce the incidence of postinfarction ventricular arrhythmias.
2. Treatment of choice for patients with torsades de pointes.
3. Digitalis-induced arrhythmias if hypomagnesemia is present.

Dosage

For acute administration during V-Tach: 1 or 2 g (2 to 4 ml of a 50% solution) of magnesium sulfate diluted in 10 ml 5% dextrose and given over 1 to 2 minutes. Administer magnesium by IV push for patients with V-fib.

For torsades de pointes: up to 5 to 10 g may be given (optimum dose not yet established).

SODIUM BICARBONATE

Actions

Sodium bicarbonate is used in the management of the metabolic component of acidosis. Metabolic acidosis results from anaerobic metabolism and the production of lactic acid during inadequate tissue oxygenation. Sodium bicarbonate buffers metabolic acidosis by reacting with hydrogen ions to form water and carbon dioxide:

$$H^+ + HCO_3^- \Leftrightarrow H_2CO_3 \Leftrightarrow H_2O + CO_2$$

As can be seen, sodium bicarbonate administration results in the rapid generation of carbon dioxide. The resultant high carbon dioxide content may worsen intracellular hypercarbia and acidosis in patients with cardiac arrest and may hinder cardiac muscle performance. Also, studies have shown that sodium bicarbonate administration during resuscitation efforts does not enhance ventricular defibrillation, improve spontaneous circulation, or facilitate survival in patients with cardiac arrest. Therefore, guidelines established by the AHA recommend that sodium bicarbonate should not be administered during the resuscitation effort; or, if it is administered, it should be performed only after defibrillation, chest compression, endotracheal intubation, vigorous hyperventilation (to reduce and correct acidosis) with 100% oxygen, and more than one trial of epinephrine have been used (see Chapter 13).

Indications

Lack of proof of efficacy of this drug has led to its not being recommended during CPR by the AHA. Its use is indicated only if preexisting metabolic acidosis, hyperkalemia, and tricyclic or phenobarbital overdose have been documented.

Dosage

If given: Initially, 1 mEq/kg by IV bolus, then a maximum of half the initial dose administered not more often than every 10 minutes. Solutions containing 8.4% (50 mEq/50 ml) sodium bicarbonate are recommended for administration during CPR.

REFERENCES/RECOMMENDED READING

Drug Facts and Comparisons. 49th ed. St. Louis: Facts and Comparisons, 1995.

Guidelines for Cardiopulmonary Resuscitation and Emergency Cardiac Care. American Medical Association, 1992;268:2171–2295.

Physicians' Desk Reference. 49th ed. Montvale, NJ: Medical Economics, 1995.

Textbook of Advanced Cardiac Life Support. American Heart Association, 1994.

APPENDICES III

STANDARD MEDICAL AND CARDIOPULMONARY ABBREVIATIONS AND SYMBOLS

A

I. SYMBOLS

Symbol	Meaning
♏	minim
℈	scruple
ʒ	dram
fʒ	fluidram
℥	ounce
f℥	fluidounce
O	pint
lb, #	pound
Rx	recipe (take)
Å	angström unit
Δ	change, heat
Ɛ	electroaffinity
mμ	millimicron, nanometer
μ g	microgram
m-	meta-
o-	ortho-
p-	para-
μm	micrometer
μ	micron
μμ	micromicron
+	plus; excess; acid reaction; positive

Symbol	Meaning
−	minus; deficiency; alkaline reaction; negative
±	plus or minus; either positive or negative; indefinite
#	number; following a number, pounds
÷, /	divided by
×	multiplied by; magnification
=	equals
~	approximate
≅	approximately equal to
>	greater than
<	less than
≮	not less than
≯	not greater than
≤	equal to or less than
≥	equal to or greater than
≠	not equal to
$\sqrt{}$	root; square root; radical
$\sqrt[2]{}$	square root

Symbol	Meaning	Symbol	Meaning
$\sqrt[3]{}$	cube root	♂	male
∞	infinity	♀	female
:	ratio; "is to"	⇔	denotes a reversible reaction
::	equality between ratios, "as"	↑	increase
∴	therefore	↓	decrease
°	degree	@	at
%	percent	[]	concentration
π	3.1416; ratio of circumference of a circle to its diameter		

II. Standard Medical Abbreviations and Meanings

Abbrev.	Meaning
ā	before
$\overline{aa}$	of each
AAA	abdominal aortic aneurysm
Ab	antibody
abd	abdomen
ABG	arterial blood gas
ABO	main blood group system
a.c.	before meals
Ac	acid
A-C	anti-inflammation corticoids
ACD	acid-citrate-dextrose
ACG	angiocardiography
ACLS	advanced cardiac life support
ACTH	adrenocorticotropic hormone
ad	to, up to
AD	right ear
ADH	antidiuretic hormone
ADL	activities of daily living
ad lib	as desired
adm	admitted, or admission
AE	above the elbow
AFB	acid-fast bacillus
AFP	alpha-fetoprotein
A/G	albumin/globulin ratio
Ag	antigen
agit	shake, stir
AGN	acute glomerulonephritis

Abbrev.	Meaning
$AgNO_3$	silver nitrate
ah (alt hor)	every other hour
AIDS	acquired immune deficiency syndrome
AK	above the knee
alk	alkaline
ALL	acute lymphocytic leukemia
ALS	amyotrophic lateral sclerosis (Lou Gehrig's disease)
ALTE	apparent life-threatening event
alt noc	every other night
a.m.	morning
a.m.a.	against medical advice
amb	ambulate, ambulatory
AMI	acute myocardial infarction
amp	ampule
amt	amount
ANA	antinuclear antibodies
ANS	autonomic nervous system
AOD	adult-onset diabetes mellitus
A-P	anterior-posterior
A & P	auscultation & percussion
approx	approximately (about)
aq	water
aq. dest.	distilled water
ARC	AIDS-related complex
ARD	acute respiratory distress
ARDS	adult respiratory distress syndrome
ARF	acute respiratory failure
ARF	acute renal failure
ARM	artificial rupture of membranes (obstetrics)
AS	left ear
AS	aortic stenosis
ASA	acetylsalicylic acid (aspirin)
asap	as soon as possible
ASD	atrial septal defect
ASHD	arteriosclerotic heart disease
ATN	acute tubular necrosis
ATP	adenosine triphosphate
AU	both ears
A-V	atrioventricular
A & W	alive and well
ax	axillary (armpit)

Abbrev.	Meaning
Ba	barium
BE	below the knee
BE	barium enema
BBB	bundle-branch block
BCLS	basic cardiac life support
bib	drink
b.i.d.	twice daily
b.i.n.	twice a night
BK	below the knee
BLL	bilateral lower lobes
BM	bowel movement
BMR	basal metabolic rate
BMT	bone marrow transplant
BP	blood pressure
BPD	bronchopulmonary dysplasia
BPH	benign prostatic hypertrophy
bpm	beats per minute, breaths per minute
BRP	bathroom privileges
BS	blood sugar
BS	breath sounds
BSA	body surface area
BSP	Bromsulphalein
BT	bleeding time
BUN	blood urea nitrogen
$\bar{c}$	with
C, °C	Celsius, centigrade
C-1	first cervical vertebra
Ca	calcium
CA, Ca	cancer
CABG	coronary artery bypass graft
CAD	coronary artery disease
cAMP	cyclic adenosine monophosphate
cap	capsule
CAT scan	computerized axial tomography scan
CBC	complete blood count
CBD	common bile duct
CBR	complete bed rest
cc	cubic centimeter
CC	chief complaint
CCF	cephalin cholesterol flocculation
CCU	coronary care unit

Abbrev.	Meaning
CD	communicable disease
CEA	carcinoembryonic antigen
CF	cystic fibrosis
cg	centigram
CGL	chronic granulocytic leukemia
CHB	complete heart block
CHD	coronary heart disease
CHF	congestive heart failure
CI	cardiac index
CK	creatine kinase
Cl	chlorine, chloride
cm	centimeter
c.m.	tomorrow morning
c/m	counts per minute
CM	competing message
cmH_2O	centimeters of water pressure
CMP	cardiomyopathy
CMV	continuous mechanical ventilation
c.n.	tomorrow night
CNS	central nervous system
CO	cardiac output, carbon monoxide
c/o	complained of
CO_2	carbon dioxide
COHb	carboxyhemoglobin
COLD	chronic obstructive lung disease
comp	compound
COMT	catechol-o-methyl-transferase
conc	concentration
COPD	chronic obstructive pulmonary disease
CP	cerebral palsy
CPAP	continuous positive airway pressure
CPD	cephalopelvic disproportion
CPK	creatine phosphokinase
cpm	counts per minute
CPR	cardiopulmonary resuscitation
CPT	chest physiotherapy
Cr	chromium
CRF	chronic renal failure
CS	cesarean section
C & S	culture and sensitivity
CSF	cerebrospinal fluid

Abbrev.	Meaning
CSR	central supply room
CST	convulsive shock therapy
CT scan	computerized tomography scan
Cu	copper
CV	cell volume
CV	cardiovascular
CVA	cerebrovascular accident
CVD	cardiovascular disease
CVI	cell volume index
CVP	central venous pressure
CW	cardiac work
CWP	coal workers' pneumoconiosis
Cx	cervix
CXR	chest x-ray
cysto	cystoscopy examination
CZI	crystalline zinc insulin
D	dose
d	day
/d	per day
DAT	diet as tolerated
db	decibels
DB&C	deep breath and cough
DC	discharge
d/c, dc	discontinue
DDX	differential diagnosis
decub	lying down
dg	decigram
Dg	decagram (dekagram)
DI	diabetes insipidus
DIC	disseminated intravasular coagulation
diff	(white cell) differential
dil	dissolve, dilute
dist	distilled
DKA	diabetic ketoacidosis
dl	deciliter
DM	diabetes mellitus
DNA	does not apply
DNA	deoxyribonucleic acid
DNAR	do not attempt resuscitation
DNR	do not resuscitate
DOA	dead on arrival

Abbrev.	Meaning
DOB	date of birth
2,3-DPG	2,3-diphosphoglycerate
DPT	diphtheria-pertussis-tetanus
dr	dram
DR	dressing room, delivery room
Dr.	doctor
DRG	diagnosis related group
drsg	dressing
DS	double strength
DTs	delirium tremens
DVT	deep vein thrombosis
Dx	diagnosis
D_5W	5% dextrose in water
EBV	Epstein-Barr virus
EC	enteric-coated
ECC	emergency cardiac compression
ECD	expected date of confinement
ECG	electrocardiogram
ECF	extracellular fluid
ECMO	extracorporeal membrane oxygenation
ECT	electroconvulsive therapy
EDC	estimated date of confinement
EDD	expected delivery date
EDTA	ethylenediaminetetraacetic acid
EDV	end-diastolic volume
EEG	electroencephalogram
EENT	eyes, ears, nose, throat
EF	ejection fraction
e.g.	for example
EGTA	esophageal gastric tube airway
EI	effort index
EKG	electrocardiogram
EL	effective level
ELISA	enzyme-linked immunosorbent assay
elix, el	elixir
EM	effective masking
EMD	electromechanical dissociation
EMG	electromyogram
EMIT	enzyme-multiplied immunoassay technique
EMS	emergency medical system
emuls	emulsion

Abbrev.	Meaning
en, enem	enema
ENT	ears, nose, throat
EOA	esophageal obturator airway
EOM	extraocular movements
eos	eosinophil
ER	emergency room
ERPF	effective renal plasma flow
ERV	expiratory reserve volume
ESP	extrasensory perception
ESR, SR	erythrocyte sedimentation rate
ESRD	end-stage renal disease
EST	electric shock therapy
et	and
ETA	estimated time of arrival
EUA	examination under anesthetic
ext	extract
F, °F	Fahrenheit
f/b	followed by
FBS	fasting blood sugar
FD	fatal dose
FDA	Food and Drug Administration
Fe	iron
FEF	forced expiratory flow
FEV	forced expiratory volume
FFB	flexible fiberoptic bronchoscopy
FH	family history
FHR	fetal heart rate
FHS	fetal heart sound
FHT	fetal heart tone
fl, fld	fluid
Fr	French (catheter size)
FRC	functional residual capacity
FSH	follicle-stimulating hormone
FTA	fluorescent treponemal antibody
FTND	full-term normal delivery
FTT	failure to thrive
FUO	fever of undetermined origin
FVC	forced vital capacity
Fx	fracture
G	gauge, gravida
g, gm	gram

Abbrev.	Meaning
GA	gastric analysis
GA	general anesthetic
gal	gallon
garg	gargle
GB	gallbladder
GC	gonococcus
GFR	glomerular filtration rate
GGT	gamma glutamyl transpeptidase
GH	growth hormone
GI	gastrointestinal
GIT	gastrointestinal tract
Gm, gm	gram
GP	general practitioner
gr	grain
GTT	glucose tolerance test
gtt	drops
GU	genitourinary
GUT	genitourinary tract
GVH	graft-versus-host
Gyn	gynecology
h, hr	hour
H	hypodermic
H_2O_2	hydrogen peroxide
HAV	hepatitis A virus
HB	hepatitis B
Hb, Hgb	hemoglobin
HBD	hydroxybutyric dehydrogenase
HBO	hyperbaric oxygen
HBV	hepatitis B virus
HCG	human chorionic gonadotropic hormone
HCI	hydrochloric acid
HCO_3	bicarbonate
HCT, Hct	hematocrit
HCVD	hypertensive cardiovascular disease
HDL	high-density lipoprotein
HDN	hemolytic disease of the newborn
hg	hectogram
Hg	mercury
Hgb	hemoglobin
hGH	human growth hormone
HI	hemagglutination inhibition

Abbrev.	Meaning
HIV	human immunodeficiency virus
HL	hearing level
HMD	hyaline membrane disease
h.n.	tonight
h/o	history of
HPI	history of present illness
hPL	human placental lactogen
HR	heart rate
h.s.	bedtime
Ht	height
HVA	homovanillic acid
Hx	history
Hz	hertz
I	radioactive iodine
IABP	intra-aortic balloon pump
IBS	irritable bowel syndrome
IBW	ideal body weight
IC	inspiratory capacity
ICD	isocitrate dehydrogenase
ICF	intracellular fluid
ICP	intracranial pressure
ICU	intensive care unit
id	the same
ID	intradermal
I & D	incision and drainage
IDDM	insulin-dependent diabetes mellitus
Ig	immunoglobulin
IH	infectious hepatitis
ILD	interstitial lung disorders
IM	intramuscular
IMV	intermittent mandatory ventilation
in.,"	inches
inf	infusion
inhal	inhalation
inj	injection
invol	involuntary
I & O	intake and output
IOP	intraocular pressure
IPPA	inspection, palpation, percussion, auscultation
IPPB	intermittent positive pressure breathing
IPPV	intermittent positive pressure ventilation

Abbrev.	Meaning
IRDS	infant respiratory distress syndrome
irrig	irrigation
IS	intracostal space
IU	international unit
IV	intravenous
IVCD	intraventricular conduction defect
IVGTT	intravenous glucose tolerance test
IVP	intravenous pyelogram
IVPB	intravenous "piggyback"
IVT	intravenous transfusion
JVD	jugular venous distention
K	potassium
K, °K	Kelvin
KCI	potassium chloride
kg	kilogram
KUB	kidney, ureter, bladder
KVO	keep vein open
L, l	liter
L	left, lumbar
L^{-1}	first lumbar vertebra
LA	left atrium, long-acting
L & A	light and accommodation
Lab	laboratory
LAD	left anterior descending
Lap	laparotomy
LAP	leucine aminopeptidase
LAP	left atrial pressure
lat	lateral
lb, #	pound
LBBB	left bundle branch block
LD	lethal dose
LDH	lactic dehydrogenase
LDL	low-density lipoprotein
LE	lupus erythematosus
LGA	large for gestational age
LH	luteinizing hormone
LHF	left heart failure
lin	liniment
liq	liquid, solution
LLE	left lower extremity
LLL	left lower lobe

Abbrev.	Meaning
LLQ	left lower quadrant
LMP	last menstrual period
LOA	left occipitoanterior
LOC	level of consciousness
lot	lotion
LP	lumbar puncture
LSD	lysergic acid diethylamide
LSK	liver, spleen, kidneys
lt	left
LTC	long-term care
LUE	left upper extremity
LUL	left upper lobe
LV	left ventricle
LVEDP	left ventricular end-diastolic pressure
LVET	left ventricular ejection time
LVF	left ventricular failure
LVH	left ventricular hypertrophy
lymph	lymphocyte
M	mix, thousand
m	minim, meter
MAO	monoamine oxidase
MAP	mean (systemic) arterial pressure
MAST	military antishock trousers
mcg	microgram
MCH	mean corpuscular hemoglobin
MCHC	mean corpuscular hemoglobin concentration
MCL	midclavicular line
MCU	maximum care unit
MCV	mean corpuscular volume
MDI	metered-dose inhaler
med	medicine
MED	minimal effective dose
MetHb	methemoglobin
m. et n.	morning and night
mEq	milliequivalent
mEq/L	milliequivalent per liter
MFD	minimum fatal dose
Mg	magnesium
mg	milligram
MI	myocardial infarction
min	minute(s)

Abbrev.	Meaning
mixt	mixture
ml	milliliter
MLC	mixed lymphocyte culture
MLD	masking level differences
mm	millimeter
mmHg	millimeters of mercury
mmole	millimole
mod	moderate
MOM	milk of magnesia
mOsm	milliosmole
MR×1	may repeat once
MRI	magnetic resonance imaging
MRSA	methicillin-resistant *Staphylococcus aureus*
MS	multiple sclerosis
MS	mitral stenosis
MS	musculoskeletal
MSL	midsternal line
MSOF	multiple systems organ failure
MSU	midstream urine
MUGA	multiple-gated acquisition scanning
MVP	mitral valve prolapse
MVV	maximum voluntary ventilation
myelo	myelocyte
N	nitrogen, normal
Na	sodium
NADH	nicotinamide-adenine-dinucleotide laced with hydrogen
$NaHCO_3$	sodium bicarbonate
NAD	no abnormality detected
NB	newborn, note carefully (note bene)
NDE	near death experience
nebul	a spray, nebulize
neg	negative
neuro	neurology
ng	nanogram
NG tube	nasogastric tube
nil	none
no. (#)	number
noct, noc	of the night
non rep	do not repeat
NPC	nodal premature complex
NPN	nonprotein nitrogen

Abbrev.	Meaning
NPO	nothing by mouth
NR	no refill, do not repeat
NS, N/S	normal saline (0.9%)
1/4 N/S	1/4 normal saline (0.2%)
1/2 N/S	1/2 normal saline (0.45%)
NSAID	nonsteroidal anti-inflammatory drug
nsq	not sufficient quantity
NSR	normal sinus rhythm
NYD	not yet diagnosed
ō	none
O_2	oxygen
OA	osteoarthritis
OB	obstetrics
OCT	ornithine carbamoyltransferase
od	once a day
OD	overdose, right eye
OGTT	oral glucose tolerance test
OHS	open heart surgery
OOB	out of bed
OPD	outpatient department
OPG	oculoplethysmography
Ophth	ophthalmology
OR	operating room
Ortho	orthopedics
os	mouth
OS	left eye
OSHA	Occupational Safety and Health Administration
Osm	one osmotically active unit per liter
OT	occupational therapy
OTC	over the counter
OU	both eyes
oz	ounce
p̄	after
P	pulse
PA	physician's assistant
PA	pulmonary artery
P-A	posterior-anterior
p.a.a.	let it be applied to the affected region
P & A	percussion and auscultation
PAC	premature atrial contraction
PALS	pediatric advanced life support

Abbrev.	Meaning
PAOP	pulmonary artery occlusion pressure
PAP	pulmonary artery pressure
Pap	Papanicolaou's smear test
Paren	parenterally
PASG	pneumatic antishock garment
PAT	paroxysmal atrial tachycardia
Path	pathology
PAWP	pulmonary artery wedge pressure
PBI	protein bound iodine
p.c.	after meals
PCG	phonocardiogram
PCN	penicillin
PCO_2	partial pressure of carbon dioxide
PCP	*Pneumocystis carinii* pneumonia, phencyclidine
PCV	packed cell volume (hematocrit)
PCWP	pulmonary capillary wedge pressure
PDA	patent ductus arteriosus
PE (Px)	physical examination
PE	pulmonary emboli
Peds	pediatric
PEEP	positive end-expiratory pressure
PEP	pre-ejection period
per	by, through
PERRL	pupils equal, regular, react to light
PET	preeclampsic toxemia
PETT	positron emission transaxial tomography
PI	present illness
PIE	pulmonary interstitial emphysema
Pg	picogram
PH	past history
PHA	phytohemagglutinin
physio	physiotherapy
PID	pelvic inflammatory disease
PKU	phenylketonuria
pl. ct.	blood platelet count
p.m.	afternoon
PMI	point of maximal impulse
PND	paroxysmal nocturnal dyspnea
PNS	peripheral nervous system
p.o.	by mouth

Abbrev.	**Meaning**
PO_2	partial pressure of oxygen
pop	plaster of paris
postop	postoperative(ly)
PPD	purified protein derivative
p.r.	through the rectum
premed	premedication
preop	preoperative(ly)
prep	preparation
p.r.n.	as needed
Prog	prognosis
pro time	prothrombin time
PSP	phenolsulfonphthalein
psych	psychiatry (psychology)
pt	pint, patient
PT	prothrombin time, physical therapy
PTH	parathyroid hormone
PTS	permanent threshold shift
pulv	powder
PUO	pyrexia of unknown origin
p.v.	through the vagina
PVC	premature ventricular contraction
PVD	peripheral vascular disease
PVR	pulmonary vascular resistance
PZI	protamine zinc insulin
q	every
q.a.m.	every morning
q.d.	every day
q.h.	every hour
q.2h., q.3h.	every 2 hours, every 3 hours, etc.
q.h.s.	every night
q.i.d.	four times a day
q.m.	every morning
q.n.	every night
q.n.s.	quantity not sufficient
q.o.d.	every other day
q.s.	sufficient quantity
qt	quart
R	right, respiration, rectal
RA	right atrium, rheumatoid arthritis
RAP	right atrial pressure
RAST	radioallergosorbent test

Abbrev.	Meaning
RBBB	right bundle branch block
RBC	red blood cells, red blood count
RD	respiratory disease
RDDA	recommended daily dietary allowance
RDS	respiratory distress syndrome
rep	may be repeated
req	requisition
RES	reticuloendothelial system
RF	rheumatoid factor
Rh	Rhesus, the Rh factor of blood
Rh Neg	Rhesus factor negative
RISA	radioiodinated serum albumin
RICE	rest, ice, compression, elevation
RL	right lateral
R & L	right and left
RLE	right lower extremity
RLF	retrolental fibroplasia
RLL	right lower lobe
RLQ	right lower quadrant
RML	right middle lobe
RNA	ribonucleic acid
ROM	range of motion
ROS	review of systems
RR	respiratory rate
RSV	respiratory syncytial virus
Rt (rt)	right
RUE	right upper extremity
RUL	right upper lobe
RUQ	right upper quadrant
RVEDP	right ventricular end-diastolic pressure
RV	residual volume, right ventricle
RVP	right ventricular pressure
Rx	prescription, take
$\bar{s}$	without
s, sec	seconds
S-A	sinoatrial (node)
SAD	seasonal affective disorder
sang	sanguineous
SaO_2	saturation of arterial oxygen with hemoglobin
sat	saturate
SB	sternal border

Abbrev.	Meaning
SBE	subacute bacterial endocarditis
SBMPL	simultaneous binaural midplane localization
SC, subcu	subcutaneous
SCAT	sheep cell agglutination test
SD	skin dose
SG	specific gravity
SGA	small for gestational age
SGOT	serum glutamic-oxaloacetric transaminase
SGPT	serum glutamic-pyruvic transaminase
SH	serum hepatitis
SHGB	sex hormone-binding globulin
SI	international system of units, seriously ill
SIDS	sudden infant death syndrome
sig	write, label
SK-SD	streptokinase-streptodornase
SL, subling	sublingual
SLE	systemic lupus erythematosus
SMR	submucous resection
SOA	swelling of ankles
SOB	short(ness) of breath
sol	solution
solv	dissolve
s.o.s.	if necessary, if needed
S/P	status post; no change after
sp, spt	spirits
spec	specimen
Sp gr	specific gravity
SR	sustained-release
SR (sed rate)	sedimentation rate
SRS-A	slow-reacting substance of anaphylaxis
SS (ss)	soap solution, soap suds (enema)
$\overline{ss}$	one half
staph	*Staphylococcus*
stat	immediately
st dr	straight drainage
STH	somatotropic hormone
STP	standard temperature and pressure
Strep	*Streptococcus*
STS	serologic test for syphilis
supp.	suppository
susp	suspension

Abbrev.	Meaning
SV	stroke volume
$S\bar{v}O_2$	saturation of venous oxygen with hemoglobin
SVR	systemic vascular resistance
SVT	supraventricular tachycardia
Sx	symptoms
syr	syrup
T	temperature
T-1	first thoracic vertebra
tab	tablet
T & A	tonsillectomy and adenoidectomy
TB	tuberculosis
TBG	thyroxine-binding globulin
Tbsp, Tbl	tablespoon
TBSA	total body surface area
TCN	tetracycline
THR	total hip replacement
TIA	transient ischemic attack
t.i.d.	three times a day
t.i.n.	three times a night
tinct, tn	tincture
TKR	total knee replacement
TLC	tender loving care
TNR	tonic neck reflex
To	telephone order
top	topically
TPN	total parenteral nutrition
TPR	temperature, pulse, respiration
tr	tincture
TSH	thyroid-stimulating hormone
tsp, t	teaspoon
TTS	temporary threshold shift
TU	toxic unit
TUPR	transurethral prostatic resection
TUR	transurethral resection
Tx	treatment
U,u	unit
UA	urinalysis
UAO	upper airway obstruction
UD	unit dose
ung	ointment
ur	urine

Abbrev.	Meaning
Ur. ac	uric acid
URI	upper respiratory infection
USP	United States Pharmacopeia
ut dict	as directed
UTI	urinary tract infection
v	vein
vag	vaginal
VC	vital capacity
VCG	vectorcardiogram
VD	venereal disease
VDH	valvular disease of the heart
VDRL	venereal disease research laboratory test
vin	wine
VLDL	very low-density lipoprotein
VMA	vanilymandelic acid
VO	verbal order
VS	vital signs
VSD	ventricular septal defect
VW	vessel wall
w/	with
WBC	white blood cells, white blood count
WDWN	well developed, well nourished
WF/BF	white female, black female
WM/BM	white male, black male
WNL	within normal limits
WOB	work of breathing
WOH	work of heart
WR	Wassermann reaction
ws	water soluble
Wt	weight
x	multiplied by

III. Abbreviations and Symbols Used in Cardiopulmonary Care

A. General Abbreviations

Abbrev.	Meaning
P	pressure in general
V	volume in general
$\bar{X}$	dash above any symbol indicates a mean value (e.g., $\bar{P}$ indicates a mean or average pressure)
$\dot{X}$	dot above any symbol indicates a time derivative, (e.g., $\dot{V}$ indicates volume per minute, or flow (LPM)

%X	percent sign before a symbol indicates percentage of the predicted normal value
X/Y%	percent sign after a symbol indicates a ratio that is expressed as a percentage (e.g., FEV_1/FEV% = 100 × FEV_1/FVC)
f	frequency of any event in time
t	time
anat	anatomic
max	maximum

B. Gas Phase Symbols and Abbreviations

Abbrev.	**Meaning**
V	gas volume
F	fractional concentration in dry gas phase
I	inspired
E	expired
A	alveolar
T	tidal
D	dead space
B	barometric
L	lung
R	respiratory exchange ratio ($\dot{V}CO_2/\dot{V}O_2$)
STPD	standard temperature, pressure, dry (O°C, 760 mmHg, without water vapor—dry)
BTPS	body temperature, pressure saturated (37°C, barometric pressure—sea level = 760 mmHg, saturated with water vapor)
ATPD	ambient temperature and pressure, without water vapor (dry)
ATPS	ambient temperature and pressure, saturated with water vapor

Note: Gas volumes in the lung are measured under BTPS conditions, whereas oxygen and carbon dioxide production are measured at STPD.

C. Combined Volume and Ventilation Measurement Abbreviations

Abbrev.	**Meaning**
V_T	tidal volume
V_A	alveolar volume
V_D	dead-space volume
V_I	inspired volume
V_E	expired volume
$\dot{V}_A$	alveolar ventilation per minute (BTPS)
$\dot{V}_{Dphy}$	physiologic dead-space ventilation per minute (BTPS)
$\dot{V}_{Danat}$	anatomic dead-space ventilation per minute (BTPS)
$\dot{V}_{Dalv}$	alveolar dead-space ventilation per minute (BTPS)
$\dot{V}_I$	inspired volume per minute (BTPS)

$\dot{V}_E$	expired volume per minute (BTPS)
$\dot{V}O_2$	oxygen consumption per minute (STPD)
$\dot{V}CO_2$	carbon dioxide production per minute

D. Blood Phase Abbreviations

Abbrev.	**Meaning**
$\dot{Q}$	volume flow of blood per minute
C	concentration in blood phase
S	saturation in blood phase
b	blood in general
a	arterial
v	venous
$\bar{v}$	mixed venous
c	capillary
c'	pulmonary end-capillary
s	shunt
t	total

E. Combined Blood Phase Abbreviations

Abbrev.	**Meaning**
$\dot{Q}c$	pulmonary capillary blood volume per minute
$\dot{Q}s$	shunted cardiac output (venous admixture portion)
$\dot{Q}t$	total blood volume per minute—cardiac output
$\dot{Q}s/\dot{Q}t$	shunted blood volume compared with the total blood volume

F. Gas Tension and Blood Gas Measurement Abbreviations

Abbrev.	**Meaning**
P_B	barometric pressure
FIO_2	fractional concentration of inspired oxygen
FEO_2	fractional concentration of expired oxygen
$FECO_2$	fractional concentration of expired carbon dioxide
PAO_2	partial pressure (tension) of oxygen in the alveoli
$PACO_2$	partial pressure (tension) of carbon dioxide in the alveoli
PaO_2	partial pressure (tension) of arterial oxygen
$PaCO_2$	partial pressure (tension) of arterial carbon dioxide
$P\bar{v}O_2$	mixed venous oxygen tension
$P\bar{v}CO_2$	mixed venous carbon dioxide tension
SaO_2	arterial oxygen saturation
$S\bar{v}O_2$	mixed venous oxygen saturation
SpO_2	oxygen saturation measured by pulse oximetry
$Cc'O_2$	oxygen content of pulmonary end-capillary blood
CaO_2	arterial oxygen content

$C\bar{v}O_2$	mixed venous oxygen content
$C(a\text{-}v)O_2$	arterial-venous oxygen content difference (also known as a-vDO_2)
$P(A\text{-}a)O_2$	alveolar-arterial oxygen pressure difference (also known as A-aDO_2)

G. Mechanics of Breathing Abbreviations

Abbrev.	**Meaning**
P_{bs}	body surface pressure (equal to P_B)
P_{aw}	airway pressure
P_{alv}	alveolar pressure
P_{ao}	pressure at the airway opening (mouth, nose, trachea)
P_{pl}	intrapleural pressure
P_L	transpulmonary pressure ($P_L = P_{alv} - P_{pl}$)
P_W	transthoracic pressure ($P_W = P_{pl} - P_{bs}$)
P_{rs}	transrespiratory pressure ($P_{rs} = P_{alv} - P_{bs}$)
P_{es}	esophageal pressure
PI_{max}	maximal inspiratory pressure (MIP)
PE_{max}	maximal expiratory pressure (MEP)
R	flow resistance (pressure/flow − cmH_2O/L/sec)
R_L	total pulmonary resistance
R_{aw}	airway resistance
G_{aw}	airway conductance (equal to $1/R_{aw}$)
sG_{aw}	airway conductance at a specific lung volume
El	elastance (equal to $1/C_{st}$)
C_{st}	static compliance (patient/ventilator system compliance is referred to as effective static compliance—C_{es})
C_{dyn}	dynamic compliance (reflection of the total ventilatory system impedance)
C/V_L	specific compliance (compliance divided by a specific lung volume; usually FRC)
W, WOB	work of breathing
WOH	work of heart

H. Pulmonary Function Abbreviations

Abbrev.	**Meaning**
TLC	total lung capacity: volume of air contained within the lung after a maximum inspiration
VC	vital capacity: maximum volume of air that can be exhaled after a maximal inspiration
IC	inspiratory capacity: maximum volume of air that can be inspired from a resting exhalation

Abbrev.	**Meaning**
IVC	inspiratory vital capacity: maximum volume of air that can be inspired after a complete expiration
FRC	functional residual capacity: volume of gas remaining in the lung at the end of a resting exhalation
RV	residual volume: volume of air remaining in the lung after a maximal expiration
ERV	expiratory reserve volume: maximum volume of air that can be exhaled from a resting exhalation
IRV	inspiratory reserve volume: maximum volume of air that can be inspired from a resting inspiration
V_T	tidal volume: volume of air inhaled or exhaled during a normal breath
FVC	forced vital capacity: volume of air that can be forcefully and rapidly exhaled after a maximal inspiration
FIVC	forced inspiratory vital capacity: volume of air that can be forcefully and rapidly inhaled after a complete expiration
SVC	slow vital capacity: volume of air that can be exhaled (or inhaled) slowly and completely after a maximal inspiration (or maximal expiration)
FEV_1	forced expiratory volume in 1 second: the volume of air exhaled in 1 second during an FVC maneuver
$FEV_1\%$	forced expiratory volume in 1 second, expressed as a percent ($FEV_1/FVC \times 100$)
PEFR	peak expiratory flow rate: the peak flow of air that can be forcefully exhaled after a maximal inspiration—L/min or L/sec
$FEF_{200-1200}$	forced expiratory flow from 200 ml to 1200 ml: measures the average flow of the early part of an FVC maneuver (formerly $MEFR_{200-1200}$—maximal expiratory flow rate)
$FEF_{25\%-75\%}$	forced expiratory flow from 25% to 75% of the FVC: measures the average flow rate during the midportion of an FVC maneuver (formerly MMFR—maximum mid-expiratory flow rate)
MVV	maximum voluntary ventilation: maximum volume of gas a patient can move in 1 minute (formerly MBC— maximum breathing capacity)
CV	closing volume: the volume of gas remaining in the lung when the small airways begin to close during a controlled complete exhalation—expressed as a percentage of the VC
CC	closing capacity: $CC = CV + RV$—expressed as a percentage of the TLC
D_L	diffusing capacity of the lung: the volume of gas per minute that crosses the alveolar-capillary membrane for a given partial pressure gradient

Abbrev.	Meaning
D_M	diffusing capacity of the pulmonary membrane
D_L/V_A	diffusion per unit of alveolar volume
V_C	average volume of blood in the capillary bed in milliliters
V/Q	ventilation to perfusion ratio: compares alveolar ventilation with the cardiac output
SBN_2	single breath nitrogen test: measures the distribution, or the evenness of ventilation after a single maximum inspiratory effort containing 100% oxygen is completely exhaled

IV. Chemical Element Abbreviations

Actinium	Ac	Gadolinium	Gd
Aluminum	Al	Gallium	Ga
Americium	Am	Germanium	Ge
Antimony	Sb	Gold	Au
Argon	Ar	Hafnium	Hf
Arsenic	As	Helium	He
Astatine	At	Holmium	Ho
Barium	Ba	Hydrogen	H
Berkelium	Bk	Indium	In
Beryllium	Be	Iodine	I
Bismuth	Bi	Iridium	Ir
Boron	B	Iron	Fe
Bromine	Br	Krypton	Kr
Cadmium	Cd	Lanthanum	La
Calcium	Ca	Lawrencium	Lr
Californium	Cf	Lead	Pb
Carbon	C	Lithium	Li
Cerium	Ce	Lutetium	Lu
Cesium	Cs	Magnesium	Mg
Chlorine	Cl	Manganese	Mn
Chromium	Cr	Mendelevium	Md
Cobalt	Co	Mercury	Hg
Copper	Cu	Molybdenum	Mo
Curium	Cm	Neodymium	Nd
Dysprosium	Dy	Neon	Ne
Einsteinium	Es	Neptunium	Np
Erbium	Er	Nickel	Ni
Europium	Eu	Niobium	Nb
Fermium	Fm	Nitrogen	N
Fluorine	F	Nobelium	No
Francium	Fr	Osmium	Os

Oxygen	O	Sulfur	S
Palladium	Pd	Tantalum	Ta
Phosphorus	P	Technetium	Tc
Platinum	Pt	Tellurium	Te
Plutonium	Pu	Terbium	Tb
Polonium	Po	Thallium	Tl
Potassium	K	Thorium	Th
Praseodymium	Pr	Thulium	Tm
Promethium	Pm	Tin	Sn
Protactinium	Pa	Titanium	Ti
Radium	Ra	Tungsten	W
Radon	Rn	Unnilhexium	Uah
Rhenium	Re	Unnilpentium	Unp
Rhodium	Rh	Unnilquadium	Unq
Rubidium	Rb	Unnilseptium	Uns
Ruthenium	Ru	Uranium	U
Samarium	Sm	Vanadium	V
Scandium	Sc	Xenon	Xe
Selenium	Se	Ytterbium	Yb
Silicon	Si	Yttrium	Y
Silver	Ag	Zinc	Zn
Sodium	Na	Zirconium	Zr
Strontium	Sr		

V. PREFIXES AND MULTIPLES USED IN THE INTERNATIONAL SYSTEM OF UNITS (SI)

Prefix	Symbol	Power
tera	T	10^{12}
giga	G	10^{9}
mega	M	10^{6}
kilo	k	10^{3}
hecto	h	10^{2}
deca	da	10^{1}
unity		1 (liter, gram, or meter)
deci	d	10^{-1}
centi	c	10^{-2}
milli	m	10^{-3}
micro	μ	10^{-6}
nano	n	10^{-9}
pico	p	10^{-12}
femto	f	10^{-15}
atto	a	10^{-18}

VI. COMMON BASE UNITS USED IN SI

Quantity	Name	Symbol
length	meter	m
mass	kilogram	kg
time	second	s
temperature	kelvin	K
electric current	ampere	amp
luminous intensity	candela	cd
amount of a substance	mole	mol

VII. SOME SI DERIVED UNITS

Quantity	Name	Symbol
area	square meter	m^2
volume	cubic meter	m^3
speed, velocity	meter per second	m/s
acceleration	meter per second squared	m/s^2
mass density	kilogram per cubic meter	kg/m^3
concentration of a substance	mole per cubic meter	mol/m^3
specific volume	cubic meter per kilogram	m^3/kg
luminescence	candela per square meter	cd/m^2

VIII. SI DERIVED NAMES WITH SYMBOLS

Quantity	Name	Symbol
frequency	hertz	Hz (s^{-1})
force	newton	N ($kg{\cdot}m{\cdot}s^{-2}$)
pressure	pascal	Pa ($N{\cdot}m^{-2}$)
energy, work	joule	J ($kg{\cdot}m^2{\cdot}s^{-2}$)
power	watt	W (J·s or J/s)
quantity of electricity	coulomb	C (A·s)
electromotive force	volt	V (W/A)
capacitance	farad	F (C/V)
conductance	siemens	S (A/V)
inductance	henry	H (Wø/A)
illuminance	lux	lx (ln/m^2)
absorbed (radiation) dose gray	Gy	(J/kg)
dose equivalent (radiation)	sievert	Sv (J/kg)
activity (radiation)	becquerel	Bq(s^{-1})
electrical resistance	ohm	Ω (V/a)

SELECTED BLOOD AND URINE STUDIES FOR THE CARDIOPULMONARY PATIENT

B

Section I: Introduction

I. Interpreting Test Results

A. The meaning of normal values is critical knowledge.
   1. Normal range varies to some degree from laboratory to laboratory. "Normal" can refer to:
      a. Normal health
      b. Ideal health state
      c. Average value
      d. Types of statistical distribution
   2. Reported reference range for a test varies with the method used as well as with the population tested.
   3. Each laboratory provides its own normal range for the specific testing method used and for the special population in which the set of values is described.

B. The meaning of abnormal values is critical knowledge.
   1. The health care provider must be able to recognize abnormal test results and the implications that pertain to the abnormal value as related to the patient's health state.
   2. The health care provider must be able to recognize "panic values" that indicate life-threatening situations.
      a. Clinical laboratories generally formulate their own critical laboratory values, and laboratory personnel are trained in the appropriate procedure for reporting critical laboratory values.
      b. Critical laboratory values must be reported immediately to the attending physician and documented.

C. Units of measurement
   1. Test results may be reported in conventional units or the International System of units (SI) (refer to Appendix A: Sections V through VIII).
   2. Many laboratories, scientific publications, and professional organizations are in the process of converting conventional units to the International System of units.
      a. In SI units, concentration is noted as amount per volume (moles or millimoles per liter) rather than mass per volume (grams, milligrams, or milli equivalents per deciliter, 100 milliliters, or liter)
      b. Numercial values may or may not differ between conventional units and SI units. For example, chloride has the same numerical value in both systems (98–108 mEq/L conventional and 98–108 mmol/L SI), whereas the normal range for calcium is 8.6–10.3 mg/dl conventional and 2.15–2.57 mmol/L SI (conversion factor of 0.2495).

II. Infection Control Issues

A. Health care providers must obtain, handle, and dispose all specimens properly according to Occupational Safety and Health Administration (OSHA) standards to minimize risks to themselves.
B. Health care providers must follow universal precautions.
   1. System of disease control that presupposes that contact with any body fluids is infectious and that each and every health care provider exposed to these fluids must be protected.
   2. Appropriate protective clothing and devices must be worn and correct handwashing must be followed.

III. Overview

A. Blood is a continuously circulating transport medium responsible for many vital bodily functions. Some of the primary functions include:
   1. Transporting oxygen (bound to hemoglobin in red blood cells) from the lungs to the body tissues and carrying carbon dioxide from the tissues to the lungs for elimination.
   2. Transporting nutrients from the intestine to all parts of the body, carrying certain waste products to the kidneys for excretion.
   3. Maintain acid-base balance via the blood buffering system.
   4. Maintain optimal temperature by distributing the heat produced from active muscles.
   5. Produce and deliver antibodies in the immune response.
   6. Maintain homeostasis with platelets and coagulation factors.
B. Composition
   1. Average person has approximately 5 L of blood (5 to 6 qt).
      a. 3 L consists of plasma.
         (1) An aqueous solution derived from the intestines and organs of the body.

(2) Normal plasma is usually thin and colorless when free from corpuscles or it may have a faint yellow tinge (straw-colored) when seen in thick layers.
(3) Consists of serum, protein, and chemical substances (electrolytes, glucose, enzymes, hormones, fats, bile pigments, and bilirubin). Also contains solids and dissolved gases.
(4) Plasma serves as the circulating transporting resource for the above-mentioned substances to various tissues and structures and also serves to transport waste products for elimination via the lungs, liver, kidneys, and spleen.

b. 2 L consists of formed elements.
(1) Primarily formed in the bone marrow and lymph (lymphocytes) and suspended in the plasma.
(2) The formed elements normally found in blood are classified as erythrocytes (red cells), leukocytes (white cells), and thrombocytes (platelets).
(3) The cells vary in size; the white cell is the largest, the red cell is next largest, and the platelets are the smallest.
(4) For every 500 red cells, there are generally approximately 30 platelets and only one white cell.

C. Types of blood samples.
1. The type of blood sample required depends on the nature of the test being analyzed.
a. Whole blood is required for blood gas analysis and hematologic studies.
b. Plasma and serum blood samples are required for most biochemical, immunologic, and coagulation studies.
2. Venous blood is used for most laboratory procedures owing to its representation of the body's physiologic status.
a. When multiple blood tests that require a good amount of blood are ordered, multiple venipunctures are avoided through the use of an evacuated tube system (Vacutainer, Corvac). This system contains interchangeable glass tubes with color-coded stoppers and enough vacuum to aspirate from 2 to 20 ml of blood. The color-coded stoppers indicate the type of additive placed within the glass tube:
(1) Red top (no additives): for tests performed on serum samples.
(2) Lavender top (contains EDTA): for tests performed on whole blood samples.
(3) Green top (contains heparin): for tests performed on plasma samples.
(4) Blue top (contains sodium citrate and citric acid): primarily for coagulation studies requiring plasma samples.

(5) Black top (contains sodium oxalate): same purpose as for blue tops (for plasma vitamin C).
(6) Gray top (contains a glycolytic inhibitor): for glucose analysis from serum or plasma samples.

3. Arterial blood is required for analysis of oxygen saturation to hemoglobin and for determination of PaO_2, $PaCO_2$, and pH.
4. Capillary blood may be obtained for studies in which laboratory microtechniques can be employed such as hemoglobin and hematocrit studies, blood smears, and certain clinical chemistry tests. Capillary blood samples may also be used in obtaining a blood gas sample, as long as the correct technique is employed (e.g., properly heating the site of puncture).

Section II. Blood Studies

IV. Hematology

A. The red blood cell (erythrocyte, red blood corpuscle).

1. The primary purpose of the red cell is to provide adequate amounts of circulatory hemoglobin.
    a. Via the hemoglobin in the red blood cell, oxygen is carried from the lungs to the tissues and carbon dioxide is transported from the tissues to the lungs.
2. Red cells also have the ability to transport large amounts of carbon dioxide for eventual absorption into the blood through the activity of its enzyme carbonic anhydrase (this red cell enzyme catalyzes the reaction of carbon dioxide and water). By this mechanism, red cells contribute to the body's acid-base balance.
3. Erythropoietin (a hormone produced primarily by the kidneys in response to hypoxia) stimulates the production of the red blood cell in the red bone marrow. This process is known as erythropoiesis.
4. The semipermeable membrane of the red blood cell permits swelling and rupture of the cell (hemolysis) when exposed to a hypotonic solution (less than 0.9% NaCl), or shrinkage of the cell (crenation) if exposed to a hypertonic solution (greater than 0.9% NaCl).
5. The mature erythrocyte has a lifespan of approximately 120 days.
6. Elimination of old or damaged red blood cells from the circulation is by the phagocytes (a type of cell that has the ability to engulf or destroy particulates in the blood) of the reticuloendothelial system (especially those cells of the spleen and liver).
7. Red blood cell count (RBC) (erythrocyte count).
    a. Determines the amount of red blood cells or erythrocytes found in a cubic millimeter of blood.
    b. Normal range:

(1) Men: 4.6–6.2 million/mm^3, or 4.6–6.2 × 10^{12}/L.
(2) Women: 4.2–5.4 million/mm^3, or 4.2–5.4 × 10^{12}/L.
(3) The average-sized person has approximately 35 trillion red blood cells.

c. Clinical implications.
(1) Anemia: reduction in circulating red blood cells, hemoglobin, and hematocrit.
(a) ETIOL: may result from excessive blood loss (acute or chronic hemorrhage), excessive blood cell destruction (hemolytic diseases), or deficient blood cell formation (defective nucleoprotein synthesis, dietary iron deficiency, loss of bone marrow, or bone marrow failure).
(2) Polycythemia: an excess of circulating red blood cells, hemoglobin, and hematocrit.
(a) Synonymous names: erythremia, erythrocytosis.
(b) ETIOL: altered production by bone marrow, chronic hypoxemia, acute poisoning, dehydration (from severe diarrhea, severe vomiting, heatstroke, massive fluid loss following extensive burns).
(3) People living in high altitudes will have high levels of red blood cells (to compensate for less atmospheric oxygen).

B. Hematocrit (HCT); Packed cell volume (PCV).
1. Determines the percentage by volume of packed red blood cells in a whole blood sample. The plasma and blood cells are separated by the process known as centrifugation.
2. Normal range:
a. Men: 42%–52% packed red cell volume.
b. Women: 37%–48% packed red cell volume.
3. Clinical implications.
a. A decreased value is indicative of anemia or hemodilution.
(1) A hematocrit less than 30% indicates moderate to severe anemia.
b. An increased value is indicative of polycythemia or hemoconcentration caused by blood loss.

C. Hemoglobin (Hb, Hgb).
1. Hemoglobin is a conjugated protein that forms the major component of the red cell (approximately 90% of the mature red cell's dry weight is hemoglobin). Hemoglobin consists of a protein (globin) to which an iron containing pigment (heme) is attached; therefore, hemoglobin synthesis is dependent on the metabolisms of heme, globin, and iron. Hemoglobin's primary function is to act as a vehicle to transport oxygen and carbon dioxide to and from the tissues, respectively. By this

mechanism, hemoglobin also serves as a buffer for regulating acid-base balance.

a. One gram of hemoglobin is able to carry 1.34 (or 1.39) ml of oxygen (resulting compound is oxyhemoglobin).
b. Hemoglobin that has given up its oxygen becomes deoxyhemoglobin, commonly known as "reduced hemoglobin."
   (1) Five grams or more of reduced hemoglobin per 100 ml of arterial blood causes cyanosis.
c. Hemoglobin activity at the tissue level:
   (1) Bohr effect: an increased $PaCO_2$ and a decreased blood pH enhances the unloading of oxygen from the hemoglobin molecule at the tissue level.
   (2) Haldane effect: oxygen unloading from the hemoglobin molecule enhances the binding of carbon dioxide to hemoglobin (resulting compound is carbaminohemoglobin).

2. Normal range:
   a. Men: 13–18 g/dl (or 13–18 g%–grams of Hb per 100 ml of blood) or 8.1–11.2 mmol/L.
   b. Women: 12–16 g/dl or 7.4–9.9 mmol/L.
   c. Critical values of hemoglobin include less than 8 g/dl (vitamin B_{12} deficiency or iron deficiency, heart failure) and greater than 18 g/dl (chronic obstructive pulmonary disease, thrombosis).
3. Clinical implications.
   a. A decreased value is associated with anemia.
   b. Panic value is less than 5 g/dl—leads to heart failure and death.
   c. An increased value indicates polycythemia.
4. Types of hemoglobin
   a. Hemoglobin A: the most common form of normal hemoglobin in the adult. Normal value is greater than 95% of the total hemoglobin content.
   b. Hemoglobin A_2: normal hemoglobin found in trace amounts in the adult. Normal value is 2.5%–4.0%.
   c. Hemoglobin F (fetal hemoglobin): normal hemoglobin in the red blood cells of the fetus and infant. Normal value is 60%–90% in newborns; 0%–4% in infants younger than 2 years of age; 0%–2% in adults. By the age of 1 year, fetal hemoglobin is replaced with adult hemoglobin (Hb A). Increased values of Hb F are associated with various types of anemia and with a condition known as thalassemia (an inherited defect in the production of hemoglobin).
   d. Hemoglobin S: a genetically inherited abnormal form of hemoglobin that causes sickle cell anemia.
   e. Hemoglobin M (methemoglobin): a form of hemoglobin that can-

not transport oxygen owing to the oxidation of ferrous iron to ferric iron in the heme portion of deoxygenated hemoglobin. Normal value is 2% of total hemoglobin content. Methemoglobinemia exists when higher than normal amounts of methemoglobin are present in the blood. Anoxia and cyanosis result.

f. Sulfhemoglobin: an abnormal hemoglobin formed by the action of hydrogen sulfide on blood. Excessive intake of phenacetin (Bromo-Seltzer), sulfonamides, and acetanilid produce sulfhemoglobinemia, which results in cyanosis.

g. Carboxyhemoglobin: formed by carbon monoxide and hemoglobin in carbon monoxide poisoning. Carbon monoxide and hemoglobin's affinity is approximately 210 times that of oxygen and hemoglobin. The result is anoxia because the carboxyhemoglobin is not able to transport oxygen to the tissues. Normal value is 0%–2.3% of total hemoglobin content; heavy smokers average 4%–5% carboxyhemoglobin levels. A toxic level is greater than 20%; 60% carboxyhemoglobin levels result in convulsion, respiratory arrest, death.

D. Reticulocyte
1. An immature red blood cell containing reticular material (network of granules or filaments in the cytoplasm).
2. Reticulocyte count.
   a. A measurement of the percentage of reticulocytes present in the total red blood cell count.
   b. Normal range:
      (1) Men: 0.5%–1.5% of the total RBC count.
      (2) Women: 0.5%–2.5% of the total RBC count.
   c. Clinical implications.
      (1) Reticulocytosis: a higher-than-normal concentration of reticulocytes.
         (a) ETIOL: hyperactive erythrocyte production is occurring, such as that which occurs after hemorrhage or during acclimatization to high altitude or by anemias caused by hemolysis or blood loss.
      (2) Reticulopenia: indicates that the bone marrow is not producing enough erythrocytes.
         (a) ETIOL: iron-deficiency anemia, aplastic anemia, chronic infection, radiation therapy, endocrine problems, untreated pernicious anemia, bone marrow tumor, myelodysplastic syndromes.

E. Erythrocyte sedimentation rate (sedrate, ESR).
1. A measurement of the rate at which erythrocytes settle out of unclotted blood in 1 hour.

2. Normal range:
   a. Men: 1–13 mm/hr.
   b. Women: 1–20 mm/hr.
3. Clinical implications.
   a. An increased sedimentation rate is noted in carcinoma, acute heavy metallic poisoning, pneumonia, severe anemia, inflammatory diseases, cell or tissue destruction, toxemia, all of the collagen diseases, infections, nephritis.
   b. A decreased sedimentation rate is noted in polycythemia vera, sickle cell anemia, congestive heart failure, hyperviscosity, or low plasma protein levels.

F. Red cell indices (erythrocyte indices, Wintrobe indices).
1. Provides important information about the size, hemoglobin concentration, and hemoglobin weight of an average red blood cell.
   a. Mean corpuscular volume (MCV): expresses the individual cell size; indicates whether the cell is normal in size (normocytic), larger than normal (macrocytic), or smaller than normal (microcytic).
      (1) Normal range: 84–99 fl/red cell.
   b. Mean corpuscular hemoglobin (MCH): a measure of the weight of hemoglobin in an average red blood cell; expressed as picograms of hemoglobin per red blood cell
      (1) Normal range: 26–32 pg/red cell.
   c. Mean corpuscular hemoglobin concentration (MCHC): measures the volume (percentage) of hemoglobin in the red cell and helps differentiate normally colored (normochromic) red cells from paler (hypochromic) red cells.
      (1) Normal range:30%–36% or 30–36 g Hb/dl RBC.
2. Clinical implications.
   a. Aids diagnosis and classification of anemias.

G. The white blood cell (leukocyte).
1. Primary function is to fight infection, defend the body against foreign organisms and transport and distribute antibodies in the immune response. The major weapon of the leukocytes is phagocytosis, a process in which the leukocytes engulf and actually digest bacteria, fragmented cells, and foreign particles. Pus, the product of inflammation, is a semiliquid mass of living and dead leukocytes and bacteria, as well as fragmented tissue cells.
2. Classification of the types of white blood cells is based on the presence or absence of granules in the cytoplasm. There are granular leukocytes (polymorphonuclear leukocytes) and nongranular leukocytes (mononuclear leukocytes).

3. Leukocytes are formed primarily in the red bone marrow (thereby known as myelogenous cells) and also in the lymphatic tissue (lymphocytes). After formation, the leukocytes are transported in the blood to the infected organ or tissue.
4. The lifespan of the leukocytes is variable, determined to some extent by the need for their services. The lymphatic system destroys the cells, and primary elimination is via fecal material.
5. White blood cell count (WBC) (leukocyte count).
   a. A measurement of the total circulating white blood cells.
   b. Normal range: 5000–10,000/ mm^3, or $5.0–10.0 \times 10^9$/L.
      (1) A white blood cell count less than 2000 is associated with bone marrow depression, whereas a leukocyte count of less than 500 indicates an extreme panic value and can be fatal because of a lack of protection against invading organisms. Patients must be placed in reverse isolation with personnel observing strict handwashing technique. A leukocyte count of greater than 50,000 indicates leukemia or severe infection.
6. Differential white blood cell count (Diff).
   a. Granulocytes (polymorphonuclear leukocytes–PMNs).
      (1) Neutrophils: comprise 60%–75% of total leukocyte count.
         (a) Band neutrophils (immature neutrophils): comprise 0%–10% of total neutrophils.
         (b) Segmented neutrophils: comprise 90%–100% of total neutrophils.
         (c) The most common type of granulocytic white blood cell; neutrophils are the body's first line of defense against infection. Neutrophils recognize foreign organisms and destroy them through phagocytosis. Each mature neutrophil can inactivate 5–20 bacteria.
      (2) Eosinophils: comprise 1%–4% of total leukocyte count.
         (a) Functions to combat parasitic infections and allergic disorders (as in asthma).
         (b) Eosinophils become active in the later stages of inflammation, detoxify foreign matter, and ingest antigen-antibody complexes before they can damage the body.
      (3) Basophils: comprise 0.5%–1% of total leukocyte count.
         (a) Essential in combating parasitic infections and to aid the nonspecific immune response to inflammation.
         (b) Tissue basophils are known as mast cells, and as with all basophils, they contain heparin, large amounts of histamine, and serotonin.
   b. Nongranulocytes (mononuclear leukocytes).

(1) Lymphocytes: comprise 20%–40% of total leukocyte count.
  (a) Essential in both the early and late stages of inflammation.
  (b) Lymphocytes function to produce antibodies and respond to a foreign antigen by neutralizing or eliminating it.
  (c) Lymphocytes B cells: after contact with a foreign antigen or infectious agent, the B cell changes into a plasma cell or a memory cell. Plasma cells produce antibodies, which then have the ability to destroy the foreign invader. Memory cells are available to produce antibodies upon reexposure to the foreign invader.
  (d) Lymphocyte T cells: mature T cells are antigen specific; each one responds to only one antigen. T cells are also responsible for regulating the activities of macrophages, B cells, and other T cells of the body, as well as aiding in tumor immunity, graft rejection, and hypersensitivity reactions. Subpopulations of T cells include:
    1. T4/helper cells: major regulatory cells that secrete interleukin-2 (IL-2), which stimulates B cells and other T lymphocytes into action. T4 cells also secrete gamma interferon, which has the ability to inhibit viral infections. The human immunodeficiency virus (HIV) in acquired immune deficiency syndrome (AIDS) primarily attacks and destroys T4 cells.
    2. T8/suppressor cells: aids the specific immune response and creates memory cells.
    3. Cytotoxic T cells and natural killer cells: directly kill other cells.

(2) Monocytes: comprise 2%–6% of total leukocyte count.
  (a) After circulating in the bloodstream, monocytes move into tissues and mature into macrophages. Through phagocytosis, monocytes and macrophages are primarily the body's second-line defense mechanism in the inflammatory response.

7. Clinical implications.
  a. Leukocytosis: an abnormally high number of white blood cells.
    (1) ETIOL: present in most bacterial infections, may also occur in unusually virulent infections such as diphtheria, pneumonia, and sepsis. Other causes include trauma or tissue injury, malignant diseases, toxins, serum sickness, tissue necrosis (caused by burns, myocardial infarcion, or gangrene) or inflammation. Unrestrained white cell production in the blood-forming organs is characteristic of leukemia, which is sometimes called "cancer of the blood."

b. Leukopenia: abnormal decrease in white blood cells.
   (1) Synonymous names: granulocytopenia, leukocytopenia.
   (2) ETIOL: failure of the bone marrow or bone marrow depression. Noted in radiation sickness, cancer chemotherapy, ingestion of mercury or other heavy metals, certain acute or chronic diseases (typhoid fever, influenza, measles, infectious hepatitis, mononucleosis, rubella).

c. Neutrophilia: an abnormally high percentage of circulating neutrophils.
   (1) ETIOL: infections (caused by septicemia, endocarditis, smallpox, chickenpox, herpes, Rocky Mountain spotted fever, gonorrhea, osteomyelitis), ischemic necrosis (caused by myocardial infarction, burns, carcinoma), stress response (caused by acute hemorrhage, surgery, emotional distress), inflammatory disease (caused by rheumatic fever, rheumatoid arthritis, acute gout, vasculitis and myositis).

d. Neutropenia: an abnormally low percentage of circulating neutrophils.
   (1) ETIOL: bone marrow depression (caused by radiation or cytotoxic drugs), deficiency of folic acid or vitamin B_{12}, collagen vascular disease (systemic lupus erythematosus), infections (caused by typhoid, hepatitis, influenza, infectious mononucleosis, measles, mumps, rubella, tularemia).

e. Eosinophilia: an abnormally high percentage of circulating eosinophils.
   (1) ETIOL: allergic disorders (as in asthma, hay fever, food or drug sensitivity, serum sickness), parasitic infections, certain skin diseases (eczema, psoriasis, dermatitis herpes), neoplastic diseases, pernicious anemia, scarlet fever, adrenocortical hypofunction.

f. Eosinopenia: an abnormally low percentage of circulating eosinophils.
   (1) ETIOL: stress response (caused by trauma, shock, burns, surgery), Cushing's syndrome.

g. Lymphocytosis: an abnormally high percentage of circulating lymphocytes.
   (1) ETIOL: infections (caused by pertussis, tuberculosis, hepatitis, mumps, German measles, cytomegalovirus, infectious mononucleosis, syphilis, brucellosis), hypoadrenalism, immune diseases, lymphocytic leukemia.

h. Lymphopenia: an abnormally low percentage of circulating lymphocytes

(1) ETIOL: severe congestive heart failure, severe renal failure, advanced tuberculosis increased adrenal corticosteroid production, immunodeficiency caused by immunosuppressives.

i. Monocytosis: an abnormally high percentage of circulating monocytes.

(1) ETIOL: infection (caused by subacute bacterial endocarditis, tuberculosis, hepatitis, malaria, Rocky Mountain spotted fever), collagen vascular disease, carcinomas, monocytic leukemia, lymphomas.

j. Basophilia: an abnormally high number of basophils.

(1) ETIOL: polycythemia vera, Hodgkin's disease, nephrosis, chronic hypersensitivity states, chronic myelocytic leukemia.

H. Complete blood count (CBC).

1. A basic screening test that gives vital comprehensive information regarding the patient's health state, includes the following tests:

a. Red blood cell count (RBC).

b. White blood cell count (WBC).

c. Differential white cell count (Diff).

d. Hematocrit (HCT).

e. Hemoglobin (Hgb).

f. Red blood cell indices.

g. Platelet count.

V. Hemostasis

A. Hemostasis and coagulation (an overview).

1. Hemostasis is the prevention of loss of blood from the blood vessels, whereby coagulation is the process that occurs to transform liquid blood or plasma into a semisolid gel: the clot.

2. Platelets, enzymes, and the protein fibrinogen are the primary components of the coagulation system.

3. Two pathways of the coagulation process exist.

a. Intrinsic pathway: coagulation occurs as a result of the activation of the clotting substances present in the circulating blood.

b. Extrinsic pathway: coagulation occurs as a result of tissue thromboplastin entering the blood.

4. Three-phase coagulation breakdown:

a. Phase I:

(1) In response to an injured site (e.g., a finger prick), platelets accumulate and disintegrate at the injured site and release a substance known as platelet factor. Activation of the platelet factor initiates the formation of thromboplastin.

b. Phase II:

(1) Thromboplastin formed in Phase I serves to initiate the conver-

sion of prothrombin (a plasma protein formed in the liver in the presence of vitamin K) to thrombin. Calcium ions and certain accelerator factors are necessary for rapid completion of the conversion.

c. Phase III:
   (1) Thrombin converts soluble fibrinogen to fibrin. Fibrin initially is a network of fine threads that eventually become denser, forming the substance of the clot: a firm but fairly elastic plug is produced at the injured site, thereby preventing the flow of blood through the injured tissue.

5. Intravascular coagulation, or thrombosis, indicates abnormal clotting of blood within the blood vessels. A thrombus (a result of thrombosis) is a stationary blood clot that may partially occlude or completely block the vessel in which it was formed. Occasionally, one of these clots may break loose and travel freely throughout the circulatory system until it plugs a vessel elsewhere in the body; the wandering clot is called an "embolus."
6. Fibrinolysis is the process in which the formed fibrin clot is dissolved through fibrinolytic enzymes.

B. Platelets (trombocytes).
   1. The smallest formed elements in the blood, platelets are fractured large white blood cells (megalokaryocytes) that function in coagulation/blood clotting. Platelets also preserve vascular integrity (platelets contain serotonin, which is liberated as platelets disintegrate and causes constriction of blood vessels and thereby further helps to control bleeding).
   2. Normal range: 150,000–350,000/mm^3, or 150–350 $\times$ 10^9/L.
      a. A panic value is a decrease in platelets of less than 50,000 and is associated with spontaneous bleeding, prolonged bleeding time, and small skin hemorrhages (petechiae or ecchymosis); when the platelet count drops below 5,000, fatal central nervous system (CNS) bleeding or massive gastrointestinal hemorrhage is possible. A platelet count greater than 1,000,000 is associated with leukemia.
   3. Clinical implications.
      a. Thrombocytopenia: an abnormally low number of platelets.
         (1) ETIOL: bone marrow disease, idiopathic thrombocytopenia purpura (ITP), pernicious, aplastic, and hemolytic anemias, HIV infection, disseminated intravascular coagulation (DIC), severe blood loss.
      b. Thrombocytosis: an abnormally high number of platelets.
         (1) ETIOL: trauma, splenectomy, heart disease, polycythemia

vera, chronic pancreatitis, myelofibrosis, chronic granulocytic leukemia.

(2) May lead to thrombosis (blood clots).

C. Thrombin time, thrombin clotting time.

1. A measurement of the time required for plasma to clot when thrombin is added to the blood sample. A clot should form almost instantly, if not, a fibrinogen deficiency exists.
2. Normal value: 10–15 seconds or control ± 5 seconds; normals vary widely between laboratories.
3. Clinical implications.
   a. Thrombin time is prolonged in the presence of anticoagulant therapy, DIC, hepatic disease, congenital abnormalities of fibrinogen, breakdown products of fibrin or fibrinogen.

D. Partial thromboplastin time (PTT); activated partial thromboplastin time (APTT).

1. A measurement of the time it takes plasma to form a fibrin clot; to determine coagulation disorders and/or to monitor heparin therapy.
2. Normal range: PTT, 30–45 seconds; APTT, 25–38 seconds.
   a. PTT greater than 60 seconds indicates anticoagulation factor deficiency, hemorrhage.
   b. APTT greater than 100 indicates spontaneous bleeding.
3. Clinical implications.
   a. Prolonged APTT noted in conditions such as hemophilia, vitamin K deficiency, liver disease, anticoagulant therapy, (DIC).

E. Prothrombin time (Pro Time, PT).

1. A measurement of the time it takes extrinsic blood factors to form a clot. Prothrombin, a protein manufactured by the liver, is converted to thrombin in the clotting process.
2. Normal value: 12–15 seconds, or less than 2 seconds from control; each laboratory has set normas, and these will vary depending on the type of thromboplastin used.
   a. Critical value is greater than 32 seconds and indicates anticoagulation factor deficiency, hemorrhage.
3. Clinical implications.
   a. Prolonged PT may indicate deficiencies in fibrinogen, prothrombin, vitamin K deficiency, hepatic disease, or ongoing anticoagulant therapy.

VI. Proteins, Protein Metabolites, and Pigments

A. Proteins (an overview).

1. Serum proteins are the most abundant compounds in the serum and primarily function to:
   a. Bind to and detoxify drugs and other toxic materials.

b. Participate in the synthesis of antibodies, enzymes, and hormones.
c. Enhance the stability of the blood.
d. Serve as a resource for tissue nutrition.
e. Maintain the acid-base balance through the blood buffering system.

2. Protein formation
   a. Albumin and the globulins (alpha$_1$, alpha$_2$, beta, and gamma) constitute the major proteins in serum.
   b. The liver produces most of the serum albumin and also the alpha and beta globulins.
   c. The reticuloendothelial system, immature plasma cells in the spleen, lymph nodes, and the bone marrow are responsible for the production of gamma globulin.
   d. Inadequate nutrition greatly inhibits the formation of proteins.
      (1) Decreased albumin levels lead to edema.
      (2) Decreased globulin levels weaken the body's defense to fight infection.
3. Protein metabolism.
   a. Proteins are degraded into amino acids, which are the reserve source for the synthesis of new proteins, hormones, enzymes, or creatine.
   b. The major metabolite from protein metabolism is ammonia, which then is metabolized in the liver to form urea.

B. Serum protein electrophoresis.
   1. Measures serum albumin and globulins by an electric charge that separates the proteins according to their size and shape. This test also evaluates the total protein content.
   2. Globulins function to carry lipids, hormones, and metals in the blood. Gamma globulin is a vital asset in the immune defense system.
   3. Albumin is a regulator of oncotic pressure, and a primary transporter of insoluble substances (bilirubin, fatty acids, hormones, drugs).
   4. The purpose of this test is to evaluate hepatic disease (the liver is the major source of protein formation), protein deficiency, blood dyscrasias, renal impairment, gastrointestinal and neoplastic disorders.
   5. Normal values:
      a. Total serum protein content: 6.6–7.9 g/dl.
      b. Albumin fraction: 3.3–4.5 g/dl (albumin constitutes approximately 50% of total serum protein).
      c. Globulin fraction.
         (1) Alpha$_1$: 0.1–0.4 g/dl.
         (2) Alpha$_2$: 0.5–1 g/dl.
         (3) Beta: 0.7–1.2 g/dl.
         (4) Gamma: 0.5–1.6 g/dl.

6. Clinical implications.
   a. Increased levels of protein content correlate with dehydration, vomiting, diarrhea, diabetic acidosis, fulminating and chronic infections, monocytic leukemia, chronic inflammatory disease.
   b. Decreased levels of protein content are associated with malnutrition, gastrointestinal disease, essential hypertension, Hodgkin's disease, uncontrolled diabetes mellitus, malabsorption, hepatic impairment, nephrosis, shock (surgical, trauma), severe burns, hemorrhage, congestive heart failure, benzene and carbon tetrachloride poisoning, hyperthyroidism, toxemia of pregnancy.

C. Ammonia
1. A measurement of the blood ammonia concentration; useful for evaluating metabolism as well as the severity of liver disease. Blood ammonia, a by-product of protein metabolism, is metabolized into urea by the liver and excreted by the kidney.
2. Normal range: 15–45 μg/dl.
3. Clinical implications.
   a. Increased blood ammonia levels occur in liver disease, hepatic coma (cirrhosis, severe hepatitis), severe heart failure, azotemia, cor pulmonale, emphysema, hemolytic disease of the newborn, acute bronchitis, pericarditis, Reye's syndrome.

D. Bilirubin
1. A measurement of the total bilirubin concentration in the blood; useful for evaluating liver function, hemolytic anemias, and hyperbilirubinemia (in newborns). Bilirubin, a by-product of hemolysis, results from the breakdown of hemoglobin in the red blood cells. Bilirubin is transported by the blood to the liver, which excretes it into the bile. Bilirubin is the predominant pigment in bile and gives bile its characteristic yellowish tinge.
2. Normal range: total bilirubin, 0.2–1.0 mg/dl; newborn, 1.5–12.0 mg/dl.
   a. Critical value in the newborn is a bilurubin level approximately 16 mg/dl; mental retardation may result if immediate exchange transfusion is not initiated.
3. Clinical implications.
   a. High bilirubin levels accompanied by jaundice may be a result of either hepatic (viral hepatitis, cirrhosis, infectious mononucleosis), obstructive (common bile or hepatic duct obstruction caused by stones or neoplasms), or hemolytic (Rh imcompatibility, ABO incompatibility, sickle cell anemia, pernicious anemia, transfusion reactions) causes.

E. Blood urea nitrogen (BUN).
   1. A measurement of the nitrogen fraction of urea; useful for evaluating renal function and as an assessment of hydration. Urea is primarily formed in the liver from ammonia and is the major nonprotein nitrogenous by-product of protein metabolism. The BUN reflects protein intake and renal excretory capability. Urea represents approximately 80%–90% of the total urinary nitrogen.
   2. Normal range: 7–18 mg/dl, or 2.5–6.4 mmol/L.
      a. Critical value of the BUN is greater than 100 mg/dl (indicates serious renal impairment).
   3. Clinical implications.
      a. Azotemia: increased BUN levels.
         (1) ETIOL: renal failure, reduced renal blood flow, shock, dehydration, infection, diabetes, excessive protein intake.
      b. Decreased BUN levels are associated with liver failure, overhydration, malnutrition.

F. Creatinine.
   1. A measurement of the concentration of blood creatinine; useful for evaluating renal impairment. Creatinine is a nonprotein end product of creatine metabolism and is found mainly in urine, muscle, and blood.
   2. Normal range: 0.6–1.2 mg/dl.
      a. Critical value is greater than 4 mg/dl and is associated with renal failure and coma.
   3. Clinical implications.
      a. Increased creatinine levels are associated with renal failure, urinary tract obstruction, muscular dystrophy, poliomyelitis, diabetic acidosis, starvation, hyperthyroidism, muscle disease (gigantism, acromegaly, myasthenia gravis).

G. Uric acid.
   1. A measurement of the uric acid concentration in the blood; useful for evaluating renal failure and gout. Uric acid is formed from purine metabolism (purine is itself a by-product of nucleoprotein digestion). More than one-half of the uric acid produced daily is excreted by the kidneys, the remaining is eliminated by the stool.
   2. Normal range:
      a. Men: 3.5–7.2 mg/dl, or 0.21–0.42 mmol/L.
      b. Women: 2.6–6.0 mg/dl, or 0.154–0.35 mmol/L.
   3. Clinical implications.
      a. Uric acid levels will be increased (uricemia) in conditions that produce excessive cell breakdown and catabolism of nucleonic acids (gout), in conditions that generate excessive production and de-

struction of cells (leukemia), or in conditions in which there is an inability to excrete bodily fluids (renal failure).

VII. Enzymes

A. Enzymes (an overview).

1. Enzymes are the catalyst in thousands of chemical reactions needed for body homeostasis.
2. Various tissue cells produce specific enzymes that are released in greater than normal amounts when these tissue cells are damaged by disease or some other defect.
3. Elevated serum enzymes may indicate the source of disease (e.g., myocardial infarction, infectious hepatitis) owing to their original source of production.
4. Some enzymes occur in multiple forms (isoenzymes) that may differ in molecular form while still retaining their basic identity.
   a. Certain organs or tissues contain more or less amounts of one isoenzyme than other tissues.
   b. Testing for isoenzymes may isolate (or pinpoint) the exact location of tissue damage rather than testing the entire group of enzymes.

B. Specific enzymes.

1. Serum glutamic-pyruvic transaminase (SGPT): the preferred current term is alanine aminotransferase (ALT).
   a. ALT is an intracellular enzyme involved in amino acid and carbohydrate metabolism. ALT is present in high concentrations in the liver; lower concentrations occur in muscle, kidneys, and the heart.
   b. Normal range: 5–35 U/L (37°C).
   c. Clinical implications.
      (1) Very high ALT concentrations (up to 50 times normal) indicate necrotic or diseased tissues and is especially indicative of hepatic disease with extensive necrosis. Marginal to moderate increases in ALT levels are noted in myocardial infarction, shock states, trauma, infectious or toxic hepatitis, severe burns, infectious mononucleosis, deliruim tremens.
2. Alkaline phosphatase (ALP).
   a. ALP is an enzyme that functions best at a pH around 9.0 ALP and its isoenzymes are primarily located in the liver, bones, and the placenta; minor activity is noted in the kidneys and intestinal lining. ALP functions to enhance bone calcification and lipid and metabolite transport.
      (1) Isoenzymes.
         (a) AP-1, Alpha 2: produced in the liver.
         (b) AP-2, Beta 1: produced by bone and placental tissue.
         (c) AP-3, Beta 2: present in small amounts in Group O and B individuals.

b. Normal range: 20–70 U/L.
   (1) Isoenzyme range is usually reported as weak, moderate, or strong.
c. Clinical implications.
   (1) Elevated ALP levels correlate with biliary obstruction and is a primary indicator of space-occupying hepatic lesions. Elevated ALP is usually associated with elevated AST and elevated bilirubin in liver disease. Other conditions that may increase ALP include pregnancy, pancreatitis, and metabolic bone disease.

3. Gamma glutamyl transferase (GGT).
   a. GGT functions in the transfer of amino acids across cellular membranes and is believed to be involved in glutathione metabolism. GGT is present primarily in the liver, kidney, prostate, and spleen.
   b. Normal range:
      (1) Men: 6–28 U/L @ 25°C.
      (2) Women: 4–18 U/L @ 25°C.
   c. Clinical implications.
      (1) Increased concentrations of GGT are noted in liver, renal, cardiac, and prostatic disease. Elevated GGT is also noted in chronic alcoholism.
4. Serum glutamic-oxaloacetic transaminase (SGOT): the preferred current term is aspartate aminotransferase (AST).
   a. Like ALT, AST is an intracellular enzyme occuring in the major organs and involved in amino acid and carbohydrate metabolism. Blood AST will rise after injury or death of cells.
   b. Normal range: 0–35 U/L (37°C).
   c. Clinical implications.
      (1) In myocardial infarction (MI), AST levels may rise 4–10 times the normal value. A secondary rise in AST indicates recurring or extensive MI. Severe arrhythmias and/or severe angina may also cause an elevated AST level.
5. Creatine phosphokinase (CPK) and isoenzymes: the preferred current term is "creatine kinase" (CK).
   a. CK is a primary heart and skeletal muscle enzyme that has three functional isoenzymes: CK_1 (BB), CK_2 (MB), and CK_3 (MM). Skeletal muscle contains primarily CK_3, whereas cardiac muscle contains both CK_2 and CK_3. CK_1 occurs in brain tissue and gastrointestinal and genitourinary tracts. Owing to the primary location of these enzymes, definitive differentiation can be made regarding where the tissue injury is. Elevation of CK_3 is an indication of skeletal muscle injury, whereas elevation of CK_2, the cardiac enzyme, indicates myocardial cell damage.

b. Normal range:
   (1) Men: 38–174 U/L.
   (2) Women: 96–149 U/L.
   (3) Isoenzymes.
      (a) CK_1: 0%.
      (b) CK_2: 0%.
      (c) CK_3: 100%.
c. Clinical implications.
   (1) A CK_2 greater than 5% is indicative of MI. Serum CK can rise as much as 10–25 times the normal level in the first few hours after MI.
   (2) Other diseases that cause an elevated CK level include acute cerebrovascular disease, progressive muscular dystrophy (levels may reach 300–400 times normal), delirium tremens, electric shock, hypokalemia, hypothyroidism, CNS trauma.
   (1) Normal values are noted in myasthenia gravis, multiple sclerosis.

6. Lactic dehydrogenase (LD, LDH).
   a. LDH is responsible for catalyzing the conversion of muscle lactic acid into pyruvic acid. This intracellular enzyme is widely distributed throughout most body tissues but essentially the kidney, heart, skeletal muscle, brain, liver, and lungs contain predominant amounts. LDH has five useful isoenzymes that aid in differentiating hepatic, pulmonary, cardiac, and erythrocyte damage.
      (1) Isoenzymes.
         (a) LDH_1 and LDH_2: primarily appear in the heart, RBCs, and kidneys.
         (b) LDH_3: present primarily in the lungs.
         (c) LDH_4 and LDH_5: in the liver and skeletal muscle.
   b. Normal range: 48–115 IU/L.
      (1) Isoenzymes.
         (a) LDH_1: 18.1%–29% of total.
         (b) LDH_2: 29.4%–37.5% of total.
         (c) LDH_3: 18.8%–26% of total.
         (d) LDH_4: 9.2%–16.5% of total.
         (e) LDH_5: 5.3%–13.4% of total.
   c. Clinical implications.
      (1) Isoenzyme analysis is necessary for differential diagnosis, because many common diseases will cause elevations in total LDH levels. LDH_1 and LDH_2 are elevated in MI and some hemolytic anemias. LDH_3 elevation is indicative of pul-

monary infarction and extensive pneumonia. LDH_2, LDH_3, LDH_4, and LDH_5 are increased in various malignancies. An increase in LDH_3 may be the first indication of cancer.

VIII. Lipids and Lipoproteins

A. Lipids (an overview).

1. Lipids, also called fats, are insoluble in water and consist mainly of total cholesterol, triglycerides, free fatty acids, and phospholipids.
2. Lipids combine with plasma proteins to form the conjugated proteins known as lipoproteins.
3. The lipoproteins are classified according to their chemical properties and densities: very low density (VLDL, has a greater ratio of lipid than protein), low density (LDL, contains more protein than VLDL, but less than HDL), and high density (HDL, contains more protein than either VLDL or LDL).
4. LDL and VLDL, owing to their low density, remain in the bloodstream and can potentially (if in high enough levels) partially occlude or occlude blood vessels; thereby, increasing the risk for coronary artery disease (CAD).
5. HDL levels are inversely proportional to the risk of coronary artery disease; high HDL levels reduce the risk for CAD, whereas low HDL levels (<35) increase the risk for CAD.
6. Lipoprotein analysis is especially useful in identifying those at risk for cardiovascular abnormalities, hypertension, atherosclerosis and/or coronary artery disease (CAD).
7. Table B.1 presents the lipids and lipoproteins.

IX. Blood Culture

A. For isolation and identification of the pathogen(s) causing bacteremia (bacterial invasion of the bloodstream) and septicemia (systemic spread of the infection).

B. Usually, three blood samples are drawn within a 24-hour time and no less than 1 hour apart.

C. The blood sample collected is incubated in a culture medium for 24–72 hours.

D. Normal blood cultures should be sterile.

E. Common blood pathogens include *Neisseria meningitides, Streptococcus pneumoniae, Hemophilus influenzae, Staphylococcus aureus, Pseudomonas aeruginosa, Brucella,* Enterobacteriaceae, Group A beta-hemolytic streptococcus, and Bacteroidaceae.

F. Antimicrobial therapy should be withheld until the blood culture series is complete (antimicrobial therapy will decrease the amount of bacteria present; making analysis difficult).

Table B.1
The Lipids and Lipoproteins

Test	Desirable Value	Purpose	Comments
Total cholesterol	140–220 mg/dl	Assess the risk of CAD[a], evaluate fat metabolism, aid diagnosis of nephrotic syndrome, pancreatitis, hepatic disease, hypo- and hyperthroidism.	Normal value varies with age and diet. A diet high in saturated fats increases the amount of fat in the liver and increases serum blood levels of cholesterol, thereby increasing the risk of CAD.
Triglycerides	Male: 40–160 mg/dl Female: 35–135 mg/dl	Screen for hyperlipemia, help identify nephrotic syndrome, assess the risk of CAD.	Values vary with age. Together with carbohydrates, these compounds provide the energy for metabolism. Increased levels of triglycerides and cholesterol greatly increase the risk of CAD.
Free fatty acids	8–25 mg/dl 0.3–1 mEq/L	Aid diagnosis of diabetes, secondary hyperlipoproteinemia.	Elevated levels may indicate diabetes, cardiac arrhythmias, or acute fasting or starvation. Free fatty acids are essential components of lipoproteins and triglycerides and account for 2%–5% of all lipids.
Low-density lipoproteins (LDL)	<130 mg/dl	Assess the risk for CAD.	Increased LDL levels correlate with a diet high in cholesterol and saturated fats. The higher the LDL level, the higher the incidence of CAD.
High-density lipoproteins (HDL)	Male: 35–70 mg/dl Female: 35–85 mg/dl	Assess the risk for CAD.	HDL is inversely related to the incidence of CAD—the higher the HDL level, the lower the incidence of CAD. Elevated HDL levels are associated with a healthy metabolic state in a person free from liver disease or intoxication of any form. HDL levels <35 increases the risk for CAD.

[a] CAD - coronary artery disease.

Section III: Urine Studies

X. Routine Urinalysis

A. Urine composition.
   1. Urine contains approximately 95% water and 5% solids.
   2. Water, urea, uric acid, and sodium chloride are primary components of urine.
   3. In disease states urine may contain protein, glucose, ketone bodies, hemoglobin, lipids, bacteria, pus, urobilinogen, or calculi.

B. Urine volume.
   1. Reflects overall fluid homeostasis
   2. Factors that affect volume output include fluid intake, concentration of the solutes in the filtrate, cardiac output, hormonal influences, fluid loss through the lungs, the large bowel, and the skin.
   3. Average adult output is approximately 1500 ml/day (an average of 40–60 ml/hr).
   4. Polyuria: urinary output exceeds 2000 ml/day
      a. ETIOL: diabetes, nervous diseases, certain types of chronic nephritis (conditions in which the kidneys fail to concentrate the urine), diuretics.
   5. Oliguria: urinary output is less than 500 ml/day.
      a. ETIOL: acute nephritis, heart disease, dehydration, fevers, eclampsia, diarrhea, vomiting, inadequate fluid intake.
   6. Anuria: urinary output is less than 125 ml/day.
      a. ETIOL: uremia, acute nephritis, metal poisoning (mercury bichloride), obstruction of biliary tract.
   7. Nocturia: urinary output exceeds 500 ml at night.
      a. ETIOL: associated with low specific gravity indicates chronic glomerulonephritis, heart failure, liver failure.

C. Routine urinalysis: normal values.

Color: pale yellow (straw) to amber	*Odor:* slightly aromatic
Appearance: clear, no solid particles visible	*Specific gravity: 1.025–1.030*
pH: 4.5–8.0 (average: about 6)	*Protein:* negative
Glucose: negative	*Ketones:* negative
Blood: negative	*Bilirubin:* negative
Urobilinogen: 0.1–1.0	*Yeast cells:* negative
Parasites: negative	*RBCs:* negative or rare
Casts: negative, occasional hyaline casts	*WBCs:* negative or rare
Epithelial cells: few	*Crystals:* negative to few

D. Significance of abnormal results.
   1. Color: changes from normal may indicate use of certain drugs, heavy metal poisoning, blood pigments, diet (certain food pigments may

change urine to a reddish color), metabolic, inflammatory, or infectious diseases.

2. *Odor:* sweet or fruity odor (smell of acetone) indicates the formation of ketone bodies as noted in diabetic states, starvation, and dehydration. A fetid odor indicates a urinary tract infection.
3. *Appearance:* a milky or turbid appearance is associated with the presence of fat globules, pus, and bacteria and reflect urinary tract infection.
4. *Specific gravity:* decreased values are associated with large dilutional volumes, acute renal failure, alkalosis, hypercalcemia, and hypokalemia. Elevated values are associated with small concentrated volumes, hepatic disorders, congestive heart failure, dehydration, and nephrosis. Fixed specific gravity is noted in severe renal failure.
5. *pH:* alkaline pH is noted in urinary tract infections, respiratory and metabolic alkalosis. Acid urine pH may result from renal tuberculosis, pyrexia, all forms of acidosis, diabetes mellitus, and starvation.
6. *Protein:* proteinuria indicates renal disease, multiple myeloma.
7. *Sugars:* glycosuria is associated with diabetes mellitus.
8. *Ketones:* ketonuria characterizes diabetes mellitus, starvation, severe diarrhea, or vomiting.
9. *Cells:* hematuria is associated with bleeding within the genitourinary tract. White cell in the urine indicate urinary tract infection. Excessive epithelial cells is indicative of renal tubular degeneration.
10. *Casts* (plugs of gelled proteinaceous matter): presence of a high number of casts indicates renal impairment.
11. *Crystals:* numerous calcium oxalate crystals indicates hypercalcemia, whereas cystine crystals (cystinuria) are associated with an inborn error of metabolism
12. *Yeast cells or parasites:* reflect genitourinary tract infection.

REFERENCES/RECOMMENDED READING

Ames Company. Factors Affecting Urine Chemistry Tests. Elkhart, IN: Ames Company, 1982.

Bryne JC, et al. Laboratory Tests: Implications for Nurses and Allied Health Professionals, Menlo Park, CA: Addison-Wesley, 1981.

Cohen JA, Pantelo N, Shell W. A message from the heart: what isoenzymes can tell you about your cardiac patient. Nursing 12(4):46, 1982.

Fischbach F. A Manual of Laboratory Diagnostic Tests. 4th ed. Philadelphia: JB Lippincott, 1992.
Gaedeke-Norris MK. Lab test tips—how to evaluate platelet values. Nursing 21(2):20, 1991.
Graff L. A Handbook of Routine Urinalysis. Philadelphia: JB Lippincott, 1983.
Grundy IM. The place of HDL in cholesterol management. Arch Intern Med 149:505, 1989.
Henry JB. Clinical Diagnoses and Management by Laboratory Methods. 18th ed. Philadelphia: WB Saunders, 1990.
Kee JL. Laboratory and Diagnostic Tests with Nursing Implications. East Norwalk, CT: Appleton and Lange, 1990.
Moss DW. Diagnostic aspects of alkaline phosphatase and its isoenzymes. Clin Biochem 20:225, 1987.
Platt WR. Color Atlas and Textbook of Hematology. Philadelphia: JB Lippincott, 1969.
Sacher RA, McPherson RA. Widmann's Clinical Interpretation of Laboratory Test. 10th ed. Philadelphia: FA Davis, 1991.
Williams WJ, et al. Hematology. 4th ed. New York: McGraw-Hill, 1990.

APPROXIMATE DOSE EQUIVALENTS C

Table C.1.
Liquid Measure

Metric	Approximate Apothecary Equivalent	Metric	Approximate Apothecary Equivalent
1000 ml	1 quart	3 ml	45 minims
750 ml	1-1/2 pints	2 ml	30 minims
500 ml	1 pint	1 ml	15 minims
250 ml	8 fluidounces	0.75 ml	12 minims
200 ml	7 fluidounces	0.6 ml	10 minims
100 ml	3-1/2 fluidounces	0.5 ml	8 minims
50 ml	1-3/4 fluidounces	0.3 ml	5 minims
30 ml	1 fluidounce	0.25 ml	4 minims
15 ml	4 fluidrams	0.2 ml	3 minims
10 ml	2-1/2 fluidrams	0.1 ml	1-1/2 minims
8 ml	2 fluidrams	0.06 ml	1 minim
5 ml	1-1/4 fluidrams	0.05 ml	3/4 minim
4 ml	1 fluidram	0.03 ml	1/2 minim

From Dorland's Illustrated Medical Dictionary, 27th ed. Philadelphia: WB Saunders, 1988.

Table C.2.
Weight

Metric	Approximate Apothecary Equivalent	Metric	Approximate Apothecary Equivalent
30 g	1 ounce	30 mg	1/2 grain
15 g	4 drams	25 mg	3/8 grain
10 g	2-1/2 drams	20 mg	1/3 grain
7.5 g	2 drams	15 mg	1/4 grain
6 g	90 grains	12 mg	1/5 grain
5 g	75 grains	10 mg	1/6 grain
4 g	60 grains (1 dram)	8 mg	1/8 grain
3 g	45 grains	6 mg	1/10 grain

Table C.2.—*continued*

Metric	Approximate Apothecary Equivalent	Metric	Approximate Apothecary Equivalent
2 g	30 grains (1/2 dram)	5 mg	1/12 grain
1.5 g	22 grains	4 mg	1/15 grain
1 g	15 grains	3 mg	1/20 grain
0.75 g	12 grains	2 mg	1/30 grain
0.6 g	10 grains	1.5 mg	1/40 grain
0.5 g	7-1/2 grains	1.2 mg	1/50 grain
0.4 g	6 grains	1 mg	1/60 grain
0.3 g	5 grains	0.8 mg	1/80 grain
0.25 g	4 grains	0.6 mg	1/100 grain
0.2 g	3 grains	0.5 mg	1/120 grain
0.15 g	2-1/2 grains	0.4 mg	1/150 grain
0.12 g	2 grains	0.3 mg	1/200 grain
0.1 g	1-1/2 grains	0.25 mg	1/250 grain
75 mg	1-1/4 grains	0.2 mg	1/300 grain
60 mg	1 grain	0.15 mg	1/400 grain
50 mg	3/4 grain	0.12 mg	1/500 grain
40 mg	2/3 grain	0.1 mg	1/600 grain

From Dorland's Illustrated Medical Dictionary, 17th ed. Philadelphia: WB Saunders, 1993.

INDEX

C

O